Handbook of Stressful Transitions Across the Lifespan

Handbook of Stressful Transitions Across the Lifespan

Edited by

Thomas W. Miller
University of Kentucky College of Medicine
Lexington, KY
USA

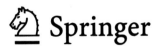 Springer

Editor
Thomas W. Miller
University of Kentucky College of Medicine,
Lexington, KY
USA
tom.miller@uconn.edu

ISBN 978-1-4419-0747-9   e-ISBN 978-1-4419-0748-6
DOI 10.1007/978-1-4419-0748-6
Springer New York Dordrecht Heidelberg London

Library of Congress Control Number: 2009931332

Printed on acid-free paper

Springer is part of Springer Science+Business Media (www.springer.com)

Life provides numerous transitions with some more stressful than others. Understanding such transitions and finding the knowledge necessary to navigate such transitions is the secret of a successful life.

It is to our grandchildren Colin, Francis, Hillarie, Derek and Heidie and to their generation that this volume is dedicated.

Foreword

This volume provides a unique and valuable contribution to our understanding of the impact of stressful life events and mass trauma on the person, the culture and society in the course of the life span. It provides a comprehensive look at our psychological state of affairs at the beginning of the twenty-first century. There are several volumes that address some or most of these areas individually but this volume is unique in that it has brought together theoreticians, researchers and clinicians who address critical challenges in our lives.

But we are now several months into the global financial crisis requiring a transition, not only for the western world but for the third world. How on earth do families in trauma zones – from Sri Lanka to Afghanistan, New Orleans to Gaza – cope with similar declining older relatives, with added traumas and zero medical resources attempt to survive? In news reports, politicians and financiers denying the inevitable and struggling for solutions that cannot be relevant to the new reality that they have yet to discover.

This must be a time for consolidation, and valuing the past. What of our old world values, principles, dreams, beliefs? Will they still be valid and functional in the new age? But even more important – what past values, principles, assumptions that we took for granted in the last 50 years have been rendered obsolete by the finance crash, and the wider collapse of finance and trading systems? These may be personal, corporate, industrial, national, and international. We are in a very real sense a global village!

So, mass transitions may be the sum of millions of individual personal revelations, and possibly of hard to identify collective values and assumptions that must be let go in order for industries, states and continents to survive and thrive. the rampant materialism that developed in the 1980s and boomed in the last 5 years was the privilege of certain groups, shared by the mass media. Since 2001, to question western values was an issue of treason. The current turmoil, and of course the shifts in leadership worldwide has led to stressful transitions in the United States and others which are scary and potentially cleansing, perhaps even cathartic.

The traumas of 9–11 seemed to have massive transformational potential. This seemed to be harnessed with amazing speed into the all-pervading international purge of the War on Terror – not quite the new age potential. I was hoping for in my optimistic scenarios. But, mass trauma transitions are more complex than I realized. The tsunami effect suggests that sudden traumas may effect individuals and communities at very different times – potentially delayed until the event impacts directly on their own lives, possibly months or years later.

My instinct is that the transition process is crucial – as the core process for individual adaptation to traumas or change. But, practical logistics and other social factors may be crucial in disseminating mass transitions from collective traumas or changes. Economic security and emotional support seemed to be the enabling factors for transition recovery. If so, the Recession scenario has a downside of extended crisis with mental health implications – and psychological distress likely to be expressed in increased violence particularly in urban settings.

In the United States, the transition timeline for the finance crisis will overlap the Presidential transition. Interesting, yet, it is hazardous for an outsider to speculate on transitions in other countries. More useful may be to offer models or templates for anticipating phases of change, with related tools e.g. scenario planning which analysts and researchers with better understanding of the local context can apply themselves. Recent events to add are aspects of the Chinese earthquake and Georgia crisis – first act of God, major transition potential in the region, national effects possibly mitigated by positive effect of the Olympics but even that with possible cycle. Combined risk period from this Oct to Feb 09. Chinese New Year could be a recovery trigger.

We must be reminded of not only the macro events, but of the micro-survival transitions in our lives that create for individuals and communities the challenges that life presents. The reader is about to encounter an extraordinary journey into understanding the several life transitions that we face in the course of the life span. One realizes how essential it is to understand how we as human being process information, the transitions that we face in education and career choices and the transitions encountered in marriage, family and sexual life cycle encounters. Unique to this volume is consideration of the legal, ethical and financial transitions which is so timely. The comprehensive nature of this volume offers an in-depth examination of the life threatening transition in maturation and health and the cultural, religious and spiritual life transitions that so many of us encounter. Finally, the volume offers a spectrum of practical interventions to stressful life transitions. Transitions in our life span are complex and require complex and multi-faceted understanding. This volume provides the opportunity for dialogue in improving our understanding and each of the authors in this book deals with a part of this complex whole. Putting the pieces together herein provides the gestalt that moves our understanding of stressful life events and the transitions we face in the life span to a twenty-first century level.

Dai Williams
Eos
Surrey, United Kingdom

Contents

About the Contributors

James D. Abbott, M.D., received a bachelor's degree in biological sciences from The Ohio State University and a medical degree from the Medical College of Ohio. He completed his residency training in orthopaedic surgery at the University of Louisville and a fellowship in orthopaedic sports medicine and partial knee arthroplasty with Dr. David N.M. Caborn at Jewish Hospital in Louisville, KY. He will enter practice in Middletown, Ohio beginning in July of 2008. Outside of medicine, he leads an active life with his wife and four sons.

Jeanine Miller Adams, Ed.D., OTR/L, CHES received her Doctor of Education degree from the University of Kentucky, Master of Science in occupational therapy from Eastern Kentucky University, and Bachelor of Arts in psychology from University of Kentucky. She has worked as an occupational therapist in the school system, taught at the collegiate level, and is currently a yoga instructor. She resides with her husband, three young children, and dog, Vino. Her love for animal assisted therapy was inspired by her certified therapy dog, Brewski, who gave 9 years of love and joy in her work as a therapy dog and to her family.

Brian Barczak, M.D., is a graduate of Indiana University School of Medicine. As a member of the University of Kentucky College of Medicine's house staff, his primary professional interests lie in divorce and its effects on children and adolescents' mental health, as well as in the interface between the fields of forensic psychiatry and child and adolescent psychiatry, in advocacy work to prevent child abuse and neglect, and in training medical students and other residents. His career aspirations involve continuing his work with youth from divorced family backgrounds, as well as his ongoing work with youth within the Juvenile Justice system.

Sarah Barczak, CSW, is a Certified Social Worker from Sunman, Indiana. After earning her Bachelors Degree in Sociology at Purdue University in 2003 she spent 2 years working with pregnant and parenting teens in a residential program in Indiana. She earned her Masters in Social Work at the University of Kentucky in 2007, focusing her graduate research on identifiable trends in divorcing parents' Minnesota Multiphasic Personality Inventory-2 (MMPI-2) personality profiles and how these trends are associated with certain child custody preferences. Sarah continues to focus her clinical work on emotionally and behaviorally disturbed youth.

Barbara L. Belew, Ph.D., is a clinical psychologist who owns and operates her own practice in south central Kentucky. A graduate of the University of Wyoming, she received her M. S. and Ph.D. degrees from the University of Kentucky. Dr. Belew has worked in several mental health settings, including inpatient, residential and outpatient programs. She is the first recipient of the Jesse G. Harris, Jr. Dissertation Award and is a Past President of the Kentucky Psychological Association. Dr. Belew initiated an APA-accredited Pre-Doctoral Internship for practice in rural areas in Eastern Kentucky, a program that continues to grow and add to the number of psychologists available in a very isolated part of the state. She has taught in the graduate psychology program at Union College in Barbourville, Kentucky.

Dorothy Ann Brockopp, RN PhD is a Professor at the University of Kentucky, College of Nursing. Her clinical and research interests are in the area of oncology. She studies the management of acute and cancer pain, the psychological well-being of women with breast cancer and the provision of comfort measures for patients receiving palliative care. In addition to her teaching and research responsibilities at the university, she is a half-time consultant at a community hospital providing guidance for research and clinical evaluation projects.

Rhonda Brownbill, Ph.D. R.D. is an instructor and foods lab manager at the University of Connecticut, Storrs, CT. She received her undergraduate and graduate degrees from the University of Connecticut. She currently teaches and has taught a variety of courses including introductory nutrition, nutrition throughout the lifecycle, research methods for health professionals, fitness for health, food safety and women's health. She has also guessed lectured for several other nutrition and foods related courses.

Jeanne Joseph Chadwick, M.P.H., M.S., Ph.D. is an Assistant Professor In-Residence in the School of Nursing at the University of Connecticut, where she teaches health policy and bio-statistics to graduate nursing students. She has significant clinical research experience and training in the Cognitive/Behavioral intervention, Mindfulness-Based Stress Reduction and received her training from the University of Massachusetts Center for Mindfulness in Medicine and Society. She has developed family-based models of mindfulness and used them to measure their effect on the quality of parent–child relationships as well as the stress associated with chronic diseases such as Type 2 diabetes, cardiovascular illnesses, and their prevention in at-risk families. She is currently adapting a mindfulness model for low-income Hispanic adults with chronic uncontrolled diabetes at Hartford Hospital to address the need for a brief, cost-effective and community-friendly program to be integrated into the existing diabetes care services at this inner-city hospital.

James J. Clark, LCSW, Ph.D. is Associate Dean for Research in the UK College of Social Work and an associate professor in the College of Medicine, Department of Psychiatry. He is co-director of the UK Center for the Study of Violence against Children which is a nationally-recognized program for the assessment and treatment of maltreated children. He has published in the areas of child maltreatment, substance misuse, professional and research ethics, forensic mental health, consumer satisfaction research, clinical decision making and psychobiography.

Catherine Cohan, Ph.D. is a Research Associate at the Penn State Population Research Institute. The broad goals of her research are to investigate predictors of change in marital satisfaction and the likelihood of divorce using psychological and sociological perspectives, multiple levels of analysis, and longitudinal designs. She focuses on personal characteristics and relationship experiences that spouses bring into the marriage, spouses' communication skills, and stressors external to the marriage. More specifically her research interests include spouses' premarital cohabitation history, observed problem solving and social support behavior, normative and non-normative stressful life events, and spouses' hormone function.

Nathan Denny, Ph.D., graduated from the University of Oregon, taught clinical psychology at Texas Tech University, and has served as a psychologist in VA medical center, Vet Center, and outpatient facilities in San Antonio, Honolulu, Houston, and Austin, Texas. Dr. Denny has participated in VA clinical studies, including the National Vietnam Veterans Readjustment Study. His current specialty integrates mental health services in Primary Care.

Janine Dewey, M.A. earned her Bachelor of Science degree in Psychology and Sociology at Eastern Kentucky University and her Master of Arts in Counseling Services at Webster University. She has worked and held management positions in adolescent treatment settings, including a psychiatric residential treatment facility, residential substance abuse treatment center, outpatient substance abuse services, community based group homes and apartment living programs and mentoring programs. Ms. Dewey is an active member of the Kentuckiana Child Care Coalition, Women's Coalition for Substance Abuse Services in Kentucky, and a founding member of Mentor Louisville. She is a strong advocate for creating new opportunities for communities to support their youth and young adults, as well as recognizing the need to enhance existing programs that assist these young people in their journey toward independence.

Cynthia Dunn, Ph.D. is the Coordinator of the PTSD Clinical Team at the Lexington, KY VAMC. In that capacity she also provides outreach clinics in central Appalachia. She obtained her Bachelor's Degree from the University of Massachusetts, M.S. and Ph.D. from the University of Kansas, Lawrence, KS. She won the Dissertation of the Year Award for her work in the area of PTSD and has presented at the American Psychological Association.

Donald Edmondson is a doctoral candidate in Psychology at the University of Connecticut. His research focuses on the existential aspects of highly stressful events such as natural disasters and life-threatening illness. Recent research has focused on the benefits of a sense of meaning and purpose in life for psychological well-being in cancer survivorship, as well as the costs associated with certain religious schemata in the terminal stage of congestive heart failure. He is currently investigating how individual worldviews are affected by traumatic events and the utility of conceptualizing PTSD as a consequence of worldview dissonance.

Jean M. Edwards received her Ph.D. from York University, Toronto, Canada. She is currently an Associate Professor of Psychology at Wright State University, Dayton, Ohio. Her research interests include individual differences in anxiety, workplace stress and job transitions.

Joseph P. Fox, Ph.D. is retired from a career in speech-language pathology spanning more than 30 years. He started as Assistant Professor and Associate Director of Speech-Language Pathology at The George Washington University. Then he was appointed Chief, Audiology & Speech Pathology Service and served the VA Medical Center in Lexington, KY for 21 years. He had adjunct teaching appointments at the University of Kentucky, the University of Louisville, and Eastern Kentucky University. After retiring from the VA he worked with rehabilitation agencies in multiple settings. He has a broad range of clinical experiences with clients of all ages.

Helene H. Fung, Ph.D. is an Associate Professor of Psychology at the Chinese University of Hong Kong. She obtained her BS from University of Washington, Seattle, and MA and PhD from Stanford University. She is the winner of the 1999 Behavioral and Social Science Pre-dissertation Research Award, Gerontological Society of America, and the 1998 Margaret Clark Paper Award, Association of Anthropology and Gerontology. She also won the 2006 Young Research Award and the 2007 Exemplary Teaching Award of Faculty of Social Science, Chinese University of Hong Kong. Currently, she is an associate editor of the Journal of Psychology in Chinese Societies.

Abbie E. Goldberg, Ph.D. received her doctorate in Clinical Psychology from the University of Massachusetts Amherst and is currently an assistant professor of psychology at Clark University, where she teaches both undergraduate and graduate courses. Her current research explores the transition to adoptive parenthood among gay, lesbian, and heterosexual parents. She has published on the topics of lesbian parenthood, adoption, the transition to parenthood, and work–family issues.

Ronald Goodman, BS, MS received his undergraduate and graduate degrees at Murray State University. His graduate training in mental health counseling led him to work with alcohol and substance abuse through community services. After suffering a brain stem stroke at the age of 34, Ron became a quadriplegic, but had some ability to write messages via computer. He loved his wife and children and shard his journey in his book entitled "In Deciding to Die, I found a Reason to Live.".

Clayton Scott Hall, D.O. graduated from the University of Kentucky in 1990 with a B.A. in Social Work and worked extensively in the Substance Abuse field with patients and their families. He graduated from Pikeville College School of Osteopathic Medicine in 2001 and completed his psychiatric training at the University of Louisville in 2005. He currently is attending psychiatrist at Three Rivers Medical Center in Louisa, Kentucky and was chief of staff in 2007. His passion is helping patients and families in Appalachia recover from problems with substance abuse, mood disorders and relational issues.

Paul J. Hershberger, Ph.D. is a licensed psychologist who earned his doctorate in counseling psychology at The Ohio State University. Currently, he is Professor of Family Medicine and Director of Behavioral Science for the Dayton Community Family Medicine Residency Program in the Department of Family Medicine, Wright State University Boonshoft School of Medicine. Prior to joining the medical school faculty in 2001, he served as a staff psychologist at the Dayton Veterans Affairs Medical Center for 12 years, practicing and conducting research in health psychology. Dr. Hershberger is a Diplomate in Clinical Health Psychology with the American Board of Professional Psychology.

Paul I Hettich, Ed.D. received his degrees in psychology from Marquette University, New Mexico State University, and Loyola University Chicago. He worked as an Army personnel psychologist, program evaluator in an education R&D lab, and applied scientist in a corporate setting. During his 35 years of mostly full-time teaching at Barat College he served also as department chair, academic dean, and grants writer. His professional work focused on teaching/learning methods, study skills, and college-to-workplace transition. In 2005 he co-authored *Connect College to Career: A Student Guide to Work and Life Transitions* and retired from Barat College of DePaul University as Professor Emeritus.

Thomas F. Holcomb, Ed.D. Dr. Holcomb is a Professor of Counseling and Chair of the Department of Educational Studies, Leadership and Counseling at Murray State University. He has been highly involved with the Kentucky Counseling Association and has held numerous leadership positions in the organization. He also served several terms on the Kentucky Board of Licensed Professional Counselors. His major interest lies primarily in the area of School Counseling and he has published numerous articles on the subject. He has been a former elementary school teacher and elementary school counselor. He has been a Counselor Educator at Murray State University since 1971.

Jasminka Ilich Ernst, Ph.D. is a professor at Florida State University, Tallahassee, FL. She received her undergraduate degrees from the University of Sarajevo, Bosnia-Herzegovina; M.S. in Nutrition from the University of Utah; and doctorate in Medicinal Sciences from the University of Zagreb, Croatia and the Ohio State University, Columbus, OH. Dr. Ilich's current research deals with investigation of the effects of various life-style modifiers, including nutrition and physical activity, on bone health, weight reduction and bone preservation in postmenopausal women. Her research has been continuously funded by federal and private agencies. Dr. Ilich is the author/co-author of numerous peer-reviewed papers and several book chapters. She presents her work on many national and international conferences, and is a recipient of several awards for her research, publications and various academic and professional functions. She is a frequently invited speaker by different organizations and forums.

Joyce E. Jadwin, Psy.D. (c) is a graduate student in the School of Professional Psychology at Wright State University. Prior to returning to school, she served as a student affairs administrator where she focused on working with first-generation college students, promoting diversity education, and improving administrative processes through technology and system redesign. She has a Master's Degree in Educational Policy and Leadership and an undergraduate degree in Business Administration.

Robert F. Kraus, M.D. is Professor of Psychiatry and Anthropology, Associate Residency Director of Training and former Chair of the Department of Psychiatry at the University of Kentucky. His career has involved clinical and academic administration, teaching, clinical practice and research. Recently he was the recipient of the Lifetime Achievement award of the Society for the Study of Psychiatry and Culture of which he is a charter member. The award was given for outstanding and enduring research contributions to the field of Cultural Psychiatry. It is the highest honor bestowed by the Society.

Clifford C. Kuhn, M.D., a native of Philadelphia, Pennsylvania, is a graduate of Ursinus College and the Jefferson Medical College. Dr. Kuhn received his psychiatric training at the University of Michigan in Ann Arbor. He is a Professor of Psychiatry at the University of Louisville, School of Medicine since 1974, where he has also served as Chief of Consultation-Liaison Psychiatry, Director of Residency Training, and Associate Chairman of the Psychiatry Department. He is the recipient of many awards and accolades for his accomplishments as an academician and teacher. He is also a humorist and a professional speaker known as the "Laugh Doctor." His latest book, *It All Starts With A Smile; Seven Steps to Being Happier Right Now,* has been described by comedian Jerry Lewis as "the best how-to book I have ever read." His company, Laugh Doctor Enterprises, Inc., teaches positive energy techniques for eliminating stress.

Katica Lackovi -Grgin, Ph.D. is professor and has lectured Life-span Psychology at University of Zadar and as Visiting Professor at University of Zagreb (Croatia), and University of Sarajevo (Bosnia and Herzegovina). She has published about hundred scientific and professional papers, as well as eight monographs. The papers and monographs are related to areas of family relationships, social interactions of adolescents, adolescent unemployment stress, the development of self-esteem, role stress and loneliness, some mechanisms of self-regulation in adult age etc. With A.Rokach, she was a senior researcher in cross-cultural study of loneliness in Canada and Croatia. She was editor – in- chief of one of Croatian journal (RADOVI), member of editorial board of national journals Revija za psihologiju and Suvremena psihologija, and she participated in a lot of conferences and symposia, at home and abroad. She was regarded from Croatian psychological association, for monograph «Stress in Children and Adolescent: Sources, mediators and effects», as exceptional scientific work.

Cassie M. Lindstrom completed her B.A. in Psychology at Niagara University in Lewiston, NY in 2003. She is currently pursuing her Ph.D. in Clinical Health Psychology at the University of North Carolina at Charlotte. Her research interests include posttraumatic growth and the aftermath of trauma, especially with respect to survivors of sexual assault and people who have sustained a Traumatic Brain Injury (TBI).

James E. Marcia, Ph.D. is currently Professor Emeritus at Simon Fraser University in Burnaby, British Columbia, Canada. He was Assistant and Associate Professor at SUNY/B from 1966–1972 and Director of the Psychological Clinic. From 1972 until 2002, he was Associate and Full Professor at Simon Fraser University and Director of the Psychological Clinic there. He has been in the private practice of psychotherapy since 1964 and has served as consultant on a number of community mental health projects. His research has been primarily in establishing construct validity for psychosocial developmental theory with a focus on ego identity.

John McKee, Ph.D. earned his doctorate in Industrial Organizational Psychology from Wright State University. McKee also received a Masters of Education in Counseling Psychology from Washington State University, a Masters of Science in Industrial Organizational Psychology from Wright State University, and a Bachelor of Arts in Psychology from The Ohio State University. In his current role as a research consultant with Kenexa, McKee is involved in a wide range of projects including job analysis, competency modeling, structured interview creation, as well as test development and validation. McKee's research interests include employee performance, turnover, job satisfaction, and work–life balance.

David T. Miller, M.D., Ph.D. is a medical geneticist and clinical molecular geneticist at Children's Hospital Boston, and an Instructor of Pediatrics at Harvard Medical School. He received his M.D and Ph.D degrees from Washington University in St. Louis. He completed a residency in Pediatrics at Yale-New Haven Hospital, and residency/fellowship in medical genetics at Harvard Medical School. He is board-certified in Pediatrics, Clinical Genetics, and Clinical Molecular Genetics. His clinical, research, and teaching activities are focused on improving patient care through genetic testing to facilitate better understanding of the molecular causes of genetic syndromes. His areas of interest include: children with developmental disabilities, especially autism spectrum disorders; neurofibromatosis; and progeroid laminopathies.

Thomas W. Miller, Ph.D. is Professor, Senior Research Scientist, Master Teacher and University Teaching Fellow through his 40 year career and tenure at the University of Kentucky, University of Connecticut and Murray State University. He received his Ph.D. from the State University of New York at Buffalo, is a Diplomate of the American Board of Professional Psychology in Clinical Psychology, Fellow of the American Psychological Association, the American Psychology Society and the Royal Society of Medicine. The American Psychological Association recognized him with a Special Achievement Award for is contributions to education, prevention and clinical services for victims of abuse. He is a Distinguished Alumnus from the State University of New York at Buffalo and the recipient of the APA Distinguished Professional Contributions to Practice Award.

Mary Alice Mills is a doctoral candidate in Clinical Psychology at the University of Connecticut. She studies various aspects of trauma, particularly the impact of trauma exposure on coping and adjustment. Recently, she has examined these issues in the context of natural disaster in a study of Hurricane Katrina survivors. Currently, she is project manager of a meaning-making writing intervention in people with PTSD.

Krista Moe, MS is a doctoral student in Counseling Psychology at the University of Kentucky. Her research seeks to identify factors that influence women's psychological well-being. In addition to specializing in women's issues in her doctoral program (i.e. counseling women with sexual trauma, low self-esteem, and with career decision-making issues) she is a member of the American Psychological Association's Society for the Psychological Study of Girls and Women. Currently, she is conducting research on the status of women for the President's Commission on Women.

Michael R. Nichols, Ph.D. received his degrees from the University of Kentucky. A licensed psychologist, he has served as a staff psychologist at Eastern State Hospital in Lexington, Kentucky and as Director of the University Counseling and Testing Center of the University of Kentucky. He is the past President of the Kentucky Psychological Association and former Editor of *The Kentucky Psychologist*. He has taught undergraduate, graduate classes and medical school classes since 1973, and has won 3 teaching awards. Dr. Nichols has published articles in a variety of areas and is a frequent presenter on the benefits of humor. He is currently serving as Visiting Professor of Psychology at his Alma Mater, Transylvania University in Lexington, Kentucky.

Steven Nisenbaum, Ph.D., J.D. is a Psychologist on the Medical Staff in the Psychiatry Department at Massachusetts General Hospital/Harvard Medical School, and a Senior Consultant at the International Negotiation Initiative at Harvard Law School. He is also the President of Family Healthy Choices, Inc., a nonprofit agency providing services to families. He has served previously as President of the Massachusetts Psychological Association, President of the Massachusetts Chapter of the Association of Family and Conciliation Courts, and President of Division 18 (Public Service Psychology) of the American Psychological Association. He was recipient of the annual Ezra Saul Award for distinguished career contributions to professional practice from the Massachusetts Psychological Association.

John Nyland, DPT, EdD ATC, CSCS, FACSM, received a bachelor's degree in physical therapy from the Medical University of South Carolina, a master's degree in athletic training from the University of Virginia, and doctorates in Kinesiology from the University of Kentucky and physical therapy from Simmons College in Boston, Massachusetts. Dr. Nyland is an Associate Professor in the Division of Sports Medicine, Department of Orthopaedic Surgery, Advisory Academic Dean in the School of Medicine at the University of Louisville, and is Adjunct Professor of Physical Therapy at Bellarmine University in Louisville, Kentucky.

Crystal L. Park, Ph.D. is Associate Professor of Psychology at the University of Connecticut. Her research focuses on several aspects of coping with highly stressful events: the roles of religious beliefs and religious coping, the phenomenon of stress-related growth, and the making of meaning from those stressful life events. In recent years, she has been examining these issues in the context of life-threatening illnesses, particularly cancer and congestive heart failure. She is currently Principal Investigator of studies of mediators of the effects of spirituality on well-being in congestive heart failure patients and of a meaning-making writing intervention in people with PTSD.

Ila Patel, M.D. is a Psychiatrist; Coordinator Mental Health Clinic, Lexington, Kentucky Veteran Affairs Medical Center; part-time private practice; Assistant Clinical Professor, University of Kentucky Department of Psychiatry. Dr. Patel is a Distinguished Fellow with the American Psychiatric Association. She obtained an MBBS in India. Her residency in psychiatry was completed at the University of Kentucky. She is also board certified in Psychiatry and Neurology. In addition, Dr. Patel provides Laughter Therapy Seminars which relates to her interest in humor and healing.

Zvjezdan Penezic, Ph.D. received his B.Sc. in psychology from University of Split in 1996. His M.Sc. in psychology from University of Zagreb was awarded in 1999. He received his Ph.D. in psychology from University of Zagreb in 2004. He is now in position of assistant professor in the field of personality psychology. He lectures Personality psychology, History of Psychology and Evolutionary psychology at University of Zadar. He has published about forty scientific and professional papers. The main interest is related to research of life satisfaction, development of self-esteem, loneliness, some mechanisms of self-regulation in adult age etc. He actively participated in numbers of Croatian and international conferences and symposia.

Emily Rosenbaum, a native of Washington, D.C., received her Bachelor's Degree in Sociology at Kenyon College in Gambier, Ohio in 2004. She has been living in Lexington, KY since early 2005. Her interests lie in clinical social work, with a focus on children and adolescents suffering from mood disorders. She is currently a full-time M.S.W. student in the School of Social Work at the University of Kentucky, and will graduate in May, 2009.

John R. Rudisill, Ph.D. is a licensed clinical psychologist who earned his Ph.D. in clinical psychology at Indiana University. Currently, he is Dean & Professor of the Wright State University School of Professional Psychology. Prior to joining the School of Professional Psychology, he was Professor of Family Medicine at the Wright State Boonshoft School of Medicine. He is a fellow of divisions 42 and 12 of the American Psychology Association and is a Diplomate in Clinical Psychology with the American Board of Professional Psychology.

Judith A. Schreiber, RN, PhD Candidate is at the University of Kentucky, College of Nursing. She has 26 years of experience as an oncology nurse and 22 of those as an Oncology Clinical Nurse Specialist (OCNS). She has a breadth of experience within community, university, and National Cancer Institute designated cancer centers. Her dissertation research, funded by the American Cancer Society and the National Cancer Institute focuses on survivorship and spirituality in cancer patients. She is actively involved at the local, regional, and national levels with the Oncology Nursing Society.

Daniel L. Shapiro, Ph.D. is founder and Director of the Harvard International Negotiation Initiative and Associate Director of the Harvard Negotiation Project. He is Assistant Professor in the Department of Psychiatry at Harvard Medical School/McLean Hospital, and is on the faculty at Harvard Law School. He has contributed to numerous scholarly and popular publications, and co-authored (with Roger Fisher)the bestseller "Beyond Reason: Using Emotions as You Negotiate." Dr. Shapiro is the recipient of numerous awards, including the American Psychological Association's Early Career Award and the prestigious "Peacemaker of the Year" award from the California Mediator's Association.

Marie-Antoinette Sossou, Ph.D. is Assistant professor at the College of Social Work, University of Kentucky. Her research interests and publications are in the areas of international social work with particular interest in Africa, feminist and gender issues, children, refugees, and social development issues. Before joining University of Kentucky as a faculty, Dr. Sossou had taught and headed the Social Work Unit at University of Ghana, Legon in Accra and also worked with UNHCR and IOM as a social work consultant and repatriation officer for refugees. Currently, she teaches social work practice, social policy and global poverty at University of Kentucky.

C.M.Y. Siu was a Master of Philosophy (in Psychology) student at theChinese University of Hong Kong when she worked on this chapter. She has worked closely with Helene H. Fung Ph.D. is an Associate Professor of Psychology at the Chinese University of Hong Kong toward the completion of the chapter which appears in this volume.

Kelli Triplett, B.A. completed her undergraduate degree in psychology from the University of North Carolina at Chapel Hill. She is currently pursuing her Ph.D. in Clinical Health Psychology at the University of North Carolina at Charlotte. Her research interests include posttraumatic growth in children and parents, coping with chronic illness, and bereavement.

Lane J. Veltkamp, MSW ACSW, B.C.D., is a Tenured Full Professor in the Child Psychiatry Division, Department of Psychiatry, College of Medicine, University of Kentucky Medical Center. He has a Joint Faculty appointment in the College of Social Work. He did his undergraduate work at Calvin College in Grand Rapids, Michigan, and his graduate work at Michigan State University. He is Board Certified. His interests over the last 35 years have focused on family violence, child abuse, and forensic issues. He has published over sixty papers, six chapters, and two books. He has given hundreds of workshops and testified in court in six states over 300 times. He developed and directed the Child and Adolescent Forensic Clinic in the Department of Psychiatry for 30 years.

Sherry Warden, Ph.D., RN is an Associate Professor in the College of Nursing at the University of Kentucky. Her clinical and research interests are in pain management and complementary and alternative therapies. Her projects have included the use of complementary and alternatives therapies for cancer pain, studying nurses' knowledge and attitudes about pain management, and elderly hospice patients' perspective on pain management.

Madelaine Claire Weiss, MSW, MBA is currently employed as a program manager at Harvard Medical School, where she has also designed and delivered mindfulness based stress management training programs for the Center for Learning and Performance. In addition to her private practice activities, she provided training for the American Immigration Lawyers Association in Washington D.C., and for Lawyers Concerned for Lawyers in Boston, MA. Ms. Weiss has spoken for the Joint Committee on the Status of Women at Harvard University, and has appeared in the Across Species Comparisons and Psychopathology newsletter on "Human Nature at Work" and "More on Territoriality."

William Weitzel, M.D. Dr. Weitzel is a physician and psychiatrist in private practice in Lexington Kentucky. He has provided expert testimony in numerous forensic cases that have included cases related to school violence and those involving school shootings by adolescent students. Dr. Weitzel is also a faculty member in the Department of Psychiatry, College of Medicine, at the University of Kentucky in Lexington, Kentucky. He has taught, provided clinical supervision and published during his career in psychiatry and psychiatric practice.

Richard Welsh, MSW LCSW is a professor in the Department of Psychiatry, College of Medicine and University of Kentucky Medical Center. He also holds a joint appointment of professor in the College of Social Work at the University of Kentucky. Mr. Welsh is licensed Clinical Social Worker and licensed Marriage and Family Therapist. Mr. Welsh is coordinator of the Hyperactive Children's Clinic and has written extensively in the area of ADHD. He has served on the Kentucky Board of Social Work and is a member of the College of Social Work Advisory Committee.

Evangeline A. Wheeler, Ph.D. (University of California, Berkeley) is Associate Professor of Psychology at Towson University in the Baltimore metropolitan area of Maryland. She is a cognitive-cultural psychologist with an interest in psychological health, a cognitivist who draws on race and gender theory in one article and health in another, but remains first and foremost a psychologist. She teaches courses in cognition, research methods and statistics. She is former Acting Director of Towson University's Multicultural Institute and a former Peace Corps volunteer. She writes on African-American women, mind-body health, pedagogy, spirituality and cross-cultural issues in psychology. She is currently at work on an edited volume of papers by African American psychologists.

Dai Williams holds an Occupational Psychology Masters from Birkbeck College, London University. He is a Chartered Occupational Psychologist in England and the founder of *Eos Life-Work Network* which offers consultation about getting the most out of life and work. It provides expertise in work and community psychology that raise challenging issues and opportunities for employers, researchers, governments and the media. Eos initially specialized in international graduate recruitment and education programmes for companies in the Far East. Clients have included Singapore Airlines, Singapore Broadcasting Corporation and Guardian Pharmacy, Shell Canada and several companies in Japan. Eos programmes were developed to help clients cope with severe career crises, stress and change – both in and out of work.

Part I

Processing Transitions in the Life Span

Chapter 1

Life Stress and Transitions in the Life Span

Thomas W. Miller

The traditional life cycle of human beings include infancy, childhood, adolescence, and adulthood. Transitions exist within each of the life cycles and such transitions produce stress. Life has many stressful life events that mark the movement from one condition or cycle to another, and they produce substantial challenges in the lives of human beings. The purpose of this volume is to focus on stressful life events associated with a spectrum of transitions in the life span.

The inspiration for this handbook of stressful life transitions across the life span has included a lifetime of research and clinical practice dealing with the transitions people had to face in very traumatic experiences along with several contributions over the last four decades. Those experiences have included working with adults and children who had been physically and/or sexually abused, victims of earthquakes and other natural disasters, veterans of combat, victims of torture, and individuals facing terminal illness and death. In addition to clinical and applied research, the recent work of Jane Goodman, Nancy Schlossberg, and Mary Anderson entitled *Counseling Adults in Transition Linking Practice with Theory* has provided our clinical research team with a clearer understanding of several of the effective strategies currently used in treating adults moving through some of life's most difficult and enduring transitions. In reviewing their contributions, I have come to realize the multiplicity of individuals worldwide who face difficult and stressful transitions in their lives. This led me to seek an international group of clinicians, researchers, and scholars to bring their illustrations of the stressful life experiences realized by human beings and interface that with the excellent work of Jane Goodman and her colleagues. In the use of this volume, one realizes that a compendium of the spectrum of the stressful transitions we face as human beings would contribute to the unique and individual transitions that we face. This handbook is intended to be a beginning toward bringing this body of knowledge to the reader, clinician, and researcher in need of this information. Among other volumes are the earlier works of Dohrwend and Dohrwend (1974), which focused on the conceptualization of stressful events and transitions, and the series on *Stressful Life Events* (Miller 1989) which provided a review of the

From: *Handbook of Stressful Transitions Across the Lifespan,*
Edited by: T.W. Miller, DOI 10.1007/978-1-4419-0748-6_1,
© Springer Science+Business Media, LLC 2010

literature and contributions of an interdisciplinary and cross-cultural spectrum of researchers and clinicians who have addressed this critical area of study. For example, this volume looks to the work of Holmes and Rahe who set the benchmark for addressing the science of measuring gradients of stressful life events (Rahe 1989; Byrne 1989; Cernovsky 1989; Fava 1989). This volume provides insights into the complexities of a highly technological world and the multiplicity of problems faced through stressful life experiences, and provides help to those involved in treating the consequences of stress in our lives.

The need to carefully assess the body of knowledge encompassing the prominent theories related to stressful life experiences was provided in *Theory and Assessment of Stressful Live Events* (Miller 1996) which brought together in one volume the current theories in studying transitions in the life span. In addition to theory, the measures for assessing stressful life events and the diagnostic nomenclature used in assessing pathology that may result from stressful life experiences were offered (McDaniel 1996; Post et al. 1996; Mollica and Caspi-Yavin 1996).

In *Clinical Disorders and Stressful Life Events* (1997), whose purpose was to examine clinical and research evidence linking stressful life events to disease and disordered functioning, the contributing authors created a comprehensive and highly current view of the rapidly evolving field or post-traumatic stress disorders (PTSD). This book provided essential information about stress-related disorders, not only for mental health professionals but also for clinicians in many areas of medicine (Engdahl and Eberly 1997; Basoglu 1997; McNally 1997). Finally *Children of Trauma* (1998) provided clinical theory and practice models for readers along with current concepts in diagnosis and treatment strategies for children. The multidisciplinary contributors to this volume included clinician-researchers from Europe, Asia, and the United States, and included physicians, lawyers, psychologists, clinical social workers, special educators, and others (Yule 1998; McNally 1998).

The transitions that we face as human beings and the impact of stressors for the infant, the child, the adolescent, and the adult, bring with them a series of events and circumstances that will define and shape the life course of each person. On the basis of that realization, analyzing the life span and the transitions human beings face, will provide yet another perspective in understanding the body of knowledge we have come to know as crucial in understanding ourselves.

In this *Handbook of Stressful Transitions across the Life Span* you will find the following areas of focus, with an international and multidisciplinary cadre of scientists and clinicians who have addressed this area of study in their research and clinical practice accepting the invitation to contribute to this handbook. Erik Erikson (1968) provides a wonderful epigenetic understanding of the sequence of psychosocial development. To address this introduction to Erikson's theory, a lifelong teacher, colleague, and friend provides a focus on life stress and stress in the context of psychosocial development; James C. Marcia, Ph.D., whose career at Simon Frazier University provides a clear understanding of Erikson and generates some new thinking as to what Erikson brings to the theoretical table, provides unique insights into developmental transitions. Professor Jim Marcia addresses the effects of life stressors and the impact of life transitions that occur within the context of overall lifespan development. In order to understand the meaning of such potentially disruptive events for the individual, it is important to understand what the general course of adult development looks like. The only developmental psychological theorist to lay out a course of expectable life cycle development is Erik Erikson. He has outlined eight psychosocial developmental periods extending from birth to old age. Each period is framed by descriptors such as "young adult," "middle age," etc. As the human life span has increased, the boundaries of these chronological periods have become increasingly elastic; however, they do provide a rough guideline as to average expectable development over the individual's life course.

The neurobiology of stress within the life cycle is the focus of Jerald Kay, M.D.'s contribution to this volume. Professor Kay is Chair of the Department of Psychiatry at Boonshoft School of Medicine Wright State University. Professor Kay examines how stressful life experiences within the life cycle influence the brain and the role of learning and memory in processing stressful life transitions. Noting that stress at times of life transitions, and other times, is often an example of poor adaptation, Professor Kay addresses an evolutionary point of view through the fight or flight reaction to danger that evoked important physiological events preservation (increased heart rate and blood pressure, production of stress hormones, increased availability of glucose to muscles) to ensure self preservation. Citing the focus of recent research that has been on the interaction between maternal separation and maternal stress, and genetics, Dr. Kay emphasizes that this body of information has led to important advances in how behaviors change genes and vice versa as well as the impact of adverse experienceson those with predisposition to depression and anxiety disorders. These advances have emerged from an appreciation of the role of genetic polymorphism in vulnerability to stress and illness.

Next, life as a source of theory is examined by James Clark, Ph.D. through his work at the University of Kentucky. Professor Clark examines Erik Erikson's contributions, boundaries, and marginalities within the context of life cycle theory as developed in *Childhood & Society* (Erikson 1950). This serves as a platform for several decades of subsequent theorizing in a wide range of domains and would help Erikson create a body of work that continues to prove meaningful for contemporary psychology and social thought. Dr. Clark addresses certain domains of concern and delineates the relevance of Erikson's theoretical approaches by discussing critical themes in his life, work, and career.

Education and Career Transitions

In considering clusters of stressful experiences in the life span, education and career transitions do certainly fall within such a domain. Professor Paul Hettich, Ed.D. at DePaul University traces the career transitions often realized by adolescents and young adults. In this chapter, one will examine several major issues encountered by some baccalaureate recipients each year who enter the workforce with inappropriate expectations, attitudes, job experiences, and levels of preparedness. The transition from college to a first full-time job is both an exciting and often stressful life event for this group of individuals. Professor Hettich through case examples supported by evidence-based decision making provides options for students wanting to improve readiness and reduce anxiety during one of life's most exciting transitions. In an effort to understand key issues and conditions that create distress for this group, two models of transition are offered. Bridges' model provides early attention to the process of making such a transition and Schlossberg's model offers direction for counseling individuals in this stressful life transition. Marcia's identity statuses and Arnett's theory of emerging adulthood reveal the dynamics of psychosocial development that underlies the thinking and behavior of individuals experiencing this transition.

Coping with the workplace and job-related transitions becomes the focus of John Rudisill, Ph.D., Wright State University. As both a common and stressful transition of modern life, examined are the factors associated with coping with job transitions. Specifically, the societal changes in the current context and the research evidence indicating job transitions can be significant life stressors. Further, examined is the role successful coping plays in the transition process, and summarized is a mediation model consisting of antecedents, coping, and outcomes necessary in successfully transitioning this life event. Case studies of job transitions are offered at four distinct points in the work-life to illustrate the model. Common themes and issues are addressed in the process of job transitions across the work-life, and questions are raised regarding how these may be uniquely played out at different points in an individual's life. The implications for the professional's role in helping individuals and organizations to facilitate transitions are discussed as are directions for future research.

Concluding this section is a contribution addressing the transition into retirement as a stressful life event. Thomas F Holcomb, Ed.D., Professor and Chair of the Department of Educational Leadership and Counseling at Murray State University offers insights into the processing of disengagement from work-life. Using Atchley's Model (Atchley and Barusch 2004) of retirement as a road map for those transition careers at various levels of the workforce, Professor Holcomb notes that preretirement planning can take many forms. What preretirement information can do to empower the individual is what Kobasa (1979) calls "Psychological Hardiness Factors." These Hardiness Factors seem to help negate detrimental effects of stress. These Hardiness Factors include viewing the change as a challenge, believing in a sense of control and that the individual does have some control and influence over things that will affect him/her, and being committed to the goals one has set. The goal of any preretirement planning should be to learn all one can about retirement and the financial, emotional, psychosocial, and transitional stressors and demands placed on the individual as he/she is experiencing this process of retirement. This seems to be especially true of married couples and their relationship, which can be stressed by being with each other 24 h a day. Several suggestions are offered. Noting that Knowledge is power if it is put to use, the author encourages a proactive mental set that keeps the end – the retirement process – in mind.

Marriage, Family, and Sexual Life Cycle Transitions

Family life cycle transition becomes the focus of the next section. Catherine L. Cohan, Ph.D., Professor at The Pennsylvania State University offers an understanding of family transitions following natural and terrorist disasters:

hurricane Hugo and the September 11 terrorist attack. This chapter recognizes that in today's world, disasters affect individuals, families, and entire communities. The majority of disaster research has been on identifying the mental health consequences for individuals following natural disasters, technological disasters, and mass violence. This chapter bridges the family as a critical unit of study during domestic and natural disasters. The unique focus on individual mental health outcomes will underestimate the full psychosocial impact of a disaster for many adults given that the consequences for adult disaster victims often unfold in the context of close relationships. The goal of this chapter broadens the focus of disaster research by considering how disasters are related to significant family transitions.

The transition to parenthood is generally regarded as a major life event that necessitates change and adjustment on the part of individuals and couples. Examined in this chapter are the transitions and challenges involved in becoming an adoptive parent. Abbie Goldberg, Ph.D., recognizes that the dyadic couple unit must evolve from a two-person to a three-person system. New parents experience change and reorganization in many aspects of their lives, which can produce both rewards and stresses. Changes within the parental relationship often emerge. While not all couples experience deterioration in their relationship quality and some couples recover relatively quickly, others experience persistent relationship instability making this a stressful life transition. The author notes that there are a number of factors that may mitigate the stress associated with the transition to parenthood. For example, possession of psychological resources (such as positive well-being and high self-esteem prior to parenthood) can help to buffer the stress associated with this significant life change. Addressing critical diversity factors and multiple resources important in transitioning, Professor Goldberg charges that various school personnel, child care workers, pediatricians, and other child/family practitioners should be familiar with the varied ways in which families are created. Specifically, they should have a basic understanding of both biological and adoptive family formation, and they should be aware of both the unique and common factors of biological and adoptive couples' transition to parenthood. Practitioners should further acknowledge the many sources of diversity in adoptive families including the type of adoption, racial makeup, and parental sexual orientation and attend carefully to the ways in which they shape the experiences of parents, children, and families.

It is recognized that one of the more stressful life events is the process of divorce in a family. The impact of divorce on children throughout the life cycle is the focus of authors Brian Barczak, M.D., Thomas W. Miller, Ph.D., ABPP, Lane J. Veltkamp, M.S.W., B.C.D., Sarah Barczak, M.S.W., C.S.W., Clay Hall, D.O., and Robert Kraus, M.D. The contributions and research of Wallerstein et al. (2001) are discussed as a basis for consideration of a case study involving a family and six children. Most significant in Wallerstein's conclusions by far is that the effects of divorce on children are not short-term and transient. They are long-lasting, profound, and cumulative. The children in Wallerstein's study view their parents differently, and they have lingering fears about their ability to commit to relationships that affect their own marriages. Children experience divorce differently from their parents, and on different schedules. Wallerstein and her clinician-researchers attribute the subsequent psychological problems in the children to the divorce itself as opposed to the psychopathology of the parents, the trauma of their parenting, and their conflicted marriage. Wallerstein began her research in the early 1970s with 131 children of divorce. She interviewed at length both the children and their parents. She has continued to follow those same families as the children have matured into adulthood and begun families of their own, continuing periodic interviews and checking their progress through life.

The "parenting process" becomes a critical element in child and family development. Jeanne Joseph Chadwick, Ph.D., University of Connecticut addresses stressful transitions in parenting through a mindfulness model. These transitions are prompted by a variety of stressful life events that tend to arise at different points in the family life cycle. For parents, these events may include pregnancy, birth of a child, divorce, remarriage, loss of job, relocation of job, or care-giving responsibilities for aging parents. For children, these events are often associated with developmental challenges that give rise to a new set of emotional needs. During such transitions, a nurturing social environment that the child experiences as occurring for his/her sake is the optimal context for healthy development. While this idea may be intuitive to parents and researchers, the kind of environment that supports families in the midst of life changes has thus far been difficult to articulate. Utilizing ecological systems theory, Dr. Chadwick notes that such a model has held promise as a conceptual framework for describing the kind of environment that incorporates many of these prescribed behaviors for parents, yet this theory is difficult to translate directly into practice and may fall short of capturing the relational complexity of the parent–child bond. This chapter uses a number of related theories to examine variables that, taken together, may be indicators of the kind of environment that is most suitable for effective developmental transitions within families. "Mindful Parenting" emerges from Mindfulness theory which promotes a skillful way of being present to children and to everyday experiences that result in greater self-awareness and clarity of purpose in communication.

Sexuality is such an essential ingredient in considering life span development and would need an entire volume to address adequately the transitions children, adolescents, the adult, and the elderly men and women are challenged to make during their lifetime. This volume has not sought to meet that expectation but has sought to provide a gateway to a better understanding of sexuality and the transitions realized through the expertise and research of Emily Koert and Judith Daniluk, Ph.D. at the University of British Columbia in their chapter on women's sexuality across the adult lifespan. The authors explain sexuality as an important and complex aspect of lives that encompasses not only the physical, but psychological, social, emotional, spiritual, cultural, and ethical domains of human experience. The spectrum of sexuality includes attitudes, beliefs, and expectations about self and others. Researchers Daniluk and Koert recognize that how women experience their sexuality changes and shifts across the lifespan, especially during key transitions such as infertility, pregnancy, mothering, menopause, and physical illness, and disability. Dr. Daniluk notes that not only do these transitions involve biological processes and changes, but the meanings that women attribute to these events and experiences also have implications for women's sexual self-perceptions, expression, and satisfaction. While focusing on women and their sexuality, men have much to gain from the take home messages in this chapter. The importance of adopting a holistic approach when considering the issues and concerns related to both male and female sexuality at key transitions must be realized as a fluid rather than a fixed process and experience.

The impact of stressful life events impacts not only the person(s) experiencing such events but the family and friends of these individuals. Family and spousal adaptation to transitioning a traumatic event is the focus of Thomas W. Miller, Ph.D., Cynthia Dunn, Ph.D., and Ila Patel, M.D., University of Kentucky and the Department of Veterans Affairs. Examined in this chapter is adaptation to change in the family that ranges from death of a spouse to Randy Pausch who entered our lives in September 2007 to returning combat veterans of wars past. The purpose and scope of this chapter is to address the transition faced by spouse and family with a nondisabled spouse who suffers a debilitating injury and loss due to a spectrum of causes. Examined are a multiplicity of issues which have been recognized through clinical research and experience as relevant to the spouse who is physically disabled. Specific issues related to life change events, their applicability to personality theory, and recent clinical research are explored. Classic case studies are offered to exemplify issues of adaptation and change. Finally, issues in the treatment of the spouse who is physically disabled and family members are explored.

Legal, Ethical, and Financial Transitions

Some of the more stressful life experiences involve legal, ethical, and financial transitions. To address these critical ingredients in our life span I turned initially to a good colleague and friend Steve Nisenbaum, Ph.D., J.D. who with Madelaine Claire Weiss, M.S.W., M.B.A., and Dan Shapiro, Ph.D., J.D. all at Harvard Law School. Their initial chapter addresses ethical and legal issues in transitioning the life span. The approach they chose was to address this topic in three parts noting that ethics and law are pivotal inventions for managing stress across the life cycle, especially at critical junctures of key life event and stage-of-life transitions. They initially examine the evolutionary origins of human capacity for law and ethics as a social institution for stress regulation. This is followed by an investigation of the scope and content of modern law and ethics for life transition and followed by a summary of some twenty-first century modernist notions of rights and entitlements for protection under the law. They conclude their treatment of this topic with an examination of the issue of formidable iatrogenic stress contributed by moral quandary and navigating legal systems with an eye toward future directions for humankind.

All of us face financial transitions across the life span and John V. Broadman, CFP, Boardman Wealth Management Associates treats this chapter with understanding and expertise. He initiates his investigation with a very recent national study that reports that as many as one-third of Americans are living with extreme stress and nearly half of Americans believe that their stress has increased over the past 5 years with financial issues being a critical factor. Most critical according to the research reported were family finances, money, and work – all identified as the leading causes of stress for three quarters of Americans. Through the use of case study methodology, Boardman provides a model for conceptualizing a client's financial life and for identifying some of the stressors associated with financial transitions, and finally, key points in managing financial stress. In his analysis, he provides the reader with personal and contextual, as well as anticipated and unanticipated, factors in financial transitions and a series of take home messages for financial transitions.

In his chapter on assessing, moderating and modifying implicit cognitive processes in alcohol and drug misuse in transitioning adulthood, Professor Marvin Krank, Ph.D., University of British Columbia focuses on the ethical and legal as well as health issues related to drug use and abuse, recognizing that adolescence is the time when individuals make the perilous journey from child to adult. Although risk-taking is natural and inevitable, adolescent development is fraught with potentially dangerous situations with choices that can lead to both short- and long-term changes with either positive or negative consequences on healthy development. The developmental imperatives of adolescence include physical, emotional, sexual, social, and cognitive change. Professor Krank notes that this early substance use occurs in a developmental and social context. In the social and developmental context of adolescence, this chapter explores social influences faced by youth through an emerging dual processing cognitive model of choice that helps to explain the vulnerability of youth to alcohol and drug use, and abuse. This chapter presents a recently developed approach to adolescent substance use that builds on dual processing models of cognition. The dual processing model is consistent with this outcome because adolescents seem to have reduced levels the executive control relative to adults. Increased vulnerability occurs because social and developmental influences on automatic memories occur before executive control matures. The dual processing approach is important because it suggests new ways of assessing vulnerability through tests of executive function and memory associations. This approach promises new tools for prevention science research.

Life-Threatening Transitions in Maturation and Health

William Weitzel, M.D. and Judith Carney, M.S. O.T. explore the stressful transitions faced by a person experiencing an unanticipated change of course in life when one receives the diagnosis of chronic progressive neurological disease. Trace with these authors the personal journey of a physician as he comes to realize the symptom onset of a neurological disease that is initially denied. His next physical exam revealed the diagnosis of Idiopathic Parkinson's Disease. Initial medications saw a reduction in symptoms for the next several years. Following that period of time, the symptoms returned with more tremors, more rigidity, and more slowness of movement. Judy Carney provides insights into treatment options and quality of life for the person with a progressive degenerative neurological disease and some essentials for patient and caregivers in transitioning this stressful life experience.

The diagnosis of cancer has affected so many through families, relatives, and friends. Transitions throughout the cancer experience that include receiving the initial diagnosis, a spectrum of treatment options, survivorship, and end of life become the essential phases in considering those transitioning the stressful sequences involved in cancer care. Dorothy Ann Brockopp, R.N., Ph.D., Krista Moe, M.S., Judith A. Schreiber, R.N., Ph.D.(c), and Sherry Warden, R.N., Ph.D., all at the University of Kentucky, College of Nursing provide a unique and compelling treatment of this stressful life transition. They note that the cancer experience, from diagnosis through treatment to survivorship, is fraught with numerous challenges and transitions. Individuals receive an anxiety-producing diagnosis and then face treatment options that are often accompanied by serious and debilitating side effects. The cancer journey is frequently long and arduous and the threat of mortality is a constant companion. The authors use the *Experiencing Transitions model* (Meleis et al. 2000) as a framework. This chapter describes the events that are likely to trigger transitions and their potential sequelae as identified in the literature and occurring in clinical forum.

Loss of the "safety signal" in childhood and adolescent trauma is examined in the next chapter by Thomas W. Miller, Ph.D. at University of Kentucky and Allan Beane, Ed.D. Bully-free programs examine the impact of losing one's safety signal as bullying is recognized as a significant problem in transitioning both childhood and adulthood in our twenty-first century. The domestic violence literature along with research associated with prisoners of war and victims of violence has known the safety signal theory since Martin Seligman wrote his book on *Learned Helplessness* (Seligman 1975). Bullying is another form of victimization that has gained considerable attention in the last quarter of the twenty-first century. Bullying experienced in the schools is something most children encounter in one form or another during school age. Children and adults struggle with being called names, being picked upon, and with being intimidated and rejected or excluded among peers and in the school, work, home, and living environment. Even though bullying has been around since time began, little attention has been given to the long-term effects of bullying behavior on both the victim and the perpetrator. Examined are research and clinical studies addressing bullying. Bullying behavior is any form of hurtful behavior toward another child that is disruptive to emotional well-being of the victim. The importance of understanding how both children and adults process and accommodate the trauma of bullying is addressed as is the importance of understanding the safety signal in coping with bullying situations. Clinical issues that need to be addressed are explored as are resources in treating victims of bullying behavior.

Among some of the most difficult transitions facing any of us is the unexpected accident that results in a traumatic change in one's life and lifestyle. Richard Welsh, M.S.W., Lane J. Veltkamp, M.S.W., and Thomas W. Miller, Ph.D. along with Emily Rosenbaum examine through theory and case example three very life-changing events resulting in serious lifestyle changes for three professionals in the health-care professions. Drawing on the theory and research of Miller and Veltkamp (1994), these authors trace the processing of three traumatic events from both a clinical and personal perspective.

Joseph Fox, Ph.D., a former Chief Audiologist and Speech Language Pathologist with the Department of Veterans Affairs offers in the next chapter important issues to consider with communicating health-related concerns and stressful markers of health critical in aging. With an emphasis on self-awareness and its importance in communication in health care, this chapter examines not only the mind–body connection and the influence of stress on the body and its functions but also the importance of communication in addressing health markers and health care.

Cultural, Religious and Spiritual Influences in Life's Transitions

Many theorists and researchers have identified the importance of "self-regulation" as an important factor across the life span and significantly important for several life transitions. Professors Katica Lackovic-Grgin, Ph.D. and Zvjezdan Penezic, Ph.D. at the Department of Psychology, University of Zadar, Croatia define through their clinical research the essential contributions of "self-regulation" in coping with and adjusting to stressful life transitions from a cultural perspective. Theories that have emerged from multiple cultures are reviewed as is research associated with cultural implications of stressful life transitions. Developmental regulation involves efforts by the individual to influence the actual development, adapting oneself psychologically to the demands of the context in which one lives. These efforts are sometimes called *volition* and according to the *volition theory* (Kuhl and Fuhrmann 1998, p. 15) volition is expressed in two ways. The first kind of volition supporting the maintenance of an active goal is called self-control or action control, and the second kind, supporting the maintenance of one's actions in line with one's integrated self, is called self-regulation. The concept that these kinds of adaptive processes in adolescence and adulthood consist of emergence, establishment, and sustaining of the equilibrium between one's intentions, goals, behavior patterns, and self, will be the analytical framework for the theoretical and empirical studies that will be employed in writing this chapter. It describes the motivational bases or the regulation of one's own development, constraints on developmental self-regulation across some life-transitions, the organizers of self-regulation, as well as the mechanisms and strategies of self-regulation.

Continuing with the cultural influence in adapting to stressful life transitions, Helene Fung, Ph.D. and Tasia M.Y. Siu, Ph.D. both of The Chinese University of Hong Kong, New Territories Hong Kong China provide theory and research on the age-related patterns in social networks among European Americans and African Americans. Specifically their research focuses on the issues and implications for socio-emotional selectivity across the lifespan. The authors review how goals change across the life cycle and the role of time perspective in the change. Empirical evidences suggest that individuals are likely to perceive time as limited (1) when they age, (2) when they have limited subjective life expectancy due to terminal illnesses or exposure to death of others, or (3) when they are facing micro- or macro-level events, such as graduation or a political transition, that symbolize an end to the life as they know it. As the finitude of future time becomes salient, they reprioritize their goals, focusing on the goals that are most important to them. The result of this reprioritization usually leads to a focus on goals that are emotionally meaningful for those facing stressful life transitions.

Often forgotten in the spectrum of groups studied are refugees' life transitions from displacement to a safe and durable resettlement. Antoinette Soussa, Ph.D. from the College of Social Work at the University of Kentucky examines the refugee experience and various life transitions as a result of armed conflicts and civil wars leading to emergency displacement in their normal everyday lives. These transitions begin at the onset of a complex emergency and last until a durable solution is found for their safety. Wars and armed conflicts are one of the main causes of forced migration leading to the creation of refugees and internally displaced persons. According to Stockholm International Peace Research Institute (SIPRI), there were 59 major armed conflicts in 48 different locations since the post cold war period.

Cultural, religious, and spiritual influences in life's stressful transitions become the focus of our next section. This chapter addresses encountering stressful events as well as normative transitions as a test of religious beliefs/coping systems. The research and clinical expertise of Crystal Park, Ph.D., Donald Edmondson, and Mary Alice Mills at the University of Connecticut provide a special and unique examination of religion and spirituality within the context of transitioning stressful life events. These authors examine two primary issues, first how religion and spirituality influence people's appraisals of, and coping with, both normative transitions and unexpected crises, and secondly as part of the coping process, how life transitions and crises influence individuals' subsequent religious and spiritual life. Employing the meaning-making framework of stress and coping (Park and Folkman 1997; Park 2005) they describe how religiousness/spirituality is a central part of this framework for many people. Then these authors use this framework to integrate theory and empirical literature on these two primary issues. The meaning making framework is broad enough to encompass the coping challenges that are considered within both the stressful life events approach and the developmental or normative transition approach. This broader framework therefore includes positive events that may be stressful, but are sought after nonetheless, as well as negative life events. While many have noted the role of religious beliefs in transforming the appraisal or interpretation of negative events, they propose that the interaction of religious and spiritual meaning systems and stressful life events is best conceptualized as an ongoing and recursive process of mutual influence. This chapter examines existing relevant empirical research and concludes with suggestions for future research.

The role of cultural and spiritual beliefs in addressing stressful life events and the transitions we face in the life span is addressed by Professor Evangeline Wheeler, Ph.D. at Towson State University. In this chapter, she offers an examination of life stress buffer as the salubrious role of African-centered spirituality. The author notes that people cope with life stress and transitions in the lifespan in myriad ways, but for many people identified with African-American culture, a primary resource is an African-centered spiritual base. While the culture of this group has been the foundation of many national artistic and cultural trends, most notable recently in the twenty-first century global youth culture, the psychological legacy commonly reflects adjustments to centuries of systemic and systematic racial bias. The analysis of the historical effect is complex and multidisciplinary, not unlike an African worldview that emphasizes connectedness and Gestalt. Evangeline Wheeler examines spirituality as a reaction to cultural oppression and finds that it is deeply embedded in the healthy life-span development of people of Africa and the African Diaspora. From a cultural perspective, spiritual issues do not wait to become pertinent in aging as some theorists have suggested. To the contrary an awareness of the spirit is instilled from a very early age and reinforced through daily practices. But for a large proportion of the African-American population, the simple "stress of living" is often magnified. Additional factors of entrenched poverty, chronic disease, juvenile crime, and societal prejudice raise questions of how people cope under such circumstances. Many African Americans find that the negative consequences of blatant prejudice ultimately manifest in issues of mental and physical well-being. The transitioning and coping process in dealing with stressful life events for African Americans and likely other cultures is found in their culture-centered spiritual base.

Directions and Interventions in Stressful Life Transitions

Dai Williams, the founder of *Eos* in the United Kingdom introduces the reader to surviving and thriving: how "transition psychology" may apply to mass traumas and stressful life events. In this chapter, the author reflects on a journey, a kind of traveller's tale that started with a Peace Corps volunteer in northern Uganda, soon after Idi Amin seized power and a cholera epidemic. Asked how he coped with these events he described a culture shock briefing that warned of a delayed crisis typically 6 months into a new assignment when volunteers were most likely to quit. Were those Peace Corps trainers aware of Elizabeth Kubler-Ross's work on stages of grief – one of the earliest descriptions of transition? Or were they acting on careful observation? In the early 1970s pioneers of transition psychology began to explore the stages of change that occur after trauma, loss, or other major life events. The author was to discover this work 7 years later from Leonie Sugarman's brilliant course on Life-Span Development in London. She alerted the author to the importance of transitions in personal development and career psychology. This author has been tracking the crises and opportunities of new leadership transitions, the collective transitions for new governments, and the wider effects of mass trauma on governments and communities from terrorist attacks like 9–11, wars, and natural disasters.

Important to the field of understanding the impact of stressful life experiences on health is the emerging literature that has focused on growth through trauma. A relatively new concept in the trauma field is "trauma growth." The focus of this chapter is on the processing of trauma after a stressful life event and what has come to be known as "trauma growth." Cassie Lindstrom and Kelli Triplett who are both in the Department of Psychology at the University of North Carolina Charlotte provide a chapter that aids in understanding the conceptualization and processing of trauma growth.

The twenty-first century has witnessed significant medical advances. What these advances mean for the diagnostics of human health is held within the genetic makeup of each of us. The capability of gaining greater insight into one's health will provide a bridge to potential prevention strategies for many illnesses and diseases and for some a stressful life transition. The influence of a growing knowledge of our genetic makeup and its potential to help us understand potential predisposition to disease offers a view of the potential psychological impact of contemporary medicine and medical genetics on transitions in the life cycle. David T. Miller, M.D., Ph.D., Boston Children's Hospital and Harvard University, provides the reader with insights as to how our genes affect many aspects of our life and health. Advances in medicine during the last decade have seen amazing progress in our understanding of human genetics. The completion of the *Human Genome Project* in 2003 brought this issue into the mainstream more than any other single event (Collins et al. 2003). Perhaps contrary to expectations, this milestone created more questions than it answered.

Certainly, knowledge of the human genome sequence has increased the pace of genetic discovery for many diseases, but translating discoveries into patient care applications is not always straightforward. One way that genetic disease information can be harnessed in clinical medicine is through genetic testing. In the coming years, information about our genes will lead to routine use of diagnostic testing on the basis of genetic markers for common diseases such as asthma, coronary artery disease, and diabetes. Genetic tests for these diseases may lead to substantive changes in medical management depending on the results.

Functional Fitness, Life Stress, and Transitions in the Life Span authored by John Nyland, D.P.T., Ed.D. A.T.C., C.S.C.S., F.A.C.S.M. and James D. Abbott, M.D., University of Louisville provides the reader with the complimentary intervention for good nutrition; the authors argue that maintaining functional fitness throughout the life cycle is essential to both independent living and to the overall quality of that life. Provided in this chapter are clinical and evidence based support for a range of physical exercises necessary and essential for health and quality of life in aging. Integration of technology with functional fitness is inherent in good health and John Nyland and Jim Abbott counsel the reader that the need to make better decisions regarding technological advances to truly harvest the specific characteristic of the technology that is desired while not damaging or marginalizing other more positive health behaviors is essential. Blending innovative technological advances with high quality real life experiences will more effectively reap some of the desired and significant health benefits sought in being functionally fit.

The influence of food on adapting to stressful life events and transitions in the lifespan is offered by Jasminka Illich, Ph.D., Florida State University and Rhonda Brownbill, Ph.D., University of Connecticut. These authors focus on a discussion of the nutritional requirements of individuals in different periods in the life cycle, spanning from infancy and childhood to old age. They begin with the pregnancy and maternal nutritional needs, which ultimately determine fetal growth and development and continue by addressing main issues in infancy, childhood, and adolescence, focusing on the critical nutrients in each period, dietary patterns, and behaviors and most common disorders associated with food intake in those periods. Adult period focuses on the balanced nutrition and life style conducive to disease prevention and maintenance of healthy state. In their discussion of the aging, the focus of this chapter is to discuss the nutritional requirements of individuals in different periods of life, spanning from infancy and childhood to old age. Their treatment of nutritional needs of older adults addresses some of the most critical nutrients for that period, as well as some chronic conditions and the ways to avoid or alleviate them.

The role of animals and animal-assisted therapy in stressful life transitions is offered in a chapter by Jeanine M. Miller-Adams, Ed.D., OTR/L, CHES. As one considers the intervention options for successfully transitioning a significant stressful life event that is marked by anxiety, depression, loss, or limited physical functioning, and that requires social contact and contact comfort, animals as well as animal-assisted therapy (AAT) is a viable and helpful option. Animals and pets have often played a significant role in the lives of humans. In this chapter the author describes AAT and how it impacts people and animals, provides three case examples of how it has affected individuals during the stressful life transitions they have experienced, and explores theoretical perspectives applicable to this form of therapy. AAT has touched the lives of many people experiencing stressful life transitions in health and illness. It is a growing form of therapy that benefits both the humans and the animals involved.

In considering the spectrum of interventions for stressful transitions in the life span, humor as a way of transitioning stressful life events has provided a vehicle for coping, adjustment, or accommodation of some of the most difficult transitions faced. Michael Roy Nichols, Ph.D., Clifford Kuhn, M.D., and Barbara Belew, Ph.D. offer a special and unique formula in their chapter. Addressed is a special understanding of humor in coping with stressful life transitions in the life span. The authors are careful in defining humor and its role in coping with difficult transitions. Their definition of humor refers to an attitude that allows one to see life in a better perspective, to transcend our current situation, to seek out and enjoy all the absurdities that present themselves to us on a daily basis, to gain control of our destinies, and to live in the present without fear of change. Humor must not be more than an arsenal of jokes, nor does it mean laughing off a situation that demands and deserves attention and action. A case example is offered of a young cancer patient who was seen by one of the authors, who used humor positively and constructively to help deal with the changes that her diagnosis produced.

Concluding comments and future directions for stressful life events and transitions across the life span is a chapter that offers the reader several current transitions and a glimpse at the next phase in understanding and researching critical issues in stressful transitions in the life span. In summary, this volume entitled *Stressful Life Events: Transitions in the Life Span* provides clinicians and researchers, students, professionals, and the general public a compendium of contributions relevant to understanding and addressing the critical issues tied to transitions in the life cycle. It offers the reader insight into critical issues related to the stresses associated with the transitions humankind faces in everyday life.

References

Atchley, R., & Barusch, A. (2004). *Social forces & aging*. Belmont: Wadsworth.

Basoglu, M. (1997). Torture as a stressful life event. In T. W. Miller (Ed.), *Clinical disorders and stressful life events*. Madison, CN: International Universities Press, Inc.

Byrne, D. (1989). Personal determinants of recent life stress and myocardial infarction. In T. W. Miller (Ed.), *Theory and assessment of stressful life event*. Madison, CN: International Universities Press, Inc.

Cernovsky, Z. Z. (1989). Refugee's repetitive nightmares. *Journal of Clinical Psychology, 54*(7), 559–633.

Collins, F. S., Green, E. D., Guttmacher, A. E., & Guyer, M. S. (2003). A vision for the future of genomics research. *Nature, 422*(6934), 835–847.

Dohrwend, B. S., & Dohrwend, B. P. (1974). *Stressful life events: Their nature and effects*. New York: John Wiley Publishers.

Engdahl, B., & Eberly, E. (1997). The course of chronic post traumatic stress disorder. In T. W. Miller (Ed.), *Clinical disorders and stressful life events*. Madison, CN: International Universities Press, Inc.

Erikson, E. H. (1950) *Childhood and Society*. New York: Norton.

Erikson, E. H. (1968). *Identity, youth and crisis*. New York: Norton.

Fava, G. (1989). Life events and distress in dermatological disorders. In T. W. Miller (Ed.), *Theory and assessment of stressful life events.* Madison, CN: International Universities Press, Inc.

Kobasa, S. (1979). Stressful life events, personality, and health: An inquiry into hardiness. *Journal of Personality and Social Psychology, 37*(1), 1–11.

Kuhl, J., & Fuhrmann, A. (1998). Decomposing self-regulation and self-control: The volitional components inventory. In J. Heckhausen & C. S. Dweck (Eds.), *Motivation and self-regulation across life span* (pp. 15–49). New York: Cambridge University Press.

McDaniel, J. S. (1996). Stressful life events and psycho-neuro immunology. In T. W. Miller (Ed.), *Theory and assessment of stressful life events.* Madison, CN: International Universities Press, Inc.

McNally, R. (1998). Measures of children's reactions to stressful life events. In T. W. Miller (Ed.), *Children of trauma: Stressful life events and their effects on children and adolescents.* Madison, CN: International Universities Press, Inc.

McNally, R. (1997). Can panic attacks produce post traumatic stress disorder? In T. W. Miller (Ed.), *Clinical disorders and stressful life events.* Madison, CN: International Universities Press, Inc.

Meleis, A. I., Sawyer, L. M., Im, E., Messias, D., & Schumacher, K. (2000). Experiencing transitions: An emerging middle-range theory. *Advances in Nursing Science, 23*(1), 12–28.

Miller, T. W. (1989). *Stressful life events.* New York: International Universities Press, Inc.

Miller, T. W., & Veltkamp, L. J. (1994). *Clinical handbook of child abuse and neglect.* Madison, CN: International Universities Press, Inc.

Miller, T. W. (1996). *Theory and assessment of stressful life events.* Madison, CN: International Universities Press, Inc.

Mollica, R., & Caspi-Yavin, Y. (1996). Assessment of events and their related symptoms in torture and refugee trauma. In T. W. Miller (Ed.), *Theory and assessment of stressful life events.* Madison, CN: International Universities Press, Inc.

Park, C. L., & Folkman, S. (1997). Stability and change in psychosocial resources during caregiving and bereavement in partners of men with AIDS. Journal of Personality, 65, 421–447.

Park, C. L. (2005). Religion and meaning. In R. F. Paloutzian & C. L. Park (Eds.), *Handbook of the psychology of religion and spirituality* (pp. 295–314). New York: Guilford.

Post, R. M., Weiss, S., & Smith, M. (1996). Impact of psychosocial stress on gene expression: Implications for PTSD and recurrent affective disorders. In T. W. Miller (Ed.), *Theory and assessment of stressful life events.* Madison, CN: International Universities Press, Inc.

Rahe, R. (1989). Recent life change and psychological depression. In: T.W. Miller (Ed.) (1996). *Theory and assessment of stressful life events,* Madison, CT: International Universities Press, Inc.

Seligman, M. E. P. (1975). Helplessness: On Depression, Development, and Death. San Francisco: W.H. Freeman.

Wallerstein, J., Lewis, J., & Blakeslee, S. (2001). *The unexpected legacy of divorce: A 25 year landmark study.* New York, NY: Hyperion.

Yule, W. (1998). Post traumatic stress disorder in children and its treatment. In T. W. Miller (Ed.), *Children of trauma: Stressful life events and their effects on children and adolescents.* Madison, CN: International Universities Press, Inc.

Chapter 2

Life Transitions and Stress in the Context of Psychosocial Development

I was discussing a movie, "The Eternal Sunshine of the Spotless Mind" with a group of clinical psychology students – psychotherapists-in-training. As we were musing about the relationship between suffering and growth, one fresh-faced student remarked that he thought that just as much growth issued from positive experiences as from negative ones and that, perhaps, negative ones weren't necessary at all for personal growth. From the perspective of 70 years, 40 of which have been spent doing psychotherapy, I was speechless, gasping inwardly at such breathtaking naivete. Then I recalled being a fresh-faced psychotherapist-in-training myself and a graduate school friend, older than I by at least 10 years, told me that he was reluctant to talk with me about his marital problems because, as he said, "You just don't have the experience necessary to understand." He was right, but I was hurt by his response. That I still remember it is important. It was a negative experience; I felt badly; and I learned from it.

Although generally optimistic, I confess to a "tragic view of life." I believe that all growth involves change, that change means loss (of a previous position, of a certain view of oneself and the world), and that loss is painful. Undergoing disequilibration and subsequent accommodation (change) is not a pleasant experience; that is why so many avoid it, preferring assimilation (remaining the same) instead. But meaningful change and growth inevitably entail some suffering. So, although this article is not intended to celebrate pain, it does recognize the necessity of some suffering as one transits life stages and stretches oneself to adapt to stressful situations.

The effects of life stressors and the impact of life transitions occur within the context of overall lifespan development. In order to understand the meaning of such potentially disruptive events for the individual, it is important to understand what the general course of adult development looks like. The only developmental psychological theorist to lay out a course of expectable life cycle development is Erik Erikson (1980). He has outlined eight psychosocial developmental periods extending from birth to old age. Each period is framed by descriptors such as "young adult," "middle age," etc. As the human life span has increased, the boundaries of these chronological

From: *Handbook of Stressful Transitions Across the Lifespan*, Edited by: T.W. Miller, DOI 10.1007/978-1-4419-0748-6_2, © Springer Science+Business Media, LLC 2010 periods have become increasingly elastic; however, they do provide a rough guideline as to average expectable development over the individual's life course (Marcia 1998a, 2002, 2004).

The basis for these stages of growth lies in body changes, social expectations concerning these changes, and social/cultural institutions within which the resolution of the crises involved in each of these stages takes place. For example, at adolescence, the individual is undergoing significant physiological, sexual, and cognitive changes. Social institutions within which these changes are more or less accommodated and supported are schools, peer groups, vocational preparation, armed forces training, religious rites of passage, etc. Such social institutions have evolved with reference to individual needs and abilities and, in the best cases, make reasonable demands and provide appropriate rewards. In Erikson's terms, there is a kind of "cog-wheeling" between the individual and the social context. Because social changes sometimes occur at a glacial pace and because individuals do differ in their needs and abilities, these institutions tend to function on a lowest common denominator basis. Hence, while many find their social context confirming, a significant number of others are discontented with the contexts furnished by their particular civilizations.

It is not just external events that impact individual growth and development, but built-in conflicts. Each Eriksonian stage consists of alternative possibilities, indicated by the term "versus" (e.g., identity vs. identity diffusion, intimacy vs. isolation, etc.) Hence, each developmental stage is a **crisis** wherein the individual may move forward, backward, or remain stuck. Below is a simple eight-stage version of Erikson's developmental scheme. Approximate chronological periods are indicated on the left perpendicular; stages of ego growth are located along the diagonal (Fig. 2-1). The resolution of each stage

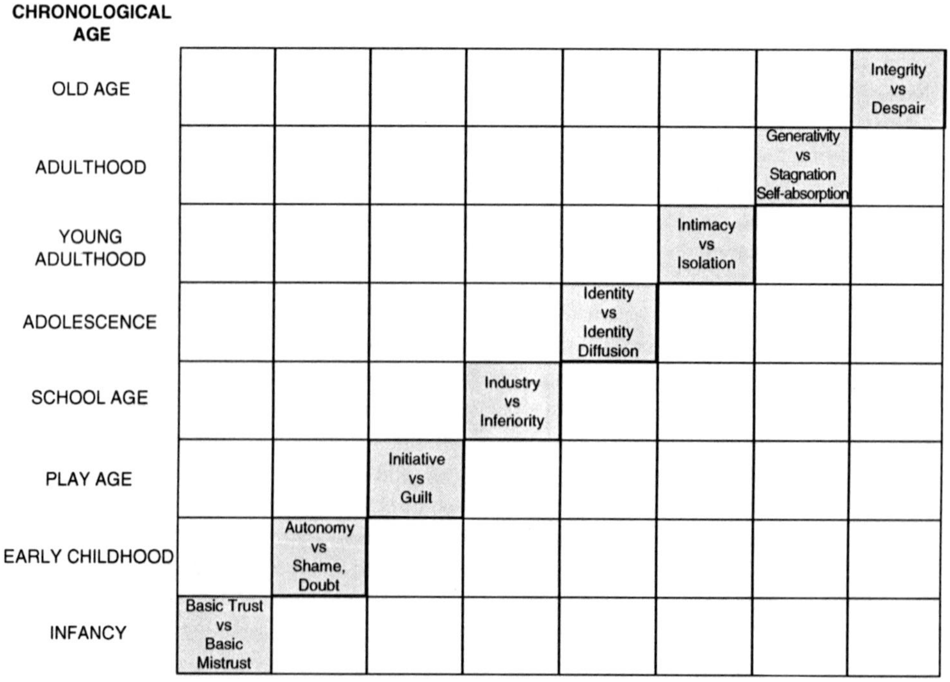

CHRONOLOGICAL AGE								
OLD AGE								Integrity vs Despair
ADULTHOOD							Generativity vs Stagnation Self-absorption	
YOUNG ADULTHOOD						Intimacy vs Isolation		
ADOLESCENCE					Identity vs Identity Diffusion			
SCHOOL AGE				Industry vs Inferiority				
PLAY AGE			Initiative vs Guilt					
EARLY CHILDHOOD		Autonomy vs Shame, Doubt						
INFANCY	Basic Trust vs Basic Mistrust							

Fig. 2-1. Simplified Eriksonian Developmental Chart

is assumed to be a necessary condition for the resolution of a succeeding stage. For example, a sense of intimacy at young adulthood is assumed to be necessary for the development of generativity at middle age; successful generativity is necessary for genuine Integrity at old age.

While this seems simple enough, the picture of adult development is more complex – just as individual human development is more complex than could be conveyed by any chart. The resolutions of stages beyond adolescence are not simple "either-or" matters. These stage resolutions take the form more of a dialectical synthesis in which the "positive" pole of a crisis becomes a thesis, the "negative" pole an antithesis, and the individual's resolution his or her own particular synthesis. Furthermore, this synthesis incorporates some elements of **both** the positive and negative elements. There is no real generativity without elements of stagnation and self-absorption and no Integrity without an abiding sense of despair. Nevertheless, the emphasis on the new integration remains on the positive pole.

In order to flesh out the meaning of these stages, I shall describe the stage content extending from adolescence through old age. I begin with adolescence because that is the time – especially late adolescence – when the most important of the post-childhood stage resolutions, identity versus identity diffusion occurs. This is the most important resolution because identity is the only truly structural component of Erikson's theory. The identity structure formed for the first time at late adolescence is a crucial component of development throughout the adult life cycle. The earlier childhood stage resolutions provide the necessary scaffolding for identity development in adolescence – especially the formation of basic trust at infancy. However, this article concerns mainly adult development, so my focus is only on psychosocial stages beginning with adolescence.

Psychosocial Stages from Adolescence Through Adulthood

Identity

The beginning of childhood's end in early adolescence sees the young person hopefully having accrued all of the psychosocial raw material needed for achieving Freud's vision of optimum development: the ability to love (basic trust, autonomy) and to work (initiative, industry). Identity formation becomes paramount during this life-cycle era because the individual is required to make a transition both physically and socially from child to adult, from receiver to provider. Until this time, the young person has made a number of part-identifications: that is, he or she has identified with some aspects of other people and with some aspects of the self, and has been generally content with playing different roles at different times without much concern for integration. The changes that are attendant upon puberty and subsequent adolescence have two effects: they disequilibrate the fairly structured life of the latency-aged child; and they require an accommodation in the form of a new integration of physique, sexuality, ideology, abilities, personal needs, and perceived social demands. Having traversed the early adolescent periods of de-structuring and re-structuring, the individual arrives at late adolescence with an identity that has become consolidated for the first time and is to be tried out in the world.

Our research (Marcia et al. 1993) indicates that two processes are important for identity formation: the *exploration* of alternative beliefs, values, and occupational goals; and a subsequent *commitment* to a selected set of alternatives. On the basis of these criteria, we have indicated four modes of identity resolution called the **identity statuses**: *identity achievement* (has undergone exploration and made commitments); *moratorium* (is currently exploring alternatives with commitments only vague); *foreclosure* (committed, but with no exploration); and *identity diffusion* (uncommitted with little genuine exploration). Described briefly, *achievements* are solid, directed, and open to identity-relevant information; *moratoriums* are struggling, interpersonally engaging (sometimes exhausting) and, usually, moving toward the commitments that will constitute an identity; *foreclosures* appear superficially content, but they maintain this through cognitive rigidity and endorse authoritarian values; and *diffusions* are scattered, without direction – at best, they are insouciant and at worst, they feel depressed and empty. More will be said about these statuses when discussing further adult development.

Intimacy

Having determined who one is, and is to be, during the previous adolescent period, the young adult now faces the task of sharing this newly minted identity with at least one other person. Intimacy refers to a relationship characterized by depth of expression of feeling, care, and concern for the other, and commitment. The risk is that in sharing oneself deeply with another, one can lose oneself unless one's new identity is sufficiently strongly flexible to permit it to be temporarily lost in merger and then recovered.

Recalling the previous statement about Eriksonian stages having a somatic basis, the prototypical situation for intimacy is sexual intercourse. This provides the occasion for merging deeply and caringly, "losing oneself in the other." It then constitutes the model for a psychological relationship in which one can suspend temporarily self-concern and self-protection, and attend to another. Clearly, sexual intercourse is neither a necessary or sufficient condition for intimacy. In fact, the most technically proficient intercourse, if it is merely "performed" can be one of life's more isolating experiences. Rather, intimacy refers to a psychological relationship, which usually does – but may not – have a physical component.

The lyrics from a now somewhat dated Simon and Garfunkel song, "I am a rock, I am an island… I touch no one and no one touches me," describe the position of the *isolate*. In the best psychosocial outcome, intimacy is integrated with isolation so that one develops one's own style of being both intimate and isolate, maintaining a sense of separate self while cherishing the mutuality of deep contact with another person.

There are two intermediate intimacy-isolation patterns that have been defined by research (Orlofsky et al. 1973; Orlofsky, in Marcia et al. 1993). One of the most common is the *pseudo-intimate* in which the individual is in a societally recognized context for intimacy, say marriage, but the content of the relationship is superficial and routine, devoid of deep contact. Commitment is superimposed on the relationship rather than emerging organically from it.

An example of pseudo-intimacy is the relationship of a man whom I am currently seeing in psychotherapy. He and his wife of 30-plus years are also in couples therapy. At ages 19 and 17, he was the quarterback and she was the cheerleader. This pattern was more or less functional as he succeeded in business and she made a home for him and their two, now adult, children. Recently, he met someone who he felt truly "listened" to him, who came to know him from the inside. He is now struggling to get his wife to "hear" him in the same way. For whatever defensive reasons, she seems unable to do this, and, in search of a deeper intimacy, he may be leaving the relationship. Not for another woman – he may likely choose to be alone for awhile – but for a level of understanding that he has felt lacking. Within the past several years, I have seen at least three men whose wives have left them, seeking the same thing. The issue is not gender-specific, nor is it about "sex"; it is about intimacy.

Two other intimacy patterns, or statuses, intermediate between *intimate* and *isolate* are the *pre-intimate* and the *stereotyped*. *Pre-intimate* individuals are similar to *intimate* ones except that, at young adulthood, they do not currently find themselves in a relationship in which their values and capacities can be realized. They are rather like the *moratorium* identity status: they are on the threshold of intimacy and are searching for the "right" relationship. *Stereotyped* persons are involved in superficial dating relationships and have no particular interest in either depth or longevity of contacts with others.

Generativity

Middle age sees the development of a predominant concern with caring for the life cycles of others. The prototypical situation for this is the generation of one's own children. Yet, *generativity* applies as well to care for any of one's valued creations, to one's relationship to the next generation as a mentor, and to contributions to one's community by establishing contexts for the growth of others. In addition, one finds one's caring directed to those older than oneself, frequently to one's own parents as they become less capable of caring for themselves. The alternative of *stagnation* suggests a kind of lying fallow, which if continued too long, becomes sterility. *Self-absorption*, the other "negative" alternative, involves treating oneself as one's one and only beloved child. Recalling earlier comments on the integration of positive and negative poles, generativity involves not just a balance but an **integration** of care for the other and care for oneself. The generative trap is that the better one becomes at it, the greater the expectations of others, and of oneself, for continued self-giving. Hence, an important aspect of authentic generativity is a generative approach to oneself as well as to others. Clearly, this involves an element of self-absorption; otherwise, continued uni-directional generativity can degenerate into drivenness and "burnout." Thus, periods of stagnation may be important in leading to a renewed generativity.

Our research (Bradley 1997; Bradley and Marcia 1998) has suggested that there are three styles of generativity intermediate between *generativity* and *stagnation, self-absorption*. These are based upon criteria of inclusivity and involvement. Inclusivity refers to the band width of one's care: Who qualifies? Just one's "own kind' or a broader spectrum of the next generation? Involvement refers to the extent of investment one makes in care-giving activity. Two styles of *pseudo-generativity* are *agentic* and *communal*. The agentic person is engaged in fostering the growth of others, but only so long as they are instrumental in aiding the agentic person in the attainment of his/her personal goals.

The communal individual is involved in the nurturance of others, but the continuance of this activity is contingent upon fairly regular expressions of gratitude on the part of the object of care. In both types of pseudo-generativity, the ultimate focus of the generative activity is more on the giver than on the recipient; and the care ceases when the giver is no longer the central beneficiary. The third intermediate generativity style is the *conventional* who restrict the scope of their caring to just those others who behave and believe consistently with the *conventional* person's own values. When others stray from these values, they are disqualified from care.

Generativity, in its most highly developed form, is independent of immediate results. Generative activity is predicated upon the benefits for generations to come, on the concern for life cycles of "children" not yet born. The generative individual is engaged presently and for the future with "growing" things: persons, projects, and communities.

Integrity

Erikson's theory is unique (save for Jung's) among psychodynamic approaches in that it posits a stage of ego growth even at the end of the life cycle. Again, the body is involved, but in a more minor key. The physical issue now is the experience of physical decline, and what this means as an omen of dying and death. The individual stands at the terminal phase of his/her one and only life cycle. Pain and loss vie with psychological strength and wisdom. *Integrity* implies a sense of wholeness and completeness even – especially – in the face of physical dis-integration. Only when the whole of the life cycle has been completed, when each stage has been resolved satisfactorally, can the developed parts be fit together in an integral way. This involves some withdrawal from the generative preoccupations of the previous period, some ceasing to "do," in order to "be," and to reflect on the meaning of what one has done.

Integrity, while referring somewhat to authenticity, has more to do with wholeness. Can the parts fit together? Is there too much missing? Are there too many risks untaken? In understanding *despair*, the words of Ibsen, interpreted as the inner self-reproaches of an aging Peer Gynt (Marcia 1998b) come to mind:

> We are thoughts, you should have formed us....
> We are watchwords, you should have proclaimed us...
> We are tears that were never shed; we might have
> melted the ice spears that wounded you... We are
> deeds, you should have performed us; doubts
> that strangle have crippled and bent us; a thousand
> times you curbed and suppressed us. In the depths
> of your heart we have lain and waited.... We were
> never called forth – now we are poison in your
> throat (Ibsen 1966).

Yet, there is no possibility of *integrity* without an awareness of *despair*. We have tried to capture this in our research (Hearn et al. in preparation) that outlines different patterns of Integrity resolution based upon commitment (to values and beliefs), continuity (from beliefs to actions), and comprehensiveness (solidarity with humankind). One of these patterns, called *pseudo-integrated* refers to persons who maintain a cheerful, but brittle, façade by means of "uplifting" slogans and bromides. Another pattern, *non-exploratory,* is composed of individuals who simply go on being who they have always been with little or no reflection on the history of their lives or the meanings of those lives in other than familiar and unexamined terms. Interestingly, we found integrity resolution to be related to identity resolution. Perhaps this is because integrity depends on the continued development of the identity structure formed for the first time at adolescence, and because both integrity and identity refer to an integration of previously developed parts into a new whole.

An important shift to universality occurs with integrity development, a shift that has been going on at least since adolescence. This is reflected in the change of referent for the pronoun "we" – from "those-similar-to-me" at adolescence, to "you-and-me" at young adulthood, to "our family" at middle age, to "all-of-humankind" (past, present, and future) at old age.

Generational Mutuality

The foregoing description of the psychosocial stages of development focuses on the individual moving through the life cycle. But, in fact, the psychosocial stages reflect interpersonal interdependency (Marcia 1993). While young children and adolescents require "good enough" parental figures in order to resolve positively their ego growth issues, parents, likewise, depend upon those for whom they care for the confirmation of their generativity. For example, a teacher, engaged in promoting a sense of industry in her/his students, looks to their confirmatory responses for her/his sense of identity and generativity. The partner looks to the significant other for confirmation of intimacy. The elder looks to the culture and to significant people in her/his life cycle for some validation (and sometimes forgiveness) for her/his life cycle commitments to persons, ideas, and achievements.

Hope and the Complete Eriksonian Chart

The simple developmental chart presented at the beginning of this article tells only a limited story of the possibilities for growth inherent in Erikson's theory. It would appear from this outline that if a stage resolution is missed, the individual is doomed to a subsequent flawed life cycle. No identity resolution, therefore, no intimacy; no intimacy, no generativity, etc. But a more complete, and, admittedly, complex view dispels this rather pessimistic outlook. There are 64, not just 8, squares in the complete diagram (Fig. 2-2). While the diagonal remains the main feature, it is important to note that every stage occurs at every other stage. For example, there is an intimacy issue at identity, and an identity issue at integrity. The vertical in this diagram represents the prefiguring of succeeding stages by preceding ones. For example, even though identity is the central issue at adolescence, it has been in development ever since infancy. The horizontal illustrates each stage's occurrence at every other stage. For example, when the central issue is intimacy at young adulthood, issues of trust, autonomy, initiative, industry, identity, generativity, and integrity are also present – all occurring within the context of young adulthood Intimacy. And, of course, the diagonal refers to the ego strength accrued from previous stages: for example, the strength of intimate connection that is so necessary to the output of care required by generativity.

Identity issue at Integrity Stage →

Autonomy issue at Trust Stage →

CHRONOLOGICAL AGE

		1	2	3	4	5	6	7	8
OLD AGE	VIII	T-M, Intg.	A-S,D, Intg.	I-G, Intg.	Ind-I, Intg.	Id-ID, Intg.	Int-Is, Intg.	G-S, Intg.	Integrity and Despair
ADULTHOOD	VII	T-M, G	A-S,D, G.	I-G, G	Ind-I, G	Id-ID, G	Int-Is, G	Generativity and Stagnation Self-absorption	Inty-D, G
YOUNG ADULTHOOD	VI	T-M, Int.	A-S,D, Int.	I-G, Int.	Ind-I, Int.	Id-ID, Int.	Intimacy and Isolation	G-S, Int.	Inty-D, Int.
ADOLESCENCE	V	T-M, Id.	A-S,D, Id.	I-G, Id.	Ind-I, Id.	Identity and Identify Diffusion	Int-Is, Id.	G-S, Id.	Inty-D, Id.
SCHOOL AGE	IV	T-M, Ind.	A-S,D, Ind.	I-G, Ind.	Industry and Inferiority	Id-ID, Ind.	Int-Is, Ind.	G-S, Ind.	Inty-D, Ind.
PLAY AGE	III	T-M, I	A-S,D, I	Initiative and Guilt	Ind-I, I	Id-ID, I	Int-Is, I	G-S, I	Inty-D, I
EARLY CHILDHOOD	II	T-M, A	Autonomy and Shame, Doubt	I-G, A	Ind-I, A	Id-ID, A	Int-Is, A	G-S, A	Inty-D, A
INFANCY	I	Basic Trust and Basic Mistrust	A-S,D, T	I-G, T	Ind-I, T	Id-ID, T	Int-Is, T	G-S, T	Inty-D, T

OLD AGE — VIII — ○ Genital / ◉ Mature instrusion-inclusion

ADULTHOOD — VII

YOUNG ADULTHOOD — VI — ○ Genital

ADOLESCENCE — V — ○ Genital / ◉ Mature instrusion-inclusion

SCHOOL AGE — IV — ○ Latent

PLAY AGE — III — ○ Phallic (oedipal) / ◉ Intrusion-inclusion / ● Individuation

EARLY CHILDHOOD — II — ○ Anal / ◉ Eliminative retentive / ● Practising

INFANCY — I — ○ Oral / ◉ Passive-active Incorporative / ● Attachment

○ Psychosexual zone
◉ Related behavioural modality
● Object relational phase

Fig. 2-2. Expanded Eriksonian Developmental Chart

For counselors and psychotherapists, this more complete diagram has special significance. It allows for both the remediation of uncompleted stages and the precocious resolution of normally unexpected ones. If an individual arrives at intimacy unprepared with a solid identity, the possibility for identity resolution still exists, albeit now in the context of intimacy. The challenge for the clinician is to handle the resolution of two (or more) psychosocial stages simultaneously. And, of course, the more incompletely resolved the previous stages are, and the earlier these stages are, the more difficult the therapeutic task becomes. But hope resides in the assumption that because each stage re-emerges in some form at every other stage, the possibility for previous stage remediation is always present – however challenging.

Similarly, the presence of each stage in nascent form before its primary period of emergence allows for premature resolution of stages. Consider the adolescent who finds herself pregnant. She must deal with identity, the "normal" adolescent task, as well as intimacy (her relationship with the baby's father), and generativity (what is the most "caring" thing to do for both the baby and herself). It is a heavy burden, indeed. But, the form of the chart suggests the possibility for some kind of precocious resolution of these future life cycle issues in the present.

Identity Throughout the Adult Life Cycle

The first identity, formed at late adolescence, is constructed both consciously and unconsciously from the part-identifications of childhood as they are experienced by the individual in his or her socialization contexts and imagined future (Erikson 1980). Because there is no organized childhood identity to deconstruct, this initial identity formation process is largely a matter of construction: of decision-making and eventual synthesis of chosen parts. However, after that first identity is formed, succeeding ones follow the disequilibrations of that and subsequent identity structures (see also Whitbourne et al. 1992).

Normal expectable disequilibrating events are associated with each of the succeeding adult life cycle stages. Each stage involves a re-formulation of identity as one responds to the demands and rewards of each developmental era. Of course, this is true only if the individual were identity achieved at late adolescence, thus remaining open to future change. If he/she is too anxious or fearful to undergo change (as in foreclosure) preferring to ignore disconfirming information or just assimilating to an existing identity structure, then a kind of psychological stasis ensues. In order to maintain un-reconstructed the identity elements based solely upon childhood identifications the individual must be selectively inattentive (Sullivan) to identity disconfirming information (Berzonsky 1989). One way of accomplishing this is to remain in a social context similar to that of one's childhood – a context that would pose little challenge to the foreclosed identity. That is a difficult task given our shifting and information-saturated world. Still, some persons are able to navigate themselves, unchanged (foreclosed), through late adolescence, young adulthood (pseudo-intimate), middle age (conventional), and old age (non-exploratory). Psychosocial stasis is a kind of death. Change or die is true both evolutionarily and psychologically.

The *expectable* changes in identity throughout the adult life cycle after late adolescence involve moving into partnership and friendship at young adulthood, mentorship at middle age, and eldership at old age. As one enters each of these psychosocial stages, an identity reconstruction can be expected. These changes in psychosocial position are not restricted in scope to one's immediate family. They refer broadly to the human family. Hence, — being a partner or a friend, a mentor or a parent, or an elder – all are descriptors referring to the quality of one's self-awareness and psychosocial stance in the world as one moves through the ages of young adulthood, middle age, and old age.

In most of our lives, there are disequilibrating circumstances *in addition to* the expectable psychosocial stage issues. These could be life events such as divorce, falling in love (sometimes with the "wrong" person), job loss, job promotion, positive and negative reversals in fortune, retirement, spiritual crises, and the loss of loved ones. As with attempts to define stress, one has to look at what is disequilibrating for the particular *individual.* Not all divorces, job promotions, and so forth are disequilibrating for all people. We must take an individual-by-individual approach. In the case of foreclosed adults, we are dealing with people who have developed a personality structure whose purpose is to prevent change. When previously foreclosed individuals do experience disequilibration in adulthood, it is likely to be a shattering experience for them. Identity diffusion individuals cannot disequilibrate because they have no solid identity structure to begin with (Kroger 2007).

The identity reconstruction process that occurs during adulthood is presented in the following hypothetical model, on the basis of the identity statuses. The figure illustrates the cycle of identity statuses one might traverse as one undergoes identity reconstruction throughout the life cycle stages of adulthood (Fig. 2-3). Identity is expected to undergo cyclical re-formulation *at least* three times following adolescence, and likely more often as the individual is confronted with identity-challenging events. These re-formulation periods are what we have referred to as moratorium-achievement-moratorium-achievement (MAMA) cycles (Stephen et al. 1992). Even though only three cycles are shown in the diagram, one would expect a new cycle every time a significant identity-challenging event occurred.

During each of these cycles, the individual may regress to earlier identity modes (Bilsker and Marcia 1990). For example, one may experience brief periods of diffusion when the current identity structure is being challenged. The person may feel confused and scattered, behave impulsively, look for support in inappropriate places, or become "irresponsible," " unreliable," and "unpredictable." This may be sufficiently distressing that the individual enters counseling or psychotherapy. However, this is regression with a purpose: to permit the previous structure to fall apart so that a new structure can emerge. So-called "*midlife crises*" ought not to be taken lightly or dismissed. They can be important developmental steps, necessary to be taken in the service of identity reconstruction.

In addition to experiencing a period of diffusion, the person may also return to previous identity contents, even to periods of preemptive commitment to them. In other words, the individual may cycle briefly through a foreclosure phase. Again, this is part of the regressive process. Ultimately, if the de-constructed identity occurred within a previously identity-achieved context, the person would be expected to enter an actively searching moratorium period wherein

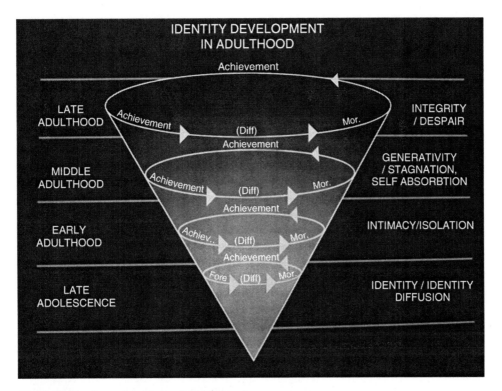

Fig. 2-3. Identity re-formulation (MAMA) cycles

she or he would begin to explore alternatives and make tentative commitments, eventuating in a new identity structure (identity achievement).

The length of these MAMA cycles may differ according to the individual and the surrounding social context. They could be as short as 6 months or as long as 10 years. Perhaps as one gets older, the cycles might be longer. One does not relinquish a hard-won identity easily. Also, there are external pressures from friends, family, and colleagues, as well as internal pressures from one's expectations of oneself, to remain the same, to be consistent. It requires more courage to re-formulate an identity when one is 40 or 60 than when one is 25.

Although the re-formulated identity is to some extent a new one, it is also continuous with, and has qualities similar to, the identity that preceded it. "Transformation" may be possible for a few individuals, but for most of us, identity change looks more like a gradual evolution of previous forms (see Flum 1990). Consistent with a cognitive developmental perspective (Kegan 1982; Piaget 1954), each reconstructed identity structure accommodates a wider range of the individual's experiences than did the previous one. Identities become broader and more inclusive. Thus, the cone shape of the diagram represents the increasingly wider range of experiences subsumed by the new identity structure (Kelly 1955). With the passage of life-time and experience, identities become deeper and richer. This is represented in the diagram by both the increase in the volume of the figure and deepening of the shading. The individual becomes more and more who she or he truly is as previous undeveloped elements of the personality are realized and new ones added.

This is similar to the processes of individuation and transcendence described by Carl Jung (1959). It is noteworthy that in one of his last articles, Erikson (1996) uses various forms of the word *numinous*, a frequently used Jungian concept, in describing the individual's sense of "I".

Psychosocial Developmental Theory and Psychotherapy

One of the most immediately apparent aspects of Erikson's theory is its basis in, and transcendence of, classical psychoanalytic theory. Its relationship to standard psychoanalytic theory is its emphasis on somatic aspects of development: there is an especially close correspondence between Erikson's first three stages of basic trust, autonomy, and initiative with Freud's oral, anal, and phallic/clitoral psychosexual stages. What Erikson added to these stages were both the ego developmental aspects and the importance of the social/cultural milieu within which these developmental issues are to be resolved.

What is the difference if a psychotherapist operates within Eriksons' psychosocial developmental framework rather than within a more orthodox analytic one? It is more a question of frame of mind, of a general outlook on the human condition, than it is of particular therapeutic techniques. However, there are some technical implications. The social context is considered to be truly meaningful; a broad and multiple network of "causes" is taken into account; and past psychological determinants (e.g., physical make-up, cultural background, family dynamics, reinforcement history, etc.) are explored within the context of individual construction. Hence, a questioning technique that is more active than the interpretation of free associations is required. Psychotherapy within this framework resembles more a mutual dialogue, a special kind of conversation, than it does a patient's production of associational material responded to with an analyst's interpretations.

Psychotherapists informed by Erikson tend to look more to issues of adaptation (see Hartmann 1964) than to repetition of early conflicts. The past is important, but of equal importance is the current level and style of coping with predominant life cycle challenges as well as the pursuit of future goals. Conflict is still important, as it is within any psychodynamic approach, but the stage on which the conflicts are played out is much expanded. Conflicts are not just internal, but between alternative ways of being in the world, of being with oneself, and of being with others. Also, the conflicts within the individual often mirror the conflicts of the culture (Erikson, 1958; 1969). Although this perspective can be derived from classical theory, it is at the heart of the Eriksonian approach, which directs the practitioner's attention to the social/cultural contexts within which an individual's development takes place. Erikson's approach *broadens* one's therapeutic perspective and techniques. If one uses Erikson's scheme as a *theoretical* developmental outline with which to formulate a patient's dynamics one may employ *techniques* borrowed from non-psychodynamic orientations (e.g., cognitive-behavioral, gestalt, client-centered, etc.) These may be used singly or in combination to further psychosocial developmental growth. While this approach may be eclectic in *technique*, it is singular in *theory*.

As discussed previously, the possibilities for the remediation of previously inadequately resolved developmental crises in ego growth, as well as the possibilities for the precocious resolution of later stages, add a note of hopefulness to the outlook of the therapist practicing within an Eriksonian framework. The social/cultural milieu is seen not solely as something against which the individual must struggle (Freud 1930) but also as the necessary matrix within which psychosocial growth takes place. That said, the earlier the difficulty lies (e.g., Basic Trust), the more difficult the therapeutic task, because subsequent stages are also likely to be flawed. Hence, the clinician is dealing not just with an age-specific issue, but all of the previously unresolved issues as well. It is difficult to expect a young adult to attain a sense of intimacy when he/she is confronting such a foundational issue as basic trust. But the possibility of doing this is suggested by the theory, and the theory also gives the practitioner some sense of direction for the level of intervention.

Another difficulty the practitioner faces within psychosocial-oriented psychotherapy is that the conditions, both individual and social, that were present when a stage was normally expected to be resolved no longer exist. Each chronological age has associated social institutions more or less keyed to individual's needs at that age. These are the "average expectable conditions" which Erikson and the ego psychologists have said are necessary for optimal crisis resolution. There are no such institutions available for, say, a middle-aged adult who, in addition to dealing with generativity and intimacy, may be confronting earlier autonomy issues. The world is not geared to provide the same kinds of supports and forgiveness for a "responsible" adult as it is for cute toddlers. The challenge facing the psychotherapist is how to deal with a toddler-age issue in the grown-up context of a middle-aged adult, without either neglecting the child-based nature of the issue, on one hand, or of infantilizing the adult patient on the other. However, because the autonomy issue exists at *every* age, one can expect to be able to help the individual to resolve autonomy (and subsequent childhood issues) within that person's adult context.

Erikson's theory is not a prescriptive theory of psychotherapy. It is a theory of ego development. It does not tell a practitioner what to do. Erikson, himself, was content to let standard psychoanalytic theory inform his clinical practice. What it does provide the practitioner is a kind of roadmap of development, of what can be reasonably expected, of where, developmentally, to intervene. The theory gives the psychotherapist a broad and reasonably optimistic framework through which to regard and to treat patients.

A Case Study: Duane (Pseudonym)

A thin, bespectacled 58 year old man faced me for his first session and said, "I think you should know that I'm planning to kill myself. What are your views on suicide?" He looked haggard as he peered up at me from underneath his large glasses, his pants' belt in its last loop. However, there was something strong and youthful in his face and he wore new, good hiking boots. While he complained of a lack of concentration, he maintained good contact with me as we spoke and displayed a "wicked," albeit self-deprecating, sense of humor. He had been referred to me by his psychotherapist who was on a 3-month leave.

Duane described his mother as depressed and "whiny." His childhood job was to listen to and comfort her. His stated main issue was with his father whom he described as distant, disapproving, and disparaging (Our research [Marcia et al. 1993] has shown a consistent relationship between identity diffusion and a lack of approval from a non-emulatible parent of the same sex). He described himself as a fat and unlovely child.

In terms of identity, he decided in college to become a social worker – in his words, "to be the opposite of his father." He said that he constructed an "upbeat, well-dressed, warm, and caring" persona. However, he was fired from his first social work job for "standing up for his principles." This unjust event was sufficient to discourage him from ever being a social worker again (One of his favorite sayings is: "You get only one chance with Duane!").

He went to an encounter group following this, which served to further confront and shatter his identity facade. However, it left him with no viable identity – a warning about the dangers of disequilibration *alone* without a fairly long period of working through the consequences. He then traversed a series of "jobs," comprising a kind of downward socio-economic spiral: computer tech assistant, fiberglass worker, machine shop operator, and, finally, security guard. In all but one of these jobs, he quit over issues of "principle."

His one major relationship, around age 45, was with a foreign-born woman. This ended when she had to return to her native country to care for her seriously ill son. She never returned and subsequently married someone else. More recently, he met and fell in love with a 33-yearold woman (25 years his junior) in his depression group. While she maintained a friendly relationship with Duane, she was in love with another man in the group, and is currently living with him – much to Duane's anger and sorrow.

Duane's current social context is a depression group in which he is a central figure, providing support and care for other members. A major part of his current identity is as a "depressed person." Much of his time is spent in seeing his GP and a psychiatrist for monitoring and regulating his medications, and two psychotherapists – myself and my colleague who has since returned from his absence. Another current identity is as a "helper" in the depression group. Others there see him as a good and caring listener. However, there is a very angry edge to him that emerges in his precipitous rejection of others ("you only get one chance with Duane") and in his dreams, many of which have to do with crime, others' incompetence, threats, assaults, and combat.

Our relationship is generally good. He seems to trust me, he has a good sense of humor, and he takes notes on sessions and seems to use these insights to at least consider making changes in his very solitary life. However, he is far too grateful, sometimes wanting to pay me extra for sessions that run a bit overtime. I'm suspicious that, at some time, the goodwill will diminish, and *my* "one chance" will get used up. However, the suicidal talk has decreased significantly.

The current challenges for us as I see them are as follows:

1. Can we loosen up his rigid ethical sense to help him to construct a more flexible and serviceable sense of values? For the psychoanalytically oriented, this is a matter of easing the superego pressures originating from his incorporated punitive, judgmental father. The task is not to shatter the superego, but to supplant it with a more flexible ethical guide.
2. Can we pick up the threads of his "social worker" identity, as currently manifested in his helper role in the depression group, to weave a new identity that would situate him generatively within the world of work?
3. Identity, intimacy, and generativity are only, at best, partially resolved. He does operate generatively within his group. But, currently, he has no really

intimate relationship. And his identity as "a depressed person" is probably not the most serviceable one. All of this raises the question of the possibility for the resolution of identity and intimacy development at a late middle age generativity period. And what are the chances for integrity resolution in the absence of these?

4. Basic Trust has been, and remains, an important issue. One way I've addressed this is to ask him to send me his dreams via email. He does this faithfully. And I, just as faithfully, acknowledge the receipt of each dream. Our sessions are also reliably accompanied by a cup of tea. As importantly as these concrete actions, I try to remain as reliably constant from session to session as I can – realistically supportive, gently challenging, and occasionally interpretive.

5. The broader theoretical/therapeutic question is to what extent a structure, identity, whose optimal time for formation has passed, can be formed? The theory suggests that it can be, but the roots of this failure go so far back developmentally that it will constitute a major effort on both our parts. It may be the case that external support will be necessary for the rest of his life: external structure provided in the absence of internal structure.

Many published case studies conclude with a happy ending. I cannot furnish one at present. We're still in the middle of the work. Some positive signs are a decrease in his suicidal talk, his willingness to participate actively in the therapeutic work, and his use of insights to re-consider his life. One of the more recent ideas he's found useful is that whenever he becomes self-destructive, or resists being self-constructive, "his father has won."

Conclusion

With respect to the theme of this book concerning life stress and life span transitions, I have tried to provide a workable theoretical outline describing normal, expectable adult life-span psychosocial issues. It is against this background that I think specific stressful events are to be considered. As contributors to this book are aware, not all stressful events are negative. Stressful events are inevitable, and built-in as part of ego development. Without them, there is no growth, only stasis. Recent research (Waterman 2007) suggests that those who undergo, and successfully resolve, identity crises have a greater sense of personal well-being than those who do not. If it is true, as I believe, that suffering, stress, and struggle are the conditions for growth, then the North American (and enlightenment) idea that all problems can be resolved or "fixed" is naïve. These "negative" events are the "night-soil" out of which we grow to become fully human. What is important for us as practitioners, social planners, and educators is to provide for ourselves and for others those *confirming contexts* which acknowledge and support crises in ego growth. After all, we're all in this together.

References

Berzonsky, M. D. (1989). Identity style: Conceptualization and measurement. *Journal of Adolescent Research, 4*(3), 267–281.

Bilsker, D., & Marcia, J. E. (1990). Adaptive regression and ego identity. *Journal of Adolescence, 14*, 75–84.

Bradley, C. L. (1997). Generativity-stagnation: Development of a status model. *Developmental Review, 17*(3), 262–290.

Bradley, C. L., & Marcia, J. E. (1998). Generativity-stagnation: A five-category model. *Journal of Personality, 66*(1), 39–64.

Erikson, E. H. (1958). *Young man Luther: A study in psychoanalysis and history*. New York: Norton.

Erikson, E.H. (1969). *Gandhi's truth*. New York: Norton

Erikson, E. H. (1980). *Identity and the life cycle: A reissue*. New York: Norton.

Erikson, E. H. (1996). The Galilean sayings and the *sense* of "I". *Psychoanalysis and Contemporary Thought, 19*(2), 291–337.

Flum, H. (1990). What is the evolutive style of identity formation? Paper presented at the meeting of the Society for Research in Adolescence, Atlanta, GA

Freud, S. (1930). Civilization and its discontents. In J. Strachey (Ed.), *The Standard Edition of the Complete Psychological Works of Sigmund Freud* (XXI). London: Hogarth.

Hartmann, H. (1964). *Essays in ego psychology*. New York: International Universities Press.

Hearn, S., Saulnier, G., Strayer, J., Glenham, M., & Koopman, R. (in preparation). *Between integrity and despair: Toward construct validation of Erikson's eighth stage*. Department of Psychology, Simon Fraser University, Burnaby, British Columbia, Canada

Ibsen, H. (1966). *Peer gynt: A dramatic poem (Translation by Peter Watts)*. London: Penguin.

Jung, C. G. (1959). Conscious, unconscious, and individuation. In *Collected Works*, (vol. 7). New York: Pantheon

Kegan, R. (1982). *The evolving self: Problem and process in human development*. Cambridge, MA: Harvard University Press.

Kelly, G. (1955). *The psychology of personal constructs*. New York: Norton.

Kroger, J. (2007). Identity development: Adolescence and Adulthood (2nd Ed.). Thousand Oaks, CA: Sage.

Marcia, J. E. (1993). The relational roots of identity. In J. Kroger (Ed.), *Discussions on ego identity* (pp. 101–120). Hillsdale, NJ: L.E. Erlbaum.

Marcia, J. E. (1998). Optimal development from an Eriksonian perspective. In *Encyclopedia of mental health* (vol. 3, pp. 29–39). New York: Academic

Marcia, J. E. (1998b). Peer Gynt's life cycle. In A. L. van der Lippe (Ed.), *Development in adolescence* (pp. 193–211). New York: Routledge.

Marcia, J. E. (2002). Identity and psychosocial development in adulthood. *Identity: An International Journal of Theory and Research, 2*(1), 7–28.

Marcia, J. E. (2004). Why Erikson? In K. Hoover (Ed.), *The future of identity: Centennial reflections on the legacy of Erik Erikson* (pp. 43–59). New York: Lexington.

Marcia, J. E., Waterman, A. S., Matteson, D. R., Archer, S. L., & Orlofsky, J. L. (1993). *Ego identity: A handbook for psychosocial research*. New York: Springer.

Orlofsky, J. L., Marcia, J. E., & Lesser, I. M. (1973). Ego identity status and the Intimacy versus Isolation crisis of young adulthood. *Journal of Personality and Social Psychology, 27*(2), 211–219.

Piaget, J. (1954). *The construction of reality in the child*. New York: Basic.

Stephen, J., Fraser, E., & Marcia, J. E. (1992). Lifespan identity development: Variables related to Moratorium-Achievement (MAMA) cycles. *Journal of Adolescence, 15*(3), 283–300.

Waterman, A. S. (2007). *Identity: An International Journal of Theory and Research, 7*(4), 263–348

Whitbourne, S. K., Zuschlag, M. K., Elliot, L. B., & Waterman, A. S. (1992). Psychosocial development in adulthood: A 22-year sequential study. *Journal of Personality and Social Psychology, 63*(2), 260–271.

Chapter 3

The Neurobiology of Stress Throughout the Life Cycle

Introduction

The study of stress is one of the most exciting areas within neurobiology and cognitive neuroscience. There has been a dramatic increase in scientific knowledge about physiological, anatomical, genetic, molecular, immuno-logical, and psychological characteristics of adversity and its extraordinary ability to influence human development throughout the life cycle. Advances in the study of learning and memory, attachment, psychological trauma, and gene X environment interaction, to name a few, have created an increasingly sophisticated appreciation of biological, social, and psychological factors comprising the response to and impact of life's challenges. This chapter will review recent contributions from studies among different fields and elucidate significant issues yet to be understood.

How Do Experiences Influence the Brain?
The Role of Learning and Memory

What is perceived as stressful is ultimately a product of the meaning attributed to an experience. Regardless of age, the meaningfulness of a current event is predicated on what has been learned and remembered in one's life. How people identify themselves, their knowledge of the world around them, ability to transmit values to their children, and capacity to adapt to novelty and challenge are the result of learning. Psychological adaptation includes the ability to utilize past experience to anticipate future events, plan, and regulate emotions. Many critical earlier events, as will be explicated, are retained outside of an individual's awareness; nevertheless, they profoundly affect contemporary life experiences. Because learning and memory are exquisitely sensitive to stress, it is prudent to review the types and neurobiology of learning and memory.

From: *Handbook of Stressful Transitions Across the Lifespan*,
Edited by: T.W. Miller, DOI 10.1007/978-1-4419-0748-6_3,
© Springer Science+Business Media, LLC 2010

35

Memory Types

Memory is classified as either short term or long term. Storage of the former generally lasts from seconds to minutes. Long term memory storage is enduring. Both types of learning are predicated on fundamental processes that alter brain structure and function. Neuronal plasticity, the capacity of the brain to change, alters synaptic transmission upon stimulation by increasing synaptic strength and the number of synapses, thereby making information processing more effective. This process is referred to as long term potentiation. Long term memory, as opposed to short term memory, also involves the creation of new genetic material. As will be discussed in detail, long term memory is intimately connected with a portion of the limbic system called the hippocampus. This structure is extraordinarily sensitive to stress hormones which may have significant impact on hippocampal size, number of cells, and the ability to learn, remember, and function psychologically

Figure 3-1 depicts the two types of long term memory. Explicit or declarative memory requires conscious awareness, sense of recollection, and sense of self and past, and is dependent on intact hippocampal function. More than 50 years ago, neurosurgical treatment of a young factory worker with intractable epilepsy demonstrated that converting short term into long term memory required effective hippocampal functioning (Penfield and Milner 1958). The recent film entitled Memento accurately depicted the plight of a young man who lived in only the present and was unable to remember that which he just experienced. It is now known that memory is consolidated through the hippocampus during sleep by going over the day's events through orchestrating multiple areas of the cortex (Ji and Wilson 2007) and by enforcing temporal sequence (Born et al. 2006). Explicit memory is traditionally defined as semantic or episodic.

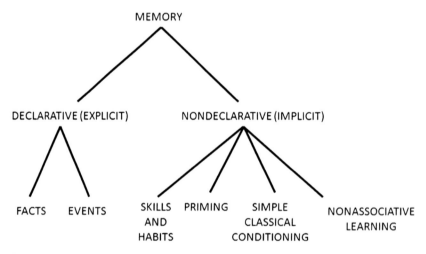

Fig. 3-1. Declarative memory refers to conscious recollection of facts and events and depends on the integrity of limbic diencephalic structures. Nondeclarative memory refers to a heterogeneous collection of abilities. In the case of nondeclarative memory, experience alters behavior nonconsciously without providing access to any memory content. Squire and Zola-Morgan (1991). Copyright by the AAAS

The former refers to knowledge of world events and general knowledge while the latter includes ongoing autobiographical facts and how a person defines him or herself.

Although implicit or nondeclarative memory in many respects is simpler than explicit memory, it is nevertheless significant in understanding many facets of behavior. Implicit memory accumulates after many trials, uses sequential stimuli, and stores information about predictive relationships. It can be studied in animals as it is based on reflexes. Indeed, Kandel (1982), whose work has been instrumental in appreciating the neurobiology of learning and memory, culminating in the 2000 Nobel Prize in medicine and physiology, employed this approach. Learning in this form of memory does not require conscious attention and does not draw upon general knowledge. Unlike explicit memory, implicit memory lacks a sense of self or the past and is not dependent on intact hippocampal function. While explicit memory requires temporal lobe information storage, implicit memory is acquired through sensory and motor systems utilized during the learning tasks. The centrality of sensory and motor contributions will become apparent shortly when the functions of the amygdala are discussed. The significance of implicit perceptual memory is that it is the basis for perceptual distortions clinically manifested in transference phenomena. Transference is the psychodynamic construct that explains why people are compelled to repeat or reenact certain emotions and behaviors that are often self defeating.

Implicit memory is the substrate for human attachment behavior. Repeated interaction between the mother and infant in affect laden experiences eventuate in the establishment of neural templates, which, in turn organize the central nervous system. In short, from a biological point of view, "neurons that fire together wire together." Attachment is the foundation upon which an infant develops a mental life and which, in turn, builds psychological structure. Attachment establishes affective regulation, a critical issue for survival, and plays an important role in the response to transitional life stresses. The enduring impact of loss and trauma early in life has great clinical relevance with respect to vulnerability and resilience. As will be discussed, early adverse experiences often place individuals at psychological and biological risk throughout a lifetime.

Another process that has become a recent focus for clinicians and researchers is mentalization, a fundamental component of empathy. Mentalization is the ability to comprehend that another person has as a different mind than one's own as well as to infer another's thoughts, ideas, motivations, and intentions (Fonagy 2001). Fonagy (2008) has argued that this capacity actually ensures social collaboration responsible for productive societies. Individuals with early life adversity and unsuccessful development of mentalization are at great disadvantage in their interpersonal relationships and their capacity to face future life challenges. Indeed, it appears that nature attempts to ensure the development of empathy by the presence of mirror neurons located in the pre-motor cortex. These mirror neurons appear to be a neural substrate for empathy and enhance the ability to perceive actions, sensations, and emotions of others (Schulte-Rüther et al. 2007).

The Neuroanatomy of Learning and Memory

The Amygdala

To appreciate the psychobiology of stress, it is necessary to highlight the central roles of two limbic system structures, the amygdala and the hippocampus. Figure 3-2 illustrates the location of these structures and their rich connections.

The amygdala serves two important functions; it is the portal for experiencing emotions and it also influences perceptions by assigning emotional valence to both implicit and explicit memories. Figure 3-3 depicts the two pathways through which events are recorded. As noted previously, the hippocampus is central to awareness of explicit memories as exemplified in both semantic and episodic types of memory. Implicit emotional memories about stressful experiences such as early childhood maltreatment often remain outside an

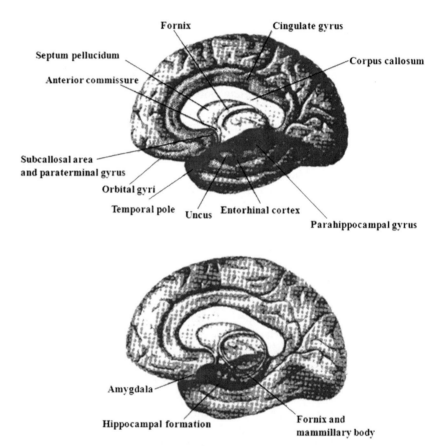

Fig. 3-2. Location of the Hippocampus and Amygdala and Surrounding Cortical Areas. The two diagrams show the medial or inside wall of the human cerebrum. The stippled area is the classic limbic lobe. The amygdala and hippocampus are found deep inside the medial part of the temporal lobe, underneath the uncus, entorhinal cortex, and parahippocampal gyrus (*top*). These cortical areas have been stripped away to show the location of the hippocampus and amygdala in the bottom illustration. (Reprinted from Figures 15-1 and 15-2 in Martin JH. (1989) Neuroanatomy: Text and atlas. New York: Elsevier. Copyright © 1989 by Appleton and Lange). LeDoux (1996)

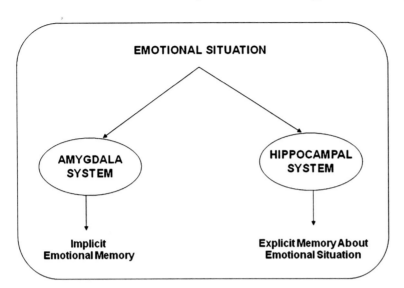

Fig. 3-3. Brain Systems of Emotional Memory and Memory of Emotion. It is now common to think of the brain as containing a variety of different memory systems. Conscious, declarative, or explicit memory is mediated by the hippocampus and related cortical areas, whereas various unconscious or implicit forms of memory are mediated by different systems. One implicit memory system is an emotional (fear) memory system involving the amygdala and related areas. In traumatic situations, implicit and explicit systems function in parallel. Later, if you are exposed to stimuli that were present during the trauma, both systems will most likely be reactivated. Through the hippocampal system you will remember who you were with and what you were doing during the trauma, and will also remember, as a cold fact, that the situation was awful. Through the amygdala system the stimuli will cause your muscles to tense up, you blood pressure and heart rate to change, and hormones to be released, among other bodily and brain responses. Because these systems are activated by the same stimuli and are functioning at the same time, the two kinds of memories seem to be part of one unified memory function. Only by taking these systems apart, especially through studies of experimental animals and also through important studies of rare human cases, are we able to understand how memory systems are operating in parallel to give rise to independent memory functions. LeDoux (1996)

individual's awareness. Dynamic psychotherapy effectively creates a new language in which the emotional memory can be verbalized and joined with new explicit memory, thereby creating a narrative of influential events previously not understood. Such people often have sensations to places and persons but have no clue to why, which is understandable as implicit emotional memory does not require cognitive mediation through the cortex. Sensory memories can elicit explicit memories stored in the cortex. Modulation of memory storage and strength is ultimately a responsibility of the amygdala.

Stress at times of life transitions, and at other times, is often an example of poor adaptation. From an evolutionary point of view, the fight or flight reaction to danger evoked important physiological events preservation (increased heart rate and blood pressure, production of stress hormones, increased availability of glucose to muscles) to ensure self preservation. Although confronting a saber toothed tiger is no longer a likely possibility, humans often respond to actual and perceived contemporary stressful situations with an outpouring of stress hormones. As fear is generated in the amygdala, this structure, as will be seen, is critical in understanding vulnerability to stress. Adverse childhood experiences can therefore produce enduring hormonal abnormalities that are significant throughout the life cycle. Arousing events can eventuate in over-activity of the amygdala (Shin et al. 2006). Inhibited childhood temperament is accompanied by increased amygdalar activity in adulthood in the presence of novelty (Schwartz et al. 2003). Abused children are also more sensitive to angry facial expressions (Masten et al. 2008).

The Hippocampus and Explicit Memory

Inextricably linked with the amygdala is the second temporal lobe memory organ called the hippocampus (See Fig. 3-2). Explicit memory cannot occur without the participation of the hippocampus (Milner 1959). The unavailability of very early memories is, by and large, a function of hippocampal immaturity and not of repression, as Freud once thought. This site matures after the amygdala and is rich in glucocorticoid receptors (cortisol and its associated stress related neurohormones). As will become clear, chronic stress has an almost toxic effect on hippocampal cells and neurons.

Some of the most exciting recent cognitive neuroscience research has focused on the hippocampus. In particular, when the author graduated medical school 30 years ago, it was axiomatic that brain cells, once lost, could never be replaced. Even considering a normal loss of brain cells during childhood and adolescence through a pruning process, adults received all of their brain cells at birth. It is now understood, that, in fact, neuroanatomy is constantly changing. As discussed earlier, the most basic of these processes, called neuronal plasticity, involves strengthening and creating new synapses during learning. Thirty years ago researchers demonstrated that stimulating learning increased both volume of the hippocampus and the number of hippocampal cells in rodents (Greenough 1975). Eriksson et al. (1998) found that as many as 1,000 new cells are created daily within the human dentate gyrus of the hippocampus and two other brain regions; however, the function of these new cells is, at present, unclear. Some have speculated that these new cells may be associated with assigning temporality to that which is learned throughout the day (Kempermann 2002). In essence this would imply learning can be anchored in time as events that occur in proximity may be encoded into the hippocampus by the new cells, or groups of cells, which, in turn, may become large numbers of overlapping patterns of new connections.

Effects of Stress on the Hippocampus

Discovery of the creation of new brain cells in the hippocampus was accompanied by a growing awareness that stress had deleterious effects in this area of the brain. It became clear stress was accompanied by increased levels of cortisol which, in turn, were responsible for long term potentiation inhibition and decreased memory performance in animals and humans. Mirescu et al. (2004) demonstrated that the stress of maternal deprivation impaired the creation of new hipppocampal cells through greater glucocorticoid hypersensitivity. Some researchers noted that when stress was relieved, memory performance improved in humans (Lupien et al. 1998; Newcomer et al. 1999). A recent study of more than 1,100 subjects between the ages of 50–70 revealed that those with elevated salivary cortisol levels had decreased performance on tasks of language, executive functioning, verbal memory, and learning (Lee et al. 2007). Nicholas et al. (2006) employed chimeric gene therapy (creating DNA made of rat glucocorticoid and human estrogen receptors) to demonstrate that memory was enhanced by the production of estrogen. Women with post traumatic stress disorder (PTSD) from childhood abuse have decreased hippocampal volume (Bremner et al. 1995, 1997).

In stressful times the neurotransmitter norepinephrine also contributes to decreased hippocampal functioning. The high levels of norepinephrine that accompany stress, for example in those that face traumatic situations, appear to consolidate emotional memories faster in the hippocampus and the memories last longer as well (Hu et al. 2007). It is as if, during these occasions, memories get laid down in concrete. Studies have demonstrated that shutting off certain enzymes related to norepinephrine results in less ability to be frightened or to recall trauma (Sananbenesi et al. 2007; de Quervain et al. 2007). Research in emergency rooms with people who have experienced trauma has demonstrated that if a drug that blocks norepinephrine (beta blocker) is given within 6 h and for the following 10 days, the number of those developing PTSD is reduced dramatically (Pitman et al. 2002).

There is one additional class of proteins, neurotrophic factors, which are remarkably sensitive to stress. The most important of these is brain derived neurotrophic factor or BDNF, which is vital in promoting long term memory and maintaining good working order of neurons through preventing cell death and facilitating growth of new neurons. BDNF is reduced in stress and in certain psychiatric disorders, the most common of which is depression. Lower levels of BDNF are associated with hippocampal volume reduction and new cell formation interference. Antidepressant medications and electroconvulsive therapy, for example, may be effective in protecting BDNF, thereby preventing hippocampal shrinkage. There is controversy whether the hippocampal volume reduction precedes depression or if depression causes hippocampal reduction. There are different genetic types (genotypes) of BDNF which appear to make some individuals more susceptible to depression (Frodl et al. 2007) and have been associated with reduced hippocampal and frontal cortex volume (Pezawas et al. 2004). The methionine or *met al*lele appears to be protective against mood disorders whereas the valine or *val* form exaggerates the negative effect of a particular form of the serotonin transporter whose function will be described shortly (Pezawas et al. 2008).

Who is More Vulnerable to Stress?

Vulnerability and resilience are the products of many contributing factors that can be subsumed under broad categories including heredity and environment. Neither is sufficient in most instances to produce vulnerability even in the presence of developmental adversity and stressful life events. However, the most exciting area in psychiatry and neuroscience is the growing appreciation for how genes and environment interact and are often expressed in the development of psychological symptoms and disorders. In short, genes are important in how people respond to their experiences and, in turn, experiences reciprocally influence genetics. Depression and anxiety, therefore, are reflections about how the brain interacts with environment.

The Enduring Impact of Attachment Issues

Vicissitudes of early infant experience are central to an understanding of psychological vulnerability to stress throughout the life cycle. According to Bowlby (1969), attachment is the process by which a child achieves an increasingly stable and sophisticated view of himself and the world. As noted previously, the mental life of infants and children is established through a process of internalization which builds psychological structure. In addition, attachment promotes the ability to regulate affect, which is essential to human survival. Trauma in early life, as will be explicated, has a profound impact on the ability to regulate affect. Early adverse experiences have an enduring effect on right brain development, which matures earlier than the left, and whose function is to defend against overwhelming situations and modulate distress through repeated soothing interactions with the primary attachment figure or caregiver. Attachment is the product of physical and emotional reciprocity between the infant and mother during communication through vocalization, gesturing, and especially facial expression. Another important component of attachment development is how the mother responds to unintended empathic failure or misreading the infant's emotions and needs. It is impossible to be empathic to one's infant on every occasion. How the mother addresses this failure is most critical as derailment resolution is a strong source for emotional growth. Also of great importance is the child's development of mentalization, defined earlier as the capacity to appreciate that someone else has a mind different from one's own. Theory of mind (ToM) has also been used to describe this process that eventuates in the child's ability to conceive another's beliefs, feelings, attitudes, and desires (Fonagy and Target 1997). This ability is the foundation for the development of empathy, a vital social characteristic of cooperative behavior necessary for survival of the species. Trauma and loss early in life have marked effects on attachment, which greatly inhibits mentalization.

Attachment Theory Research

The scientific support for John Bowlby's attachment theory was established by Mary Ainsworth and colleagues (1978) in the development of the strange situation paradigm, which, through a separation experience, assesses a child's attachment patterns between 1 and 2 years of age. This research differentiated three distinct childhood patterns of response to separation from the mother: secure, anxious/resistant, and anxious/avoidant. A fourth category, disorganized attachment, has been the focus of most recent research and has the most supporting evidence (Main and Solomon 1990). These anxious children lack a strategy for addressing separation from the caregiver. Often, they respond with strong denial or hiding. Contradictory behavior is the hallmark of disorganized attachment frequently manifested by both clinging and hitting or a freezing posture, to name a few. As expected, these children have abnormalities in their representational processes and tend to view themselves and others very negatively. Disorganized attachment has a remarkable predictability of future psychopathology not only in childhood but throughout adolescence and into adulthood.

Disorganized attachment and maternal vulnerability have been associated with the following behavioral patterns:

- higher childhood aggression levels and externalizing behavior problems (Lyons-Ruth 1996)
- aggression, controlling behavior, and poor peer relationships in middle and high school (Shaw et al. 1996; Sroufe 2005)
- dissociative symptoms at four points in time over a 19 year period (Ogawa et al. 1997)
- dissociation and behavioral problems in preschool, primary school, and high school (Carlson 1998)
- hostile behavior toward classmates (Lyons-Ruth et al. 1993)

The impact of disorganized attachment is evident in adulthood as well though an in depth review of this rich topic is beyond the scope of this chapter. To summarize, however, without treatment, disorganized attachment colors the nature of interpersonal relationships by limiting intimacy, effects of which are evidenced in marital partner choice, psychotherapy outcome, and doctor–patient relationships to name a few areas.

Unresolved parental loss and disorganized attachment together can explain the transmission of intergenerational conflict and psychopathology. Although not discussed yet, genes provide an inextricable contribution as well. It is important to recall that neither trauma nor biology is sufficient to explain childhood difficulties and resultant vulnerability and psychopathology. However, from a psychological point of view, there have been a number of models that elucidate how early parent trauma or loss is instrumental in producing disorganized attachment. Women who have unresolved trauma and or loss can be categorized as either frightening or frightened mothers. In the first case, mothers behave toward their child with hostility. When their mothering skills are challenged at times, for example, when the infant cannot be easily soothed, this becomes a threat to their sense of being an adequate mother. On the other hand, frightened mothers are anxious and worried about their ability to care for an infant and often are overprotective, which hinders the infant's move toward increasing separateness and autonomy. In both cases, irresolvable, repeated interactions engender attachment problems. Figures 3-4 and 3-5 depict two explanatory models for how disorganized attachment is transmitted from one generation to another. Passing on this vulnerability is an important contribution to how life transitions are addressed.

Neurobiological Aspects of Animal Attachment: Separation Studies in Rodents

How disrupted attachment produces profound and often enduring stress-related biological changes has been demonstrated through maternal separation studies in non-human primates and rodents. This effect has been termed programming (Lupien et al. 2009) and refers to experiences or environmental events during a sensitive developmental period that impacts both brain function and structure which persists throughout an animal's life. To summarize a vast scientific literature, maternal separation in rodents and non-human primates has been associated with the following changes:

- emotional and behavioral regulation
- coping style
- neuroendocrine response to stress

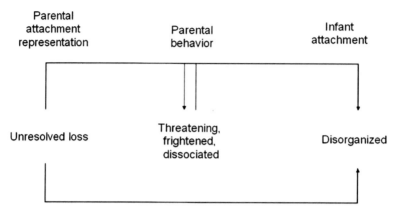

Fig. 3-4. Theory of Main and Hess linking unresolved loss and infant disorganization. From Schuengel et al. (1999). Unresolved loss and infant disorganization: links to frightening maternal behavior. In J. Solomon, C. George (Eds.), *Attachment disorganization*. New York: Guilford

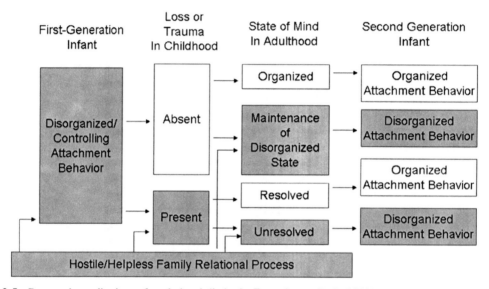

Fig. 3-5. Proposed contributions of a relational diathesis. From: Lyons-Ruth (1999)

- brain morphology (hippocampal changes from synaptic inefficiency)
- destructive cellular changes
- receptor decreases
- cognitive impairment

Three representative studies will be described that illustrate the significant impact of maternal separation on offspring. Suomi's (1999) highly influential work with monkeys demonstrated that infants reared apart from the mother exhibited signs of what might be called depressive behavior. The infants were anhedonic, withdrawn, anxious, unable to socially or sexually interact, isolative, and frightened. When their sibs, who were not separated, were introduced, they served as "therapist monkeys" and were instrumental in advancing the socialization process for the affected littermates. Nevertheless, despite the social gains, those separated monkeys responded to stress with a greater outpouring of stress hormones. This increased production of stress hormones has been replicated by Sapolsky et al. (1990), Rosenblum et al. (1994), Kraemer and Clarke (1996), and Barr et al. (2004) among others.

The Emory group (Heim et al. 2004) also demonstrated that early experiences produce enduring changes in the brain. They separated rat pups from the dam for 3 h each day between days 2 and 14 after birth. These rats had disrupted eating, sleeping, and reproductive behavior. Like Suomi's monkey, the rats were anhedonic, restless, and withdrawn. At 90 days, a stressor was introduced (puff of air on the cornea) which produced a dramatic increase in stress hormones as well as double the concentration of one stress hormone precursor in the amygdala. An unpredicted finding however was that mothers treated the separated rat pups with more hostility.

Essex et al. (2002) designed an elegant human study that demonstrated the impact of maternal stress on infants. In this study, salivary cortisol levels were obtained from 282, 4.5-year-old children (and 154 of their control sibs). The mothers of these children were assessed for stress when the children were 1, 4, 12, and 78 months. High levels of cortisol among the children were associated with a documented history of maternal stress when the children were infants. This was not true of children whose mother was stressed only at the time of the cortisol measurement. Maternal depression beginning in their children's infancy was the most potent predictor of high child cortisol levels and mental health symptoms in the first grade. Maternal depression has also been implicated in elevated cortisol levels in adolescents (Halligan et al. 2004).

Rodent studies have also demonstrated the positive aspect of nurturing altering nature. Different mothering styles alter the activity of specific genes in the offspring that in turn govern the response to stress that persists into adulthood. For example, adult rats, which received adequate licking and grooming from their mothers, recover much faster from stress, are more explorative, and have less anxious behavior (Weaver et al. 2004). Moreover, these effects are transmitted from one generation to the next (Francis et al. 1999). Rodent studies have also delineated the significance of the peptide oxytocin in maternal behavior and attachment (Insel 1997). This work has lead to recent investigations in humans regarding the role of maternal depression and decreased oxytocin levels (Heim et al. 2008).

Gene–Environment Interaction and Vulnerability to Stress

Two significant human studies will serve as an introduction to gene X environment interaction. The first demonstrated the interplay between abuse, violence, and genes and how early experiences influenced the expression of behavior. In the Dunedin study, Caspi et al. (2002) examined 442 subjects with histories of child abuse and identified those with high and low concentrations of the enzyme monoamine oxidase A (MAOA). This enzyme is an important component in the intracellular metabolism of epinephrine, norepinephrine, and serotonin. Low levels of MAOA have been associated with aggression in mice and humans. Subjects abused as children with reduced MAOA levels, but not subjects abused as children with normal levels of MAOA, had dramatically more antisocial behavior. This included conduct disorder diagnosis in childhood, a precursor to adult antisocial personality disorder, three times the conviction of violent crimes by the age of 26, and four times the rate of robbery, rape, and assault. Men with low MAOA appear to have less ability to control aggressive urges. Imaging studies have shown greater activity in the amygdala and hippocampus and less activity in the frontal lobes that control impulses when subjects recall emotional experiences (Meyer-Lindenberg and Weinberger 2006). The Dunedin study supports the critical concept that, by themselves, neither experience nor genes is sufficient to explain behavior.

Kendler et al.'s work (1999) has been instrumental in elucidating contributions of stress in triggering genetic vulnerability. He studied 2,164 pairs of female twins over a 17 month period of time (Kendler et al. 1999). In the presence of a stressor, such as the loss of a loved one, assault, marital problems, and separation/divorce, subjects at low risk for depression increased their probability for major depression from 0.5% to 6.2%. Twins at highest risk increased their probability of major depression from 1.1% to 14.6%. This study demonstrates the role of gene—environment interactions at times of life transitions such as those involving marital stages and interpersonal loss.

Genetic Polymorphism

A focus of recent research in rodents, primates, and humans has been the interaction between maternal separation and maternal stress, and genetics. This body of information has lead to important advances in how behaviors change genes and vice versa, as well as in how the impact of adverse experiences affects those with predisposition to depression and anxiety disorders. These advances have emerged from an appreciation of the role of genetic polymorphism in vulnerability to stress and illness. Genetic polymorphism refers to the existence of more than one allele or form of a portion of a gene. In two particular conditions, these polymorphisms are functional in both animals and humans. The first is that of the clinical consequences of different forms of the serotonin transporter (5-HTTP), which facilitates the utilization of serotonin (5-HT). This neurotransmitter is densely distributed throughout the brain and is intimately involved in neurobiology of depression. (In the treatment of depression the most frequently prescribed medications increase serotonin concentration in the brain often decreased in this disorder, by blocking its reuptake in the synaptic cleft.) The second has addressed an enzyme called catechol-O-methyltransferase or COMT, equally essential in appreciating some related aspects of stress and cognition.

It is important to note that while knowledge about genetics will play an increasingly important role in understanding human normal and abnormal development, there is no single gene responsible for any specific psychiatric disorder. The focus, rather, is on how genomic variations contribute to the development and functioning of brain circuitry which then influences behavior. Each of these variations however, is responsible for only small contributions, perhaps 2–3%, to an individual's psychological vulnerability. Stress during life transitions becomes overwhelming or disabling when risk factors seem to outweigh protective ones (Insel 2008; Moran 2008).

Studies of the Serotonin Transporter Gene

There are both maternal and paternal contributions to the serotonin transporter gene. The polymorphism of this gene is illustrated in the following manner.

There are three forms of long (*l*) or short (*s*) alleles possible: *ll*, *ls*, and *ss*. The *ll* configuration in humans was thought to confer the highest level of resilience in the face of both stress and in the subsequent development of psychiatric disorders. The *ss* form, on the other hand, was thought to be associated with the greatest stress vulnerability while the *ls* type was intermediate. Serotonin transporter activity and the expression of serotonin are lowest in those animals and humans with the *ss* allele.

Maternal separation studies in monkeys have shown that those with the *ls* genotype reared apart have higher stress hormone levels compared to monkeys with the *ll* form (Barr et al. 2004; Suomi 2003) as well as having a greater alcohol preference (Barr et al. 2004). Another way to study the effect of the serotonin transporter is to remove or knock out the responsible gene. This has been done in knockout mice which then show a serotonin uptake impairment accompanied by increased anxiety (Holmes et al. 2003).

Human studies have also confirmed the clinical importance of the serotonin transporter polymorphism. Figure 3-6 illustrates this with respect to depression.

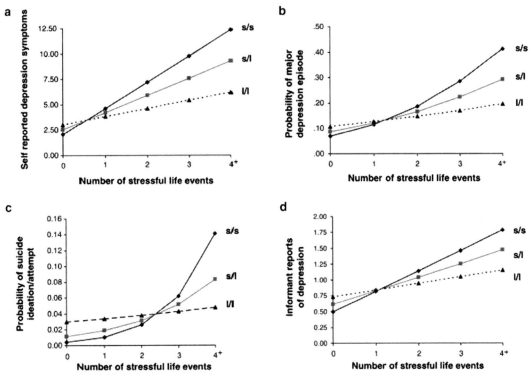

Fig. 3-6. Results of multiple regression analyses estimating the association between number of stressful life events (between ages 21 and 26 years) and depression outcomes at age 26 as a function of 5-HTT genotype. Among the 146 s/s homozygotes, 43 (29%), 37(25%), 28 (19%), 15 (10%), and 23 (16%) study members experienced 0, 1, 2, 3, and 4 or more stressful events, respectively. Among the 435 s/l heterozygotes, 141 (32%), 101 (23%), 76 (17%), 49 (11%), and 68 (16%) experienced 0, 1, 2, 3, and 4 or more stressful events. Among the 264 l/l homozygotes, 79 (29%), 73 (28%), 57 (21%), 26 (10%), and 29 (11%) experienced 0, 1, 2, 3, and 4 or more stressful events. (**a**) Self-reports of depression symptoms. (**b**) Probability of major depressive episode (**c**) Probability of suicide ideation or attempt). (**d**) Informant reports of depression. Caspi et al. (2003)

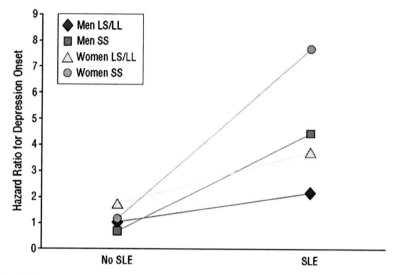

Fig. 3-7. The hazard ratio of onset of major depression within a 2-month period as a result of (1) sex (men vs. women), (2) genotype at the 5-HTT polymorphism (SS vs. LS and LL), (3) the occurrence, in the first month, of a stressful life event (SLE). A hazard rate of unity was defined as the risk level for a male with an SS genotype and no life-event exposure. S indicates short allele; L indicates long allele. Kendler et al. (2005). The interaction of stressful life events and a serotonin transporter polymorphism in the prediction of episodes of major depression: a replication. *Archives of General Psychiatry, 62,* 529–535

Similarly, the interaction of stressful life events and serotonin transporter polymorphism in the prediction of depression was documented by Kendler et al. (2005). In 549 adult twins, only those with the two short alleles (*ss*) showed greater negative responses to stressful life events leading to major depression. Variation in the transporter gene, therefore, appears to moderate sensitivity to the depressogenic effects of stressful life events. Figure 3-7 illustrates a gender effect as well.

Recently, an important meta-analysis of 14 human studies failed to confirm the clinical importance of the interaction between the serotonin transporter gene, stressful life events, and the risk of depression (Risch et al. 2009). This study was disappointing to psychiatry and neuroscience because the serotonin transporter gene has been the model par excellence for the gene–environment theory regarding psychiatric disorders (Caspi et al. 2003). Numerous questions however, have been raised about the methodology of this study and included the fact that 11 important studies were excluded from the meta-analysis, which examined nine negative investigations but only five positive ones. Moreover, the largest negative study utilized phone interviews by non-clinicians to determine depression. Although this one meta-analysis failed to support the relationship of the 5-HTTLPR genotype to stressful life events and depression, it does not invalidate the gene–environment approach for understanding human development and psychopathology. It did emphasize the enormous challenge of looking for specific, or candidate, genes with very small effects and reinforced the wisdom of whole-genome association studies.

The *ss* alleles, however, are clearly associated with twice as rapid turnover of serotonin in those with depression (Barton et al. 2008). Recall that depression is associated with lower concentrations of serotonin. This effect can be reduced by antidepressants that promote greater availability of the neurotransmitter. Neuroimaging correlates of the 5-HTTP polymorphism also demonstrate that in the *ss* genotype there is decreased gray matter volume and less interactivity between the amygdala and other areas implicated in the biology of depression and anxiety (Pezawas et al. 2005). As the *ss* allele has been associated with increased amygdala reactivity and decreased prefrontal cortical regulation, it is not surprising that decision making around positive and negative choices (the framing effect) appears to be influenced by having the *ss* form (Risch et al. 2009; van den Bos et al. 2009; Roiser et al. 2009). Last, the *ss* configuration has been shown to predict side effects to the selective serotonin reuptake inhibitors (Murphy et al. 2004).

Recently, Hayden et al. (2008) compared non-depressed and depressed 7-year-old children exposed to sad movies or asked to imagine a sad experience. Children with the *ss* form of the 5-HTTP had more negative self-referential responses on an encoding task. As depression is associated with negative information processing as well as increased activity in the amygdala, it may help explain the concept of negative automatic thoughts, from a neurobiological stance, as described in CBT. (Beck 2008). Although speculative at this time, perhaps heightened activity in the amygdala may be responsible for negative cognitive distortions so common in depression. At this time, it is fair to say that the association of 5-HTTP gene with increased vulnerability to psychiatric disorders requires further elucidation.

The Role of COMT

According to Weinberger (2009), catechol-*O*-methyltransferase (COMT) functions as a "tuner" of the frontal lobes of the cortex. This enzyme, which has been studied less than the serotonin transporter gene, is critical in the degradation of key neurotransmitters hypothesized to influence human cognitive function, motivation, and attention, as well as sensitivity to stress. The COMT gene on chromosome 22 contains a functional polymorphism (val-met) that determines high and low activity of this enzyme. Recent evidence suggests the met allele is associated with superior performance on measures of prefrontal cortical function (Malhotra et al. 2002). The val form is associated with more efficient processing of emotional information. This polymorphism does not intimate that one variant is superior to another; rather, the different configurations may account for normal cognitive variability. For example, the val configuration appears to make individuals less stress sensitive than the met form. On the other hand those with the latter appear to have better memory than individuals with the val form. The potential for human survival in early times may have been aided by the val configuration, which favored activity over introspection. In short, the role of COMT brings yet another genetic contribution to understanding stress throughout the life cycle.

Toward an Understanding of Stressful Life Transitions

What may be considered within a normal realm of responses to life transitions is predicated upon biological factors (genetic), psychological factors (previous experience, including meaning attributed to events, as well as psychopathology),

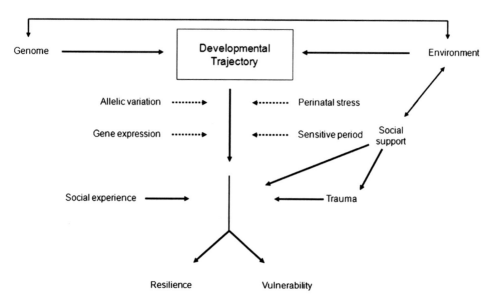

Fig. 3-8. Responses of Life Transitions. Modified from Nemeroff, C.B. (2008). *Gene-environment interactions in the pathophysiology of depression: Implications for treatment selection.* American College of Psychiatrists 2008 Annual Meeting and Pre-meeting

and social factors (culture and social support to name but two). Figure 3-8 depicts the interplay of these factors.

It is vital to recall that the majority of individuals traversing the challenges of life transitions do not become dysfunctional. These challenges, in a sense, define normal human development. Attention will now shift to appreciation of the variability of experience in life transitions within the framework of the gene-environment paradigm. To varying degrees, successful transitions are predicated on the accommodation to stress and the meaning of change. It is beyond the scope of this chapter to address each possible response to stressful life transitions throughout the life cycle; however, the vulnerability to stressful life transitions such as individuation, marriage, separation and divorce, illness, retirement, and object loss appear to be influenced by earlier mastery of challenges. A very recent study demonstrated that long-term grief selectively activates, through yearning for lost loved ones, certain neurons related to the reward system, possibly coloring the memories of lost loved ones and giving them an almost addictive like property (O'Connor et al. 2008). The power of early negative experiences upon human development can be summarized through an examination of misfortune early in life.

Some Consequences of Childhood Adversity

The review of attachment and its disorders established the promise and the disappointment of childhood. The experience of growing up within the confines of a safe and empathic family environment in which the child experiences self-affirmation eventuates in the development of talents and skills which are critical in the consolidation of self cohesiveness. On the other hand, the youngster who is a victim of neglect or abuse experiences himself or herself as inadequate in many dimensions, while perceiving the environment as generally untrustworthy. The enduring emotional valence of explicit and implicit memories is a vital contribution to the organization of the developing brain. Persistent biological vulnerabilities as expressed in the hyperreactivity of the neuroendocrine system, for example, affect life experience throughout childhood, adolescence, and adulthood. This is especially true, as was reviewed earlier in animal and human studies, with respect to stress response. It is the sensitization to the stress response that appears to be related to the development of psychiatric disorders in adulthood (Heim et al. 2000; Bradley et al. 2008).

Childhood maltreatment has been associated repeatedly with diminished resilience in overcoming stress. Moreover, it has been solidly linked with psychological maladaptation and psychiatric disorders throughout the life cycle. A large study of more than 17,000 adult health maintenance organization members demonstrated, for example, that those having adverse childhood experiences including, but not limited to, emotional, physical, and sexual abuse as children, were two to five times more likely to have attempted suicide as children, adolescents, and adults (Dube et al. 2001). In another large study of nearly 2000 women, 22% with a history of childhood physical or sexual abuse, had more physical symptoms, depression, anxiety, low self esteem, alcohol abuse, suicide attempts, and psychiatric admissions (McCauley et al. 1997). An examination of depressed women with and without a history of childhood sexual abuse found that those in the former group became depressed earlier in life, had attempted suicide, were more likely to have panic disorder, and in general, displayed many more self defeating coping strategies (Gladstone et al. 2004). Heim et al. (2008) have found that men with depression and histories of childhood abuse, but not those with depression and no childhood maltreatment, also demonstrate hyperreactivity of the neuroendocrine system. Another study of personality disordered men with a history of childhood trauma demonstrated that these subjects had higher concentrations of stress hormones directly correlated with the extent of emotional neglect (Lee et al. 2005). Obesity in middle-aged adults has been linked to childhood physical abuse (Thomas et al. 2008). Moreover, adults who experienced physical abuse as children were recently found to have 49% higher cancer risk than those without an abuse history (Fuller-Thomson and Brennenstuhl 2009).

Recently the question of how early life stress may interact with the immune system especially in those with depression has been addressed (Pace et al. 2006; Danese et al. 2008; Gimeno et al. 2008). It is highly probable that inflammation may be an underlying biological correlate of depression and perhaps be associated with early life stress.

A Developmental View of Stress Across the Life Cycle

In closing, an overarching conceptualization of the effects of stress throughout human development is in order. Examining what is known about **prenatal** stress, the following stand out:

- maternal stress, anxiety, and depression have been associated with increased HPA activity in offspring at different ages in childhood
- maternal stress has been linked with smaller size for gestation or low birth weight

- maternal stress and depression are associated with behavioral disturbances in childhood and selected psychiatric disorders in childhood and adulthood such as anxiety, mood, and substance abuse disorders

With respect to **postnatal** stress, these findings have been demonstrated:

- maternal emotional unavailability that characterized depression, often results in heightened HPA axis activity in children and depression when they become adolescents
- behavioral problems and insensitivity to others in children of depressed mothers are common
- severe early maltreatment, as experienced by those in traumatizing orphanages, can produce a lifelong hypocortisolism that mimics PTSD in adulthood.
- The post mortem examination of brains of suicide completers who had histories of child abuse revealed increased methylation (associated with decreased resilience) of a gene responsible for glucocortioid receptor expression (McGowan et al. 2009) This same gene was incriminated in a study of newborns, with follow up at 3 months, who had been exposed to increased maternal anxiety and depression in their mothers' third trimester (Oberlander et al. 2008).

Adolescence and **early adulthood** are characterized by significant frontal lobe development which appears to confer additional sensitivity to stress and elevated gulcorticorticoid levels especially germane to the increasing challenges in college mental health issues regarding anxiety, mood, trauma, and eating and substance abuse disorders (Kay and Schwartz in press).

Regarding the effects of stress in **aging,** the following are significant:

- elevated levels of cortisol in the elderly have been associated with decreased hippocampal volume and related memory problems
- prefrontal cortical functioning appears to be particularly sensitive to elevated levels of cortisol and therefore may be related to less efficient executive processes.

To summarize, at times of heightened sensitivity to cortisol, as is the case especially in the prenatal, adolescent, and aging periods of development, stress is likely to have significantly more impact. As Lupien et al. (2009) have noted, it is helpful to conceptualize the effects of stress following a neurotoxicity and/or vulnerability hypothesis. Although neither is mutually exclusive, the former refers to the damage to the hippocampus from excessive HPA activity as occurring in PTSD, and the latter postulates that there may be increased hippocampal sensitivity to stress because of genetics or early childhood experience. Similarly, increased amgydala volume and sensitivity could be the result of chronic stress. As well, they note that early stress may manifest much later in development when the brain matures as in late adolescence and early adulthood.

Conclusion

The chapters in this book address the vicissitudes of specific transitions throughout the life cycle. This chapter however, has attempted to elucidate the neurobiological mechanisms that underlie responses to these stressful transitions. The magnitude of such stress must be appreciated in terms of gene-environment interaction. Adverse childhood and adult experiences, when accompanied by genetic vulnerability, may have profound consequences on human development. Moreover, even in the absence of genetic challenges, such negative events have remarkable impact on memory and the physiological and anatomical organization of the brain. There is a wide variability in how developmental tasks are approached and integrated. Yet it is clear that one central component to weathering these challenges is the meaning assigned to them which is highly influenced by previous experience in adaptation.

References

Ainsworth, M. D. S., Blechar, M. C., Waters, E., & Wall, S. (1978). *Patterns of attachment: A psychological study of the strange situation.* Hillside, MJ: Erlbaum.

Barr, C. S., Newman, T. K., Shannon, C., Parker, C., Dvoskin, R. L., Becker, M. L., et al. (2004). Rearing condition and rh5-HTTLPR interact to influence limbic-hypothalamic-pituitary-adrenal axis response to stress in infant macaques. *Biological Psychiatry, 55,* 733–738.

Barton, D. A., Esler, M. D., Dawood, T., Lambert, E. A., Haikerwal, D., Brenchley, C., et al. (2008). Elevated brain serotonin turnover in patients with depression: Effect of genotype and therapy. *Archives of General Psychiatry, 65,* 38–46.

Beck, A. T. (2008). The evolution of the cognitive model of depression and its neurobiological correlates. *American Journal of Psychiatry, 165,* 969–977.

Born, J., Rasch, B., & Gais, S. (2006). Sleep to remember. *Neuroscientist, 12,* 410–424.

Bowlby, J. (1969). Attachment and Loss, Vol. 1 Attachment. London: Hogarth Press and Institute of Psycho-Analysis; New York: Basic Books.

Bradley, R. G., Binder, E. B., Epstein, M. P., Tang, Y., Nair, H. P., Liu, W., et al. (2008). Influence of child abuse on adult depression: Moderation by the corticotropin-releasing hormone receptor gene. *Archives of General Psychiatry, 65,* 190–200.

Bremner, J. D., Randall, P., Scott, T. M., Bronen, R. A., Seibyl, J. P., Southwick, S. M., et al. (1995). MRI-based measurement of hippocampal volume in patients with combat- related posttraumatic stress disorder. *American Journal of Psychiatry, 152,* 973–981.

Bremner, J. D., Randall, P. R., Vermetten, E., Staib, L., Bronen, R. A., Mazure, C. M., et al. (1997). Hippocampal volume reduction in PTSD. *Biological Psychiatry, 41,* 23–32.

Carlson, E. A. (1998). A prospective longitudinal study of attachment disorganization/disorientation. *Child Development, 69,* 1107–1128.

Caspi, A., McClay, J., Moffitt, T. E., Mill, J., Martin, J., Craig, I. W., et al. (2002). Role of genotype in the cycle of violence in maltreated children. *Science, 297,* 851–854.

Caspi, A., Sugden, K., Moffitt, T. E., Taylor, A., Craig, I. W., Harrington, H., et al. (2003). Influence of life stress on depression: moderation by a polymorphism in the 5-HTT gene. *Science, 301,* 386–389.

Danese, A., Moffitt, T. E., Pariante, C. M., Ambler, A., Poulton, R., & Caspi, A. (2008). Elevated inflammation levels in depressed adults with a history of childhood maltreatment. *Archives of General Psychiatry, 65,* 409–415.

De Quervain, D. J., Kolassa, I. T., Ertl, V., Onyut, P. L., Neuner, F., Elbert, T., et al. (2007). A deletion variant of the alpha2b-adrenoceptor is related to emotional memory in Europeans and Africans. *Nature Neuroscience, 10,* 1137–1139.

Dube, S. R., Anda, R. F., Felitti, V. J., Chapman, D. P., Williamson, D. F., & Giles, W. H. (2001). Childhood abuse, household dysfunction, and the risk of attempted suicide throughout the life span: Findings from the Adverse Childhood Experiences Study. *The Journal of the American Medical Association, 286*, 3089–3096.

Eriksson, P. S., Perfilieva, E., Bjork-Eriksson, T., Alborn, A. M., Nordborg, C., Peterson, D. A., et al. (1998). Neurogenesis in the adult human hippocampus. *Nature Medicine, 4*, 1313–1317.

Essex, M. J., Klein, M. H., Cho, E., & Kalin, N. H. (2002). Maternal stress beginning in infancy may sensitize children to later stress exposure: effects on cortisol and behavior. *Biological Psychiatry, 52*, 776–784.

Fonagy, P. (2001). *Attachment theory and psychoanalysis*. New York: Other Press LLC.

Fonagy, P. (2008). The mentalization-focused approach to social development. In F. N. Busch (Ed.), *Mentalization: The theoretical considerations, research findings, and clinical implications* (Vol. 29, pp. 3–43). New York: Taylor & Francis.

Fonagy, P., & Target, M. (1997). Attachment and reflective function: Their role in self-organization. *Development and Psychopathology, 9*, 679–700.

Francis, D., Diorio, J., Liu, D., & Meaney, M. J. (1999). Nongenomic transmission across generations of maternal behavior and stress responses in the rat. *Science, 286*, 1155–1158.

Frodl, T., Schule, C., Schmitt, G., Born, C., Baghai, T., Zill, P., et al. (2007). Association of the brain-derived neurotrophic factor Val66Met polymorphism with reduced hippocampal volumes in major depression. *Archives of General Psychiatry, 64*, 410–416.

Fuller-Thomson, E., & Brennenstuhl, S. (2009). Making a link between childhood physical abuse and cancer: results from a regional representative survey. *Cancer, 115*(14), 3341–3350.

Gimeno, D., Kivimäki, M., Brunner, E. J., Elovainio, M., De Vogli, R., Steptoe, A., et al. (2008). Associations of C-reactive protein and interleukin-6 with cognitive symptoms of depression: 12-year follow-up of the Whitehall II study. *Psychological Medicine, 4*, 1–11.

Gladstone, G. L., Parker, G. B., Mitchell, P. B., Malhi, G. S., Wilhelm, K., & Austin, M. P. (2004). Implications of childhood trauma for depressed women: an analysis of pathways from childhood sexual abuse to deliberate self-harm and revictimization. *American Journal of Psychiatry, 161*, 1417–1425.

Greenough, W. T. (1975). Experiential modification of the developing brain. *American Scientist, 63*, 37–46.

Halligan, S. L., Herbert, J., Goodyer, I. M., & Murray, L. (2004). Exposure to postnatal depression predicts elevated cortisol in adolescent offspring. *Biological Psychiatry, 55*, 376–381.

Hariri, A. R., Mattay, V. S., Tessitore, A., Kolachana, B., Fera, F., Goldman, D., et al. (2002). Serotonin transporter genetic variation and the response of the human amygdala. *Science, 297*, 400–403.

Hayden, E. P., Dougherty, L. R., Maloney, B., Olino, T. M., Sheikh, H., Durbin, C. E., et al. (2008). Early-emerging cognitive vulnerability to depression and the serotonin transporter promoter region polymorphism. *Journal of Affective Disorders, 107*, 227–230.

Heim, C., Newport, D. J., Heit, S., Graham, Y. P., Wilcox, M., Bonsall, R., et al. (2000). Pituitary-adrenal and autonomic responses to stress in women after sexual and physical abuse in childhood. *The Journal of American Medical Association, 284*, 592–597.

Heim, C., Plotsky, P. M., & Nemeroff, C. B. (2004). Importance of studying the contributions of early adverse experience to neurobiological findings in depression. *Neuropsychopharmacology, 29*, 641–648.

Heim, C., Mletzko, T., Purselle, D., Musselman, D. L., & Nemeroff, C. B. (2008). The dexamethasone/corticotropin-releasing factor test in men with major depression: role of childhood trauma. *Biological Psychiatry, 63*, 398–405.

Heim, C., Newport, D. J., Mletzko, T., Miller, A. H., & Nemeroff, C. B. (2008). The link between childhood trauma and depression: Insights from HPA axis studies in humans. *Psychoneuroendocrinology, 33*, 693–710.

Holmes, A., Murphy, D. L., & Crawley, J. N. (2003). Abnormal behavioral phenotypes of serotonin transporter knockout mice: Parallels with human anxiety and depression. *Biological Psychiatry, 54*, 953–959.

Hu, H., Real, E., Takamiya, K., Kang, M. G., Ledoux, J., Huganir, R. L., et al. (2007). Emotion enhances learning via norepinephrine regulation of AMPA-receptor trafficking. *Cell, 131*, 160–173.

Insel, T. R. (1997). A neurobiological basis of social attachment. *American Journal of Psychiatry, 154*, 726–735.

Insel, T.R. (2008, July 7). Psychiatric News.

Ji, D., & Wilson, M. A. (2007). Coordinated memory replay in the visual cortex and hippocampus during sleep. *Nature Neuroscience, 10*, 100–107.

Kandel, E. R., & Schwartz, J. H. (1982). Molecular biology of learning: Modulation of transmitter release. *Science, 218*, 433–443.

Kay J. & Schwartz, V. (eds). The Textbook of College Mental Health. Chichester, England, John R. Wiley and Sons, in press.

Kempermann, G. (2002). Why new neurons? Possible functions for adult hippocampal neurogenesis. *The Journal of Neuroscience: The Official Journal of the Society for Neuroscience, 22*, 635–638.

Kempermann, G., Gast, D., & Gage, F. H. (2002). Neuroplasticity in old age: sustained fivefold induction of hippocampal neurogenesis by long-term environmental enrichment. *Annals of Neurology, 52*, 135–143.

Kendler, K. S., Karkowski, L. M., & Prescott, C. A. (1999). Causal relationship between stressful life events and the onset of major depression. *American Journal of Psychiatry, 156*, 837–841.

Kendler, S., et al. (2005). The Interaction of Stressful Life Events and a Serotonin Transporter Polymorphism in the Prediction of Episodes of Major Depression: A Replication. *Archives of General Psychiatry, 62*, 529–535.

Kraemer, G. W., & Clarke, A. S. (1996). Social attachment, brain function, and aggression. *Annuals of the New York Academy of Sciences, 794*, 121–135.

LeDoux, J. (1996). *The emotional brain: The mysterious underpinnings of emotional life*. New York: Simon & Schuster.

Lee, R., Geracioti, T. D., Kasckow, J. W., & Coccaro, E. F. (2005). Childhood trauma and personality disorder: Positive correlation with adult CSF corticotropin-releasing factor concentrations. *American Journal of Psychiatry, 162*, 995–997.

Lee, B. K., Glass, T. A., McAtee, M. J., Wand, G. S., Bandeen-Roche, K., Bolla, K. I., et al. (2007). Associations of salivary cortisol with cognitive function in the Baltimore memory study. *Archives of General Psychiatry, 64*, 810–818.

Lupien, S. J., de Leon, M., de Santi, S., Convit, A., Tarshish, C., Nair, N. P., et al. (1998). Cortisol levels during human aging predict hippocampal atrophy and memory deficits. *Nature Neuroscience, 1*, 69–73.

Lupien, S. J., McEwan, B. S., Gunnar, M. R., & Heim, C. (2009). Effects of stress throughout the life span on the brain, behavior and cognition. *Nature Reviews Neuroscience, 10*, 434–445.

Lyons-Ruth, K. (1996). Attachment relationships among children with aggressive behavior problems: The role of disorganized early attachment patterns. *Journal of Consulting and Clinical Psychology, 64*, 64–73.

Lyons-Ruth, K. (1999). A relational diathesis model of hostile-helpless states of mind expression in mother-infant interaction. In J. Solomon & C. George (Eds.), *Attachment disorganization* (p. 44). New York: Guilford.

Lyons-Ruth, K., Alpern, L., & Repacholi, B. (1993). Disorganized infant attachment classification and maternal psychosocial problems as predictors of hostile-aggressive behavior in the preschool classroom. *Child Development, 64*, 572–585.

Main, M., & Solomon, J. (1990). Procedures for identifying infants as disorganized/disoriented during the Ainsworth Strange Situation. In M. Greenberg, D. Ciccetti & E. M. Cummings (Eds.), *Attachment during the preschool years: Theory, research, and intervention* (pp. 121–160). Chicago, IL: University of Chicago Press.

Malhotra, A. K., Kestler, L. J., Mazzanti, C., Bates, J. A., Goldberg, T., & Goldman, D. (2002). A functional polymorphism in the COMT gene and performance on a test of prefrontal cognition. *American Journal of Psychiatry, 159*, 652–654.

Martin, J.H. (1989). Neuroanatomy: Text and Atlas. Elsevier, New York.

Masten, C. L., Guyer, A. E., Hodgdon, H. B., McClure, E. B., Charney, D. S., Ernst, M., et al. (2008). Recognition of facial emotions among maltreated children with high rates of post-traumatic stress disorder. *Child Abuse & Neglect, 32*, 139–153.

McCauley, J., Kern, D. E., Kolodner, K., Dill, L., Schroeder, A. F., DeChant, H. K., et al. (1997). Clinical characteristics of women with a history of childhood abuse: unhealed wounds. *The Journal of the American Medical Association, 277*, 1362–1368.

McGowan, P. O., Sasaki, A., D'Alessio, A. C., Dymov, S., Labonte, B., Szyf, M., et al. (2009). Epigenetic regulation of the glucorticoid receptor in human brain associates with childhood abuse. *Nature Neuroscience, 12*(3), 241–243.

Meyer-Lindenberg, A., & Weinberger, D. R. (2006). Intermediate phenotypes and genetic mechanisms of psychiatric disorders. *Nature Reviews: Neuroscience, 7*, 818–827.

Milner, B. (1959). The memory defect in bilateral hippocampal lesions. *Psychiatric Research Reports: American Psychiatric Association, 11*, 43–58.

Mirescu, C., Peters, J. D., & Gould, E. (2004). Early life experience alters response of adult neurogenesis to stress. *Nature Neuroscience, 7*, 841–846.

Moran, M. (2008). Isnel: 'Different kind of science' poised to transform psychiatry. *Psychiatric News, 43*(13), 6.

Murphy, G. M., Jr., Hollander, S. B., Rodrigues, H. E., Kremer, C., & Schatzberg, A. F. (2004). Effects of the serotonin transporter gene promoter polymorphism on mirtazapine and paroxetine efficacy and adverse events in geriatric major depression. *Archives of General Psychiatry, 61*(11), 1163–1169.

Nemeroff, C.B. (2008). *Gene-environment interactions in the pathophysiology of depression: Implications for treatment selection.* American College of Psychiatrist 2008 Annual Meeting and Pre-meeting

Newcomer, J. W., Selke, G., Melson, A. K., Hershey, T., Craft, S., Richards, K., et al. (1999). Decreased memory performance in healthy humans induced by stress-level cortisol treatment. *Archives of General Psychiatry, 56*, 527–533.

Nicholas, A., Munhoz, C. D., Ferguson, D., Campbell, L., & Sapolsky, R. (2006). Enhancing cognition after stress with gene therapy. *The Journal of Neuroscience: The Official Journal of the Society for Neuroscience, 26*, 11637–11643.

Oberlander, T. F., Weinber, J., Papsdorf, M., Grunau, R., Misri, S., & Devlin, A. M. (2008). Prenatal exposure to maternal depression, neonatal methylation of human glucorticoid receptor gene (NR3C1) and infant cortisol stress responses. *Epigenetics, 3*(2), 97–106.

O'Connor, M. F., Wellisch, D. K., Stanton, A. L., Eisenberger, N. I., Irwin, M. R., & Lieberman, M. D. (2008). Craving love? Enduring grief activates brain's reward center. *Neuroimage, 42*, 969–972.

Ogawa, J. R., Sroufe, L. A., Weinfield, N. S., Carlson, E. A., & Egeland, B. (1997). Development and the fragmented self: longitudinal study of dissociative symptomatology in a nonclinical sample. *Development and Psychopathology, 9*, 855–879.

Pace, T. W., Mletzko, T. C., Alagbe, O., Musselman, D. L., Nemeroff, C. B., Miller, A. H., et al. (2006). Increased stress-induced inflammatory responses in male patients with major depression and increased early life stress. *American Journal of Psychiatry, 163*, 1630–1633.

Penfield, W., & Milner, B. (1958). Memory deficit produced by bilateral lesions in the hippocampal zone. *AMA Archives of Neurology and Psychiatry, 79*, 475–497.

Pezawas, L., Verchinski, B. A., Mattay, V. S., Callicott, J. H., Kolachana, B. S., Straub, R. E., et al. (2004). The brain-derived neurotrophic factor val66met polymorphism and variation in human cortical morphology. *The Journal of Neuroscience: The Official Journal of the Society for Neuroscience, 24*, 10099–10102.

Pezawas, L., Meyer-Lindenberg, A., Drabant, E. M., Verchinski, B. A., Munoz, K. E., Kolachana, B. S., et al. (2005). 5-HTTLPR polymorphism impacts human cingulate-amygdala interactions: a genetic susceptibility mechanism for depression. *Nature Neuroscience, 8*, 828–834.

Pezawas, L., Meyer-Lindenberg, A., Goldman, A. L., Verchinski, B. A., Chen, G., Kolachana, B. S., et al. (2008). Evidence of biologic epistasis between BDNF and SLC6A4 and implications for depression. *Molecular Psychiatry, 13*(7), 709–716.

Pitman, R. K., Sanders, K. M., Zusman, R. M., Healy, A. R., Cheema, F., Lasko, N. B., et al. (2002). Pilot study of secondary prevention of posttraumatic stress disorder with propranolol. *Biological Psychiatry, 51*, 189–192.

Risch, N., Herrell, R., Lehner, T., Liang, K. Y., Eaves, L., Hoh, J., et al. (2009). Interaction between the serotonin transporter gene (5-HTTLPR), stressful life events, and risk of depression: a meta-analysis. *JAMA, 301*(23), 2462–2471.

Roiser JP, de Martino B, Tan GC, Kumaran D, Seymour B, Wood NW, Dolan RJ (2009). *Journal of Neuroscience, 29*(18), 5985–5991

Rosenblum, L. A., Coplan, J. D., Friedman, S., Bassoff, T., Gorman, J. M., & Andrews, M. W. (1994). Adverse early experiences affect noradrenergic and serotonergic functioning in adult primates. *Biological Psychiatry, 35*, 221–227.

Sananbenesi, F., Fischer, A., Wang, X., Schrick, C., Neve, R., Radulovic, J., et al. (2007). A hippocampal Cdk5 pathway regulates extinction of contextual fear. *Nature Neuroscience, 10*, 1012–1019.

Sapolsky, R. M., Uno, H., Rebert, C. S., & Finch, C. E. (1990). Hippocampal damage associated with prolonged glucocorticoid exposure in primates. *The Journal of Neuroscience: The Official Journal of the Society for Neuroscience, 10*, 2897–2902.

Schuengel, C., Bakermans–Kranenburg, M. J., & Van Ijzendoorn, M. H. (1999). Frightening maternal behavior linking unresolved loss and disorganized infant attachment. *Journal of Consulting and Clinical Psychology, 67*, 54–63.

Schulte-Rüther, M., Markowitsch, H. J., Fink, G. R., & Piefke, M. (2007). Mirror neuron and theory of mind mechanisms involved in face-to-face interactions: A functional magnetic resonance imaging approach to empathy. *Journal of Cognitive Neuroscience, 19*, 1354–1372.

Schwartz, C. E., Wright, C. I., Shin, L. M., Kagan, J., & Rauch, S. L. (2003). Inhibited and uninhibited infants "grown up": Adult amygdalar response to novelty. *Science, 300*, 1952–1953.

Shaw, D. S., Owens, E. B., Vondra, J. I., Keenan, K., & Winslow, E. B. (1996). Early risk factors and pathways in the development of early disruptive behavior problems. *Development and Psychopathology, 8*, 679–699.

Shin, L. M., Rauch, S. L., & Pitman, R. K. (2006). Amygdala, medial prefrontal cortex, and hippocampal function in PTSD. *Annals of the New York Academy of Sciences, 1071*, 67–69.

Squire, L. R., & Zola-Morgan, M. (1991). The medial temporal lobe memory system. *Science, 253*, 1380–1386.

Sroufe, L. A. (2005). Attachment and development: A prospective, longitudinal study from birth to adulthood. *Attachment & Human Development, 7*, 349–367.

Suomi, S. J. (1999). Attachment in rhesus monkeys. In J. Cassdy & P. R. Shaver (Eds.), *Handbook of attachment: theory, research and clinical applications* (pp. 181–197). New York: Guilford.

Suomi, S. J. (2003). Gene-environment interactions and the neurobiology of social conflict. *Annuals of the New York Academy of Sciences, 1008*, 132–139.

Thomas, C., Hyppönen, E., & Power, C. (2008). Obesity and type 2 diabetes risk in midadult life: the role of childhood adversity. *Pediatrics, 121*, 1240–1249.

van den Bos, R., Homberg, J., Gijsbers, E., den Heijer, E., & Cuppen, E. (2009). The effect of COMT Val158 Met genotype on decision-making and preliminary findings on its interaction with the 5-HTTLPR in healthy females. *Neuropharmacology, 56*(2), 493–498.

Weaver, I. C., Cervoni, N., Champagne, F. A., D'Alessio, A. C., Sharma, S., Seckl, J. R., et al. (2004). Epigenetic programming by maternal behavior. *Nature Neuroscience, 7*, 847–854.

Weinberger, D.R. (2009, July 17). How do genes cause mental illness? The good, the bad, and the ugly. Second Annual Chairs in Psychiatry Summit, Charleston, SC

Chapter 4

Life as a Source of Theory: Erik Erikson's Contributions, Boundaries, and Marginalities

James J. Clark

The boundary is the best place for acquiring knowledge.
   – Paul Tillich, *Religiose Verwirklichung*

We become ourselves by entering with open eyes into the boundary situations.
   – Karl Jaspers, *Philosophy, vol. 2, Existential Elucidation*

So, it is true, I had to try and make a style out of marginality and a concept out of identity-confusion. But I also have learned from life histories that everything that is new and worth saying (or worth saying in a new way) has a highly personal aspect. The question is only whether it is also generally significant for one's contemporaries. That I must let you judge.
   – Erik Erikson, *Autobiographical notes for Robert Coles*

Introduction: Psychobiography and Theory

Psychobiography and the study of lives – an area of specialized study in the discipline of psychology – asserts that it is often clarifying and sometimes essential to analyze the life histories of intellectual leaders whose ideas have shaped social and cultural life. Psychobiographies can help us understand the personal and historical contexts of theory construction, dissemination, and reception, while providing interpretive clues to the complex process of theory development and institutionalization (Anderson 2005). In fact, William Runyan (2006) has argued that studying how the lives of scientists have influenced their scientific projects can help steer observers away from misleading causal abstractions. Uncovering the connections between lives and theories has great heuristic value. The study of lives can advance the study of ideas.

Erik Erikson understood these possibilities and spent much of his long, productive life writing about the lives of historical figures who fascinated him: Hitler, Gorky, Jefferson, Luther, Gandhi, and of course, Sigmund Freud. Erikson saw the study of lives as critical to understanding historical events (e.g., The rise of Nazi Germany, the Protestant Reformation, India's Independence Movement) and he believed that persons influencing important social changes were leaders precisely because they were "working out"

From: *Handbook of Stressful Transitions Across the Lifespan,*
Edited by: T.W. Miller, DOI 10.1007/978-1-4419-0748-6_4,
© Springer Science+Business Media, LLC 2010

personal conflicts that were psychosocial in origin. In brief, these leaders were able to navigate personal, developmental transitions in ways that were relevant to their sociohistorical contexts, and they were able to engage and powerfully influence the public and political conflicts of their times – for good and ill. In advancing and developing such ideas, Erikson reformulated and sometimes implicitly repudiated the central ideas of his professional mentors, Sigmund and Anna Freud. While considering himself personally and professionally "loyal" to the founders of psychoanalysis, he nonetheless tried to expand the focus of psychoanalysis from its "vertical," geological drilling for the riches of intrapsychic toward an additional exploration of those dense surfaces of interpersonal, historical, and social geographies that contextualize human development.

Erikson's unique "ways of seeing" led to innovative psychological constructs such as "identity," "identity crisis," "epigenetic development," "psychohistory," "pseudospeciation," and "adult development" – constructs now absorbed into the daily lexicon of psychology and American culture. Unlike many of his psychoanalytic colleagues, Erikson's epistemology was grounded in direct observation and visual-configural thinking, which he found more trustworthy than verbal-analytic rumination (Friedman 1999). He was a thinker who tackled the problem of how personal selfhood shapes and is shaped by the movement of putatively impersonal historical transitions. This required an intrepid intellectual courage, because as he repeatedly chose to grapple with these larger social, cultural, and historical realities, his stage theory of the human life cycle became more tenuous, flexible, and problematic (Smelser 1998). Indeed, in his middle and older years he appeared to generously and enthusiastically embrace the risks of grappling with the complexities of the world, even if this meant privately revising his renowned theoretical positions (Hoare 2002).

This chapter examines the connections between Erik Erikson's life history and the development of his theoretical approaches. Erikson's life cycle theory emphasizes the transitions across the human life span, and the ongoing tensions (crises) facing persons as they age. I argue that Erikson's personal life history was an important source of his theoretical focus on transitions, marginalities, and ambiguities in human experience. Indeed, the "growth of his work" represented a series of geographical and intellectual emigrations over the course of nine decades during twentieth century (Coles 1970). The life cycle theory as developed in *Childhood & Society* (Erikson 1950) would serve as a platform for 30 years of subsequent theorizing over a wide range of domains and would help him create a body of work that continues to prove meaningful for contemporary psychology and social thought. This chapter briefly explores these domains of concern and delineates the relevance of Erikson's theoretical approaches by discussing critical themes in his life and work.

Origins

Erikson's life history helps explain his intellectually risky decision to give central importance to the contingent, historical, and contextual dimensions of human existence. In addition to providing greater clarity for specifically understanding his work, thinking about Erikson's biography provides fresh

Table 4-1. Phases of Erikson's Life as described by Erik Erikson in his own Autobiographical Writings as analyzed by L. Friedman (2004a, b).

1. Childhood and extended adolescence (1902–1926)

2. Six years with the Freud Circle in Vienna (1927–1933)

3. Emigration to and professional settlement in the U.S. (1933–1949)

4. Publication of *Childhood & Society* (1950)

5. McCarthy "loyalty oath" crisis, Austen Riggs, *Young Man Luther* (1951–1960)

6. Harvard professor, *Gandhi's Truth*, studies in ethical development (1960–1975)

7. "Galilean Sayings," old age, cognitive decline (1976–1994)

ways of understanding how significant theoretical and empirical investigations are developed and established in the behavioral sciences. Such an endeavor also creates the opportunity for contemporary workers to think about how they conduct their own intellectual projects. As William Mckinley Runyan has observed, the study of lives can have "... a power to meet us deeply, to help us imagine what it must have been like to live in different social and historical circumstances, to provide insights into the workings of lives, and perhaps, to provide a frame of reference for reassessing our own experience, our fortunes, our possibilities of existence" (1982, p. 3) (Table 4-1).

The most important "actuality" to know about Erikson's origins is that while his father was always a powerful presence in his life, he never knew his father's actual identity. Remarkably, his mother refused to meaningfully assist Erikson's search for him – even when Erik appealed to her on her deathbed. Karla Abrahemsen was a Jewish woman from a respected Copenhagen family. She had an artistic spirit and enjoyed reading and discussing Christian thinkers such as Kierkegaard and Emerson. Lawrence Freidman (1999) believes that shortly after a very brief, failed marriage to a different man, Karla became involved with a Danish photographer and became pregnant with Erik. He was born in June 1902, and spent several years living with his mother in northern Germany. Erikson remembered his mother as a beautiful, sad, and intelligent woman with whom he shared an intimate attachment, especially during his toddler years. Recently, Friedman (2004b) has become convinced that Karla's association with the artistic community might have reflected a quasi-bohemian approach to relationships as a young woman, so she herself might have not known the identity of Erikson's father. If true, this mitigates previous biographical criticisms of her decision not to name him. However, the majority of observers believe that Karla knew, and moreover, that Erik knew that she knew, with all the encumbrances and ramifications this implies.

In 1905 Karla married Theodor Homburger, a successful pediatrician who promised redemption from social disgrace and long-term economic security for her young son. Karla agreed that Erik would be raised as his biological son in a Jewish household. This culturally plausible but phenotypically absurd plan was foiled as Erik Homburger developed into a latency age child with Nordic features and grew "flagrantly tall" (Erikson 1975, p. 27). Although he was *bar mitzvahed*, he was called "goy" by his peers at synagogue, and grew into adolescence with a sense of being cut off from his true heritage. He reveled in intricate fantasies of being rescued by his unknown, artistic Danish birth-father. While the Homburger family treated them well, both mother and son identified more with their Danish heritage than with their German-Jewish community. This created ongoing tensions that, while rarely erupting into open conflict, would lead Erik to a more solitary, introspective, and eventually rebellious adolescence. He was a bright child, but soon proved ill-suited for the kind of technical-scientific training required to become a medical doctor. In late adolescence, Erik took up the life of the wandering *Kunstler*, much like those young men romanticized by Goethe and Schiller. After a brief stint in a Munich art academy, at age 22, Erik began what he would later conceptualize as his "psychosocial moratorium."

In the respectable world of the German burghers, Erik had become a misfit – apparently unemployable, melancholic, and determined not to give into the ambitions held on his behalf by the well-meaning adults who were financially supporting him. He clumsily extended the socially acceptable period of his *Wanderschaft*, even to the extent that he began to secretly doubt his own capacity to find a way to live with sufficient sanity, commitment, and independence. Irving Alexander (2005) has argued that Erikson's identity crisis was the result of his parentage, his adoption into a Jewish family, and the internalization of this "…demanding situation, which he seemed to bear mostly in silence, inwardly, to maintain the good graces of his mother, his only anchor in the world" (p. 274). This coping approach may have contributed to extended periods of his psychological confusion and misery as he approached young adulthood. Indeed, Friedman sees this period as characterized by "a rather profound and unresolved identity crisis rooted in early parental aggression against his sense of selfhood" (2004a, p. 262).

The German literary and cultural milieu of those years might also provide clues about Erikson's inner experiences. One example of this can be found in Walter Sokel's description of the writer *in extremis* after World War I:

….the traditional peripheral social existence of the German intellectual.… [tended] to incline him toward a greater subjectivism and rebelliousness than his more integrated Western colleagues. While the French high-school student already tended to look on himself as part of society, and on his misery as something in the nature of things, a necessary passing phase, the German adolescent did not see himself as part of society and was more prone to resort to violent anarchic rebellion in his daydreams and fantasies (1959, p. 97).

If this is an accurate description of the cultural milieu in which Erikson had immersed himself during his *Wanderschaft*, then his psychological responses to the dilemmas he faced as a young adult had some social sanction. In fact, Erikson (1968) would later devise the theoretical concepts of "identity diffusion" and "negative identity" as expectable psychosocial outcomes for adolescents struggling with significant developmental impasses. As we shall see, he developed clinical strategies to address psychosocial states characterized by high levels of anxiety which sometimes included psychotic process. His clinical students would remember his remarkable empathy for such patients.

While many biographers note the dangerous psychological vulnerabilities of Erikson's late adolescence, Friedman's (1999) research into these years revealed a countervailing intellectual resilience. During his wandering, Erikson had assembled notebooks filled with his poetry, prose, and sketches, which prefigured many of his later, formal, and theoretical concerns:

....'Manuscript von Erik' consisted of some fascinating and unique notations....including the human life cycle, the same of 'self,' "I," and identity: the masculine balancing the feminine in the human personality; the importance of the leader in political trans-formations; and the conflict between pseudospeciation and human specieshood. To be sure Erik drew heavily from several German intellectuals, especially the works of Nietzsche, Goethe, and Hegel, even as he formulated his most original and unique perspectives. Like Schiller, Rilke, and Goethe, he anchored his thoughts to a respect of the free individual and displeasure with nationalism's pressure to conform. Freud, too, had drawn from these same German thinkers, and had embraced cosmopolitan values. *But it is well to keep in mind that in 1923 and 1924 Erik knew almost nothing about the founder of psychoanalysis....*(p. 55–56, emphasis added).

Despite such intensive intellectual experimentation, Erikson's return to the family home seemed to verify his immaturity, marginality, and inability to blaze a clear developmental path into young adulthood. Salvation from this identity confusion came in 1927 when Erikson received an invitation from his childhood friend, Peter Blos, to join him in Vienna. Blos was teaching in a Montessori school sponsored by Dorothy Burlingham and Anna Freud, which hosted the children of American analysands who had entered treatment with Sigmund Freud. Observing his talents for teaching and relating with (if not disciplining) his students, Anna Freud soon offered to supervise and train Erik in the new field of child psychoanalysis. Education in child analysis – which required multidisciplinary and intensive training for work with adults and children – brought him into a course of studies that deepened his intellectual skills, promised him a viable profession, and helped him cross the heretofore elusive psychosocial bridge from interminable adolescence to adulthood. This accident of fate and friendship would draw Erikson into the intense, inner circle of psychoanalysis, and help establish his adult identity.

Erikson was admitted to the International Psycho-Analytical Association in 1933, which entitled him to practice anywhere in the world. During his training analysis, Erik married Joan Serson, a Canadian national who had come to Vienna to study dance and art. She was to become the most important person in Erikson's life, and the true nature of her extraordinary influence on and involvement with his intellectual work is currently being explored by biographers. Joan's dissatisfaction with her own experiences as an analysand, her perceptions of the intellectual stultification characterizing the inner circle of psychoanalysis, and her conviction that Anna Freud's influence was too controlling of her husband's decisions were all instrumental in Erikson's decision to return to Denmark.

There was another important reason for considering emigration. Erikson's first major experience of how lives could be transformed by historical events came with Adolph Hitler's ascension as German Chancellor. He would later reflect that when he raised the impending danger of a Nazi encroachment into Austria, the Freud circle – inured by decades of relative prosperity in anti-Semitic Vienna – considered this as Erik's "rationalization" for flight as opposed to "insight" (Coles 1998). In fact, Freud and his family would escape by the skin of their teeth only in 1938, finally awakened by personal experi-ences of detention by the Gestapo. Freud's emigration was engineered by representatives of the American government and underwritten by the massive bribes proffered to the Nazis by his European friends. Their alarm was well-founded as many members of the extended Freud family would spend their final days in the death camps (Edmunson 2007). More than simply a story of extraordinary political naïveté, Erikson came to see this is as a historical parable about the danger of exclusively holding any focus on the "inner world" that is maintained at the expense of carefully analyzing the power of the "outer world" – a dialectic and problem that he continued to explore as a theorist.

After failing to settle in Copenhagen, the Eriksons entered the United States in 1933. Erikson was a 31-year-old husband and father immersed in a foreign culture, struggling with a new language, and plying a little understood profession. After an unsuccessful New York meeting with A. A. Brill, he brought the family to Boston where he was able to develop a successful analytic practice treating children and young adults. Erikson was a stunningly effective therapist, and his subsequent appointments to research posts at Harvard, Yale, and Berkeley were partially due to his remarkable treatment successes, which included the children of powerful university administrators and faculty (Friedman 1999; Roazen 1976).

Erikson's Life Cycle Theory

Erikson's great revision of psychoanalytic theory (or heretical rejection of it, as often argued by his Viennese elders and colleagues) was his insistence that human development was qualitatively different from that of other animals because of the action of complex cultural and social forces shaping the trajectories of an extended life cycle. Instead of an organism whose development was the sole product of instinctual drives targeting maternal figures as "objects" of those drives, Erikson emphasized that the caregivers, family, and culture into which an infant began life shaped, evoked, and constrained development. Unlike Freud, who conceptualized human development as essentially located in the individual and as the product of an evolutionary, pre-programmed unfolding, Erikson's developmental theory pointed to a process that heavily relied on relationships with caregivers and was extraordinarily impacted by the historical and sociocultural "factualities" into which the person was born.

He designed a schedule of psychosocial crises, which occurred at eight points of the life cycle and were composed of stepwise experiences and tasks marked by dialectical, psychosocial crises. Like Heinz Hartmann, Melanie Klein, and Heinz Kohut, he was a personality theorist who experienced personal and professional formation through psychoanalysis as it developed in the first decades of the twentieth century in Vienna, but who would later come to understand Freud's classical metapsychology as insufficient for explaining human development. He is rightfully credited with extending and revising Sigmund Freud's work by identifying and including important developmental events occurring during adulthood, and by postulating the complex transactional relationships between individual human organisms and the overwhelming social forces that shaped their lifelong development as persons.

In fact, Erikson argued, that while Freud's "discoveries" were critical breakthroughs for understanding the structure and action of the human mind, classical psychoanalytic theory was never intended to be a complete theory of human personality (Evans 1967). In contrast, Erikson saw his own work as providing the necessary theoretical extensions for a psychosocial theory of personality that was informed by Freud's more limited psychosexual developmental scheme. This understanding is evident when examining his charts of the human life cycle, first presented in *Childhood and Society* (1950) and finally presented in the summing up of his life's work in a concise text sponsored by the U.S. National Institute of Mental Health, *The Life Cycle Completed* (1989). Erikson's scheme was biologically grounded in Freud's architecture of oral, anal, phallic, and genital psychosexual stages of childhood and early adolescent development. In this sense, Freud's depiction of the human lifespan was in line with classical biology's understanding of adulthood as the attainment of reproductive capacity. As Frank Sulloway (1979) and others have shown, Freud drew on a nineteenth century Darwinian framework as he developed his theory of mind, and thereby understood human psychosexual development as necessarily completed by early adolescence. This developmental timeline, which was so fundamental to Freud's metapsychology, led to his explanations for adult patients' psychopathologies as the ramifications of remote childhood developmental events and processes, rather than as problems with contemporary origins (Table 4-2).

In contrast, Erikson's stage theory depicted a lifelong process driven by the physiological processes of aging itself and by the operation of historical events and sociocultural forces impinging at particular developmental periods. This epigenetic approach was drawn from the model of the in vitro human fetus developing each organ system – e.g., a brain or a heart – during critical periods of ascendancy and opportunity. Erikson utilized this analogy for psychosocial development, but stipulated that unlike embryonic development, psychosocial development sometimes offered "second chances" for repair and new development.

Along with ego psychologist Heinz Hartmann (1951), he emphasized the adaptive aspects of ego functioning as the best way for understanding normal human development, and in contrast to Freud's pessimistic view, Erikson asserted a philosophical anthropology that argued for developmental creativity and flexibility. Erikson would summarize this in *Childhood and Society* as the "triple bookkeeping" of somatic, ego, and social processes that were required to explain the complexities of human development and behavior (Erikson 1950). This approach provided exponentially greater degrees of explanatory freedom than those available to Freud, whose metapsychological power

Table 4-2. Erikson's eight psychosocial stages of the human life cycle.

Age	Psychosexual stage (Freud)	Psychosocial crisis	Associated virtue
1. Infancy	Oral	Trust vs. mistrust	Hope
2. Early childhood	Anal	Autonomy vs. Shame and doubt	Will
3. Childhood (play age)	Phallic	Initiative vs. guilt	Purpose
4. Childhood (school age)	Latency	Industry vs. inferiority	Competence
5. Adolescence and young adulthood	Genital	Identity vs. role confusion	Fidelity
6. Young adulthood		Intimacy vs. isolation	Love
7. Mature adulthood		Generativity vs. stagnation (or self-absorption)	Care
8. Old age		Ego integrity vs. despair	Wisdom

relied on reductive, instinctual explanations for normal and pathological development – an approach that Erikson would later criticize as the "originology fallacy." Instead, Erikson would map multiple sources of causality and influence to explain developmental outcomes and behaviors, which could occur at many points along the human life cycle. He would use the theoretical flexibility inherent in this configural approach as he turned to a wide range of interdisciplinary concerns throughout his life, which ultimately included ethical, religious, social, and historical problems.

Erikson's decision to stand on the boundary where Freudian drive theory bordered newly developing psychosocial, political, and cultural psychologies was conceptually confusing. While David Rapaport attempted to demonstrate Erikson's allegiance to psychoanalytic ego psychology by showing that his work had clear lines of agreement and continuity with Hartmann (Gill 1967), Erikson and most observers agreed this proved a futile effort (Friedman 1999). Roy Schafer wrote critically about what he considered troubling, non-systematic, theoretical, and clinical obfuscations generated by Erikson's continued if partial adherence to Freud's metapsychology. At the same time, he appreciated how Erikson's approach to "identity," if considered outside of a rigid ego psychology framework, had the potential to advance clinical theory:

.... [In] a deeper way, this use of identity is only a breath away from saying "the person" or "the agent." Moreover, I believe it to be true that, as Erikson uses it, and despite his own lapses into reification, identity is more phenomenological and existential-analytic that Freudian-metapsychological. Identity is very similar to the existential-analytic concept of *being-in-the-world* in that both are used to attempt a basic thematic characterization of a person's way of creating arranging, and experiencing his or her life. Identity is the theme of significant personal actions (1976, p. 114)

It is intriguing to consider how Erikson's biography influenced his central theoretical concerns. We know that he laid out a developmental scheme that looks at life from infancy to old age. His conceptualization of childhood and adolescence involves an epigenetic process in which the human being moves through life in a series of critical, developmental periods, each driven by biological changes and pulled by a psychosocial crisis – the dialectical tensions between trust and mistrust; autonomy and shame; initiative and guilt; industry and inferiority – with identity and diffused identity in adolescence. Adult psychosocial crises include the tensions between intimacy and isolation, and then between midlife generativity and rejectivity/stagnation; old age brings the struggle of retrospective meaning-making, which Erikson identified as the tension between integrity and despair (Meissner 2000). Erikson's life history is quite suggestive of the types of crises and struggles depicted in the model. Note that there are no terminal resolutions of these dialectics. He believed his theory could be clinically applied if the psychotherapist was also cognizant and tolerant of the discontinuity of life. Unfortunately, Erikson's theory – in the hands of secondary interpreters – is sometimes parodied into rigid prescriptions that offer only limited clinical and theoretical utility.

Further, because psychosocial crises are never finalized, the clinician is always required to develop a particular, historical understanding of how any life cycle is specifically experienced – this is the key to understanding how a person develops an identity. The details of that struggle reveal the person's "ego strengths" and their capacities for managing danger and opportunities.

If fortunate, he or she will be able to robustly engage the challenging task of identity formation – a capacity that depends on the cumulative developmental resources in place available for this effort.

During this critical psychosocial crisis – the period characterizing adolescence and young adulthood – long resisted regressions may appear, and can include tremendously frightening and disorganizing mental experiences. But when such regressions are directed into the service of development, these can serve as the adolescent's way of communicating through words, behaviors, gestures, dreams, and silences about what remains damaged or incomplete. Such gaps and inconsistencies in the person's narratives offer important clues about conflicts and gaps in development that may be preventing movement into healthy adulthood. Given a supportive setting, the young person can safely regress, and work to repair what is insufficient. The unsuccessful alternative is to hobble along and age with truncated understanding, skills, and affects, resulting in a set of compromised abilities for loving others, enjoying intimate relationships, developing a lifework, raising healthy children, and striving for the best interests of the next generation.

Identifying this vulnerable bridge between adolescent identity development and the ongoing process of adult development is one of Erikson's most important contributions. The formation of the generative adult (as opposed to one who is rejected and rejecting), is crucial for Erikson's envisioned "cogwheel" of the generations. Culture can only be inherited if its most important dimensions are transmitted through childrearing practices enacted by adults who choose to consistently focus on the well-being of children – including birth children, foster children, adoptive children, abandoned children, and imprisoned or institutionalized children.

These processes usually occur in the family but are significantly shaped by how a particular society and its political establishment impact family and neighborhood life. Such institutional practices globally and concretely shape the identities of young citizens who prepare to take up the positions of parents, teachers, therapists, employers, and religious, cultural, and sociopolitical leaders in that society. A contemporary example may serve to illustrate Erikson's concerns. Almost 800,000 traumatized, drug-addicted, and violent child soldiers currently fight in armed conflicts across failed nation-states in Asia and Africa (Betancourt et al. 2008; Brett and Specht 2004; Macha 2001). In response, the United Nations has launched major campaigns for the demobilization, rehabilitation, and reintegration of these children back into their civil societies, with an Eriksonian realization of the otherwise disastrous consequences for future economic, religious, social, and political institutions in the developing world.

Another way to appreciate Erikson's theory is to see how he applied it as a clinician treating his young patients. For example, Friedman (1999) gives us a fascinating account of Erikson's treatment of marginalized children in Boston at the Judge Baker Clinic – many who had suffered maltreatment. Erikson encouraged children to play, draw, and manipulate building blocks; he then analyzed these enactments and configurations, allowing him to interpret the central internal conflicts and the external dangers the child was experiencing. His collateral use of home visits, field trips, shared meals, and warm conversations created powerful therapeutic relationships characterized by trust and realistic optimism. Erikson's own credentials as a lonely, introverted child who became an adult who was more comfortable with *looking and drawing* rather than *talking* gave him special capacities for such relational approaches.

Edward Shapiro and M. Gerard Fromm (2000) – Erikson's colleagues and students – provide an insider's view of how Erikson actually worked as a clinician with privileged adolescent and young adult patients at Austen-Riggs in the 1950s, and how he captured the "configurations" he saw at the interface of the person and the environment:

In Erikson's thinking, the surface (i.e., the ego) revealed the depth. When he listened to patients, he listened with an artist's ear – he heard the words, saw the spatial relationships, and made temporal links between the somatic, affective and interpersonal parts of the personality. He listened to texture and saw configuration. He paid attention to the whole life context of any immediate situation. He asked a number of questions. What is the immediate stimulus for the patient's reaction? What is the acute life conflict, the current developmental stage, the issues that are manifest? In what developmental context did the patient's reaction first occur? Is it now manifest in the relationship to the therapist, in a repetitive conflict, in a characteristic way that the individual solved earlier developmental struggles? In what social context is the individual embedded, what roles are available? What are the typical stereotypes, particular opportunities and barriers? What are the characteristic ways the person takes in information? What defenses does the individual use? What are the individual's deepest psychological investments?...Like his contemporary, Donald W. Winnicott, Erikson had a family perspective. He recognized that children react to the shared family unconscious, reading their parents' vulnerabilities and unexpressed wishes with clarity. Studying seriously disturbed patients, he saw that their breakdowns occurred during times of developmental separation or individuation (e.g., physical intimacy, occupational choice, or identity formation)....He saw social recognition as providing defenses against impulses, and he saw work as a means to consolidate conflict-free achievements (p. 2201).

Erikson believed that developmental and historical understanding offers the clinician information about the sources of current problems, as well as an opening to understanding the kinds of relationships patients have with others, including the clinician. Rather than a rigidly prescribed protocol, the clinician utilizes "disciplined subjectivity," the use of the total self – reason and intuition, theory and experience, the patient's symptoms, and the clinician's own reactions – to understand the patient's experience of self and world in the context of his/her biography. Erikson lays out the argument for the therapeutic value of disciplined subjectivity in *Insight and Responsibility* (1964), which offers us important insights into his approach to treatment and research, as well as into his thinking about the organization of the human sciences. Note his use of Albert Einstein's terminology in his implied critique of orthodox psychoanalytic theory and behavioral theory:

The relativity implicit in clinical work may, to some, militate against its scientific value. Yet, I suspect, that this very relativity, truly acknowledged, will make the clinicians better companions of today's and tomorrow's scientists than did the attempts to reduce the study of the human mind to a science identical with traditional natural science. ....[S]cientists may learn about the nature of things by finding out what they can do to them, but....the clinician can learn of the true nature of man only in the attempt to do something for and with him (p. 80).

Erikson also argued that patients' "times" – their historical and cultural actualities – must be part of this understanding. History and culture shape the ego, and for some individuals (especially exceptional "cases" like Luther and Gandhi) the personal struggle to respond to the times will transactionally influence the unfolding of social change and history itself. In sum, Erikson's clinical approaches give us clues as to how he built on the life cycle theory to construct the psychohistorical studies for which he would later receive so much acclaim and criticism.

Adult Transitions and Marginalities

For reasons that in many ways defy explanation, Erikson found himself embraced by his adopted country, and he enthusiastically fell in love with America in a wholehearted and uncritical manner that was very different from the highly critical European émigrés who would flee Hitler later in the 1930s (Heilbut 1983). (Erikson would sober up after being asked to sign a loyalty oath during the McCarthy era and later when confronted with the realities of American racism and military policies in the 1960s.) He was determined to learn to speak and write English (with Joan's considerable editorial collaboration), and he learned many American colloquialisms from his patients. He grew fond of punning and making jokes in English.

When he became a citizen in 1939 he changed his name to "Erikson" with the consent and collaboration of his wife and children – a symbolic embrace of his suspected paternal origins and the self-designation of a new American identity (Heinze 2004). He would forever be called "Homburger" by the Vienna crowd. He spent his early academic career on the East coast and traveled west to study Native Americans (the Yurok and Sioux), which provided rich cross-cultural perspectives that he never forgot. He joined the war effort by providing psychoanalytic portraits of Hitler, German youth, and other aspects of Nazi psychology. He consulted with the U.S. government regarding what would be necessary for America to successfully occupy and then transform Germany into a democratic state after the war was won, and wrote a 1945 memorandum that has remarkable implications for the contemporary international situation, especially in its analysis of the complexities involved in wide scale ideological and political transitions:

It is obvious only history can change people. The question is not what discipline alone or what disciplines combined could solve the historical dilemma but rather: What combination of disciplines is now well enough integrated to present the Germans with a total situation which must convince them that their history, as they see it and saw it, is over? Only an unequivocal change in its total historical situation will convince a people that its common panics and its traditional enthusiasms are outlived and that its habitual forms of self assertion do not pay any longer. Only after such conviction has had time to sink in can changes in those family patterns and attitudes of child training be expected. (Schlein 1987, p. 368).

In other words, no discipline or profession can readily apply technologies to rapidly change an aggressive empire into a peaceable nation. Historical change drives personal change, Erikson argued, and only adults with successful experiences with democratic governments will raise children who grow to become new leaders with democratic ideals.

Erikson held appointments at Harvard (where he worked for Henry Murray who became a crucial mentor), subsequently at Yale, and then at the University of California. Not surprisingly, this solitary man was a poor team player, and was sometimes seen by colleagues as preferring to pursue research in his isolated, idiosyncratic, and perhaps selfish manner. Erikson presented himself in his typically marginal way – as an entitled rebel pursuing the research questions that engaged him, but also as undereducated, and therefore lacking the necessary credentials to play a competent part in the high-pressure world of competitive social science research. This conflict would consistently unfold throughout his adulthood and, as we shall see, contribute to serious personal and public dilemmas.

While he valued the prestige of academic posts, Erikson almost always maintained a private practice to augment the initially limited salaries he earned through research and teaching. In the 1950s he left academia and worked primarily as an analyst and consultant at the Austen Riggs Center in Massachusetts where he trained a new generation of American psychoanalytic clinicians.

In another important career move, he decided to write a psychoanalytic study of Martin Luther, which signaled his first sustained project in psychobiography. *Young Man Luther* (1950) would further demonstrate Erikson's intellectual originality and generate invitations into prestigious academic circles. Characteristically, he would continually remain insecure in such settings. For example, despite special appointment as a university professor at Harvard in 1960, he would confide to Robert Coles that he was constantly amazed and bemused by his mysterious "success," as if never fully understanding how he had achieved this level of academic and social status (Coles 2004). Such accounts, as gathered from friends, students, and Erikson's own autobiographical writings, indicate that throughout his life Erikson struggled with a powerful sense of being marginal, and that this experience of identity probably intensified when finding himself at the pinnacle of academic celebrity. While such marginality offered Erikson interdisciplinary freedoms unavailable to specialist colleagues, it exacted psychosocial and emotional costs.

A Theory of Adulthood

Erikson was the one of the first psychoanalytic thinkers to assert that human adulthood could no longer be understood as attained with the capacity to biologically reproduce. Instead, adulthood was an unfolding psychosocial process of transition and development unto death, even into an eighth or ninth decade of life. This was a radical departure from Freud's "hard determinism" and might be seen as severing adult development from its psychosexual moorings in childhood. Some have claimed that this limited biological grounding was a weakness in Erikson's system. However, in recent years biological research has turned to investigating the complex processes of human aging that occur after adolescence and that extend into old age. These investigations – still in their nascent phase – have suggested that the aging process involves much more than simple cell deterioration unto death. For example, the recent breakthroughs of neuroscience have discovered the lifelong plasticity of the brain, including unforeseen capacities for repair, reconstruction, and adaptation during adulthood. Therefore, it appears that previous biological demarcations of the human life cycle are open to revision as neuroscientists develop theories of adult brain development that extend beyond the traditional focus on childhood and adolescence (Kirkwood 2008).

Erikson's former student, Howard Gardner (1999), has described Erikson's four great intellectual projects. The first two – the replacement of Freud's originology with a new epigenetic approach, and his subsequent development of the concept of "identity" – (already discussed above) were essentially in place by 1960. The third project – a cultural analysis through psychohistory – was undertaken primarily through his psychobiographies of Luther and Gandhi. In these psychohistorical investigations he sought to discover how the personal psychosocial crises faced by two powerful religious, political, and cultural leaders interfaced with the fundamental crisis of their historical periods. Interestingly, *Young Man Luther* (1958) is a story of adolescent identity formation – of finding a "voice" through individuation from the father (and holy mother church). His study of Gandhi's development of the "truth-force" (satyagraha), an ascetic and intellectual strategy for personal freedom and non-violent resistance, led to further explorations of generativity – the ultimate responsibility of adults to their children, their nation, and their species (Erikson, 1969).

Gardner identifies Erikson's fourth project as his formulation of a new, psychologically based morality. Profoundly influenced by his intensive study of Gandhi, Erikson sought to delineate emergent psychosocial strengths and weaknesses that were correlated to sociocultural rituals and ritualizations. Carolyn Hren Hoare's recent examination of unpublished papers from Erikson's Harvard archives has revealed that his developing conceptions of the wise, ethical, and spiritual adult were inextricable from the capacity to care for the next generation. In fact, according to Hoare (2002), Erikson would later see such generative activity as integral to the achievement of "integrity" – the positive dimension of old age – and as also necessary to successful *midlife* development. Erikson saw the mature adult as the person who embraced his or her identity and used moral, psychological, and religious energies for the good of others – including those extending far beyond the biological family.

Ultimately, Gardner sees Erikson's study of adult morality as the exploration of species identity and the danger of pseudospeciation. This latter concept provides the framework for understanding the genocide and ethnic violence that plague late modernity despite (and in many ways shaped by) its technological achievements. When humans (through their conscious and unconscious enactments of harmful psychosocial ritualisms) select rejectivity instead of mutuality, the consequences include socially sanctioned violence against and even extinction of marginalized groups. These "others" will be defined as sub-humans, monsters, or as evolutionary accidents. The phenomenon of "ethnic cleansing" suggests such a deep-rooted, psychosocial justification of instrumental and political violence to maintain personal identity and social cohesion (Muller, 2008; Sen, 2006).

Erikson believed that mature adults must be engaged in the fight against pseudospeciation and do not have the option of retreating into a psychologically well-adjusted private life.

What does happen, we may well ask in conclusion, to adults who have "found their identity" in the cultural consolidation of their day? Most adults, it is true, turn their backs on identity questions and attend to the inner cave of their familial, occupational, and civic concerns. But this cannot be taken as an assurance that they have either transcended or truly forgotten what they have once envisaged in the roamings of their youth. The question is: what have they done with it, and how ready are they to respond to the identity needs of the coming generations in the universal crisis of faith and power? In the end, it seems, psychoanalysis cannot claim to have exhausted its inquiry into man's unconscious without asking what may be the inner arrest peculiar to adulthood – not merely as a result of leftovers of infantile immaturity, but as a consequence of the adult condition as such. For it is only too obvious that, so far in man's total development, adulthood and maturity have rarely been synonymous. The study of the identity crisis, therefore, inexorably points to conflicts and conditions due to those specializations of man which make him efficient at a given stage of economy and culture at the expense of the denial of major aspects of existence. Having begun as a clinical art-and-science, psychoanalysis cannot shirk the question of what, from the point of view of an undivided human race, is "wrong" with the "normality" reached by groups of men under the conditions of pseudo-speciation. Does it not include pervasive group retrogressions which cannot be subsumed under the categories of neurotic regressions, but rather represent a joint fixation on historical formulae perhaps dangerous to human survival? (Erikson 1972, p. 31).

Theoretically, Erikson struggled with the problem of whether the genocide and violence that he conceptualized as pseudospeciation involved elements of drive theory (instinctual regressions) or whether such violent actions represented the powerful seduction of violent ideologies. Biographically, Erikson seems to reflect on his own struggle with the temptation to enjoy living a comfortable, politically low-risk, private life, with his intensifying moral realization that this could indicate an insidious if socially sanctioned immaturity. Note the suggestive autobiographical references ("roamings of their youth") of Erikson-the-elder in the foregoing discussion of species survival and moral responsibility.

Reversals of Fortune

Erikson enjoyed his successful, if brief, tenure at Harvard as a popular teacher and mentor – years which had also included consistently positive critical reviews and bestselling public receptions of his books, satisfying interdisciplinary work with the American Academy of Arts and Sciences, an iconic portrait by Norman Rockwell, an appreciative biographical profile published in the *New Yorker* by his student and friend, Robert Coles, and his reception of the Pulitzer Prize and the National Book Award for *Gandhi's Truth*. Following a cascade of popular and professional successes during the 1960s, Erikson would subsequently endure the 1970s as a time to be criticized as a patriarchal, monocultural, historically naïve, politically conservative, methodologically unscientific, theoretically fuzzy, theological dilettante – a pseudo-Christian utopian, and a sociological eclectic who had irreversibly diluted psychoanalysis. Most grievously, in 1975, he was depicted by Leftist critic, Marshall Berman, in the *New York Times Book Review* as a man who had engineered a cowardly flight from Jewish origins by changing his name from Homburger to Erikson.

By the late-seventies, Erikson faced intellectual assaults from all sides: the analytic community, academic psychology, biological psychiatry, influential feminists like former student Carol Gilligan, and postmodern theorists. The period from 1964 through 1976 (an era where the nation exploded with political assassinations, the Civil Rights and Women's movements, the Viet Nam War, and Watergate) was one of the most polarized in American history.

It was an era that saw the *ad hominem* attack as a viable tool for the public intellectual – and especially damning was the accusation of being "a phony" or of demonstrating "bad faith." These personal assaults were realizations of Erikson's deepest fears. The rapidity of this public decline was confusing to him as he saw his own biographical history quite differently – an agonizingly hard-won, incremental emergence from obscurity and marginality.

Berman's public attack also raised a personal issue that had long been speculated upon by even Erikson's admirers, namely, his Jewish heritage. The so-called "Jewish Question" (Bein 1990) did not only concern the political fate of European Jews at the hands of the Nazis, but also encompassed the personal matter of an individual's acceptance or rejection of Jewish background. For some, Erikson could be considered a self-hating Jew who had covered up his true identity in exchange for rapid assimilation as an ethnically-ambiguous American citizen, admission into WASPish, quota-driven academic institutions, and uncomplicated public idealization. Despite the fact that hundreds of foreign-born Jewish intellectuals, businessmen, politicians, artists, and celebrities who had prospered in America had changed their names to effectively assimilate, many observers did not find that the psychoanalyst and moralist who had developed the concept of "identity" should enjoy any right to exercise such an option. Stephen Whitfield suggests that Erikson held a more complex set of personal motives:

He liked living at the edge of boundaries that he ignored or surmounted as he chose. He shared the American proclivity to want to combine options, to have it all, or maybe to split the difference. Erikson wanted to be gentile or Jew, psychoanalyst and artist and historian and prophet, explorer of both the inner world of children freely at play and the outer world of men who fantasized that they could make history itself their plaything – and then, like Martin Luther and Mahatma Gandhi, proceeded to do so. Out of such ambiguities, his biographical and psychoanalytical work on identity could be forged.... But how he related to...Judaism, or how he even understood it, remains a mystifying subject (2002, pp. 163–164).

Berman's attack caught Erikson by surprise, and while he tried explaining his position to selected friends and colleagues, he proved unwilling and perhaps incapable of publicly defending himself. This was not only due to his probable underestimation of the impact of such criticisms, but also because he had not achieved his American celebrity and its concomitant rewards by plunging into public controversy. He was fragile in many ways and shielded from the world in a quasi-monastic lifestyle that Joan fiercely maintained. He was constitutively unable to strike back decisively and brutally in the manner of a battle-hardened, public intellectual.

Additionally, because of his introversion and his intense resistance to psychoanalytic institutes of all types, he never developed a school of "Eriksonians" who might have been deployed on his behalf. In many ways, Erikson's entire life was about living at the margins, rebelling, wandering, and not buckling under psychoanalytic dogmatics or academic constraints – he effectively "de-institutionalized" himself whenever he could manage this. Solitary rebels don't build institutions. Unlike Freud, Erikson preferred to launch students rather than to convene and direct them. Paradoxically, this *modus vivendi* made him more vulnerable to the marginalization of his work. Psychoanalyst Peter Lomas noted this decision to be a "loner" as cutting both ways for Erikson and his readers:

.....Erikson tends to follow his own line of thought and pay little attention to the theories of others. This is both his strength and weakness. Without this inclination he would, I'm sure, never have given his illuminating account of crises during the life-cycle. The disadvantage is that he has not made use of the ideas of these colleagues, who are, like him, working toward a less mechanistic interpretation of personal experience (1970, p. 67).

Lomas might have overstated the case. Close readings of Erikson's work reveal that he was employing ideas from many classical and contemporary quarters. Much like Freud, who avoided reading Nietzsche and Schopenhauer for fear of being "influenced," Erikson prized his sense of individuality and originality. At the same time, the informed reader can discern Erikson weaving in many important ideas from literature, cultural and film criticism, philosophy, biology, sociology, and psychologies friendly and unfriendly to psychoanalytic perspectives. These works and authors are sometimes cited but many times were incorporated without explicit acknowledgement. This dichotomous view of being original versus being derivative sometimes blocked him from the intellectual generosity and synergy he often displayed when personally meeting with other intellectuals. So in addition to lacking disciples, he deprived himself of important scholarly alliances which might have enriched his work and shored him up when under assault by enemies who caricatured his ideas.

In addition to considering his personal characteristics, Erikson's writings require that we recognize the historical forces that contributed to these reversals of fortune. Chief among these was the overall decline of psychoanalysis as the Nation's metapsychology and clinical theory of choice. Erikson's professional ascent after his emigration to the United States in the early 1930s paralleled the ascent of psychoanalysis as the premier psychiatric theory in U.S. medical schools, the mental health professions, literary theory, art criticism, etc (Coles, 2000a). Hence, W. H. Auden (1940, p. 93) memorialized the newly deceased Freud as "...no more a person now/ but a whole climate of opinion/ under whom we conduct our different lives...."）

Erikson prospered under psychoanalysis' reign, and his personal fate was a harbinger of the profession's fall which would soon follow. By 1980, the analytic paradigm was replaced by a distinctly American biomedical, atheoretical approach, manualized as *DSM-III*, and officially voted (after fierce debates in the American Psychiatric Association) as the new "bible" of American psychiatry. Advocates argued that the neurobiological approach to psychopathology afforded psychiatry a re-entry into scientific medicine proper. Emerging brain imaging technologies, accompanied by ambitious philosophies and psychologies of mind, promised empirical rigor.

The financing of mental health also changed, shifting reimbursement from long-term to brief treatment, from talk to pharmacologic therapies, from approaches based on case studies to those putatively confirmed by randomized controlled trials, from long-term recovery at Menninger or Austen Riggs to the 3-day stay in crisis stabilization units, from privileged communication to routinized managed care disclosures. While there were many positive developments flowing from these new approaches, there were also grievous assaults on the ethics of care. Furthermore, the intellectual and professional insularity of psychoanalysis and its endless internecine warfare rendered it ineffectual in stemming this tide which nearly eclipsed psychoanalysis's meaningful scientific, clinical, and theoretical contributions (Prince 1999; Malcolm, 1983; Shapiro and Carr 1993).

In 1994 Erik Erikson died in a Massachusetts nursing home after a decade of suffering Alzheimer's disease. He had lived a long life as an accomplished thinker, clinician, teacher, and husband. His qualities as a father were more problematic, nowhere more so than in regard to the decision to institutionalize his fourth child, Neil, who was born in 1944 with Down's syndrome. Friedman (1999) gives a sensitive rendering of the dilemmas that Joan and Erik faced when making decisions about Neil, who essentially disappeared from the family after placement – a not unusual fate for that era. However, he also believes that the trauma that cascaded from that decision changed Erik and Joan forever. Teetering close to divorce, the couple eventually began to heal as they developed the life cycle schema that laid out "healthy" developmental lines, even as they looked to the impact that Neil (the referent of negative development) had created for their family.

This is a powerful, troubling, and profoundly psychobiographical reading of the development of Eriksonian theory. "Manuscript von Erik" notwithstanding, Friedman's interpretation suggests that the life cycle theory itself was an act of preserving the identity and intimacy of the Eriksons, even as it was later developed to emphasize the centrality of generativity over rejectivity in healthy and ethical adult development. The paradox (or travesty) of the theory of adult generativity as emerging from this experience of parental rejectivity is unsettling indeed.

Some critics will see this new historical evidence as simply one more piece of data to support those who claim Erikson was a fraud. Without going that far, it is reasonable to speculate that such critics were able to wound the Eriksons so deeply, precisely because of the negative ramifications of this hidden but corrosive family secret which resounded long after Neil's death in 1965. Certainly it is easy to characterize Erikson's decision to institutionalize Neil, his 20 year exclusion from the family, and the deception of two of his three children (Sue and Jon) regarding these actions as amazingly selfish and hypocritical for a thinker who postulated parental generativity as the gold standard of psychosocial maturity.

Now with such recent biographical accounts at hand, it proves even more provocative to think about Erikson's massive but unpublished efforts in his last decade of productive and private theorizing. The hundreds of sketches, colored-pencil diagrams, and self-edited and profusely annotated texts of his previously published work recently "discovered" by Friedman (1999) and Hoare (2002) in the archives of Harvard's Houghton Library depict an elderly and now more isolated theorist who criticized, deconstructed, and reformulated his own intellectual positions on maturity, ethics, and religious identity.

Shortly after the publication of Friedman's biography, Erikson's daughter, Sue Bloland (2005), published a poignant account of Erik's emotional distance and shortcomings as an adult and as a father, providing further questions about the connection between the man and his work. Her account of her parents' refusal to return from a European trip when notified of Neil's death and the delegation of his burial to Kai, Jon, and Sue is troubling and defies easy explanation. It is reasonable to believe that Erikson's psychological struggle with an absent father had much to do with his own compromised generativity and heartbreaking reenactments of parental absenteeism. Yet Bloland ends her memoir with gratitude that Erik and Joan were able to parent as well as they did, given their own childhood struggles. Additionally, it is important to note that Erikson shared the financial fruits of his American successes with his family in Europe and Israel, and in adulthood worked hard to develop a closer relationship with his aging stepfather.

It is difficult to dispute Friedman's (2004b) recent argument that Erikson's life did not neatly fit into the eight psychosocial stages of his life cycle theory. However, our discussion seems to confirm the grounding of his human development theory in the exigencies, possibilities, and fragilities of epigenetic development. Indeed, another way of seeing Erikson's life suggests the ancient image of the "wounded healer," whose personal errors, tragedies, blind-spots, selfishness, and failures nevertheless opened up possibilities for recovery, healing, endurance, and creativity for the healer and his patients. The transformations of suffering into insight, and insight into theory are important sources of psychoanalytic thought (Borden 2009).

This kind of knowing is quite consistent with the German cultural tradition that had shaped Erikson as a young man. For example, we can turn to R.M. Rilke – a poet both fearful of and sympathetic toward psychoanalysis. Rilke's *Duino Elegies*, composed over the period of 1910–1922, evoked the crucial personal struggles of living in the early twentieth century, while providing commentary on the unstable and fragmented institutions reeling from the social, political, and economic ramifications of the Great War. In the "Tenth Elegy" Rilke wrote of the necessary and enduring relationship between suffering and insight in the powerful metaphors of time and place: "We wasters of sorrows! How we stare away in sad endurance beyond them,/ trying to force their end!/ Whereas they are nothing else than our winter foliage, our somber evergreen, *one*/ of the seasons of our interior year – not only/ season – they're also place, settlement, camp, soil, dwelling." (1939/1963, p. 79).

This is not a romantic perspective. Acquiring knowledge through adverse life experiences involves magnitudes of personal and social suffering, endured and inflicted. But this vision is congruent with Erikson's developmental theory which acknowledged the inevitability of moving through life confronting and re-confronting the existential, dialectical, psychosocial crises that are integral to the human condition. If this image of the wounded healer is justified, we can further understand how losses and mistakes endured in the intimacies of family life also made these significant domains for psychological probing, moral attention, and theoretical formulation. Erikson's life and work raises questions about how such connections between "biography" and "theory" contribute to the development of meaningful theories of human behavior and psychotherapy in ways that are distinct from the empirical methods advanced by the social sciences (Lachman 2004; Vaillant and Milofsky 1980).

Erikson's Generativity

Resilience and hope are dominant themes in Erikson's writings, and they seem to now apply to future consideration of his work. Recent essays, articles and books have appeared that offer fresh and more sophisticated appraisals of Erikson's life and ideas. Interestingly, some "old" actors have reappeared on stage to soften their earlier, more critical treatments of his work (e.g., Roazen 2000). And new anthologies of his most important publications and previously unpublished manuscripts have probably assured that Erikson's important work will be in print for many years to come (Coles, 2000b; Schlein 1987; Wallerstein & Goldberger, 1998).

However, it remains to be seen how Erikson's work will ultimately contribute to human development theory. Investigators have found the identity construct as particularly robust, developing psychometric and other empirical studies to trace its development in young people and endurance in adulthood (Marcia 2004). Some scholars have found Erikson's approach to generativity as a helpful framework for examining adulthood and midlife, especially as the impetus for legacy development and sociocultural achievement (De Aubin et al. 2004; Kotre 1996). Still others have followed his lead in "….studying in the lives of religious innovators that border areas where neurotic and existential conflict meet and where the "I" struggles for unencumbered awareness" (Erikson 1972, p. 30), including Robert Coles (1987a, b) and James Fowler (1981, 1984). Kai Erikson helped develop the sociology of war and disaster which also reflected moral considerations of the importance of human solidarity and adaptation (Erikson 1994), while Neil Smelser (1998) worked to conceptualize the relationship between psychoanalytic theory and methods with the social sciences. Erikson's friend and collaborator, Robert Jay Lifton (1986), explored the implications of Erikson's concerns about pseudospeciation and genocide, generating important new insights about human capacities for evil and destructiveness. Erikson's work has also been instrumental for the development of psychohistory and psychobiography, as well as enriching more traditional approaches to historical and biographical scholarship (Schultz 2005). In sum, his work continues to inspire and open up important areas of inquiry (Table 4-3).

I would like to close this chapter by suggesting another area where his work will continue to resonate – the moral imperative for professionals and, in fact, all adults to vigorously address the worldwide phenomenon of violence against children. More than most psychoanalysts, Erikson recognized that the constraints of traditional psychotherapy often prevented (and protected) clinicians from confronting the actualities of their violent world, and he worried about the impact of this on the development of psychoanalytic theory and practice:

Table 4-3. Representative selection of significant intellectual figures influenced by Erik Erikson.

Robert Coles	Moral resilience of children; Spiritual biography (Coles, 2003; 1987a,b)
Robert Jay Lifton	The psychohistory of genocide (Lifton & Olson, 1974)
James Marcia	Empirical studies of identity development (Marcia, 2004)
Jane Kroger	Process of identity formation (Kroger, 2004)
James Fowler	Stage theory of faith development (Fowler, 1984)
John Kotre	Aging and generativity (Kotre, 1996)
M. Gerard Fromm and Edward Shapiro	Contemporary clinical theory (Shapiro, Fromm, 2000)
Carol Gilligan	Feminist psychology and moral development (Gilligan, 2004)
Howard Gardner	Theory and research of multiple intelligences (Gardner 1993a,b; 1995; 1997)
de St. Aubin and Dan McAdams	Adult generativity (De Aubin & McAdams, 2004)
Kai Erikson	Sociology of disaster and community solidarity (Erikson, 2004)
Neil Smelser	Psychoanalysis and social science theory and methods (Smelser, 1998)

A close study of the original clinical setting as a laboratory would, incidentally, also reveal the fact that, together with locomotion, one elemental aspect of life – namely, violence – systematically escapes the treatment situation, as if the individual would participate in any uses of direct violence (from personal assault to aimless riot to armed force) only when absorbed in the unenlightened and uncivilized mass that makes up the "outer world." But then, as pointed out, the clinical laboratory channels all impulse to act or even move into introspection, so that the cured patient may be prepared for rational action. Thus, the clinician learns much more about the nature of inhibited, and symptomatic action than about that of concerted action in actuality – with all its rationalizations and all its shared a-rationalities (Erikson 1975, p. 106).

Erikson believed that their primary focus on professional prestige, a value-free epistemological stance, and the relentless pursuit of institutional power had blocked too many psychoanalysts from "seeing" their responsibilities to use the power of psychoanalysis to serve the vulnerable and oppressed of the world. In the book that first introduced him as an important thinker, Erikson declared that this refusal to "see" was an ethical and developmental failure of the highest magnitude:

In analogy to a certain bird, [the psychotherapist] has tried to pretend that his values remained hidden because his classical position at the head of the "analytic couch" removed him from the patient's visual field. We know today that communication is by no means primarily a verbal matter: words are only the tools of meanings. In a more enlightened world and under much more complicated historical conditions the analyst must face once more the whole problem of judicious partnership which expresses the spirit of analytic work more creatively than does apathetic tolerance or autocratic guidance. The various identities which at first lent themselves to a fusion with the new identity of the analyst-identities based on Talmudic argument, on messianic zeal, on punitive orthodoxy, on faddist sensationalism, on professional and social ambition-all these identities and their cultural origins must now become part of the analyst's analysis, so that he may be able to discard archaic rituals of control and learn to identify with the lasting value of his job of enlightenment. Only thus can he set free in himself and in his patient that remnant of judicious indignation without which a cure is but a straw in the changeable wind of history (Erikson 1950, p. 442).

It would be tempting to consider this closing passage of *Childhood & Society* as specific to a particular profession operating in a distant historical context. However, Erikson continually emphasizes the human proclivity to deny the darker elements of personal development (generated early in the repressed terrors of vulnerable childhoods) which lead otherwise good people to shirk engaging the unique challenges of their times (Erikson, 1956). This is one aspect of his work that Erikson's critics routinely miss. He argued that such responsibilities lay not only at the feet of extraordinary leaders, but are also integral to the healthy development of every reasonably functional adult. Elegant psychotherapy research projects rendering positive clinical outcomes are meaningless if the professions do not also address damaging incursions into the life cycles of "others."

Pseudospeciation is the unconscious and deliberate negation of the identity of another human as a *person*. Instead, others are conflated into inferior, undesirable, and evil categories. As Lifton (1986) has shown, when such cognitive and emotional processes are popularized, it becomes easy and even morally justified for "good people," professional healers, and legitimate institutions to pervert the unfolding of others' life cycles – through war, genocidal murder, ethnic cleansing and exile, imprisonment, slavery, etc. For Erikson, ethical integrity requires adults to mount a vigilant and fierce opposition to pseu-dospeciation in its global and local presentations. Such a commitment is not only a crucial developmental milestone for those struggling with midlife and old age, but also an essential process for the survival of humane cultures.

Human evolution has produced civilizations that create discontent and constraints for those craving absolute freedom, and Erikson like Freud, saw those inherent losses as justified for avoiding the Hobbesian nightmare of life as *homo homini lupus est.* (Indeed, Freud and Erikson had seen such a social catastrophe unfold during the 1930s.) Unlike Freud, Erikson additionally believed that ethical maturity involved many conscious, active, and individual choices for the pursuit of possibilities and generativities that could engender personal and social integrity. This seems to be at the heart of what he consid-ered adult "wisdom" (Table 4-4).

Erikson saw that childhood must be protected because those sociohistorical, political, cultural, religious, economic, scientific, and "therapeutic" decisions that insult the epigenetic development of basic trust, autonomy, purposiveness, and competence also destroy the possibilities of identity development and the psychological and moral energies necessary for the continuation of the human species and the maintenance of culture. Such destructive forces must be faced down, analyzed, and opposed, even as the adults attempting to do this strug-gle with their own lifelong, recurrent vulnerabilities, turbulent life cycles, and unforeseeable midlife and elder transitions. Much will still go terribly wrong. That is why hope and the other psychosocial strengths derived from the earli-est years of the life cycle must constantly be in play and available to sustain adults in midlife and old age, as well as the important psychological gains made through achieving adult intimacy. As Jerome Wakefield has pointed out, "For Erikson, love was in effect a psychological laboratory for the develop-mental capacities critical to generativity" (1997, p. 139).

Erikson would have us remember that the integrity born of exercising "judi-cious indignation" is essential for adults striving to live lives characterized by psychosocial maturity and wisdom. He chose to develop as an adult who pur-posely embraced such moral and religious struggles while sometimes failing egregiously to meet his own standards for adult wisdom and maturity. Erikson was neither a hero nor a saint, but he grappled with some of the most impor-

Table 4-4. Erikson's legacies

I.	Psychoanalytic innovator (Human Life Cycle)
II.	Founder of contemporary psychohistory
III.	Exemplar of "exuberant" adulthood
IV.	Advocate for the engaged self in service of humankind
V.	Advocate for civil rights, multiculturalism and gender respect
VI.	Clinical theory emphasizing the patient's strengths and the power of the thera-peutic relationship
VII.	Co-founder of twentieth century American humanism
VIII.	Exemplar of a postmodern life – living across borders, boundaries, and limits
IX.	Fierce intellectual resistance to pseudospeciation and genocide

See appraisals by Coles 1970, Friedman 1999, 2004a , Gardner 1999, Heinze 2004, Hoare 2002, Kinnvall 2004, Monroe 2004

tant problems of his time, and his professional work moved from attempting a comprehensive, descriptive, and naturalistic view of human development to one that emphasized its moral and religious dimensions – moves which made a grand theoretical system impossible. In doing so he came to appreciate Paul Tillich's autobiographical conclusions about what it felt like "on the boundaries"

> This is the dialectic of existence; each of life's possibilities drives of its own accord to a boundary and beyond the boundary where it meets that which limits it. The man who stands on many boundaries experiences the unrest, insecurity, and inner limitation of existence in many forms. He knows the impossibility of attaining serenity, security, and perfection. This holds true in life as well as in thought…. (Tillich 1966, pp. 97–98).

Now as we survey his life and work following the "decade of the brain," and as we stand at the brink of the "century of the mind," we see that Erikson's perspective is not the dominant paradigm for understanding human development. However, his relevance for contemporary theorists must be found, in part, in his enduring insight that even the scientific study of *human* beings cannot, in the final analysis, exclude matters of ultimate concern.

Acknowledgment: The biographical "facts" discussed in this chapter are drawn from what the *New York Times* (Lomas 1970) described as the seminal and "spiritual biography" written by Robert Coles (1970); the authorized, exhaustive, and historical biography written by Lawrence Friedman (1999); and the important British biographical perspectives provided by Kit Welchman (2000). As I never had the privilege of personally knowing Erikson, I have relied for the most part on the texts described above, which include Erikson's autobiographical writings as well as those by others cited in the chapter. I am also very grateful for my conversations with Robert Coles and Lawrence Friedman who shared personal memories and impressions of this complex man whom they came to know so well at very different points in Erikson's life cycle. In addition, William Borden, Wiliam MacKinley Runyan, Robert Walker, and Thomas Miller provided generative suggestions and criticisms. Finally, because each life is ultimately a mystery, I hope that the reader will see my claims as grounded in reasonable inferences as opposed to definitive conclusions. I am deeply indebted to Robert Coles for directing my attention to childhood society's closing insights regarding "judicious indignation" by purposefully quoting it from memory to me on many occasions, finally clarifying for this occasionally obtuse listener that this text reflects Erik and Joan Erikson's moral core.

Evidence for Erikson's affinity for Paul Tillich's perspectives can be found in the essay written for Tillich's memorial service in 1966. (See Erikson 1987.)

References

Alexander, I. (2005). Erikson & psychobiography, psychobiography & Erikson. In W. T. Schultz (Ed.), *Handbook of psychobiography* (pp. 265–284). New York: Oxford University Press.

Anderson, J. W. (2005). The psychobiographical study of psychologists. In W. T. Schultz (Ed.), *Handbook of psychobiography* (pp. 203–209). New York: Oxford University Press.

Auden, W. H. (1940/1979). In memory of Sigmund Freud. In E. Mendelson (Ed.), *W. H. Auden: Selected Poems, New Edition* (pp. 91–95). New York: Vintage

Bein, A. (1990). *The Jewish question: Biography of a world problem*. New York: Herzl.

Berman, M. (1975, March 30). Review of *Life History and the Historical Moment. New York Times Book Review*, pp. 1–2

Betancourt, T. S., Borisova, I., Rubin-Smith, J., Gingerich, T., Williams, T., & Agnew-Blais, J. (2008). *Psychosocial adjustment and social reintegration of children associated with armed forces and armed groups: The state of the field and future directions*. Austin, TX: Psychology Beyond Borders.

Bloland, S. E. (2005). *In the shadows of fame: A memoir by the daughter of Erik Erikson*. New York: Viking.

Borden, W. (2009). *Contemporary psychodynamic theory & practice*. Chicago: Lyceum.

Brett, R., & Specht, I. (2004). *Young soldiers: Why they choose to fight*. Boulder, CO: Lynne Rienner.

Coles, R. (1970). *Erik Erikson: The growth of his work*. Boston: Little, Brown.

Coles, R. (1987a). *Dorothy day: A radical devotion*. Reading, MA: Addison-Wesley.

Coles, R. (1987b). *Simone Weil: A Modern Pilgrimage*. Reading, MA: Addison-Wesley.

Coles, R. (1998). Psychoanalysis: The American Experience. In M.S. Roth (Ed.) *Freud: Conflict and Culture*. Newyork: Knopf.

Coles, R. (2000a). Psychoanalysis: The American experience. In M. Roth (Ed.), *Freud: Conflict and culture* (pp. 140–151). New York: Vintage.

Coles, R. (2000b). *The Erik Erikson reader*. New York: Norton.

Coles, R. (2003) Childern of Crisis: Selections from the Pulitzer Prize-Winning five volume, Children of Crisis Series. Boston: Back Bay.

Coles, R. (2004). Remembering Erik. In K. Hoover (Ed.), *The future of identity: Centennial reflections on the legacy of Erik Erikson* (pp. 17–23). Lanham, MD: Lexington.

St De Aubin, E., McAdams, D. P., & Kim, T.-C. (2004). *The generative society: Caring for future generations*. Washington, DC: APA.

Edmunson, M. (2007). *The death of Sigmund Freud: The legacy of his last days*. New York: Bloomsbury USA.

Erikson, E. H. (1950). *Childhood and society*. New York: Norton.

Erikson, E. H. (1956). The first psychoanalyst. *Yale review, 46,* 40–62.

Erikson, E. H. (1958). *Young man Luther*. New York: Norton.

Erikson, E. H. (1964). *Insight & responsibility*. New York: Norton.

Erikson, E. H. (1968). *Identity, youth and crisis*. New York: Norton.

Erikson, E. H. (1969). *Gandhi's truth: On the origins of militant nonviolence*. New York: Norton.

Erikson, E. H. (1972). Autobiographical notes on the identity crisis. In G. Holton (Ed.), *The twentieth century sciences: Studies in the biography of ideas* (pp. 3–32). New York: Norton.

Erikson, E. H. (1975). *Life history and the historical moment*. New York: Norton.

Erikson, E. H. (1976). Reflections on Dr. Borg's life cycle. *Daedalus, 105,* 1–31.

Erikson, E. H. (1980). Themes of adulthood in the Freud-Jung correspondence. In N. J. Smelser, ed., *Themes of work and love in adulthood* (43-74). Cambridge, MA: Harvard University Press

Erikson, E. H. (1981). The Galilean sayings and the sense of "I." *Yale Review* 9(8). (Reprinted (1998) In R. Wallerstein, & L. Godlberger (Eds.), *Ideas and identities: The life and work of Erik Erikson* (pp. 277–322). Madison, CT: International Universities Press

Erikson, E. H. (1987). Words for Paul Tillich (1966). In S. Schlein (Ed.), *A way of looking at things* (pp. 726–728). New York: Norton.

Erikson, K. T. (1994). *A new species of trouble: The human experience of modern disasters*. New York: Norton.

Erikson, K. T. (2004). Reflections on generativity and society: A sociologist's perspective. In St E. de Aubin, et al. (Eds.), *The generative society: Caring for future generations* (pp. 51–62). Washington, DC: APA.

Evans, R. (1967). *Dialogue with Erik Erikson.* New York: Harper & Row.

Fowler, J. (1981). *Stages of faith: The psychology of human development and the quest for meaning.* San Francisco: Harper & Row.

Fowler, J. (1984). *Becoming adult, becoming Christian: Adult development and Christian faith.* San Francisco: Harper & Row.

Freud, S. (1930). *Civilization and its discontents* (J. Strachey, Trans., 1974 ed., vol. 21). London: Hogarth

Friedman, L. J. (1999). *Identity's architect: A biography of Erik Erikson.* New York: Scribner.

Friedman, L. J. (2004a). Erik Erikson on generativity: A biographer's perspective. In E. de St Aubin, et al. (Eds.), *The Generative society: Caring for future generations* (pp. 257–264). Washington, DC: APA.

Friedman, L. J. (2004b). Erik Erikson: A biographer's reflections. In K. Hoover (Ed.), *The future of identity: Centennial reflections on the legacy of Erik Erikson* (pp. 17–23). Lanham, MD: Lexington.

Gardner, H. (1993a). *Creating minds: An anatomy of creativity seen through the lives of Freud, Einstein, Picasso, Stravinsky, Eliot, Graham, and Gandhi.* New York: Basic.

Gardner, H. (1993b). *Multiple intelligences: The theory in practice.* New York: Basic.

Gardner, H. (1997). *Extraordinary minds: Portraits of exceptional individuals and an examination of our extraordinariness.* New York: Basic.

Gardner, H. (1999). The enigma of Erik Erikson. *The New York Review of Books, 46*(11), 51–56.

Gardner, H., & Laskin, E. (1995). *Leading minds: An anatomy of leadership.* New York: Basic.

Gill, M. M. (ed). (1967). *The collected papers of David Rapaport.* New York: Basic.

Gilligan, C. (2004). Recovering psyche: Reflections on life-history and history. *Annual of Psychoanalysis, 32,* 131–147.

Hartmann, H. (1951). Ego psychology and the problem of adaptation. In D. Rapaport (Ed.), *Organization and pathology of thought* (pp. 362–396). New York: Columbia University Press.

Heilbut, A. (1983). *Exiled in paradise: German refugee artists and intellectuals in America, from the 1930s to the Present.* New York: Viking.

Heinze, A. R. (2004). *Jews and the American soul: Human nature in the twentieth century.* Princeton, NJ: Princeton University Press.

Hoare, C. H. (2002). *Erikson on development in adulthood: New Insights from the unpublished papers.* New York: Oxford University Press.

Kinnvall, C. (2004) Globalization, identity, and the search for chosen traumas. In K. Hoover (Ed.), The future of identity: centennial reflections on the legacy of Erik Erikson (pp. 111–136). Lanham MD: Lexington.

Kirkwood, T. B. L. (2008). A systematic look at an old problem. *Nature, 451,* 644–647.

Kotre, J. (1996). *Outliving the self: How we live on in future generations.* New York: Norton.

Lachman, M. E. (2004). Development in midlife. *Annual Review of Psychology, 55,* 305–331.

Lifton, R. J. (1986). *The Nazi doctors: Medical killing and the psychology of genocide.* New York: Basic.

Lifton, R., & Olson, E. (eds). (1974). *Explorations in psychohistory: The Wellfleet papers.* New York: Simon & Schuster.

Lomas, P. (1970, November 22). Review of *Erik Erikson: The growth of his work. New York Times Book Review.* vol. 1, pp. 66–67

Macha, G. (2001). *The impact of war on children.* London: Hurst.

Malcolm, J. (1983). *The impossible profession.* New York: Knopf.

Marcia, J. (2004). Why Erikson? In K Hoover (Ed.), The future of identity: Centennial reflections on the legacy of Erik Erikson (pp 43–60) Lanham MD: Lexington.

Meissner, W. W. (2000). *Freud & psychoanalysis.* Notre Dame, IN: University of Notre Dame Press.

Monroe, K.R. (2004). Identity and choice. In K. Hoover (Ed.), The Future of identity: Centennial reflections on Erik Erikson (pp. 77–96). Lanham MD: Lexington.

Muller, J. Z. (2008). Us and them. *Foreign Affairs, 87*(2), 18–35.

Prince, R. M. (ed). (1999). *The death of psychoanalysis: Murder? Suicide? Or rumor greatly exaggerated?.* Northvale, NJ: Jason Aronson.

Rilke, R. M. (1963). *Duino Elegies.* (J. B. Leishman, & S. Spender, Trans.) New York: Norton (Original work published 1939)

Roazen, P. (1976). *Erik Erikson: The power and limits of a vision.* New York: Free.

Roazen, P. (2000) Political theory and the psychology of the unconscious. London: Open Gate Press.

Runyan, W. M. (1982). *Life histories and psychobiography.* New York: Oxford University Press.

Runyan, W. M. (ed). (1988). *Psychology & historical interpretation.* New York: Oxford University Press.

Runyan, W.M. (2006). Psychobiography and the psychology of science: Understanding relations between the life and work of individual psychologists. *Review of General Psychology, 90*(2), 147–162.

Schlein, S. (ed). (1987). *Erik Erikson: A way of looking at things: Selected papers.* New York: Norton.

Schultz, W. T. (2005). *Handbook of psychobiography.* New York: Oxford University Press.

Sen, A. (2006). *Identity and violence: The illusion of destiny.* New York: Norton.

Shapiro, E., & Carr, A. W. (1993). *Lost in familiar places: Creating new connections between the individual and society.* New Haven: Yale University Press.

Shapiro, E., & Fromm, M. G. (2000). Eriksonian clinical theory and psychiatric treatment. In B. J. Sadock & V. S. Sadock (Eds.), *Kaplan & Sadock's Comprehensive Textbook of Psychiatry* (7th ed., pp. 2200–2206). Philadelphia: Lippincott Williams & Wilkins.

Smelser, N. J. (1998). *The social edges of psychoanalysis.* Berkeley: University of California Press.

Sokel, W. H. (1959). *The writer in extremis: Expressionism in twentieth century German literature.* Stanford, CA: Stanford University Press.

Sulloway, F. (1979). *Freud, biologist of the mind: Beyond the psychoanalytic legend.* New York: Basic.

Tillich, P. (1966). *On the boundary.* New York: Collins.

Vaillant, G. E., & Milofsky, E. (1980). Natural history of male psychological health: IX. Empirical evidence for Erikson's model of the life cycle. *American Journal of Psychiatry, 137*(11), 1348–1359.

Wakefield, J. C. (1997). Immortality and the externalization of the self: Plato's unrecognized theory of generativity. In D. P. McAdams & St E. de Aubin (Eds.), *Generativity and adult development: How and why we care for the next generation.* Washington, DC: American Psychological Association.

Wallerstein, R., & Goldberger, L. (eds). (1998). *Ideas and identities: The life and work of Erik Erikson.* Madison, CT: International Universities Press.

Welchman, K. (2000). *Erik Erikson: His life, work and significance.* Buckingham: Open University Press.

Whitfield, S. J. (2002). Enigmas of modern Jewish identity. *Jewish Social Studies: History, Culture & Society, 8*(2–3), 162–167.

Part II

Education and Career Transitions

Chapter 5

College-to-Workplace Transitions: Becoming a Freshman Again

This chapter explores major issues encountered by many of the 1.5 million baccalaureate recipients each year (National Center for Educational Statistics 2006) who enter the workforce with inappropriate expectations, attitudes, job experiences, and levels of preparedness. Transition from college to a first full-time job is an exciting and much anticipated event, but it creates distress as well as eustress. Unlike the transition from high school to college, entry to the workplace represents a relatively clear demarcation from the past in one's identity, sense of responsibility, independence, intellectual activities, relationships, and life-style. Consequently, this transition is also a period of incredible uncertainties and insecurity. After introducing the topic with four contrasting approaches to reporting on transition stress, I summarize models of transition and psychosocial and cognitive development that serve as a framework for understanding organizational and related factors that contribute to stress. I conclude with recommendations for increasing workplace readiness.

Experiencing College-to-Work Transition

Case in Point

Brad seemed to have everything going for him his senior year: a perfect 4.0 G.P.A, strong interpersonal skills, a reputation as a team-player well-liked by peers and teachers, and the luxury of not having to work part-time his last 2 years. But life changed drastically after graduation. In spite of working with a personnel service, his first interview was a disaster: Questioners asked how he would handle situations he had never been part of nor read in textbooks. After weeks of managing overwhelming self-doubts, carefully researching organizations, and completing several interviews, he was finally hired by a strategic sourcing organization to recruit employees for finance positions. Excited and confident, he expected his first week to be special. It was! Brad quickly learned he was in an environment that squelched self-expression and individuality, made minimal use of his college knowledge, and dictated what he would wear when he would eat and how he would answer his phone.

From: *Handbook of Stressful Transitions Across the Lifespan,*
Edited by: T.W. Miller, DOI 10.1007/978-1-4419-0748-6_5,
© Springer Science+Business Media, LLC 2010

Over the weeks, excitement turned to resentment and resentment to anger. The creativity, critical thinking, charisma, and interpersonal skills that helped him score in college seemed like liabilities. The impulsiveness and occasional loss of emotional control that emerged from his anger soon alienated him from his boss and co-workers; he was branded a "difficult employee." After reaching a psychological nadir a few months into his job, Brad sought support from family and friends, reassessed his strengths and weaknesses, and realized that a key component of his college success was relating well to teachers. Gradually, he established better relations with peers and began to excel in his duties to the level of receiving performance awards. In addition, Brad began a productive mentoring relationship with his supervisor which he maintains today and holds a position where one of his major responsibilities is to build internship programs with client companies.

Brad had become a freshman again. He began a new chapter in his life, one filled with high expectations, a dependence on old assumptions, and new challenges in a new setting with new roles, responsibilities, and relationships that generated frustration, self-assessment, change, and ultimately, new growth. The sense of control and mastery he felt about his world as a college senior disappeared totally; he had to start over again. Brad's story may not reflect *the* typical experience of college grads entering the workplace, but it illustrates key issues that contribute to the stress and angst many undergo: (a) Graduates with a high G.P.A. and sterling personal qualities do not necessarily excel when they begin their first full-time job; they may fall victim to expectations and work strategies that worked in college but are counter-productive in the workplace. (b) Unlike Brad, many new graduates do not possess the personal resources to recover from entry shock; he lived at home, had ready access to support from family and friends, and stuck with the job. (c) Graduates with limited prior work experience (Brad held only part-time jobs during his freshman and sophomore years) are vulnerable to the types of organizational practices he encountered. (d) As his high grades generated generous tuition grants during college, Brad's loan debt was lower than most graduates. These dimensions of college-to-workplace transition (expectations and attitudes, support networks, prior work experience, and debt) are the more significant but not the only challenges new hires confront as they cross the ocean between the college and corporate continents. In general, graduates from science and technical programs will have benefited from relatively high starting salaries and a curriculum that requires internships, cooperative education, or other forms of "hands-on" learning; most liberal arts graduates do not experience such opportunities.

Unfortunately, the scientific literature describing graduates' first-job experiences is sparse. Polach (2004) reports that studies describing the work experience of new graduates are generally limited to surveys of their socialization experiences of their first-year, and "few have captured the feelings, frustrations, and challenges of the experiences from the individuals' perspectives" (p. 6). The data from a qualitative study consisting of 2 hour-long interviews of eight college graduates' first year of "real work" at a medical device company generated nine themes that Polach grouped into three categories: *work environment, performance,* and *friendship.* Of the two themes in the work environment category, one was positive and one negative: Surprise and relief that the work environment of this particular organization was easy going (the company's socialization process was very informal); and "Frustration with so much to learn and no structures to follow" (p. 12). The performance category was defined by four themes: Graduates (a) were unsure of their performance due to a lack of feedback; (b) experienced guilt when they were not producing; (c) felt satisfied when they were contributing; and (d) derived satisfaction and growth in their overall experience. The third category, friendship, revealed three themes important to the new hires: (a) Establishing friendships is critical to belonging and feeling settled; (b) the process of making friends in college and that in the workplace differs; and (c) moving is often necessary to establish a better sense of belonging. Polach concludes that Human Resources Development professionals can facilitate a successful first-year experience by providing emotional support, feedback, and mentoring to new graduates.

In contrast to the Case in Point about Brad and the Polach qualitative study, Saks and Ashforth (2000) investigated via a survey the role of personal dispositions (negativity and general self-efficacy), plasticity theory, and entry-level stressors (role conflict, role ambiguity, role overload, and unmet expectations) in predicting the adjustment of 297 business students (60% female, mean age = 23.5 years). They were surveyed during the final semester before beginning a full-time job and again after 4 and 10 months on the job. Although the authors hypothesized that dispositions and plasticity would predict adjustment, the results revealed weak effects for these constructs. Instead, the four entry-level stressors consistently predicted, although not equally, the adjustment measures employed, namely, job satisfaction, organizational commitment, organizational identification, intention to quit, frustration, stress symptoms, and performance. The findings "indicate that the newcomers' affective and behavioral reactions are largely the result of the situation they encounter during the first 4 months of organizational entry" (p. 58). Saks and Ashforth recommend that organizations monitor the problem of unmet expectations and try to reduce the level of stressors newcomers encounter and/or train them to cope effectively with stress. Newcomers are encouraged to be proactive by seeking information and feedback to counter the effects of role ambiguity and role conflict and improve the accuracy of their expectations.

One of the more illuminating descriptions of transition to the "real world" is the pioneering work of two young college graduates who faced many of the issues presented in Brad's case. In *Quarterlife Crisis: The Unique Challenges of Life in Your Twenties* (2001), Robbins and Wilner interviewed a hundred diverse college graduates about their post-college experiences. The most widespread and difficult manifestation of the twentysomethings' "quarterlife crisis," regardless of their levels of self-confidence or overall wellbeing, were their self-doubts, especially about decisions, readiness, adulthood, abilities, and the past, present, and future. The great majority felt they were alone in harboring these feelings. In addition, the expectations that they had developed and the guidelines they had mastered in college seemed to have no counterparts in an often sterile and non-nurturing workplace that did not recognize their college achievements. Robbins and Wilner view these and similar experiences analogous to Charlie Brown's feelings when Lucy removes the football at the crucial moment. In addition, the nature of friendships and other relationships change, and individuals must become more proactive in their search for persons who share common interests. Many twenty somethings experience a shift from having close relationships during college to having acquaintances in the workplace.

As the years pass after graduation, many twentysomethings feel the pressures from not reaching their goals, not having the position or income they had expected, witnessing peers moving upward rapidly, and having to delay marriage, family, and home ownership. The coping mechanisms the twenty somethings used were diverse and generally included a combination of determination, the right attitude, and open-mindedness. At least one twenty something attended graduate school because they did not know what to do; and after completing her program, she still did not know what to do. As depression is often a factor in this age group, some sought therapy. The extent to which any interviewees used drugs or alcohol to cope appears undetermined.

Although the methodology and analysis reported in *Quarterlife Crisis* may not meet the criteria for a scientific study (the book was written for a broad audience), and the use of the term "quarterlife crisis" may be debated, Robbins and Wilner contribute significantly to the understanding of the post-college life for young adults in the midst of a critical life transition. They responded to their audience's search for guidance in Wilner and Stocker's *The Quarterlifer's Companion* (2005) and Robbins' *Conquering Your Quarterlife Crisis* (2004). Some readers may dismiss the findings of Robbins and Wilner as typical young-adult apprehension, an unwillingness to cut the proverbial umbilical cord, or whining by a spoiled younger generation. For the great majority of these young adults, however, the problems and concomitant stresses were perceived as real. The inability of some new graduates to resolve transition issues healthily and early can lead to failure at work, continued self-doubt, and the incapacity to live up to the personal and professional goals they worked to achieve during college.

Perspectives on Transition

A transition is a passage or movement from one situation or condition to another. Using the 2002 General Social Survey (GSS), Smith (2003) surveyed about 1,400 American adults to assess the importance of seven youth-to-adult transitions. The 1,350 respondents stated that to become an adult it was "extremely," "quite," or "somewhat" important for young people to complete their education (97%), achieve financial independence (97%), obtain full-time employment (95%), support a family (94%), not live with parents (82%), get married (55%), and have a child (52%). About 80% of the respondents believed these transitions ought to occur by the age of 26; many should be completed by age 21 (Smith 2003; Hettich and Helkowski 2005). In short, most adults in this sample expect young people to complete most major life transitions within a 5-year period and by the age of 26. Although current societal expectations are becoming less rigorous than those reported in this survey, college graduates enter the workplace carrying the burden (correctly or not) of such expectations. How can models of transition inform workplace transition?

The Bridges Model

William Bridges (2003) describes three overlapping phases or processes that characterize transition. In the *ending* phase, an individual breaks away from the old identity or ways of doing things. In the *neutral zone*, a person is between two ways or habits of doing or being. The old ways may be gone, but new beliefs, attitudes, or habits have not yet been firmly established. In the *new beginning*, an individual is productive and goal-oriented in the new ways and possesses a new identity that corresponds to the new situation. "Because transition is a process by which people unplug from an old world and plug into a new world, we can say that transition starts with an ending and finishes with a beginning" (p. 5).

If we apply Bridges' model to college students, we might quickly conclude: (a) Graduation is the student's disengagement from the way things were in college – the ending phase; (b) the time between graduation and the first few weeks of a new full-time job is the neutral zone; and (c) the new beginning occurs after the first weeks or months on the job. Given the experiences of Brad (Case in Point) and others, however, this conclusion is unwarranted. Students and educators should view graduation as the ceremonial conclusion of the ending phase, not the ending itself. Graduation is the point of physical departure from the institution with diploma in hand and the inspiring words of the commencement speaker mostly forgotten. Instead, students should *begin* the ending phase much sooner if they are to avoid problems described by Robbins and Wilner (2001) and Brad. *When students carefully plan the last four semesters of coursework and activities as essential components of their ending phase, the neutral zone and new beginning phases are likely to be satisfying* (Hettich and Helkowski 2005).

Obviously, students cannot disengage completely when courses remain. However, disengagement should include an early and thoughtful analysis of how to connect, integrate, and apply one's knowledge, experiences, and resources to future plans while still in college. For example, when is the best academic term to complete an internship or study abroad? What campus organization does the student wish to join in order to hold a leadership position by the senior year? How far into the sophomore or junior year should the student begin working with the life/career planning office? What opportunities exist for conducting research with a professor and possibly having the results presented or published? Many graduates with whom I have spoken, quick to admit what they should have done differently their last 2 years, mentioned these kinds of activities.

Why is it difficult to disengage from college? Students operate on long entrenched assumptions nourished by an education culture dominated by specified student-teacher roles, expectations, reward structures, and repetitious schedules of academic terms that are far different from most workplace environments. The subject matter may change from term to term, but the processes of learning, performing, and receiving feedback remain essentially unchanged. Extinguishing highly engrained expectations and behaviors and substituting new ones in a different and often unsympathetic environment is the major challenge during Bridges' neutral zone phase of transition. If Brad had begun his ending phase in the manner described above, his journey through the neutral zone could have been much less frustrating.

Graduates enter the workplace unprepared for other reasons. Many lack sufficient work experience and observation skills to understand and act upon the differences between college and corporate cultures and practices. Few, if any, of their teachers articulated these differences or explained how classroom skills do or do not transfer to the real world (Apparently, many professors, especially in liberal arts, have limited experience with traditional full-time jobs).

Finally, many individuals are first-generation graduates who were never coached by college-educated parents or siblings on interview skills, workplace attitudes, and office politics. Some persons do slip comfortably into a new organization and pass through the neutral zone in a timely manner; others discover the neutral zone is a "hot zone" – challenging and painful. Bridges views the neutral zone as a limbo, a psychological no-man's-land between the old and new ways of doing things. Students should know about the neutral zone so they do not rush through it (and become frustrated), escape from it (and become job-hoppers), or miss opportunities to apply their interests and skills creatively early in their career (Bridges 2003; Hettich and Helkowski 2005). At the end of the neutral zone is the new beginning when the new hires reflect a new identity compatible with their new organization; they are comfortable with their new role and productive. "Letting go, repatterning, and making a new beginning: together these processes reorient and renew people when things are changing all around them" (Bridges 2003, p. 9).

Schlossberg's Transition Framework

In contrast to Bridges' model that guides students productively through their final academic terms is a systematic framework developed by Schlossberg for clinicians, counselors, and social workers whose clientele may represent a wide array of transition circumstances. The Transition Framework is described in Goodman Schlossberg, and Anderson (2006), but only its major components are summarized below. The first of the model's three major parts is labeled *approaching transitions*; one of its subcomponents is *transition identification* (the specific transition impending). The counselor determines if the transition is anticipated, unanticipated, or a non-event transition (i.e., an expected transition that never occurred, for example, a promotion). Factors such as relativity (how the person defines the transition), context, and impact (degree to which it alters the person's daily life) are explored at this point. *Transition process*, the second subcomponent of approaching transition, seeks to locate the person in the process over time (Goodman et al. 2006). For instance, is the new graduate unsure about what career to enter, has held a frustrating first job for 6 weeks, or is in his sixth job in 6 months?

Taking stock of coping resources, the second major part of the transition framework involves the 4 S System to identify potential resources (variables) the client possesses: *Situation* (the trigger, timing, control, role change, duration, prior experience, concurrent stress, and assessment factors of what is happening), *self* (characteristics and resources of the client), *support* (the types and extent of help available), and *strategies* (how this individual copes). The 4 S System collectively represents the person's potential assets and liabilities; the counselor must understand how these resources are interrelated and assess them. The coping resources of a 22-year-old sociology grad who worked in a fast-food restaurant and is seeking a business position will differ from those of the 28-year-old single-parent accounting major who worked part-time as a bookkeeper for several years.

Taking charge: Strengthening resources, the final part of the transition framework, is the application of new strategies to managing the transition and strengthening the individual's resources. The authors devote chapters to individual and group counseling and a chapter to consultation, program development and advocacy to explain taking charge (Goodman et al. 2006). The transition framework may best be summarized in the authors' words:

> The transition model provides a framework, a conceptual lens if you will, for counselors to use as they help their adult clients look within themselves, their relationships, and their work. Our approach is simple: help clients enhance their resources for coping by assessing their Situation, Self, Support, and Strategies (p. 179).

Psychosocial Development

Marcia's Identity Statuses

The research of James Marcia on identity statuses and Jeffrey Arnett on emerging adulthood provide helpful psychosocial development contexts for understanding college-to-workplace transition. Pursuing Erikson's belief that occupation (a person's work role in society) and ideology (fundamental beliefs especially as they relate to religion and politics) are at the core of identity, Marcia and his associates classified young persons on the basis of structured interviews into four identity statuses that represent particular developmental positions held by an individual: *identity achievement, moratorium, foreclosure, and identity diffusion* (McAdams 2001). Young adults who actively question their career and values decisions and have made commitments to an occupation and ideology that were thoughtfully developed have reached identity achievement, the most advanced of the statuses. Identity achievers are typically self-reliant, have internalized their goals, and make decisions in an autonomous and principled way. Young adults in moratorium status are exploring the questions of work and values but have not made commitments yet. College is generally regarded as the preferred institutionalized venue for such exploration. While a lack of commitment can and often does lead to an identity crisis, Marcia viewed moratoriums as mature. Young adults may not have the answers yet, but they are asking the necessary questions. In contrast, individuals in foreclosure have committed to career and values without exploring them, perhaps yielding to the pressures of authority figures or media models. Identity diffusions, on the other hand, have neither searched for answers to questions about occupation and ideology (or are overwhelmed by the possibilities) nor made any commitments and often appear as aimless drifters. Marcia believed that today's moratoriums are usually tomorrow's identity achievers. Foreclosures and identity diffusions do not typically move up the developmental ladder as young adults. While foreclosures avoided an early identity crisis, they are ripe for one at a later point. Identity diffusions may go through life without the identity anchors that offer them a true sense of self (McAdams 2001; Hettich and Helkowski 2005).

Marcia's work is not without its critics. Research suggests: (a) The four statuses do not operate in a developmental sequence as Marcia believed; (b) conscious exploration is not required for and often does not occur in identity achievement; and (c) numerous studies conducted in support of the statuses focus less on developmental concerns and more on classification issues (Cote 2006).

Nevertheless, the Marcia *framework* is relevant to understanding the journey of many new graduates. Numerous students enter college foreclosed, i.e., they have chosen their academic direction and life's work based on parental expectations, the careers of role models, a valued teacher's occupational suggestion, or their favorite television shows. As an aside, this assertion does not deny that some apparently foreclosed individuals will ultimately succeed in a career that may have begun as a dream or from a special experience in elementary or secondary school. Although the foreclosed freshman is not new on campuses, the fact that institutions of higher education seem to prefer students this way is not only surprising, but it is also alarming. Admissions counselors are trained to ask prospective students about major and program interests. If the student states a preferred program or major, the admissions representative provides the appropriate information and contact persons. With a career decision firmly made without sufficient exploration, the entering student can move on to the more important aspects of college, like making friends and finding decent food on campus. Parents are pleased their child has a direction, and the school is pleased because it is easier to advise and plan for "declared" students. The student may never be asked "Why this program?" or "What other areas have you thought about?" in spite of the fact that college has become the predominant means for exploring identity (Hettich and Helkowski 2005). For many in the foreclosed status, the problem with their choice of major or career reveals itself before graduation. The psychology major who wants only to "help people" must complete seemingly inappropriate courses in statistics and research methodology. Some foreclosures get through college and into their first jobs before they realize that asking "why" and "what else" years earlier would have been helpful.The application of Bridges' model and Marcia's foreclosure status to workplace transition may create a dilemma for some readers and students. On one hand, it is important to *begin* preparing for transition midway through college (the point where a major is usually declared) to avoid entry shock, yet foreclosure should be avoided. While the solution to this dilemma depends on the individual, many suggestions for improving readiness presented later in this chapter are not major-specific. For example, career counseling, study abroad, co-curricular activities, and monitoring a part-time job can facilitate readiness regardless of the major chosen. Nevertheless, for some students the line between acting foreclosed and deciding on a major thoughtfully is tenuous and will create uncertainties which they must confront.

Arnett's Emerging Adulthood

Marcia's research helps explain the connection between exploration and career choices, but it does not speak of the social context in which contemporary young people mature. From his qualitative studies of 300 young people ages 18–29 in San Francisco, Los Angeles, New Orleans, and rural Missouri, Jeffrey Arnett (2000) argues that the period between18 and 25 in contemporary industrialized countries is neither adolescence nor adulthood, but emerging adulthood. Emerging adulthood is distinct demographically (median age for marriage and childbirth has risen since the 1960s; higher rates for attending college and moving) and subjectively (uncertainty about when adulthood is reached; accepting responsibility for self, making independent decisions, and financial independence as criteria) from adolescence and young adulthood. Emerging adulthood is characterized by five features (Arnett and Tanner 2006).

Age of Identity Exploration

Emerging adulthood is the age of identity explorations in the sense that it is the period when people are most likely to be exploring various possibilities for their lives in a variety of areas, especially love and work, as a prelude to making the enduring choices that will set the foundations for their adult lives (p. 8).

By age 25 about 70% of emerging adults have obtained at least some college or university education (Arnett 2004). More than 45% of today's undergraduates are over 21, compared to 25% 30 years ago. In addition, the median time required to complete the baccalaureate has risen from 4 to 5 years; the proportion of students finishing in 6 years has risen from 15% to 23% (Fitzpatrick and Turner 2006). Although identity exploration characterizes the search of many emerging adults, Arnett maintains that there are many others in their late teens and early twenties who move during college from major to major and subsequently from job to job, often unsystematically, searching for what best fits their identity; they meander. "*Meandering* might be a more accurate word, or maybe *drifting* or even *floundering*. For many emerging adults working simply means finding a job, often a McJob that will pay the bills until something better comes along (Arnett 2004, p. 150)." According to Levit (2004), U.S. Department of Labor estimates indicate the typical American holds approximately nine jobs between the ages of 18 and 32. In addition, "the median length of time workers stay on the job has shrunk by half since 1983 – from 2.2 years to 1.1 years now (p. 12)." Further support of these results comes from Farber (2006) who analyzed changes in long-term employment and concluded that *churn* (a series of jobs lasting less than a year) is to be expected in an industrialized society where new employees, even those in their thirties, are searching for the right person-job fit. These findings help explain the second characteristic of emerging adulthood, instability.

Age of Instability

By instability Arnett refers to changing of residences, i.e., from home to residence halls and then to apartments. Such moves are in part a response to identity exploration in work-related changes as well as relationship changes (e.g., marriage and cohabitation).

The Self-Focused Age

Emerging adults are self-focused in so far as they leave the structures of home and have relatively few social obligations, duties, and commitments to others. Most have only themselves to worry about, but Arnett maintains this form of self-focus is not equivalent to self-centeredness.

The Age of Feeling In-Between

In response to the question "Do you feel you have reached adulthood?" "Yes," "No," or "Yes and no," about 60% of Arnett's sample between the ages of 18 and 25 responded "Yes and no," and about 60% of those between 26 and 35 responded "Yes." Apparently, the slow journey to feeling like an adult is based on the emerging adults' belief that adulthood is defined primarily as accepting responsibility for themselves, making independent decisions, and becoming financially independent.

The Age of Possibilities

Two phenomena characterize 18–25 as the age of possibilities. Emerging adults have high expectations and high levels of optimism and hope for the future perhaps in part, because these beliefs and feelings have not been tested by the realities of life and the workplace. "Before people settle into a long-term job, it is possible for them to believe they are going to find a job that is both well-paying and personally fulfilling, an expression of their identity rather than simply a way to make a living" (Arnett and Tanner 2006, p. 13). Emerging adulthood is also the age of possibilities for those who wish to transform their lives, whether they experienced difficult or normal family conditions, before making commitments to intimate relations and jobs that structure adult life.

What picture does Arnett's emerging adulthood paint of typical graduates transitioning into the world of work? As the number of college graduates in Arnett's sample could not be determined, his findings should be generalized with caution to that population. It is likely however, that a majority of graduates are still engaged in self-exploration, but there are many foreclosures and meanderers. Graduates are mobile, self-focused, have high expectations, and believe they will reach adulthood when they achieve financial and decision-making independence and accept responsibility for themselves.

Given Arnett's five defining characteristics of emerging adults, what do these individuals look for in a job? In a survey conducted by MonsterTRAK (Chao and Gardner 2007), 9,000 young adults aged 18–25 were asked to rate 15 common job characteristics on the importance of each in a job search. In the rank order of their importance, respondents named: interesting work, good benefits (e.g., health insurance), job security, chances for promotion, opportunity to learn new skills, geographical location, annual vacations of a week or more, high income, flexibility of work hours, regular hours (no nights/weekends), being able to work independently, limited job stress, travel opportunities, prestigious company, and limited overtime. The order of these rankings seems to reflect respondents' general preferences for jobs that promote long-term success and quality of life issues as well as continued self-exploration. High income was ranked in the middle, contrary to a popular belief that income is the primary job motive for this age group. The report indicates relative consistency in responses across gender, ethnic affiliation, and academic major (Chao and Gardner 2007).

Baxter Magolda's Epistemic Model of Knowing

Growth in psychosocial development during and after college is usually paralleled by changes in an individual's epistemology, i.e., the assumptions the person holds about the process of knowing. These assumptions often influence how an individual approaches work. In a longitudinal study begun in 1986 on a homogeneous sample of 101 college freshmen (51 women and 50 men) in a Midwestern university, using interviews and questionnaire data, Marcia Baxter Magolda (1992) observed four discernible levels of knowing: *absolute, transitional, independent,* and *contextual.*

Advancement through each level is characterized by changes in students' progressively more complex beliefs regarding the certainty of knowledge and the roles of authority, self, and peers in the process of knowing. In the first stage, absolute knowing, students believe that knowledge is certain, absolute answers exist in all areas, ideas are either right or wrong, good or bad, and authorities have the answers. Transitional knowing serves as a transition between the perceived certainty of absolute knowing and the high level of uncertainty characteristic of independent knowing. Still passive learners, transitional knowers recognize the existence of multiple perspectives; but if knowledge still seems uncertain, it is only because authorities have not yet found *the* answer. Classmates have little or nothing to do with the learning process. For independent knowers, knowledge is mostly uncertain. Teachers and texts are no longer *the* authorities; an individual's beliefs are equally valid as those of authorities, regardless of the evidence. Yet, independent knowers begin to think for themselves, *construct* knowledge from experience, and start to value the opinion of peers as a source of knowledge. Contextual knowers are aware that knowledge is mostly uncertain but realize that some claims to knowledge are better than others if evidence exists to support them relative to a particular situation. They enjoy thinking through issues, comparing perspectives critically, integrating new with existing knowledge, and applying it to new contexts (Baxter Magolda 1992; Hettich and Helkowski 2005).

The four stages of knowing, unfortunately, do not correspond to the 4 years of college. Absolute knowing dominates the first year, and transitional knowing the second, third and fourth years. Transitional stage assumptions remain through most of college for several reasons, including: (a) the unwillingness or inability of students to accept the challenges of intellectual and personal growth, (b) students' entry to that vast storehouse of knowledge – the academic major – much of which must be memorized, and (c) the failure of some academic environments to promote independent and contextual knowing. Independent knowing was the predominant mode for only 1% of the sophomores, 5% of the juniors, and 16% of seniors in her sample. Contextual knowing was observed in only 1% and 2% of the juniors and seniors, respectively. (Baxter Magolda 1992; Hettich and Helkowski 2005).

Of what importance is Baxter Magolda's study for college graduates in transition? She conducted post-college interviews with 70 of her original 101 participants during the fifth year of the study and with 51 participants during the sixth year. Most graduates had accepted jobs in such areas as insurance, sales, accounting, teaching, mental health, airlines, and government; others entered graduate or professional school. Her interviews revealed independent knowing rapidly increased to 57% and 55% during the fifth and sixth years, respectively, while contextual knowing improved to 12% and 37%, respectively.

What did employment accomplish that college did not? Three themes emerged from the interviews that appear to account for the growth of independent knowing. As employees, the graduates were expected to *function independently, use peers as sources of information and models*, and l*earn by direct, hands-on experience* in situations that required decision-making – no more vicarious learning through teachers and textbooks. Similarly, three major themes emerged from interviews with contextual knowers that likely explain the increases from 1% to 2% during the junior and senior years to 12% to 37% respectively after college. Contextual knowers were frequently required to make *subjective decisions involving uncertainties*. Gone was the transitional knowing assumption that sooner or later *the* answer will be found. Contextual knowers were also in positions that offered them *independence and authority*, including authority over their schedule and that of others (e.g., in manager or assistant manager positions). Finally, contextual knowers were required to *collaborate* with coworkers, especially in the exchange of ideas. Gone was the transitional knowing assumption that peers play little or no part in the learning process. In short, part of workplace stress new graduates encounter is likely due to work demands that force changes in their epistemological assumptions from predominantly transitional to increased levels of independent and contextual knowing (Baxter Magolda 1994; Hettich and Helkowski 2005).

There are no magic bullets to move students from transitional to independent and contextual knowing during college, but they can actively pursue several options which collectively may increase the complexity of their assumptions. Among these options are to: (a) seek and actively participate in student-centered courses where critical thinking, discussion, debate, and thoughtful group projects are central activities that contribute heavily to the final grade; (b) complete at least one internship that thrusts the student into realistic workplace situations requiring some autonomy, independent thinking, subjective decision making in ambiguous contexts, and collaboration (but not all internships provide these elements); (c) spend an academic term abroad, in an intense immersion experience, or in an unfamiliar culture directly experiencing its different structures, customs, and ambiguous situations that often demand subjective decision-making in the absence of familiar authorities or rules; (d) join co-curricular activities and faculty research opportunities that promote collaboration, hands-on experience, and the other aspects of independent and contextual knowing; and (e) critically examine those aspects of a part-time job that do and do not promote higher level knowing. For example, Brad, like many students, believed that his education could be achieved only through coursework; he never left the classroom to participate in the array of educational experiences that collectively enrich a person's epistemological assumptions.

In summary, the work of Marcia, Arnett, and Baxter Magolda reveals that college graduates entering the workplace are very much a work-in-progress psychosocially and epistemologically. They leave the security of a familiar and structured academic environment and must now apply their knowledge and skills to new and often highly ambiguous situations where they have less control and where, once again, they are freshmen.

Organizational Aspects of Transition

Holton's Taxonomy of New Employee Development Learning Tasks

At our college's alumni reunions, I frequently asked graduates to comment on the education we provided. Often I heard responses such as "I received an excellent liberal arts education here, but it didn't prepare me well for what I had to learn in my job." Ed Holton and Sharon Naquin (2001) refer to this phenomenon as the paradox of academic preparation.

College and work are fundamentally different. The *knowledge* you acquired in college will be critical to your success, but the *process* of succeeding in school is very different from the process of succeeding at work. Certain aspects of your education may have prepared you to be a professional, but evidence from the workplace indicates that this is not enough for professional success. (p. 7).

Some scholars view the process of breaking-in to a new job in a three-stage model such as prearrival, encounter, and metamorphosis (Robbins 2005), but this perspective does not directly address the new learning employees must accomplish nor identify the sources of stress that they experience. Table 5.1 outlines Holton's taxonomy of new employee development learning tasks which consist of four domains: *individual, people, organization,* and *work tasks.*

Mastery of the individual domain is heavily influenced by the values, beliefs, and prior experiences graduates bring to the job; this domain is most critical for new employees. If the graduate's attitudes, expectations, and breaking-in-skills (e.g., work ethic, willingness to learn, flexibility) match those of the organization's, the new employee is on the correct trajectory for success in the other domains and, perhaps, a relatively smooth neutral zone phase of transition. However, "at risk" graduates who enter with unrealistically high expectations of their education, salary, job challenge, or advancement opportunities will likely experience entry shock (also known as reality or role shock): the dramatic discrepancy between personal expectations and workplace reality (Ashforth 2001). Furthermore, if the new employee had jumped through numerous hoops more successfully than the other 50 or 100 job applicants, chances are that the recruiting process reinforced high expectations. New employees must realize (and recruiters should remind them) that being hired is one achievement, but being accepted by others is a new and different hurdle. Ashforth (2001) reports "individuals who felt their position was not what they had anticipated having (despite its career appropriateness) reported more stress and difficulty with the role transition and lower job satisfaction and organizational commitment" (p. 159). Brad experienced reality shock: He triumphed over a large pool of candidates, experienced a sharp change in roles (his intellectual skills were underutilized; his attire, lunch hour and phone responses were dictated), and depended on previously successful learning processes fueled by a weak work record and no internship experience. What Brad expected versus what he encountered shocked him.

Table 5.1. Holton's taxonomy of new employee development learning tasks.

Domain	Learning task
Individual	Attitudes
	Expectations
	Breaking-in-skills
People	Impression management
	Relationships
	Supervisor
Organization	Organizational culture
	Organizational savvy
	Organizational roles
Work Tasks	Work savvy
	Task knowledge
	Knowledge, skills, and abilities

Source: Holton 1998, Chapter 7 (p. 103)

Mastering Holton's second domain (people domain) is primarily a social learning process that focuses on establishing favorable impressions and strong relationships with supervisors and coworkers, including coworkers from the Baby Boomers to the Millennials. The quality of the employee-supervisor relationship is critical because the supervisor has the major role in determining the organizational socialization of the new hire. The new employee must not only be aware of the importance of favorable relationships but also possess the appropriate skills to create them. For instance, the informal manner a student used to communicate with teachers and peers in person or via e-mail may not be acceptable or ethical (e.g., hacking into a fellow student's files) on the job. Major (2000) contends that effective relationships with supervisors and coworkers are not only the heart of successful organizational socialization, but also the quality of these relationships is likely to influence future career development. Brad's long-term mentoring relationship with his supervisor is a case in point.

The extent new hires learn the tasks of the individual and people domains will influence their success in Holton's organizational domain. Mentoring is an important tool for helping new hires learn those tasks, including internalizing the organization's values and traditions (organizational culture), its informal practices (organizational savvy), and the roles expected of them. Role learning is often accompanied by a myriad of stressors including role stressors (resulting from multi-tasking or multi-roles), role ambiguity (situations where an employee is unclear about the specific behaviors expected in a role), role conflict (when demands from different sources collide), work-family conflict, and role overload (when the employee is expected to fill too many roles simultaneously) (Landy and Conte 2004). Students are exposed to all or most of these role stressors during college, so their challenge is how to perceive the stressfulness of new situations and cope successfully. Solid prior work experience can facilitate the learning of roles. An organization's commitment to socializing new employees also plays an important role in Holton's third domain – organizational domain. Considerable research has been conducted on socialization and its variables as a means of helping new employees through Bridges' neutral zone and new beginning. Readers are encouraged to consult Ashforth (2001) for an understanding of the types of socialization and their outcomes and Holton (1999) for a longitudinal investigation of the interplay of organizational entry constructs and newcomer characteristics.

When we ask college seniors what they intend to learn or do in their new job, they typically say little or nothing about the individual, people and organization domains. Instead, they describe activities comprising the work task domain: Work savvy (applying their knowledge and skills, especially those gained in the academic major); task knowledge (learning the specific activities that define their daily work); and knowledge, skills, and abilities (opportunities to acquire additional knowledge and skills to perform current and future work). For some newcomers, the match between task demands and their skill sets will be satisfying because of their academic or job preparation; others must learn everything from scratch.

Holton's taxonomy is a useful road-map for understanding the dynamics of organizational entry, but most students will never learn about it in their coursework. It is not the mission of a university to teach students about the organizational cultures of Motorola, Boeing, or United Way. Graduates who begin their first full-time job with significant prior work experience that includes attention to the organization's culture and socialization processes will have an edge over those who do not.

Differences Between College and Workplace

College and corporate cultures certainly differ, but what are those specific differences? Holton (1998) reports on a survey of graduates regarding specific differences between college and workplace; from the results he created a list that comprises Table 5.2.

When I have shown this list to students enrolled in an Organizational Behavior course, those with full-time jobs quickly affirm the accuracy of these contrasts; those "at risk" students with little or no work experience look puzzled. For instance, a full-time student may receive a minimum of 20 specific measures of learning each academic term (e.g., five measures for each of four courses), but a full-time employee has a performance review perhaps twice each year. The uncertainty created by a lack of concrete feedback (see Table 5.1, item 1) and, implicitly, lack of control, is highly stressful to those who have depended on it for years. Whereas students may have substantial control of their schedule (item 2), the employees' time is controlled primarily by a supervisor, as Brad discovered. A student may choose to perform at the "A" level in one course and the "C" level in another course (item 4), but an employee is expected to perform at the "A" level in all tasks. And while some teachers may offer "makeup" work for badly performed assignments, supervisors do not. Whereas defined course structures and clear assignments (item 10) are common to most classrooms (and important to teachers for gaining high course evaluations), there is no syllabus in the workplace; uncertainty often rules. Holton's list is illuminating but not complete. For example, individuals accustomed to retiring at 2:00 A.M. and rising at 10:00 A.M. may have to adjust to an early rising, a tense commute, and a long work day. In college, learning occurs mostly by reading; in the workplace learning occurs mostly

Table 5.2. Graduates' perceived differences between college and workplace.

College	Workplace
1. Frequent and concrete feedback	Feedback infrequent and not specific
2. Some freedom to set a schedule	Less freedom or control over schedule
3. Frequent breaks and time off	Limited time off
4. Choose performance level	"A" level work expected continuously
5. Correct answers usually available	Few right answers
6. Passive participation permitted	Active participation and initiative expected
7. Independent thinking supported	Independent thinking often discouraged
8. Environment of personal support	Usually less personal support
9. Focus on personal development	Focus on getting results for organization
10. Structured courses and curriculum	Much less structure; fewer directions
11. Few changes in routine	Often constant and unexpected changes
12. Personal control over time	Responds to supervisors' directions
13. Individual effort and performance	Often, team effort and performance
14. Intellectual challenge	Organizational and people challenges
15. Acquisition of knowledge	Acquisition and application of knowledge
16. Professors	Supervisors

Source: Holton 1998, Chapter 7 (p. 102), Adapted with permission by Wiley, Inc

by doing. In college, a student can choose partners for a group project, but the employee may be required to work closely with someone disliked by all. As noted in the Polach (2004) study, establishing friendships often differs in the two settings. Part of Brad's poor adjustment in his early months was his inability to adapt to the distinctive practices of his workplace.

Transferable Skills

One of the major sources of anxiety for new graduates centers on skill development, identification, and application. Graduates of technical programs enter the workforce with a good idea of the types of knowledge and skill sets required in their field, qualities that are typically augmented by internships, cooperative learning, or other hands-on experiences. Liberal arts graduates, although prepared in a variety of academic work competencies, are often deficient in the people-related applied skills required in the workplace such as those Holton addressed in his taxonomy of new employee development learning tasks (Holton 1998) and described by Gardner (1998). The Conference Board report "Are They Really Ready to Work?" (Casner-Lotto and Barrington 2006) identified deficiencies among college graduates in written communications, writing in English, and leadership. The U.S. Department of Education's Spellings Report (2006) named critical thinking, writing, and problem-solving skills as deficits among college graduates.

According to the National Association of Colleges and Employers (NACE, 2008), the 14 most important skills and qualities employers seek (each received a mean rating of at least 3.9 on a 5.0 scale) include, in descending order of importance: communication skills, strong work ethic, teamwork skills, initiative, interpersonal skills, problem-solving skills, analytic skills, flexibility/adaptability, computer skills, technical skills, detail oriented, organizational skills, leadership, and self-confidence. Although employers were not asked to rank the importance of GPA, 62% screen candidates for grade point average and 61% use 3.0 as the cut-off. The areas of major deficiencies employers identified in new college graduates included communications skills (i.e., writing, face-to-face, interview, presentation, phone, and interpersonal), workplace conduct (i.e., work ethic, analytical and problem-solving skills, business acumen, flexibility, computer skills, and professionalism), and lack of workplace experience.

A significant aspect of the competency issue is the student's failure to translate coursework to skill sets. Recruiters show little or no interest when an applicant speaks proudly of A's received on term papers; they want to know if the individual can articulate what skills were strengthened during the course and how those skills can be applied to the job. As most instructors do not translate course content to transferable skills, it is up to students to create the comparisons. Career counselors who help students develop job resumes can serve as excellent resources for the articulation of academic and co-curricular activities into skills and qualities employers seek. Many university career centers help students create an electronic skills portfolio for use in career planning and job searches. If Brad had worked with his college's career planning services during his senior year to translate his academic accomplishments into workplace skill sets, chances are his interviews would have been more productive than they were.

Another way of illustrating the importance of organizational and skills issues during transition is to identify factors that cause new hires to be promoted or fired. Gardner (2007) queried the employers responding to his annual college hiring survey about the reasons new hires were fired or promoted and then categorized their responses. The top ten reasons (with the corresponding percentage of occurrence at the high end of the scale) as to why new hires are fired included lack of work ethic/commitment (52%), unethical behavior (46%), failure to follow instructions (41%), ineffective in teams (41%), failure to take initiative (26%), missing assignments/deadlines (33%), unable to communicate effectively – verbally (32%), inappropriate use of technology (34%), being late for work (28%), and unable to communicate effectively – writing (28%). Six of these reasons are also bases for terminating new hires (in descending order of frequency): unethical behavior, lack of motivation/work ethic, inappropriate use of technology, failure to follow instructions, late for work, and missing assignment deadlines. Most of the behaviors and attitudes that lead new college hires into conflict with their supervisors are identical to those that have negative consequences in the classroom. Neither size of company or geographical region were significant factors, but the economic sector was important (e.g., construction, utilities, retail, financial and business services companies reported more discipline problems). Similarly, companies heavily involved in campus recruiting reported higher occurrences of discipline related to motivation and integrity.

What factors contribute to promoting new hires? After sorting through 1,500 characteristics, Gardner compiled a list of the seven most frequently mentioned qualities: taking initiative (16%), self-management (13%), personal attributes (9%), commitment (9%), leadership (8%), show and tell (7%), and technical competence (7%). Organizational savvy, learning, and critical thinking were mentioned about 5% each, and willingness to follow, perspective, and prior assignments about 3% each (Gardner 2007). At this point, the reader may wish to compare the reasons new hires are fired and promoted with the NACE list of skills and Holton's taxonomy of new employee development tasks.

Other Aspects of Transition

Health

Health is an important dimension of workplace transition to which college graduates are highly vulnerable. They leave behind the safety net of the insurance provided by parents and school only to encounter a decreasing number of organizations that offer affordable health care plans. About one out of three young adults ages 18–34 (about 18 million) do not have health insurance, yet even a single day in a hospital may cost thousands of dollars (Draut 2005). In a comprehensive review of electronic databases, articles, and reports since 2000, Park, Mulye, Adams, Brindis, and Irwin (2006) discovered that health issues among young adults (ages 18–24) received much less attention than adolescents, in spite of the similarity of health problems between the two groups: substance abuse, mental health, injury, reproductive health, obesity, and access to health care. Their analysis revealed the prevalence in this group of problems such as motor vehicle injuries, substance abuse, STIs, and homicides – problem behaviors that peak during the early twenties, though large disparities exist among some ethnic groups (Park et al. 2006).

Individuals who have experienced mental disorders as adolescents may be vulnerable to facing them again as young adults at a time when services are less available. According to Tanner, Arnett, and Leis (2009), grouping adolescents according to their mental health problems and subsequently following them into emerging adulthood "indicates that some adolescents afflicted by serious psychopathology are likely to experience persistence into emerging adulthood, but those with low levels of mental health problems are unlikely to experience mental health problems in emerging adulthood" (p. 46). In their analysis of studies of mental health issues during emerging adulthood, Schulenberg and Zarrett (2006) observed: (a) Mental health and problem behaviors are relatively stable; (b) an individual's well-being tends to increase from ages 18 to 26; but (c) the incidence of psychopathology also increases. Problem behaviors such as binge drinking and marijuana use tend to increase after high school but decrease during the early twenties. They believe the increases in well-being and depressive disorders reflect, in part, "the multiple transitions, the increased individual agency, and the drop in institution structure that comes for most with emerging adulthood" (Schulenberg and Zarrett 2006, p. 162). The general improvement in well-being is likely to be the result of the emerging adult's opportunities to choose from a variety of activities and contexts that match their goals and desires. Increases in depressive disorders may be due to the overwhelming of coping capacities, the reduction of structure and support, or to a decline in person-context match (Schulenberg and Zarrett 2006). Their conclusions were drawn from data on emerging adults, but they may also apply to college graduates. The new graduate is free to search for and choose a job (when offered) that best matches the individual's background and interests. Once on the job however, the new hire, like Brad, must cope with discrepancies between expectations and reality, and the fact that, like it or not, the job was freely accepted. Given these and other factors, it is understandable why depression may affect this group. To conclude, because there is little data available specific to recent college graduates, assessment of health issues is understood within the context of emerging adulthood. Clearly, research is needed to better understand the relationship between transition and health, especially mental health issues.

Finances

As the lifetime earnings of a person with a college degree is on average 73% higher than individuals with only a high school diploma, it is no surprise that approximately two of every three students are willing to go in debt to pay college costs. The average graduate leaves college owing about $19,000 in loans and an additional $3,000 in credit card debt (Marksjarvis 2007). Graduates of private universities can easily owe twice the average college debt or more, and those continuing in professional or graduate programs can readily incur debt of $30,000 or more annually. Brad was fortunate to graduate with only a $10,000 debt obligation. Many students never finish college because they cannot afford its costs, but then they have loans to repay. Furthermore, graduation from college is the time in most families when an individual is expected to become self-sufficient, financially and emotionally. Debt affects decisions in many ways. Marksjarvis reports on a survey conducted by Mathew Greenwald and Associates. Of 1,508 college graduates between the ages of 21 and 35, debt caused 32% to move back home with parents or live at home longer, 27% to skip medical or dental procedures, 44% to delay buying a house, and 28% to delay having children. A Nellie Mae survey of graduates revealed that 54% wished they had borrowed less for college (Marksjarvis 2007).

In an analysis of data obtained from an institution that introduced a "no loans" policy (all financial aid was in the form of grants), Rothstein and Rouse (2007) discovered the accumulation of debt causes some students to choose jobs with higher salaries and avoid "public interest" jobs that pay lower salaries. Debt also reduced alumni donations years after graduation. It is essential for students and their families to carefully consider the impact of debt before decisions are made about a school, to carefully monitor debt accumulation throughout college, and to prepare for the possibility that it may be several years before the graduate is earning a comfortable living.

Recommendations to Students

What can students do to improve readiness and reduce anxiety during one of life's most exciting transitions? In his analysis of emerging adulthood as an institutionalized moratorium, Cote (2006) emphasizes that "emerging adults more than ever need a repertoire of personal resources – some of which I call *identity capital* – to successfully integrate themselves into mainstream adult society, if they so wish" (p. 91). We have explored a variety of factors that help explain why the process of moving from college-to-workplace is stressful. Several recommendations – forms of identity capital – were stated directly or indirectly in the previous sections and are reiterated below in the form of recommendations to students. Some suggestions below may be viewed as stressors by students, but each represents an opportunity for personal growth.

1. Get a job, and if you have a job, pay close attention to it. Even a mundane and boring job shares some similarities to your dream job: a supervisor, co-workers (usually), roles and responsibilities, an organizational culture, tasks to perform, and other characteristics. Examine the attitudes and expectations you hold (Holton's individual domain) and their appropriateness if you held a higher level, full-time job in the organization. Ask yourself about the extent you can deal with people you do not like, delegate tasks, work productively under stress and boredom, demonstrate initiative, respond maturely to criticism, and the way you respond to stressful events. Examine the job for transferable skills using the NACE list. Search for jobs related to your career interests. In a survey of human resources managers, Foreman (1996) reported 77% of the respondents consider an applicant's part-time employment when hiring; 86% viewed part-time employment as potentially important as a student's G.P.A.; and, if given two applicants academically equal, 94% would choose the candidate with part-time work experience. Even if a student's college costs are covered by grants, scholarships, and family support, it behooves many students to hold a job on a regular basis. Without substantial work experience that includes thoughtful analysis of the organization's culture, the new graduate can expect entry shock.
2. Search carefully for and complete at least one internship which contains opportunities for assuming significant responsibilities, developing beneficial workplace skills and attitudes, and applying course concepts. The internship is not simply about completing tasks related to your academic major but also about learning the tasks of the individual, people, and organizational domains.

3. Enroll in courses that focus on process and organizational issues, such as small group and interpersonal communication, management, business communications, leadership, technology, organizational behavior, and similar courses.

4. Join campus organizations, sports, and other co-curricular activities that promote collaboration, competition, and leadership. Consider becoming a resident hall assistant. Plan to become an officer of a campus organization by your senior year. Attend workshops and seminars that focus on conflict management, leadership, communication and related "soft-skills" development.

5. Work with a career counselor by the junior year to create a plan that helps identify your goals, strengths, weaknesses, interests, and potential career fields. Create a skills-based portfolio of your academic, job, and co-curricular activities during your senior year. Network! Network!

6. Complete study abroad, immersion, service learning, and similar activities that place you in culturally unfamiliar environments which require problem-solving in unstructured, ambiguous situations.

7. Use these and other experiences to establish realistic expectations about your first job, avoid the "entitlement mentality," and learn to embrace uncertainty.

It should be noted that opportunities for travel abroad may not be open to students with limited financial resources, and internships and co-curricular activities may be out of reach for some students with commitments to jobs and families.

What can institutions do to improve the readiness of their graduates?

(a) Expand the availability of challenging internship opportunities throughout the institution and promote them as an essential tool of a successful transition. Continue to encourage study abroad and other experiential learning activities that help students explore their identity and challenge their assumptions about knowing. (b) Encourage employers on and off campus, teachers, advisors, and student personnel professionals to help students translate their responsibilities and tasks into transferable skill sets. (c) Encourage career planning professionals and departments that sponsor career events to view career planning, not as an end, but as an essential component of Bridges' ending phase. Support courses that focus on career and transition planning, including the nuts and bolts of post-college money management. Solicit alumni and members of the profit and not-for-profit organizations in your community to speak at career planning events.

Concluding Remarks

Transition to the workforce is an exciting and maturing but inherently stressful phase of development, especially for those unprepared for its challenges. In an effort to understand key issues and conditions that create distress, two models of transition were summarized, Bridges' model to facilitate early attention to transition and Schlossberg's for counseling individuals in transition. Marcia's identity statuses and Arnett's theory of emerging adulthood reveal the dynamics of psychosocial development that underlie the thinking and behavior of young people. Baxter Magolda's study suggests an individual's assumptions about knowing, especially beliefs about authority and certainty, can attain greater complexity as a result of workplace demands. Regarding organizational influences, Holton's taxonomy of new employee development learning tasks and his survey of college versus corporate cultures and practices discloses a body of knowledge, skills, attitudes, and behaviors graduates must master in a radically different environment. Finally, health and financial concerns intersect with organizational and developmental issues to further complicate the graduate's new life. Perhaps the common denominator shared by these diverse concepts is the graduates' relinquishing of routine, the feeling of certainty, and control to the demands of their new environments – they are freshmen again facing new challenges in a post-college world.

The study of college-to-workplace transition poses challenges to educators and counselors who work in this area. In spite of the numerous concepts and studies presented in this chapter, the research and clinical literature does not reveal nearly enough about the more than one million college graduates who enter the work force annually and strive, with various levels of success, to adjust. It seems we are left with more questions than answers. Research is needed that tests hypotheses generated by the theories and models presented here as they related to transition. For example, what percent of college graduates actually encounter serious problems adjusting to the workplace? What particular academic and non-academic activities contribute most to a successful transition and in what types of work environments? What aspects of successful organizational socialization programs can be incorporated in classrooms, career planning courses, or experiential learning settings? How can we best help persons whose first full-time experience in the world of work ended in frustration and failure? What can we learn from those who succeed?

"Success is measured not so much by the position one has reached in life as by the obstacles which he has overcome while trying to succeed."

Booker T. Washington

Acknowledgment: The author gratefully acknowledges the comments and observations of Camille Helkowski and the critical reading and recommendations provided by Christine Anderson, Jerry Cleland, and Dee Konrad.

References

Arnett, J. J. (2000). Emerging adulthood: A theory of development from the late teens through the twenties. *American Psychologist, 55*, 469–480.

Arnett, J. J. (2004). *Emerging adulthood: The winding road from the late teens through the twenties.* New York: Oxford University Press.

Arnett, J. J., & Tanner, J. L. (eds). (2006). *Emerging adults in America: Coming of age in the 21st century.* Washington, DC: American Psychological Association.

Ashforth, B. E. (2001). *Role transitions in organizational life: An identity-based perspective.* Mahwah, NJ: Lawrence Erlbaum.

Baxter Magolda, M. B. (1992). *Knowing and reasoning in students: Gender-related patterns in students' intellectual development.* San Francisco, CA: Jossey-Bass.

Baxter Magolda, M. B. (1994). Post-college experiences and epistemology. *The Review of Higher Education, 18*(1), 25–44.

Bridges, W. (2003). *Managing transitions: Making the most of change* (2nd ed.). Cambridge, MA: Perseus.

Casner-Lotto, J., & Barrington, L. (2006, October). *Are they ready to work? Employers' perspectives on the basic knowledge and applied skills of new entrants to the 21st century U.S. workforce.* The Conference Board, Partnership for 21st Century Skills, Corporate Voices for Working Families, Society for Human Resource Management. Retrieved October 1, 2007, from http://www.conference-board.org/pdf_free/BED-06-Workforce.pdf

Chao, G. T., & Gardner, P. D. (2007, Winter). *Important characteristics of early career jobs: What do young adults want?* White paper prepared for MonsterTrak. East Lansing, MI: Michigan State University Collegiate Employment Research Institute. Retrieved October 17, 2007, from http://ceri.msu.edu/publications/publications.html

Cote, J. E. (2006). Emerging adulthood as an institutionalized moratorium: Risks and benefits to identity formation. In J. J. Arnett & J. L. Tanner (Eds.), *Emerging adults in America: Coming of age in the 21st Century* (pp. 85–116). Washington, DC: American Psychological Association.

Draut, T. (2005). *Strapped: Why America's 20- and 30- somethings can't get ahead.* New York: Anchor.

Farber, H. S. (2006, December). Is the company man an anachronism? Trends in long term employment in the U.S. between 1973 and 2005. *Network on Transitions to Adulthood Policy Brief, 38,* pp. 1–2

Fitzpatrick, M. D., & Turner, S. E. (2006). September). *The changing college experience for young adults. Network on Transitions to Adulthood Policy Brief, 34,* 1–3.

Foreman, R. (1996). UPS study relates student employment to job-hunting success after graduation. In R. Kincaid (Ed.), *Student employment: Linking college and the workplace.* Columbia, SC: National Resources Center for the Freshman Year Experience & Students in Transition.

Gardner, P. (2007). *Moving up or moving out of the company? Factors that influence the promoting or firing of new college hires.* Research Brief 1-2007. Michigan State University Collegiate Employment Research Institute

Gardner, P. D. (1998). Are college seniors prepared to work? In J. N. Gardner, G. Van der Veer, et al. (Eds.), *The senior year experience: Facilitating integration, reflection, closure and transition* (pp. 60–94). San Francisco, CA: Jossey-Bass.

Goodman, J., Scholssberg, N. K., & Anderson, M. L. (2006). *Counseling adults in transition: Linking practice with theory* (3rd ed.). New York: Springer.

Hettich, P. I., & Helkowski, C. (2005). *Connect college to career: A student's guide to work and life transitions.* Belmont, CA: Thomson Wadsworth.

Holton, E. F., III. (1998). Preparing students for life beyond the classroom. In J. N. Gardner, G. Van der Veer, et al. (Eds.), *The senior year experience: Facilitating integration, reflection, closure and transition* (pp. 95–115). San Francisco, CA: Jossey-Bass.

Holton, E. F., III, & Naquin, S. S. (2001). *How to succeed in your first job: Tips for new college graduates.* San Francisco, CA: Berrett-Koehler.

Holton, E. F., III, & Russell, C. J. (1999). Organizational entry and exit: An exploratory Longitudinal examination of early careers. *Human Performance, 12*(3–4), 311–341.

Landy, F. J., & Conte, J. M. (2004). *Work in the 21st century: An introduction to industrial and organizational psychology.* Boston, MA: McGraw Hill.

Levit, A. (2004). *They don't teach corporate in college: A twenty-something's guide to the business world.* Franklin Lakes, NJ: Career.

Major, D. A. (2000). Effective newcomer socialization into high-performance organizational structures. In N. M. Ashkanasy, C. P. M. Wilderom & M. F. Peterson (Eds.), *Handbook of organizational culture and climate.* Thousand Oaks, CA: SAGE.

Marksjarvis, G. (2007, April 29). For many, loans pay off in trouble. *The Chicago Tribune,* section 5, p. 5

McAdams, D. P. (2001). *The person: An integrated introduction to personality psychology.* Orlando, Fl: Harcourt College Publishers.

National Association of Colleges and Employers. (2008). *Job outlook 2008*. PA: Bethlehem.

National Center for Educational Statistics (2006). *Digest of educational statistics*.

Park, M. J., Mulye, T. P., Adams, S. H., Brindis, C. D., & Irwin, C. E. (2006). The health Status of young adults in the United States. *Journal of Adolescent Health, 39*, 305–317.

Polach, J. L. (2004). Understanding the experience of college graduates during their firstyear of employment. *Human Resource Development Quarterly, 15*, 5–23.

Robbins, A. (2004). *Conquering your quarterlife crisis: Advice from twentysomethings who have been there and survived.* NY: Berkeley.

Robbins, A., & Wilner, A. (2001). *Quarterlife crisis: The unique challenges of life in your twenties.* New York: Penguin Putnam.

Robbins, S. P. (2005). *Organizational behavior* (11th ed.). Upper Saddle River, NJ: Pearson Prentice Hall.

Saks, A. M., & Ashforth, B. E. (2000). The role of dispositions, entry stressors, and behavioral plasticity theory in predicting newcomers' adjustment to work. *Journal of Organizational Behavior, 21*, 43–62.

Schulenberg, J. E., & Zarrett, N. R. (2006). Mental health during emerging adulthood: Continuity and discontinuity in courses, causes, and functions. In J. J. Arnett & J. L. Tanner (Eds.), *Emerging adults in America: Coming of age in the 21st century* (pp. 135–172). Washington, DC: American Psychological Association.

Smith, T. W. (2003). *Coming of age in 21st century America: Public attitudes toward the importance and timing of transitions to adulthood (GSS Topical Report No. 35).* Chicago, IL: University of Chicago, National Opinion Research Center.

Tanner, J. L., Arnett, J. J., & Leis, J. A. (2009). Emerging adulthood: Learning and development during the first stage of adulthood. In M. C. Smith, & N. DeFrates-Dench (Eds.), *Handbook of research on adult development and learning.* NY: Routledge/Taylor & Francis.

U.S. Department of Education. (2006). *A test of leadership: Charting the future of U.S. Higher education.* Washington, DC: U.S. Department of Education.

Wilner, A., & Stocker, C. (2005). *The quarterlifer's companion: How to get on the right career path, control your finances, and find the support network you need to thrive.* New York: McGraw Hill.

Chapter 6

Coping with Job Transitions over the Work Life

John R. Rudisill, Jean M. Edwards, Paul J. Hershberger,
Joyce E. Jadwin, and John M. McKee

A job transition is a process involving a number of steps, including thinking about goals and skills, evaluating the potential job market, conducting the job search, managing personal reactions, and negotiating entry into the new organization. As both a common and impactful transition of modern life, it is important to examine the factors associated with coping with job transitions. Specifically, we would like to consider the societal changes in the current work context, and the research evidence indicating job transitions can be significant life stressors. We then examine the role that coping plays in the transition process, and outline our mediation model of antecedents, coping and outcomes. Case studies of job transitions at four points in the work-life are presented to illustrate the model. We search for common themes and issues in the process of job transitions across the work-life, and raise questions regarding how these may be uniquely played out at different points in an individual's life. The implications for the professional's role in helping individuals and organizations facilitate transitions are discussed. Finally, we present directions for future research.

The Changing Context of Job Transitions

The context of job transitions has changed dramatically over the last decade. In response to the competitive pressures of the global economy, deregulation, technological innovation, and profitable quarterly returns, many employers have emphasized productivity and reduction of costs at the expense of employee stress and strain. Major changes include the following:

The Number of Job Transitions Individuals make over their Careers has Increased

Changing social and economic conditions are forcing employees to undergo job transitions as a result of increased mergers, downsizing (rightsizing), and corporate restructurings. Downsizing and restructuring have become common strategies designed to increase profit.

From: *Handbook of Stressful Transitions Across the Lifespan*,
Edited by: T.W. Miller, DOI 10.1007/978-1-4419-0748-6_6,
© Springer Science+Business Media, LLC 2010

In the United States, one-third of American Management Association firms downsized their workforce in the period 1990–1995 (American Management Association 1997). By 2004, the American Management Association survey of executives revealed that 52% anticipated increases in the number of employees. The remaining either anticipated a decrease or consistency in their workforce size. While just under half indicated that the size of the work force would remain the same or decrease , this percentage is down from 2003 when 62% anticipated a decrease or steady state. The top three explanations for job eliminations included organizational restructuring, automation or technological improvements, and re-engineering of business processes (American Management Association 2004). From 1990 to 1999, the number of mergers and acquisitions tripled. Downsizing often follows mergers and acquisitions by about 6–9 as a result of the duplication of functions and staff resulting from mergers and acquisitions. Corporate downsizing and restructuring following mergers result in significant employee displacement and transition. Nearly 40% of the 120 large revenue companies responding to an American Marketing Association survey, reported they had cut jobs in three or more years since 1990, and that about one-third of the positions cut in the past year were at the managerial level (Shapiro and Kitaeff 1990). From 1979 to 1995, 43,000,000 jobs were erased in the US while 236,000 were added per month creating a tumultuous job market. During recent years, the manufacturing sector of our economy has been especially hard hit by downsizing initiatives and continues to constrict as a segment of our economy. Studies of the personal impact of downsizing show that 27% of US citizens report no personal impact, 33% report downsizing happening to a family member, and 40% report downsizing happening to a relative, friend, or neighbor. Only 35% of replacement jobs after downsizing result in higher paying jobs (NIOSH 2002). Reflecting the increasing instability and insecurity of jobs, the percentage of employees with lay-off concerns doubled (22–46%) in the period 1988–1995.

People born at the end of the baby boom held an average of 10.2 jobs between the ages of 18 and 38 (Bureau of Labor Statistics 2004). On average, only 4.4 jobs were held in their earlier years (18–22) suggesting a number of continued changes beyond early adulthood (Bureau of Labor Statistics 2004). The duration of the jobs increased with the age of the person. Workers in this cohort between the ages of 33 and 38 experienced 39% of their jobs lasting less than a year and by 5 years 70% of the jobs ended (Bureau of Labor Statistics 2004).

In a 2004 report, the US Department of Labor indicated that 10.1 million workers between 2001 and 2003 lost jobs due to plant or company closings, elimination of the job or cut backs within the organization. Of these employees, 5.3 million had been employed for 3 or more years at the time of the job loss with 32% coming from professional and managerial fields and another 33% from the manufacturing segment. The remaining people were employed in wholesale and retail trade and professional service positions. Though many workers found reemployment in 2004, 57% of those working were making less than their prior salary (Bureau of Labor Statistics 2004).

Frequent Reduction in Personnel Costs

This has resulted in increased expendability of workers – more temporary, part-time, contingent workers, and a decrease in the number of unionized employees (Tetrick and Barling 1995). Layoffs are no longer tools of the last resort for desperate economic situations. Most corporations are asking, "How can we restructure the organization to find the smallest number of employees we need to run this business effectively?" Eighty percent of companies downsized in profitable years. The recent economic slowdown, has resulted in additional cost cutting measures to maintain corporate profitability.

The Diversity of the Workplace is Increasing

Numbers of female and minority workers are on the rise (Keita and Hurrell 1994). Participation of racially and ethnically diverse people in the workforce has doubled since 1970 (Foner and Fredrickson 2004) and represents 33% of the workforce (Moss 2005). Given the increasing diversity of the United States, the diversity of the workplace will continue to grow.

Issues of child care, aging parents, and balancing multiple work/nonwork roles are growing in importance. The increasing diversity of the workplace creates challenges for employers to deal with issues of fairness and accommodation. Recent changes in government policies and economic climate have brought a number of individuals who may have multiple needs and challenges transitioning into the workforce and into the labor market. These individuals may require additional support services to be successful.

Increased Demands for Worker Productivity

This trend has resulted in longer work hours and increasing demands to do more with less. Companies often demand higher levels of performance as evidenced by an increase in work hours for all occupations in the US since 1985 (Rones and Ilg 1997). The percentage of the salaried workforce who worked "long" hours (in excess of 48 h weekly) grew 30%, to over 21 million workers from 1985 to 1993 (Rones and Ilg 1997). The increase in work activity has placed increasing stress (job stress-related disorders have mushroomed, National Counsel of Compensation Insurance 1985, Northwestern National Life Insurance Company 1991) and has decreased the discretionary time resources of individuals, couples, and families. Safety and health issues may result from increased levels of stress and fatigue. The "Do more with less" philosophy has resulted in increased concern over job strain and burnout. Concerns about safety and health resulting from increased organizational demands have given impetus to the new psychological specialty of occupational health psychology (Sauter et al. 1999).

The Relationship between Employers and Employees has Weakened

A decrease in company loyalty toward employees and the erosion of the ideals of lifelong employment have been noted (Hakim 1994). Employees are less loyal to their employers and often view themselves as working for themselves as "free agents" rather than for an employer. This fundamental change in the contractual basis of employment has caught some employees unaware and unprepared for unemployment and job transition. Recent scandals such as those involving Enron and WorldCom have emphasized the uncertain benefits from company employment and the growing distrust of highly paid company officials. In turn, employees are adopting attitudes emphasizing self-preservation and abandoning company loyalty. Some employees have united to file class action suits against what are perceived as unfair company practices.

New research into employability suggests a continuation of the trend of thinking of workers as "free agents" (Fugate et al. 2004). While not a formal construct at this point, Fugate and his colleagues suggest employability is based on the intersection of career identity, personal adaptability, and social and human capital. Given the number of job changes most individuals will face in a lifetime, a model for predicting opportunities in the workplace and a method to help individuals be vigilant regarding career ownership is appropriate. Other approaches to managing employment uncertainty include being adaptive in thinking and planning, understanding contextual challenges of the workplace, and understanding the job transition process (Ebberwein et al. 2004).

Many Employees undergo Transitions Despite Excellent Job Performance

The old dictum of "to keep your job, simply do a good job," is no longer sufficient to maintain employment and employability. In previous times, many of the employees who were terminated or the first to go in a slow down had performance problems warranting the company's action. Now many employees undergo transition multiple times despite quality performance.

Many Companies "Outsource" Functions Originally Assigned to Permanent Employees

The trend to outsource functions (Gowing et al. 1998) contributes to lowered worker opportunity and attainment. Many employees experience a gap between their expectations of job security, opportunities for advancement and the ability to use their creative and problem-solving skills. Leiter and Maslach (2000) have identified six areas to assess in determining if a position meets an employee's expectations for degree of control over their workload, degree of reward for work, sense of community, perceptions of fairness, and degree of fit between personal and organizational values. Outsourcing and the decreased use of permanent employees makes the realization of these career expectations less available.

More Employees Are Working from Home than Before

Working from home opens up a whole new set of issues for organizations, employees, and mental health workers. The confusion of how to define an employee who works from home makes the research more elusive. The actual calculation of people working from home ranges from 10 to 12% of the working population according to the Census Bureau (Mokhtarian et al. 2005). The numbers change based upon the definition of working from home and the organizations calculating it: US Census, Bureau of Labor Statistics, American Housing Survey, or private researcher firms. Issues of work/home balance, coping, and job transitions are only just beginning to be studied (Kossek et al. 2006). The lack of mentoring, informal learning, and interpersonal networking are among three issues which specifically face telecommuters and may result in professional isolation (Cooper and Kurland 2002). The isolation may have short and long term consequences for the employee. Not being considered for promotions, being unaware of other opportunities within or outside the organization and remaining stagnant in the approach to work are just three potential negative outcomes. Job loss would be a harsher reality for someone professionally isolated.

Job Search Mechanisms Have Developed to Facilitate Mastery over Job Transition

Outplacement firms are consulting agencies hired by companies who are terminating employees. The goal of the outplacement firm is to help terminated employees find jobs or careers outside of the company. Since the 1960s, corporations have turned to outplacement firms in increasing numbers. Corporations may provide outplacement internally or contract for services externally though outplacement service agencies. Companies turn to outplacement firms to provide (a) coaching and support regarding termination of the employee, (b) career guidance and placement assistance, and (c) emotional support in dealing with the demoralization frequently associated with unemployment. Often, outplacement benefits differ depending upon the status of the employee and can be more easily negotiated and provided off-site. The organizational objectives for using such services include (a) presenting a public image of an organization that cares about its employees; (b) maintaining morale by rapidly removing and finding employment for terminated workers; (c) saving unemployment expenditures; (d) reducing lawsuits and legal costs; and (e) reducing the "people problems" associated with corporate reductions and mergers (Brammer and Humberger 1984). Outplacement agencies typically offer services such as information on potential employment options, résumé development, instruction in job seeking, interview skills training, networking advice, assistance in developing job search strategies, career counseling, emotional support, and facilities for conducting one's job search including an appropriate business address and secretarial services. Outplacement gives the displaced executive an office to get up and go to each day. Their new job is "to find a job."

A recent trend is the development of job centers through public funding. The job center functions as the public equivalent of an outplacement agency. Due to its size and the multiple needs of the population it serves, it features multiple agency involvement and a wide variety of services. Job centers serve as resources for labor-market exchange and workforce development while providing individuals and families with financial, medical, and other support services essential to reducing and preventing dependence while strengthening the quality of life. It features a one-stop shopping career system with a single point of contact. It aims to reduce welfare recipients and help job seekers find jobs on their own, be matched to jobs and placed into subsidized employment, or be placed in a work experience position that can lead to paid employment. It also provides a single place where employers can access a pool of qualified, job-ready workers. Multiple support services are available to help the multiple-needs of the unemployed worker.

Stress Is Associated with Job Transitions

Job loss has long been recognized as a significant stressor (Bartley 1994; Holmes and Masuda 1974), and a diverse research literature indicates that occupational stressors affect well-being, performance, and health (Harkness et al. 2005; Kahn and Byosiere 1992; Keita and Hurrell 1994; Quick et al. 1992; Quick et al. 2003).

Strains experienced by unemployed workers and their families include increased anxiety, depression, somatic complaints and self-evaluated ill health, and decreased self-esteem and self-efficacy (Claussen et al. 1993; Hamilton et al. 1993; Iversen and Sobroe 1988; Kalil 2005; Kessler et al. 1989; Schwarzer et al. 1994). During the job transition period, many employees face family strain, conflicts with co-workers and supervisors, financial and legal problems, and substance abuse. For others, the prolonged stress of unemployment can cause physical problems. Brewington et al. (2004) explore the relationship between involuntary job loss and grief. They found similarities in grief patterns between bereaved individuals and individuals with involuntary job loss especially regarding anger, guilt, and social isolation. Hopefully, the commonplace nature of job displacement may eventually ease the sense of failure, stigma, and shame traditionally associated with job loss.

The end result of these socio-economic trends is that employees are dealing with an increasing number of periods of transitional unemployment in their career. At the same time, employees are burdened with developing and managing their own career plan and direction.

Coping with Job Transitions

Much of the early research on job transitions focused on documenting the negative effects of unemployment. A meta-analytic study of job search literature from 1987 to 2002 reviewed psychological factors and well-being during unemployment (McKee-Ryan et al. 2005). Not surprisingly, the analysis showed negative impacts on mental health during job loss periods. They also noted that researchers had rarely studied positive affect variables.

In the past decade increased research attention has examined the role of coping in the job transition process. Coping has been a widely investigated component of the stress process since the seminal work of Lazarus and his colleagues in the 1980. They (Laza and Folkman 1984) defined coping as the cognitive and behavioral efforts to manage stressful internal and external demands, and proposed that coping is a key component of the stress process. The literature shows how people manage their stress and expectations during job loss and how it impacts their overall well-being (McKee-Ryan et al. 2005). There have been a number of definitions of coping proposed, and the antecedent and outcomes of coping with a variety of stressors have been examined (Zeidner and Endler 1996; Prussia et al. 2001). The model of coping with job transitions that has guided our research is shown in Fig. 6-1.

Coping as a Part of a Self-Regulatory Process

Carver and Scheier's (1999) definition of coping as a process of self-regulation under duress strongly influenced our model of job transition coping. In their theory, stress is a discrepancy between one's desired state and one's current state. Coping is part of the regulatory system that attempts to resolve or manage stressful interactions, and facilitates movement toward one's goals. We define job transition coping as cognitive and behavioral efforts to manage specific external and internal demands related to the job transition, to preserve

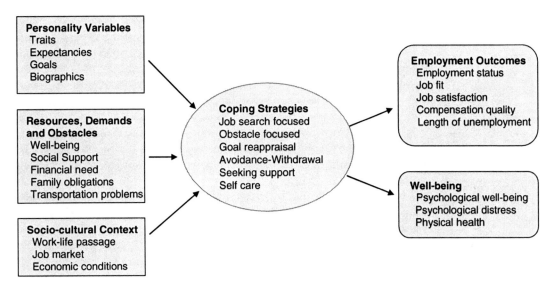

Fig. 6-1. A model of coping with job transitions

resources, and to create conditions allowing one to progress toward desired goals. This definition restricts coping to conscious cognitive and behavioral activities directed toward self-regulation with regard to the experienced stress. It implies that coping involves multiple strategies.

Laza and Folkman (1984) suggested that although coping strategies could be categories in terms of problem-focused and emotion-focused strategies, more differentiated strategies may be useful in understanding the stress process. Their research indicated individuals typically use multiple strategies in coping with specific stressors. There is still considerable disagreement over the level, number and content of coping strategies that are needed to best represent the conceptual definition, and predict the relevant outcomes (Ben-Zur 1999; Carver et al. 1989; Endler and Parker 1990; Lyne and Roger 2000; Schwarzer and Schwarzer 1996; Vinokur and Schul 2002).

Research on job transitions has assessed a variety of relevant coping strategies. These strategies can be roughly divided into those focused specifically on job search activities and those focused on coping in other life areas. Blau's (1994) coping measures focused on the job search and assessed: (1) preparatory job search behavior, including planning, thinking about what needs to be done, developing information on job leads, and (2) active job search behaviors, including preparing one's résumé, completing applications, and interviewing for positions. Networking intensity, that is contacting friends and associates regarding job opportunities and openings, has also been included in assessments of job search coping (Wanberg et al. 2000). One of the most extensive measures of coping with job transitions was developed by Latack and her colleagues (Kinicki and Latack 1990; Latack et al. 1995). In addition to proactive job search they assessed: non work organization (i.e., efforts to control one's life situation); positive self assessment (i.e., favorably evaluating one skills and abilities); distancing (i.e., efforts to avoid the reality of the job loss or to escape the situation); and job devaluation (i.e., reassessing the importance of other aspects of one's life). A number of other researchers have used this or similar measures, (Gowan et al. 1999; Kinicki et al. 2000; Wanberg 1997). Vinokur examined the relationships among job search motivation, job search intensity, financial strain, job search efficacy, mastery and depressive symptoms made to reemployment at 6 months and after 12 months within different demographic variables (Vinokur and Schul 2002). The negative impact of elevated depressive symptoms on reemployment within the 6 to 12 month time frame was critical. Vinokur's model also attempted to predict the quality of reemployment related to the prior factors. Other coping strategies that have been proposed include seeking support, seeking retraining, considering relocating, and engaging in community activism (Leana and Feldman 1990; Leana et al. 1998).

Clearly it is important to assess strategies directly aimed at problem solving and obtaining one's goals (e. g., job search planning and activities). Other dimensions of coping, including reappraisal and revaluation of one's goals, are also part of self-regulation. Similarly, strategies directed toward protecting and enhancing one's resources (e.g., seeking support for one's job search and self-care activities) are important aspects of coping from this theoretical perspective. The self-regulatory function of some dimensions of coping may appear less clear. Avoidance and withdrawal may contribute to self-regulation by allowing one to ameliorate one's emotional reactions or to protect scarce resources, but over time may contribute to distress. Emotional venting may be a cost resource early on but over time may allow one to process the impact of the event, and provide for the renewed investment in the transition process. Our work with clients of a publicly funded job agency has suggested multiple strategies of coping with job transitions may be used by the job seeker.

Antecedents of Coping

The antecedents of coping impact the self-regulatory process. The antecedents considered in the current model include (1) resources, demands and obstacles, and (2) individual differences. Consistent with Hobfoll's (1998) theory, resources are defined as means for responding to events, for example, investing in attempts to change one's circumstances and progress toward one's goals (Hobfoll 1998). Demands represent needs or requirements for the expenditure of resources. Demands both tax and motivate the individual. Obstacles may block or impede goal progress. For employees making job transitions, obstacles may be a crucial determinant of the coping process. Previous research indicates that social support is a resource that facilitates coping with job transitions (Vinokur and Caplan 1987; Wanberg et al. 1996), and that financial need represents a demand that is positively related to job transition coping (Blau 1994; Gowan et al. 1999; Vinokur and Caplan 1987; Vinokur and Schul 2002; Wanberg et al. 1999). Our recent work suggests that obstacles to job transitions, such as difficulties with transportation, family obligations, or health issues, may influence coping and perhaps outcomes. Resources, demands, and obstacles to job transitions may vary over the different passages in one's work-life.

Individual differences include both relatively stable personality variables such as traits as well as context specific cognitive affective variables. There is a growing recognition of the strong conceptual link between personality and coping strategies, and Bolger's (1990) assertion that "coping is personality in action under stress" (p. 525) has gained support over the last decade.

For example, Watson and Hubbard (1996) found that the dimensions of the Five-Factor Model are differentially related to coping styles, with neuroticism and conscientiousness being strongly related, extroversion being moderately related, and openness and agreeableness being modestly related. Studies have also found significant relations between neuroticism, extraversion, openness, and a variety of coping dimensions (McCrae and Costa 1986; Costa et al. 1996). Results from diary studies indicate that neuroticism, extraversion, and openness are associated with coping with daily stressors and significant evaluation stressors (Bolger 1990; David and Suls 1999).

There is some support that personality is associated with coping with job transitions. A recent meta-analytic review concluded that the extraversion and conscientious dimensions of the Five-Factor Model are moderately positively related to active job search coping. A modest positive relationship was found for openness and agreeableness and job search activities as well as a small negative relationship with neuroticism. Cognitive affective personality variables including appraisals of what is at stake in a situation and whether one has the competencies necessary in the specific situation have also been examined as predictors of coping (Laza and Folkman 1984). For example, the meaning of the job transition, including what goals are at stake (Gowan and Gatewood 1997) may influence coping responses. Research indicates a positive association between commitment to one's career and job search intensity (Leana et al. 1998; Wanberg et al. 1999), and between one's efficacy expectations and coping strategies in job transitions (Blau 1994; Kanfer et al. 2001; Saks and Ashforth 1999, Wanberg et al. 1999). Wanberg (1997) found that personal resilience, a composite variable assessing self esteem, global perceived control and optimism, predicted coping by engaging in nonwork organization, and positive self assessment but did not predict proactive job search coping. Leana and Feldman (1990) did not find support for their hypothesis that Type A, locus of control and self-esteem influence problem focused coping. There are mixed results regarding the relationship of individual differences in biographical variables and the coping process and the outcomes of the job transition process. A recent meta-analysis (Kanfer et al. 2001) reported that age and tenure show small negative association with job search behaviors.

The Consequences of Coping

Coping is primarily intended to affect adaptation outcomes (Laza and Folkman 1984). How a person copes may influence both well-being and the outcome of the stressful situation. Much of the outcome research has focused on psychological well-being or level of distress. Yet, which coping strategies reduce distress and increase well-being or, indeed, whether any means of coping consistently influence well-being, remains uncertain. For example, Holohan et al. (1996) concluded that active, approach coping is associated with less concurrent distress and fewer relevant problems in the future, whereas, coping strategies based on avoidance are associated with greater concurrent and future distress. Aspinwall and Taylor (1992) found that active coping was associated with better adjustment to a new environment whereas avoidance coping was associated with poorer levels of adjustment. In contrast, Bolger (1990) found that wishful thinking, self-blame and problem-focused coping were all positively associated with anxiety, whereas, distancing coping was negatively associated with anxiety. Aldwin and Revenson (1987) found that coping, particularly emotion focused coping, tended to increase distress.

Within the literature about coping with job loss the research examining the impact of coping on distress and well-being has been inconclusive. Studies have reported that job search activities are negatively correlated with concurrent well-being (Leana and Feldman 1990; Wanberg 1997). However, found a negative relation between problem focused coping and distress and a positive relation between emotion focused coping and distress. Gowan et al. (1999) found no relation between job search activities and level of distress, and a negative association between distress and both distancing and participation in nonwork activities. Coping may be related to well-being in several ways. The costs of coping may impact well-being. In addition, the relation between coping and goal progress may be associated with changes in well-being. Also, the relation between coping and outcomes is that outcomes (e.g., well-being) usually develop over time during the stress process, making it important to examine both concurrent and prospective relations between coping and well being.

Several studies have examined the association between reemployment status and coping dimensions (Gowan et al. 1999; Kanfer and Hulin 1985; Leana and Feldman 1995; Wanberg et al. 1996, Wanberg 1997). A recent meta-analysis (Kanfer et al. 2001) concluded job search behaviors were associated with employment status, number of offers, and duration of unemployment, however, few studies noted coping strategies and employment related outcomes and were not included in the meta-analysis. Wanberg (1997, 1999) reported an association between job search activities and employment. Leana et al. (1998) found that both problem focused job search strategies and symptom focused coping strategies (i.e., seeking social support, seeking financial assistance, and community activism) were associated with reemployment. Gowan et al. (1999) found no association between satisfactory reemployment and either job search or non work activities (participating in community, church, and leisure activities), however positive association between reemployment and distancing coping exists. Similarly, Leana and Feldman (1995) found a positive association between distancing and reemployment, although those who used distancing were also more likely to be dissatisfied with their new jobs. Wanberg (1997) found a positive association between distancing and reemployment for participants who believed they had control over their situation. Saks and Ashforth (1999) found that active job search by university seniors was associated with employment upon university graduation, whereas preparatory job search was associated with future employment. The career stage at which the transition occurs may affect the impact of the antecedents on the coping process and the outcomes of the job transition both in terms of well-being and employment status.

In summary, the literature suggests personality, motivational and biographic variables are predictors of some strategies of coping with job transitions (Hanisch 1999; Kanfer et al. 2001). Job search coping activities are associated with employment outcomes, however, it is unclear how other coping strategies are related to employment and whether coping is related to quality of employment or socialization into the new job. Results of the research on coping and well-being during job transitions are inconsistent. Coping may change over the course of the job transition and perhaps with the career stage and life stage at which the transition occurs.

Case Studies of Job Transitions Across the Work-life

Four case studies are presented that represent job transitions at different passages of the work-life. Work entry represents the individual's first work experience. In the current socio-economic climate this often occurs before the individual has completed education or training and perhaps before the job seeker has clearly identified career options. Launching the vocation represents transitions to jobs that are related to long-term goals for support and work-life identity. Mid-career transitions represent changes that occur after one's work-life identity has been established, and may significantly impact that identity. Later career transitions occur as the job seeker approaches the conclusion of the work-life and may frequently involve significant changes in work-life identity or a reduced commitment to career. The four case studies are based on job seekers that were either part of our research or consulting practice. While the basic antecedents, coping issues and outcomes are representative of these job seekers, details of the cases have been changed to protect anonymity. An overview of each case is presented and then specific aspects of the case that illustrates the components of the model are highlighted.

Work Entry

Tina, a 19 year old, single Hispanic female comes to a publicly funded job search center. Tina has continued to live with her mother since dropping out of high school in the 10th grade 2 years ago. She has recently been asked by her mother, a working single parent, to find her own place and move out on her own. She wants a place of her own and has been working toward her GED. She does not have a car and her small city does not offer adequate public transportation. Although jobs are available at a freight company outside the city, she is unable to find consistent transportation to take this job. She is currently healthy but she has no health insurance. Tina is in the early stages of her work life and is facing considerable financial pressures. She approaches the job center with a friend, jovially engaging others as she looks for any and all jobs available with little focus on her own abilities and interests. She rapidly flips through the pages of a book with openings for any position. She only has a vague idea of future career development and how current employment opportunities may lead to future career opportunities. Her job search activities are diffuse and unfocused and eventually she fails to return to the center.

Antecedents
Tina has a number of resources including youth and health. She has access to training and education through the job agency. She has a close, supportive friend who will accompany her during her job transition. The absence of a potential obstacle, having children to care and provide for, also is an asset. She has obstacles associated with her social-economic class including transportation problems and lack of health insurance. She lacks job-related skills, education and experience. Her mother's unwillingness to continue to provide housing serves as both an obstacle and a demand. Her mother also provides a model of a working person who has not engaged in career planning and is still working at an entry level position. In terms of demands, she needs financial support to provide herself an adequate living situation. Tina's personality is characterized by a minimal sense of self-efficacy in her job skills or her ability to search for a job.

She is not proactive, although her extroversion and optimism appear to sustain her motivation for a time. She is high in extroversion and openness to experience and low in both neuroticism and conscientious while being intermediate in agreeableness.

Coping Issues

The quality of Tina's employment and her psychological well-being are all at stake here. She has been a waitress which fits her extroversion and ability to deal with stress but offers little opportunity for advancement. She has an opportunity to advance her socio-economic status but her problems with planning and delay of gratification stand in her way. Ideally, she will choose a career that builds on her strengths and minimizes her weaknesses.

Tina has a goal of getting a job and so uses reappraisal of goals as a coping strategy. Although she is engaging in problem focused coping, whether she will end up with a good fit in a position is questionable. Her search is arbitrary and unsystematic. Ideally, she might have finished her GED prior to the job search which then would have opened up a larger array of career possibilities. Tina's case raises questions about the quality of her coping strategy and the mixed results that her coping yields.

Outcomes

Tina failed to return to the job agency after quickly becoming discouraged in her job search. After several months of babysitting and increasing conflict and demands from her mother to move out, she moved in with a new boyfriend. Later, Tina began taking GED classes and eventually hoped to enter the work arena by becoming a licensed practical nurse.

Launching a Vocation

Wendell is a 26 year old, African-American, married, college graduate. On sponsorship from an alumnus booster of his college, he came for career counseling regarding his future vocational choice. He is well known to the local community as a "star" basketball player who has been playing in Europe and South America since his graduation from college. Recently, his wife had an affair during one of his frequent absences from home. He felt betrayed and was deeply disturbed by the "damage to his name" caused by the affair and decided that it was time to quit his basketball career (he had also had nagging injuries) and begin a new career. He wanted to be home to "keep a better eye on his son and wife." Although deeply distracted by the affair and at a loss to cope with it, he has a deep concern about giving back to his local community after growing up "in the projects and being on welfare." He and an old neighborhood friend have been talking to the alumnus booster about starting their own business.

Antecedents

Wendell's case illustrates how one transition impacts and helps create another. To cope with the threat to the integrity of his family, he feels a change in his vocation is required. Wendell has a number of resources including his community support and "fame." In terms of his personality, he is high on conscientiousness, and low in neuroticism (although his situational anxiety is quite high), whereas his extroversion, agreeableness and openness to experience are intermediate. He is an energetic person with strong leadership qualities but is also 'planful' and deliberate. In terms of obstacles, will he be able to focus on his career or will he become preoccupied with his family issues? Has he picked the right business partner? Will he be able to obtain capital to start a business? Will he be able to give up the glamour of basketball stardom to a more mundane work role? How will he deal with ending the extended adolescence that basketball has provided?

Coping Issues

There is reason to be optimistic about the quality of Wendell's occupational outcomes given his thoughtful approach of looking at his own abilities, interests, and personality to find a suitable job match. His networking skills coupled with his leadership ability suggest that he will get an opportunity to manage a business. He appears to be engaged in problem focused coping. The ambivalence he has towards his wife is very distracting and distressing for him and diverts energy from the launching of his career.

Outcomes

Wendell spent several sessions with a therapist devoted to the resolution of his marital problems prior to being able to focus on his career transition. After career exploration and with the sponsorship of the college booster, he decided to go into business with a neighborhood friend and to try to use the leadership skills that he had developed from basketball. His plan is to "make as much money as possible" in order to help his local community. The success of his business career will partially hinge upon his performance in this start up business venture.

Mid-Career

Timothy is a 43 year old, Caucasian, married male with two children at home. He started college with a major in business but left it in his 3rd year to get married and to work fulltime at an auto dealership. He is the CFO of an auto dealership owned and run by his father in a small town. His brother and sister are also in the family business. He came for career counseling when he realized that "he couldn't do it anymore." His father and brother frequently criticize him for being "too soft" in the business. He is distressed about the way he is treated by customers who relate stereotypically to him like a "used car salesman." He often feels hurt deeply by the comments of his family and customers. Feeling mismatched with his career but also feeling hopelessly trapped by his family's expectations and the monetary requirements of his family lifestyle, he tentatively approached this career transition at mid-life. The career counseling confirmed the mismatch of his abilities, interests, and personality with car sales but going back to school to train for a professional role that did fit him seemed totally unrealistic given the amount of schooling required and his family context.

Antecedents

One resource that Timothy had was the consistent support of his wife who told him "you don't have to do this" and her willingness to fight with his family in a way that Timothy was unable to assert himself. An obvious obstacle and pressure were the needs of his family of origin and the well designed script he was supposed to follow in the family business. The forcefulness of his father created an obstacle only removed by his death. Timothy's personality is high in introversion, neuroticism, agreeableness, and conscientiousness.

His openness to experience is low. His shaken self-esteem and self-confidence in himself are also issues.

Coping Issues

In a narrative sense, Timothy rewrote his script. His coping strategies included goal appraisal, avoidance, and social support (his wife providing positive social support and his family negative social support). His self care coping strategy was not adequate and gave rise to increasing levels of tension and dissatisfaction. His problem focus changed when his goal reappraisal took place. When situational change modified the obstacles he faced, he was able to engage in a creative resolution to the problem. His well being was significantly increased when he was able to deal with his job transition.

Outcomes

Timothy was unable to get unstuck from his career dilemma and grew increasingly depressed until his father died suddenly and at which point Timothy took over management of the car dealership. Timothy redesigned the dealership from its previous emphasis on marketing, merchandising, selling, and negotiating to a retail store in which each buyer was offered a fair price with no haggling or surprises and the costs of marketing were minimal allowing him to offer a low, fair price that sustained the dealership but pleased the customer. This type of dealership, later emulated by others, wasn't perfect for him but matched his abilities, interests, and personality much better and resolved his career transition. Conflict with his brother over this direction eventually led to Timothy buying out his brother's share of the business.

Late Career

Allen is a 57 year old married male with an MBA. He is a displaced executive who came into outplacement from a large manufacturing company. He was released in a company initiative to reduce the costs of North American operations. At the time of his release he was earning a large salary and was well integrated into his existing community. He felt a considerable sense of loss of work identity and faced a sizeable effort in finding fulfilling employment and maintaining the family lifestyle. He wanted to continue to work and felt he needed to work to maintain his financial plan. His family encouraged him to continue to work fearing boredom since his only hobby was golf. During his period of outplacement, he went to the ER fearing that he was having a heart attack. After medical evaluation, his personal physician concluded that he had had a panic attack. He saw a clinical psychologist for a few sessions of therapy that evolved into couples counseling.

Antecedents

Allen has a number of resources including a supportive, working wife. Outplacement and the support of his old work colleagues provided support and allowed him to contemplate his future. His personal resources were also considerable. He had knowledge of and status in the community. A barrier to significant change is the presence of his family including his grandchildren in the local community. He also had aging parents who were beginning to face possible long term care. This barrier prevented him from leaving the local community. His personality was characterized by high levels of neuroticism and conscientiousness and low levels of agreeableness and openness to change, whereas extroversion was intermediate.

Coping Issues

His strong work commitment and reliance on work for identity resulted in adjustment challenges for Allen. His commitment to career versus his ties to the existing community resulted in considerable conflict and anxiety for him. His coping strategies included venting, self-care, and goal clarification.

Outcomes

Allen's case reminds us of the impact of stress and coping on health outcomes. After several months of being unable to find a desirable position in the local area, Allen continued to reject the idea of a national search and decided that maintaining his existing family and community ties was more important to him than continuing his career. He sold his vacation home and retired to his local community. Initially, he and his wife had increased conflict, particularly around territorial and boundary issues in the home. After a period of transitional adjustment, he reported enjoying his new lifestyle. Later, he began teaching night classes in a local junior college.

Common Themes

At any point in the adult life cycle or career trajectory, coping with a job transition is affected by a complex interplay between multiple antecedent variables. The coping process involves recognition and utilization of available resources, while developing strategies to address the obstacles that are present. An individual's personality and biographic characteristics contribute to one's coping repertoire and problem-solving options. The socio-cultural context of any job transition dictates to a great extent the choices that are available to the individual in transition. As an example, the coping strategy of goal re-appraisal is affected by one's financial circumstances, the personality trait of conscientiousness, and the availability of jobs or training in the marketplace. The extent to which any person is able to make an adaptive job transition largely depends on the effective management of antecedent variables in the coping process.

In our case studies, we have elucidated factors that affect coping as they pertain to career passages in the life cycle. While there may be general tendencies in how the meaning of work changes for persons as they progress through adulthood, any job transition is dramatically affected by socio-cultural factors. For example, the change from an era in which one could expect to spend an entire career with the same company to an age of "free agent" workers impacts both younger and older individuals, albeit with differing experiences and perspectives.

For several decades, the focal work-family concern was finding care providers for children of working parents. Today's work-family issues include providing long term care for aging parents and the spillover of work into family life through electronic mail, pagers, and cellular phones. Familial responsibilities and quality of life factors now affect middle and late career job transitions in ways unknown to those making late career changes in previous generations.

As persons live longer, more individuals experience a "retirement" that includes a job. Thus, the transition to retirement may involve changing jobs rather than the adjustment to no longer working. Furthermore, increasing numbers of individuals now make a transition from retirement back to the workforce due to financial necessity or for a better quality of life.

Theories of adult development and the adult life cycle contribute to our understanding of individuals making job transitions at different points in adulthood, but they cannot account for the myriad of other factors that ultimately impact the coping for a given individual. Life stage can best be viewed as a contextual variable, but only in relation to the other individual and sociocultural features that impact a job transition.

Intervention with Job Transitions

There are opportunities for intervention at both the corporate and individual level to help manage the psychological challenges of job transition. Employees/executives may need assistance in learning the "new process of career progression" and in the need to constantly develop a "skill set," for the benefit of thinking developmentally about career assignments, and not depend on the paternalism of any given company. Employees/executives need support in being proactive in the process of moving into another position. Sometimes employees/executives need help in reading the "handwriting on the wall." The danger signs of management dissatisfaction often include not making target numbers, the arrival of a new boss or a change to a new reporting official, changes in the old management team, philosophy or direction, or changes in one's duties that require a different type of person to fulfill. More subtle signs of dissatisfaction with the employee/executive often include conflict with or withdrawal by the boss, isolation from the remainder of the executive team, lack of communication from the executive's superior, and loss of authority, power, and influence in decision-making. Unfortunately, in some companies the use of a coach is a "bad sign" in terms of the employee/executive's long-term viability. Inability to "read the tea leaves" often results in the employee/executive being completely surprised and blindsided by the meeting in which the employee/executive's boss and the human resource director offer a severance package and introduce the employee/executive to the outplacement official. Although many employees/executives prefer to wait and get a "package" (severance and outplacement benefits) rather than leave a position voluntarily, today's employee/executive must be consistently aware of their next career move.

Coaching is a venue for helping the employee/executive in transition. Coaching the unemployed employee/executive involves listening carefully for the sense of loss generated by the event and helping the employee/executive repair their battered sense of themselves and their efficacy. If an employee/executive is unable to learn from the experience, or becomes immobilized and unable to move on, the coach may have to help in the creation of legitimate defenses against the personal sense of threat (e.g., externalizing the blame). The coach also needs to listen carefully to the individual coping strategies of the employee/executive. If the coach separates "feelings" from how one "copes with feelings" a profitable discussion can often be generated. By validating feelings and helping the executive see what their intended coping strategies will produce, employees/executives can sometimes get unstuck and break a destructive pattern of search avoidance.

Consultants are often used to assist the organizational change process resulting from downsizing (e.g., Quick 1992). Charlie Klunder, PhD, a psychologist, consulted with Kelly Air Base officials when it closed. He identified gaps in the delivery system for casualties and hired transition life advisers (TLAs) to provide services. They conducted discussion groups and stress-management workshops, and helped employees individually. They referred workers to job training, financial and family counseling, and a host of other services, and then followed up with employees to make sure that they were getting the help that they needed. Kelly had positive results compared to other base closures. There were no increases in violence, no suicides once the TLA program was implemented, a decreased number of employee complaints and no litigation. The way downsizing, mergers and acquisitions are implemented may be as important as whether they occur or not (Sauter et al. 1999). Concerns about ways to address the growing human problems resulting from changes in work organization challenge the consultant. There is also concern that the financial consequences of downsizing are not necessarily positive. Employee attitudes (e.g., trust in management, loyalty) and health may suffer serious negative effects (New York Times 1996). More recently clinicians have been offering workshops for downsized workers based on dealing with the trauma of downsizing (Noer 1993). Psychologists need to be sensitive to address issues that may underlie work stress such as lack of control, as indicated by Karasek and Theorell's job strain model (Karasek and Theorell 1990). A variety of consultant roles are available to assist organizations and individuals deal with transition.

Research Directions

The effort to characterize adaptive coping with job transitions is an ongoing challenge as the majority of pertinent variables are dynamic. Individuals now tend to make more job transitions over their careers than did workers in the past (Bureau of Labor Statistics 2004), and employees are burdened with the responsibility to develop and manage their own career path and direction. The health and well being of individuals, families, and communities are affected by how effectively individuals cope with job transitions. Learning how best to help people cope with job transitions has the potential to be of great benefit. Viewing other critical issues such as physical health and other nonpsychological variables can illuminate the experience of the worker in transition (McKee-Ryan et al. 2005).

Research in this area provides important guidance to applied interventions. For coaches and consultants, knowledge about the changing demographics of the new workplace is essential in working with the displaced worker and their families. Frequently, terminations are no-fault terminations in today's market. Helping workers and families to deal with the guilt and blame associated with frequent worker displacements is a key supportive aspect of counseling. Erosion of institutional support and loyalty, force the new worker to develop a sense of career responsibility, direction, and planning independent of the company for which they are employed.

More work needs to be focused on the moderators to well-being during employment: the unemployment rate at the time of the study, the length of unemployment, benefits provided during unemployment, and differences between those leaving school and those losing jobs (McKee-Ryan et al. 2005). Learning whether there are differences in how employees from different generational cohorts (e.g., Baby Boomers, Generation X-ers, etc.) cope with job transitions, given reported differences in work values, will help inform and guide interventions (Smola and Sutton 2002). Additional factors of socioeconomic status, disability status, and race or ethnicity would give further insights into the factors influencing coping in job transition.

Research aimed at identifying high risk workers and identifying useful coping mechanisms to master unemployment experiences will prove useful to coaches, outplacement counselors, and organizational consultants. Job finding mechanisms such as outplacement agencies and job centers will continue to employ professional consultants in a variety of roles (Rudisill et al. 1992). Such mechanisms need further study to evaluate their effectiveness. Finally, in today's changing work context, such research can provide information to facilitate job transitions in such a way as to promote the health of the organization as well as the individual.

References

Aldwin, C., & Revenson, T. (1987). Does coping help? A reexamination of the relation between coping and mental health. *Journal of Personality and Social Psychology, 53*(2), 337–348.

American Management Association (2004). *AMA 2004 job outlook survey*. Retrieved April 26, 2006, from http://www.amanet.org/research/pdfs/job_outlook04.pdf

American Management Association (1997). *Job creation, job elimination, and downsizing*. http://www.amanet.org/research/archive_1998_1995.htm#1997

Aspinwall, L. G., & Taylor, S. E. (1992). Modeling cognitive adaptation: a longitudinal investigation of the impact of individual differences and coping on college adjustment and performance. *Journal of Personality and Social Psychology, 63*, 989–1003.

Bartley, M. (1994). Unemployment and ill health: Understanding the relationship. *Journal of Epidemiology and Community Health, 48*(4), 333–337.

Ben-Zur, H. (1999). The effectiveness of coping meta-strategies: Perceived efficiency, emotional correlates and cognitive performance. *Personality & Individual Differences, 26*(5), 923–939.

Blau, G. (1994). Testing a two-dimensional measure of job search behavior. *Organizational Behavior and Human Decision Processess, 59*, 288–312.

Bolger, N. (1990). Coping as a personality process: A prospective study. *Journal of Personality and Social Psychology, 59*, 525–537.

Brammer, L., & Humberger, F. (1984). *Outplacement and inplacement counseling*. Englewood Cliffs, NJ: Prentice-Hall.

Brewington, J. O., Nassar-McMillan, S. C., Flowers, C. P., & Furr, S. R. (2004). A preliminary investigation of factors associated with job loss grief. *Career Development Quarterly, 53*(1), 78–83.

Bureau of Labor Statistics (2004, July 30). *Displaced workers summary*. Retrieved April 24, 2006, from http://www.bls.gov/news.release/disp.nr0.htm

Bureau of Labor Statistics (2004, August 25). *Numbers of jobs held, labor market activity, and earnings growth among younger baby boomers: Recent results from a longitudinal survey*. Retrieved April 24, 2006, from http://www.bls.gov/nls/

Carver, C. S., & Scheier, M. F. (1999). *Stress, coping, and self-regulatory processes*. New York, NY, USA: Guilford Press.

Carver, C. S., Scheier, M. F., & Weintraub, J. K. (1989). Assessing coping strategies: A theoretically based approach. *Journal of Personality and Social Psychology, 36*, 267–283.

Claussen, B., Bjorndal, A., & Hjort, P. F. (1993). Health and re-employment in a two year follow up of long term unemployed. *Journal of Epidemiology and Community Health, 47*(1), 14–18.

Cooper, C. D., & Kurland, N. B. (2002). Telecommuting, professional isolation and employee development in public and private organizations. *Journal of Organizational Behavior, 23,* 511–532.

Costa, P. T., Jr., Somerfeld, M. R., & McCrae, R. R. (1996). Personality and coping: A reconceptualization. In M. Zeidner & N. Endler (Eds.), *Handbook of coping: Theory, research and applications* (pp. 44–61). New York: Wiley.

The downsizing of America: New York Times special report (1996). New York: Time Warner

David, J. P., & Suls, J. (1999). Coping efforts in daily life: Role of big five traits and problem appraisals. *Journal of Personality, 67,* 265–294.

Ebberwein, C. A., Krieshok, T. S., Ulven, J. C., & Prosser, E. C. (2004). Voices in transition: Lessons on career adaptability; voices in transition: Lessons on career adaptability. *Career Development Quarterly, 52*(4), 292–308.

Endler, N., & Parker, J. (1990). Multidimensional assessment of coping: A critical evaluation. *Journal of Personality and Social Psychology, 58,* 844–854.

Foner, N., & Fredrickson, G. (eds). (2004). *Not just black and white.* New York: Russell Sage Foundation.

Fugate, M., Kinicki, A. J., & Ashforth, B. E. (2004). Employability: A psycho-social construct, its dimensions, and applications. *Journal of Vocational Behavior, 65*(1), 14–38.

Gowan, M. A., Gatewoood, R. D. (1997). A model of response to the stress of involuntary job loss. *Human Resources Management Review, 7*(3): 277–298.

Gowan, M., Riordan, C. M., & Gatewood, R. (1999). Test of a model of coping with involuntary job loss following a company closing. *Journal of Applied Psychology, 84,* 75–86.

Gowing, M. K., Kraft, J. D., & Quick, J. C. (1998). *A conceptual framework for coping with the new organizational reality.* Washington, DC: American Psychological Association.

Hakim, C. (1994). *We are all self-employed: The new social contract for working in a changed world.* San Francisco: Berrett-Koehler.

Hamilton, V., Hoffman, W., Broman, C., & Rauma, D. (1993). Unemployment, distress and coping: A panel study of autoworkers. *Journal of Personality and Social Psychology, 65,* 234–247.

Hanisch, K. A. (1999). Job loss and unemployment research from 1994 to 1998: A review and recommendations for research and intervention. *Journal of Vocational Behavior, 55,* 188–220.

Harkness, A. M. B., Long, B. C., Bermbach, N., Patterson, K., Jordan, S., & Kahn, H. (2005). Talking about work stress: Discourse analysis and implications for stress interventions. *Work and Stress, 19*(2), 121–136.

Hobfoll, S. (1998). *Stress, culture and community: The psychology and philosophy of stress.* New York: Plenum.

Holmes, T., & Masauda, M. (1974). Life Changes and Susceptibility in B.S. Dohrenwend and B.P. Dohrenwend (eds.), *Stressful Life Events.* New York: John Wiley & Sons.

Holohan, C. J., Moos, R. H. & Schaefer, J. A. (1996). Coping, stress resistance, and growth: Conceptualizing adaptive functioning. In M. Zeidner & N.S. Endler (Eds.), *Handbook of Coping.* New York: Wiley.

Iversen, L., & Sobroe, S. (1988). Psychological well-being among unemployed and employed people after a company closedown: A longitudinal study. *Journal of Social Issues, 44,* 141–152.

Kahn, R. L., & Byosiere, P. (1992). Stress in organizations. In M.D. Dunnette & L.M. Hough (eds.), *Handbook of Industrial and Organizational psychology* Vol. 3 (pp. 571–651). Palo Alto, CA: Consulting Psychology Press.

Kalil (2005). Unemployment and job displacement: The impact on families and children. *Ivey Business Journal, 69*(6), 1–5

Kanfer, R., & Hulin, C. L. (1985). Individual differences in successful job searches following lay-off. *Personnel Psychology, 38*, 835–846.

Kanfer, R., Wanberg, C. R., & Kantrowitz, T. M. (2001). A personality motivational analysis and meta-analytic review. *Journal of Applied Psychology, 86*, 837–855.

Karasek, R., & Theorell, T. (1990). *Healthy work: Stress productivity and the reconstruction of working life.* New York: Wiley.

Keita, G. P., & Hurrell, J. J. (1994). *Job stress in a changing workforce: Investigating gender, diversity, and family issues.* Washington: American Psychological Association.

Kessler, R. C., Turner, J. B., & House, J. S. (1989). Unemployment, reemployment, and emotional functioning in a community sample. *American Sociological Review, 54*(4), 648–657.

Kinicki, A. J., & Latack, J. C. (1990). Explication of the construct of coping with involuntary job loss. *Journal of Vocational Behavior, 36*(3), 339–360.

Kinicki, A. J., Prussia, R. E., & McKee-Ryan, F. M. (2000). A panel study of coping with involuntary job loss. *Academy of Management Journal, 43*, 90–100.

Kossek, E. E., Lautsch, B. A., & Eaton, S. C. (2006). Telecommuting, control, and boundary management: Correlates of policy use and practice, job control, and work-family effectiveness. *Journal of Vocational Behavior, 68*(2), 347–367.

Latack, J. C., Kinicki, A. J., & Prussia, G. E. (1995). An integrative process model of coping with job loss. *Academy of Management Review, 20*(2), 311–342.

Laza, R., & Folkman, S. (1984). *Stress, appraisal, and coping.* New York: Springer.

Leana, C. R., & Feldman, D. C. (1990). Individual responses to job loss: Empirical findings from two field studies. *Human Relations, 43*, 1155–1181.

Leana, C. R., & Feldman, D. C. (1995). Finding new jobs after a plant closing: Antecedents and outcomes of the occurrence and quality of reemployment. *Human Relations, 48*, 1381–1401.

Leana, C. R., Feldman, D. C., & Tan, G. Y. (1998). Predictors of coping behavior after a layoff. *Journal of Organizational Behavior, 19*, 83–97.

Leiter, M., & Maslach, C. (2002), Beating burn-out. *Human Resource Management International Digest, 10*(1), 6–9.

Lyne, K., & Roger, D. (2000). A psychometric re-assessment of the COPE questionnaire. *Personality & Individual Differences, 29*, 321–335.

McCrae, R. R., & Costa, R. T. (1986). Personality, coping and coping effectiveness in an adult sample. *Journal of Personality, 54*, 385–405.

McKee-Ryan, F., Song, Z., Wanberg, C. R., & Kinicki, A. J. (2005). Psychological and physical well-being during unemployment: A meta-analytic study. *Journal of Applied Psychology, 90*(1), 53–76.

Mokhtarian, P.L., Salomon, I., & Choo, S. (2005). Measuring the Measurable: Why can't we agree on the numbers of telecommuters in the US. *Quality and Quantity, 39*, 423–452

Moss, D. (2005, Anniversary Issue 13). Diversifying demographics. *HR Magazine, 50*, 37–37

Noer, D. M. (1993). *Healing the wounds: Overcoming the trauma of layoffs and revitalizing downsized organizations.* San Francisco: Jossey-Bass.

Northwestern National Life Insurance Company. (1991). *Employee burnout: America's newest epidemic.* Minneapolis, MN: Author.

Prussia, G. E., Fugate, M., & Kinicki, A. J. (2001). Explication of the coping goal construct: Implications for coping and reemployment. *Journal of Applied Psychology, 86*, 1179–1190.

Quick, J. C., Cooper, C. L., Nelson, D. L., Quick, J. D., & Gavin, J. H. (2003). *Stress, health, and well-being at work.* Mahwah, NJ: Lawrence Erlbaum Associates, Publishers.

Rones, P. L., & Ilg, R. E. (1997). Trends in hours of work since the mid-1970s. *Monthly Labor Review, 120*(4), 3.

Rudisill, J. R., Painter, A. F., & Pollock, S. K. (1992). Psychological consultation to outplacement (job finding) firms. In L. VandeCreek & S. Knapp (Eds.), *Innovations in clinical practice: A source book* (Vol. 11, pp. 425–430). Sarasota, FL: Professional Resource Press.

Saks, A. M., & Ashforth, B. E. (1999). Effects of individual differences and job search behaviors on the employment status of recent university graduates. *Journal of Vocational Behavior, 54,* 335–349.

Sauter, S.L., Hurrell, J.J., Fox, H.R., Tetrick, L.E., & Barling, J. (1999). Occupational health psychology: An emerging discipline. *Industrial Health, 37,* 199–211

Schwarzer, R., Hahn, A., & Fuchs, R. (1994). *Unemployment, social resources, and mental and physical health: A three-wave study on men and women in a stressful life transition.* Washington, DC: American Psychological Association.

Schwarzer, R., & Schwarzer, C. (1996). A critical survey of coping instruments. In M. Zeidner & N. Endler (Eds.), *Handbook of coping: Theory, research and applications* (pp. 107–132). New York: Wiley.

Shapiro, A., & Kitaeff, R. (1990). Downsizing and its effect on corporate marketing research. *Marketing Research, 2*(4), 56–59.

Smola, K. W., & Sutton, C. (2002). Generational differences: Revisiting generational work values for the new millennium. *Journal of Organizational Behavior, 23,* 363–382.

Tetrick, L.E. I., & Barling, J. (Eds.). (1995). *Changing employment relations: Behavioral and social perspectives.* Washington, DC: American Psychological Association

Vinokur, A., & Caplan, R. D. (1987). Attitudes and social support: Determinants of job-seeking behavior and well-being among the unemployed. *Journal of Applied Social Psychology, 17,* 1007–1024.

Vinokur, A. D., & Schul, Y. (2002). The web of coping resources and pathways to reemployment following a job loss. *Journal of Occupational Health Psychology, 7,* 68–83.

Wanberg, C. R. (1997). Antecedents and outcomes of coping behaviors among unemployed and reemployed individuals. *Journal of Applied Psychology, 82,* 731–744.

Wanberg, C. R., Kanfer, R., & Rotundo, M. (1999). Unemployed individuals: Motives, job-search competencies, and job-search constraints as predictors of job seeking and reemployment. *Journal of Applied Psychology, 84,* 897–910.

Wanberg, C. R., Kanfer, R., & Banas, J. T. (2000). Predictors and outcomes of networking intensity among unemployed job seekers. *Journal of Applied Psychology, 85,* 491–503.

Wanberg, C., Watt, J. D., & Rumsey, D. J. (1996). Individuals without jobs: An empirical study of job-seeking behavior and reemployment. *Journal of Applied Psychology, 81,* 76–87.

Watson, D., & Hubbard, B. (1996). Adaptational style and dispositional structure: Coping in the context of the five-factor model. *Journal of Personality, 64,* 737–774.

Zeidner, M., & Endler, N.-S. (Eds.). (1996). *Handbook of Coping: Theory, research, applications.* New York: John Wiley and Sons.

Chapter 7

Transitioning into Retirement as a Stressful Life Event

Thomas F. Holcomb

Retirement can be for some a very stressful life experience. To get the idea, one needs only to witness the press conference on March 6, 2008, of Bret Farve, the Green Bay Packers quarterback who tearfully announced his retirement. It was very difficult for him to give up a career that he loved and that had lasted so long. As a matter of fact, it was so stressful that he eventually came out of retirement and played the 2008 season for the New York Jets.

Many individuals find themselves in a similar situation concerning their retirement if they really enjoyed their work and the many positive aspects of self-esteem that work brought them. Most individuals spend their early life gearing up for a career, acquiring a work ethic and becoming a contributing member of society. A great many aspects of the self are grounded in one's occupation and acquired work ethic and skills. When the time to transition from ones work life into retirement comes, it is a whole new journey of life. This chapter examines retirement as a stressful life transition in that it is a common developmental challenge faced by maturing adults and as such it brings with it many new and unique demands, challenges and opportunities.

Bossé et al. (2008) suggest that the stressfulness of retirement is both a transitional event and also a life stage or phase. In their investigation, transitional stress was assessed using a life events approach, and phase stress using a "hassles" approach. Respondents were 1,516 male participants in the "Normative Aging Study" of the Department of Veterans Affairs (Bossé et al. 2008), 45% of whom were retired. Among those retiring in the past year, respondents' own and spouses' retirement were rated the least stressful from a list of 31 possible events. Only 30% found retirement stressful. Retirement hassles were also less frequently reported and were rated less stressful than the work hassles of men still in the labor force. The only consistent predictors of both the transitional and retirement stress were poor health and family finances; personality did not predict retirement stress.

From: *Handbook of Stressful Transitions Across the Lifespan,*
Edited by: T.W. Miller, DOI 10.1007/978-1-4419-0748-6_7,
© Springer Science+Business Media, LLC 2010

Nearly one and a half million people who are due to retire over the coming year admit they feel stressed and depressed about the prospect (Bossé et al. 2008). About 40% of people who are planning to retire said they felt apprehensive about the future, while 36% said they were anxious, according to the insurance giant Prudential. Another 22% said they felt depressed about the prospect of giving up work, and 19% said they were nervous about what the future held.

At the same time, nearly a third of the people who had already retired said life was financially harder than it had been while they were working. Four out of 10 people who are due to retire in the near future said that they planned to return to work. But the research found that nearly one million pensioners who had wanted to continue working had been unable to get the job they wanted because of their age.

Far from being a chance to relax after their working life, many pensioners also found that retirement had brought other problems. About 3% of the people said that they had experienced relationship problems with their partner once they had given up work; nearly a third said that they missed being part of a team; and 17% said that they felt lonely. However, 55% said that they now enjoyed a better social life and were able to spend more time with their family. The research also found that two-thirds of the people had failed to take financial advice about retirement planning while they were still working; this rising to 75% among women.

So What Is Retirement?

Retirement has been defined by Webster (1974) as "withdrawal from work, business etc., because of age" (p. 1214). This paradigm of retirement as a withdrawal from work because of age has been etched into the cultural landscape of America for some time. This social paradigm has held a perspective that there is a single point in time-65-when a person needs to retire or should retire. This paradigm has been in existence since Social Security was established in 1935 (Kail and Cavanaugh 2004).

The twenty-first century paradigm of retirement is being forged. This new paradigm proposes that retirement is not simply a single event or point in time connected to a specific age, but that retirement is a process. This process is theorized as consisting of numerous phases. Each of these phases is unique and requires coping and adapting over time (Atchley and Barusch 2004; Schlossberg 2004).

Because of these unique phases and the multiple demands placed on the individual undergoing the retirement process, each phase can present its own transitional stressors. These stressors must be managed and they require good coping skills and flexible adaptations to master. Many of these stressors will be quite transitory and short lived. But, if the demands of retirement transitional stressors outweigh the individuals capacity to adequately cope, this can cause emotional distress and can lead to anxiety, depression and other negative feelings. Consequently, this chapter will examine this unique developmental time of life from a multi-dimensional and multifaceted perspective. To do this, several critical areas will be examined: cultural context and ageism; transitional stressors and phases of the retirement process; financial stressors and personal empowerment by de-stressors of the body, mind, spirit and heart.

Cultural Context and Ageism

How a society views age and aging is very critical to a discussion of retirement. What a society thinks is appropriate and what they expect from a certain age population has profound cultural implications. Our culture's perception of the older worker has been highly influenced by a long-standing paradigm of a specific set age for retirement. According to Atchley and Barusch (2004), age 65 is the most used age to categorize someone as old or aged. Sixty-five has been embedded as America's paradigm for retirement since Social Security was first founded in 1935. This paradigm of age 65 as old, has contributed to age bias and stereo typical beliefs about older workers. This concept of age 65 and a done work life was supported by many companies and government agencies with mandatory retirement policy set at age 65. According to Schlossberg et al. (1978) as they looked at age bias, they believed society thought that around 60 people were supposed to be old and ready to retire from work into some un-described fuzzy future. This stereotype of being put out to pasture or retiring to the front porch rocker was the paradigm that society held and believed about older workers. This was a very limiting perspective and as such could be very toxic to older individuals who could feel rejected by society and consequently question their own value and usefulness. This could be especially true for those who loved their job and wanted to continue working.

Today this paradigm of retirement age as well as that of the older worker is undergoing a genuine makeover. While age bias is still prevalent the old perceptions and stereotypes are giving way to a much more energized vibrant paradigm of the older worker and retirement in general. Individuals are coming into this younger older developmental age group-60 plus- with greater health and wellness as well as a greater and longer life expectancy (Kail and Cavanaugh 2004). Consequently this calls for a new view and a more realistic vibrant societal paradigm of this retirement age group.

Age bias has been defined as the last of the civil rights areas to receive attention. With the passage of the Discrimination in Employment Act of 1967 age could not be used as a reason for firing or not hiring an individual. This act was amended in 1978 to also include doing away with mandatory retirement. While age discrimination toward the older worker was prohibited by law there was still an age bias. But things were changing. As early as the 1980s some of the futurist writers were cautioning companies about the necessity of keeping the older worker. Toffler (1980) cautioned companies to reconsider policies on retirement and look for more flexible approaches to keep older workers employed in roles society values. Nesbit and Aburdene (1985) also were cautioning companies and organizations to take a new look at older workers because their expertise was needed.

While age bias still exists, Sklody (2007) believes that age bias towards older workers is entering its own slow phased out retirement. According to Sklody, employer attitudes are changing towards the older worker. Employers were very willing to be flexible to keep older workers employed. In his research he found 36% of employers believed age bias was declining. Statistics from Employee Benefit Research Institute (2007) seem to support this perspective. Full time employment for the 65–69 age group has had an increase from 36.4% in 1987 to a 48.9% increase in 2005 statistics. Part time workers have remained the same.

This cultural paradigm of the usefulness of the older worker is important because there is a big difference in being forced to retire because one is too old vs. being able to decide for oneself when it is time to retire. Plus some older workers may choose to keep working or work part-time. A society's paradigm of aging and retirement does make a big difference. It can have an impact on how individuals views themselves and their ability to have a meaningful retirement life.

This paradigm of the more vibrant energized younger older person has also been touted by AARP and the 76 million baby boomers who are just now beginning to hit early retirement age – age 62. Numerous advertisements are being shown on TV that portray very vibrant retirement communities. These communities feature a very wide variety of activities in which individuals can become engaged. The emphasis is on a vibrant active life style. The cultural concept of aging and what is possible is shifting and with this paradigm shift comes many more options about work, retirement, aging and life for this segment of the population. As a matter of fact, because this new orientation to retirement is occurring, Boles and Nelson (2007) have identified a wide variety of new names with which retirement has been labeled. These include: The New Retirement; Re-Firement; Re-Wirement; Rest-of-Life; The Second Half of Life; The Third Age; and Unretirement (p. 17).

Transitional Stress and Phases of Retirement

Atchley's Phases

As with other normal developmental phases, there is a certain amount of adapting to change that goes with the process of retirement. The social gerontologist, Robert Atchley has been studying retirement for many years and has developed and refined a series of phases that exemplify this specific stage of the life cycle. These phases of retirement are: pre-retirement; honeymoon; immediate retirement routine; rest and relaxation; disenchantment; re orientation; retirement routine and the transition from retirement (Atchley and Barusch 2004, pp. 258–260). These phases of retirement seem to have had wide acceptance. However, these authors caution that all these phases are not inevitable nor are they sequential but serve only as a framework to help conceptualize the fact that retirement is not a single entity but a series of phases that makes retirement a process. These phases can help shed light on all the dimensions and possibilities that are faced as one transitions into and out of this developmental stage of life. The importance of these specific phases is that they can help in organizing ideas, services and methods of helping those undergoing this transition. To reiterate, transitions are always a part of change. According to Holmes and Rahe (1967) change is stressful no matter whether it is a positive or a negative change. Consequently, each of these previously mentioned phases will be discussed and examined with regard to transitional stressors that could be faced in each of these phase of retirement.

Pre-retirement

Retirement is something that individuals think about and look forward to someday. They are not there yet but they start the process of thinking about it. They conjure up what it will be like. They may even envision and set in motion self expectancies of this future time. They may think about trips they would like to take. To help with this pre-retirement phase, workshops can be designed to allow individuals to look at all the different aspects of retirement that they will face. But the focus is on the future. In addition, when it involves the question "can you afford to retire" it may even mean more serious financial planning.

What are the stressors here? Financial matters are usually the first area that individuals think about. Will there be enough money to live comfortably? Will a comfortable lifestyle have to change significantly? What will one do with one's time? Will part-time work be available or will it be necessary to work at all? Where should one live? Should one sell their house and move into something smaller? Should one move to a new location or a retirement community? All of these things could be very stressful because they may involve some very major changes. Just thinking about some of these things may cause some individuals to be overwhelmed. But some good retirement workshops would really help individuals look at these issues and try to answer these questions for themselves. Plus they would also help delve into the emotional and psychosocial aspects of retirement which accompany such major decisions.

The Honeymoon

This is a time of excitement and new experiences. The newness of not having to go to work and be able to do whatever one wants to can be exciting. The excitement in the honeymoon phase requires that one has a positive attitude towards retirement and financial resources to enable an individual to do some of the things they desire and have looked forward to, like travel. It is a time of doing things. Eventually the excitement or enthrallment subsides.

What exactly are the stressors of this honeymoon phase? Positive stressors here could be travel. Going to new places and being out of one's routine. This could be stressful for some individuals. Even moving to a new retirement community or home and the adjustments this calls for can be very demanding. On the negative side there is always the stress of a lack of sufficient financial resources. If this is the case, there is no honeymoon. Financial distress may already have a person in the disenchantment phase.

Immediate Retirement Routine

Routines provide a sense of stability to human beings. Work or employment provided a sense of stability for what one did for 40 or more hours a week. If an individual had many other things going on in their life besides work before retirement, they probably could find other activities or causes to engage their time and attention. Such individuals could settle into a routine rather quickly. These types of routines seem to be fairly satisfying. Consequently, transition stressors here would be rather transitory and of a short duration. However, if one only had work as their major focus of their life, this transitional phase would need much more effort and work. Time would need to be spent re-creating and re-focusing on areas of enjoyment and new areas for possible engagement. Managing this phase would be much more demanding of a total makeover.

Rest and Relaxation

In comparison to the active phase of the honeymoon this phase is exemplified by low activity. Rest and relaxation is a time to not do much. It is like a long leisurely vacation. This phase is in until the individual becomes tired of relaxing and resting and begins to seek other forms of something to do. To become active again, stressful transitions here only become an issue when the individual is bored with inactivity. Then it becomes an issue of what the individual wants to do and can do; that which will bring some excitement or make a difference in their life, which will take away the boredom. The individual will need help to see that there can be too much of a good thing. Engagement in relevant activities can provide some meaning and activity into one's life. But the individual will have to make some effort and look for it.

Disenchantment

Some individuals become disenchanted as soon as the honeymoon is over. Some individuals may not have planned well for retirement. Other individuals may have created a pre-retirement picture for themselves that was terribly unrealistic. Disenchantment then can begin quite soon after retirement. Transitional stressors at this stage are mostly cognitive distortions. Consequently these stressors would require re thinking or cognitive restructuring of expectations. If one was not happy or somewhat pessimistic before retirement, retirement could not possibly make one happy. It would take lots of work to bring this attitude around. Depression and malcontent can also be present and that would require even more work. This is probably the most critical phase to help an individual recover from. Lots of work would need to be accomplished in helping the retiree find some meaning and value for themselves in their life at this time. This would only come if one would take some action and get in motion. It might even be necessary to help the individual rethink of going back to work on a part time basis. This would be especially true for those who were disenchanted because of financial stress and pressure.

Reorientation

This is a time of real soul-searching. It is a time when individuals can take stock and actively engage in real re-engineering or re-creating themselves. While this phase can come after the rest and relaxation phase or the disenchantment phase, the focus is on exploring and defining what one will do. Establishing a real routine and rewarding stable retirement can be developed. Transitional stressors here would center around having to engage in real soul-searching and taking stock of core values and defining what really gives one a sense of purpose and fulfillment. This can be very stressful because it involves risks. Risks, while stressful also have the greatest possibility for rewarding payoffs. This also could be a time to really brainstorm and try to reconnect to former hopes, dreams and real possibilities.

Retirement Routine

This is a phase where individuals have really settled into acceptance of their role in retirement. It is a time of stability and is based on individuals making good choices and decisions about themselves and their retirement. There are no transitional stressors here because the individual has made a good adjustment and has mastered the previous transitional stressors. They have stabilized their retirement with their meaning full routines. However, this does not mean that individuals can't continue to re-create themselves or seek other opportunities for extended growth or to make meaningful contributions.

Termination of Retirement

This phase according to Atchley, is transitioning into the final stages of life. Poor health, major illnesses and even disability have become the permanent focus of life at this time. Thus the retirement period is over.

Schlossberg's Phases

Schlossberg (2004) has also conceptualized the retirement transition process. According to her model there are three basic phases: moving out; moving through and moving in. Each of these transitions has certain identifiable tasks that must been mastered. She also highlights the fact that each individual is unique. While individual adjustment to retirement will be uniquely different, there is a great amount of common challenges. Slosberg has also highlighted roles, routines, relationships and assumptions as playing a part in relevant transitions of retirement.

Moving Out

The task here is letting go! To be able to transition into something new like a retired person, one has to let go and become an ex. This demands a letting go, which may or may not be easy. It is all unique to each individual. A lot has to do with how grounded and tied each individual really is to their work role, routines and relationships.

Transitional stress here comes in the form of giving up something of value. She suggests grieving and letting go. Identifying as an ex and grieving can be very exhausting but necessary to complete the disengagement process. That can be fairly depressing but working through it can help accept that this phase of one's life is over. But there is still more to come, after becoming an ex.

Moving Through

The task here is searching for the new life and new something since one let go and became an ex. The transitional stress here is what does the individual do? It is a time to search and seek. It is a time to take the time to ask lots of self searching questions. It is the time to explore new possibilities and what might be available to help the individual invest time, energy and talent. Exploration and awareness are keys to finding ones direction. But there will be uneasiness and tension because of this not knowing.

Moving In

The task here is committing to roles, relationships, routines, and assumptions about oneself and retirement. It is a time of re-engaging who and what one is. The transition stress here could be a lack of reaching this stability. If one is not comfortable and engaging in satisfying experiences that have some meaning for the individual, then more recycling of self-exploration would be necessary. Some individuals may take longer and have to search harder to eventually settled into a satisfying routine. Over time most individuals do make peace with this adjustment.

Schlossberg (2004) also categorized individuals into five paths that they undertook to get a retirement life. Retirees could fall into more than one category and could change categories as the situation demanded. These identifiers are used to highlight the process and dynamic aspect of retirement.

It reinforces the fact that retirement is a process and not a static one time phenomenon. These categories are: continuers-utilizing past skills in a modified way; adventurers-starting new ventures and skills; searchers-learning by trying a hit or miss approach to one's place; easy gliders-enjoying their easy go with the flow approach; and retreaters-get emotionally down and withdraw or give up trying and never move in (pp. 88–89).

Financial Matters

Financial planning is one of the major areas that are usually talked about with regard to one's future retirement. Without adequate financial means things can look and be bleak. Many individuals may even believe that they will never be able to afford to retire. Others may be fearful and have grave worries if they will have enough to sustain 20–30 years of retirement. According to an on-line poll by Life-Care conducted in the month of June, 2006 finances were the biggest concern at 59%.

Also, Boles and Nelson (2008) have raised questions about the old three legged stool for retirement-employer pension, social security and personal savings account as being inadequate. They propose the new model should include: employer pension, social security, personal savings, real estate and keep working. No matter if one believes they have planned well or if one has great worries about money in retirement, planning and managing this aspect of life is always necessary.

Financial stressors may indeed be tough to overcome. Some may have increased anxiety and depression as a result of worrying about this area of life. Consequently some may need some cognitive behavioral interventions to manage the emotional aspects of this state. Plus when that gets under control there is still the problem of what to do. Some individuals may need career help in looking at working part time or going back to work full time. The more skilled one's job or work has been, the greater the likelihood one can make some type of arrangement to work.

Another very critical aspect of retirement financial planning has to do with married couples. It is essential to do this financial planning together. Sometimes one spouse may handle all the money matters. However when considering retirement, it is important for couples to work collaboratively on this. Each must know all about the financial plan. Financial matters can be a genuine source of conflict especially if a tight retirement budget is involved. Working, planning, together is essential.

Personal Empowerment: Mind, Body, Heart and Spirit

One thing to remember is that while there are common challenges and transitional stressors associated with the retirement process each individual brings whatever they were with them into this transitional process of change. While there will be vast individual differences and uniqueness for each person, there are some common areas that can enhance each individual's ability to cope and manage transitional stressors more effectively. Each person can work at empowering themselves. Empowerment is a do-it-yourself job. Retirement is also a do-it-yourself venture. There are numerous things the individual can do to help cope more adequately and create a retirement that one truly desires and that can bring meaning, purpose and satisfaction to their life. Like Helen Keller said, "Life is either a grand adventure or it is nothing at all." Consequently personal empowerment areas of mind, body, heart and spirit can help act as stress busters and de-stressors (Holcomb et al. 1994).

Where Do I Go from Here?

Specific recommendations to enhance each of these potential empowerment areas for the individual are provided.

Empowering the Mind/Cognitive Components

Expectations and self-efficacy are cognitive beliefs that can help each unique individual adjust and transition into retirement. As a part of these beliefs it is imperative that the individual engages in pre-planning of the retirement process. Pre-retirement planning and planning while in retirement are both critical empowerment tools. To reiterate it is most important for couples to actively engage in pre-planning collaboratively.

Pre-retirement planning can take many forms. But the goal is to learn all that one can about retirement and the financial, emotional, psycho-social and transitional stressors and demands placed on the individual as they are experiencing this process of retirement. This seems to be especially true of married couples and their relationship, which can be stressed by being with each other 24 hrs a day. Consequently, read books, pamphlets and do Google searches. Attend pre-retirement seminars and workshops. Gather as much relevant information as possible. This would include as much information on all aspects of retirement as possible. Knowledge is power if it is put to use. Be pro-active and keep the end-the retirement process-in mind.

What pre-retirement information can do to empower the individual is what Kabossa calls "Psychological Hardiness Factors" (Kobasa 1979). These Hardiness Factors seem to help negate detrimental effects of stress. These Hardiness Factors are as follows: viewing the change as a challenge; believing in a sense of control and that individuals do have some control and influence over things that will affect them; and being committed to and involved in what they have decided to do. Consequently these seem an ideal cognitive orientation for individuals to take towards the process of retirement. An individual can view retirement as a challenge-an understanding reached from all the reading and workshop information on the emotional, psychosocial and financial challenges retirement brings. An individual can believe that it is possible to create one's own unique retirement perspective and control it. Plus an individual can make a strong commitment to accomplishing their unique retirement by following up with directed action. Thus the individual is highly engaged, committed and actively living their retirement that they created, plus is adaptable if other changes need to be made.

The idea of projecting forward with regard to future planning is something well supported by Covey (1989). In his Seven Habits of Highly Effective People he poses his very first habit as being pro-active. This implies an active orientation to one's life. In regards to retirement, being proactive means looking at that future and having a plan and goal as to what one wants and can create, rather than just letting retirement happen to one.

Covey's second habit "begin with the end in mind," also exemplifies the need for being pro-active. Planning a successful retirement demands some tough decision-making. According to Covey individuals create something twice; once in their mind and then in reality. The reality of retirement demands many tough decisions and of being an active creator and developer of the retirement one seeks. This holds true not just at the pre-retirement level but also while one is undergoing the processes of retirement. If what one is creating is not providing the meaningful experience that one desires, then one must re-create, re-design and recommit. The individual may have that power. These are indeed "Hardiness Factors." Besides planning and pre-planning it is important to each individual to keep their mind engaged in a wide variety of activities. The old saying, "the mind is a terrible thing to waste" is really true for retirees. Staying mentally alert and utilizing one's mind brings payoffs. This could mean taking classes-most states allow senior citizens 65 and older to take classes free. Also there is Elderhostel. This is a great way to learn and spend time on a college campus studying a wide variety of topics. Furthermore an individual should keep up on the latest technology. Many community colleges and universities have community or short classes that teach new computer applications and technologies. Technology will only keep developing and staying engaged with it will help to make the individual feel contemporary and up to date.

Reading and being in book clubs also can help stimulate and activate the mind, let alone meet new interesting people. Also information on every aspect of retirement is as close as the computer. Google in "retirement issues" and literally hundreds of thousand responses pop up. Lifelong learning and the engagement of the mind is a great stress buster.

Humor is also a great de-stressor and helps individuals cope (Recker 1996). Laughter helps to manage difficult times. There are many DVD seasons of such shows like Golden Girls, Seinfeld, and M*A*S*H, for example that are good for a laugh. Laughter is good medicine for the soul. Look for the humor in the retirement process and learn to laugh at incidence of growing older and other aspects of oneself. Laughter is therapeutic and helps individuals keep their perspective. Plus it is great medicine for the soul.

The mind can also be engaged in easing the transition stress and tension by learning and practicing meditation and the Relaxation Response (Benson and Klipper 2000). In addition prayer can also help because it too, is a form of meditation. The point is that the mind can ease the tension the body feels but one has to learn to use these tools.

Another key to surviving and thriving on change is the utilization of the mind in what Wonder and Donavan (1991) call the Flexibility Factor. The gist of this is that the individual should use both sides of their brain-whole brain thinking- to examine and explore aspects of retirement or any change. The left side of the brain is the rational sequential thinker while the right side is the more creative holistic thinker. These authors identify four types of thinking that relate to ones style of change: risker-very decisive about change and action oriented and impatient to gather details; relator-seeks out other individuals and gets their perception and opinions; refocuser-practical with great concentration and strongly held beliefs but can miss essential details; and reasoner-very analytical, cautious and may overplan (pp. 21–23). They suggest utilizing all four types of thinking to help the individual manage and adapt to change. This is especially important since most individuals may rely on only one pattern of thinking. Flexibility in thinking and acting can be learned. Flexibility does help the individual view things from different points of view and allows for adapting and accommodating to life and living-especially with all the transitions of retirement. Plus, since some individuals may seek to recreate or reinvent themselves in retirement, there are also creative "outside the box" possibilities if one looks for them. An interesting example of this is suggested by Zelinski (2007) in his *The Get-a-Life Tree* which is a variation of mind mapping. It does challenge the individual to brainstorm about possibilities and does provide lots to think about.

Since there may be some anxiety and depression connected to the different phases of retirement it is important for the individual to be able to utilize some cognitive behavioral techniques to help them manage and cope. A great source for this that the individual can read and get some very good tips from is the 'Feeling Good' Handbook by Burns (1999). This has been used as a self-help book with great success. It would be another great way that the mind could be utilized to help manage negative thinking and stressors.

Empowering the Body/Physical Components

Nothing ruins retirement more than poor health. There are many pro-active things individuals can do to strengthen and improve their physical well being. Good physical health helps fight the effects of stress on the individual's immune system. Exercise and nutrition are two areas that individuals can concentrate on both in retirement and more importantly in the pre-retirement phase of the process. This seems even more important when according to Lucas (2003), the first year of retirement seems to make individuals more prone to emotional and physical problems because of inactivity and a sedentary lifestyle.

Exercise is crucial to have the body functioning properly. Even small increase in exercise seems to help promote health. Walking, biking, swimming, doing water aerobics, jogging or other aerobics all can help contribute to a feeling of wellness and cardio fitness. The main thing is to get moving and keep moving. Weight gain in retirement can be a problem because of inactivity. Consequently, nutrition is also crucial. Watching what one eats can also contribute to heart and cardio health. Practice good health habits by scheduling regular doctor visits. With the high incidence of overweight Americans diabetes is on the rise as well as heart disease and high blood pressure. Plus prevention approaches with pap smears and mammograms as well as prostate screening and colonoscopies are necessary parts of practicing good health habits. Also the body can be utilized to relax the mind and stressors. This can be done through learning and practicing yoga as well as systematic relaxation. Both of these approaches engage the body and seem to provide a deep sense of relaxation and invigoration. Plus they seem to help with blood pressure control.

Empowering the Heart/Commitment, Passion and Social Relationships

Typically when the word heart is mentioned most individuals think of love and relationships. Empowering the heart is attained by both interpersonal relationships and an individual's network of friends and family. Individuals need social support systems and to feel that they belong and are bonded to others.

They also need love with this belonging according to Glasser's Choice Theory (1998) Social support and love helps individuals navigate through tough and difficult times as well as transition stressors. Man is a social being and as such the psychological need for others is a true genuine and real need that cannot be overlooked or taken for granted. Maslow (1970) also reinforces this idea and has belonging as one of mans major hierarchy of needs that must be met if the individual is to move toward self-actualization.

Erickson (1968) and his psychosocial stages of development identifies generativity vs. stagnation as a later life developmental challenge of which retirees could take full advantage. Generativity is described as seeking to be productive in a caring way. This special psychosocial time strengthens the individual if they reach out to others. Every individual can take something they love to do and have a passion for-like sports, fishing, golf or sewing and quilting and teach that love and passion to someone else. Caring is sharing. This could be a cross generational type of activity. Big Brothers and Big Sisters, community parks and recreation and Boys and Girls Clubs are always looking for volunteers just to mention a few examples. If there are individuals who have a love of reading, math or English, there are schools that could use volunteers to help teach children these or other subjects that the children are having trouble with. But caring about others and giving of time and talent is therapeutic and does strengthen the individuals' psychosocial aspects of their development.

Another unique type of sharing and caring could come from a passion an individual has with animals such as dogs or horses. Pet therapy is widely used in hospitals. Individuals and their dog could get training and then provide hours of comfort to others in the hospital. There is also equine therapy where horses are used as a therapeutic intervention with disabled children. Again this would take some training but this sharing and caring would pay dividends for all concerned.

Nothing assassinates the spirit like loneliness and isolation. Consequently this is something individuals need to really be aware of and work at. If an individual and their spouse retire and move to a new community several miles away, they will be leaving their network of friends that they may have built over a lifetime. Or for many individuals their work life may also have been their social support life. If an individual or their spouse have not had much of a social life and they are a little reluctant to meet and greet new people then it may be wise not to do to many changes all at once. Instead of choosing to move to a new retirement community or a new location right after retirement it may make more sense to wait on that move till the individual has adjusted to some of the major transitions of retirement.

Since relationships are so crucial to one's overall well being, individuals need to actively explore new possibilities for themselves. This means extending and reaching out to others. Explore where and how to meet new friends. This will take some time but look first at places that the individual may go to. Church and church groups always have aspects of fellowship connected to them. One can take part in them. Community service groups and organizations always look to recruit new members to join them. By trying many activities there will be some that will offer more promise for developing social contacts and even friendships. But the emphasis must be on reaching out and taking action. Otherwise an individual may be in what Erickson (1968) calls the psychosocial stage of stagnation.

Empowering the Spirit/Purpose and Meaning Components

The spirit of an individual is that which provides true direction and purpose to life. Retirement can have a definite power of purpose. At a very basic sense, work provided a focus and purpose that took up at least 40 h or more a week not counting the time getting ready in the morning and getting to work. Work may have also been an individual's entire life. Retirees can provide themselves a great buffer to transitional stressors by refocusing on or recreating their sense of purpose and meaning of their retirement life. Purpose and meaning may or may not have a religious focus. But the bottom line is that every individual needs to have a higher purpose than themselves to serve. What an individual values and what they stand for is critical to this. It helps as a focus for living and for directing one's time, attention and actions. The individual creates this meaning, nurtures it and grows this into something even more unique and an inner source of joy by acting upon it.

If an individual had this before retirement then it is a matter of continuing on with it. If not, then the individual would have to spend time in thoughtful exploration of things in his/her life that he/she felt had value. Meaning for life comes from a focused purpose in such life. Covey (1989) suggests imagining that the individual is at their own funeral. What would they want people to say about them? How would they want to be remembered? One thing that is true, value and meaning come from a purpose that is more than self serving or something financial. It comes from caring and being enthusiastic about life, living and engaging in activities that one chooses because they do fit with ones larger life philosophy, and values! Life is a verb and engaging in activity that is in the service of a greater good does bring a true sense of joy and a meaning to life. Retirement is an opportunity at a new life with endless possibilities. It is about the purposeful life an individual has left in their years and what they choose to create!

Personal Journaling/Reflecting

To take full advantage of developing an individual's personal empowerment skills does take thought and action. Taking time for reflection and personal inventory on the dimensions of empowerment and life is a necessary component for growth. Since there are so many transitional stressors and phases to retirement, Journaling is a great way to keep track of things. Just like a photo album holds a wide array of pictures that are a snapshot in time, so too is journaling a picture in time of one's thinking, feeling and behavior. Remember that retirement could last 15–20 years. Consequently, this journaling activity helps review the retirement process for the individual. It allows the individual to see where he/she has cognitively, affectively and behaviorlly chosen to truly create a unique retirement life!

References

Atchley, R., & Barusch, A. (2004). *Social forces and aging*. Belmont: Wadsworth.

Benson, H., & Klipper, M. (2000). *The relaxation response*. New York: HarperCollins.

Bossé, R., Aldwin, C. M., Levenson, M. R., & Workman-Daniels, K. (2008). *How stressful is retirement? Findings from the Normative Aging Study*. Boston, Massachusetts: Veterans Administration Outpatient Clinic.

Burns, D. (1999). *The feeling good handbook*. New York: Plume.

Boles, R., & Nelson, J. (2007). *What color is your parachute for retirement*. Berkeley: Ten Speed Press.

Covey, S. (1989). *The 7 habits of highly effective people*. New York: Free Press.

Erickson, E. (1968). *Identity: Youth and crisis*. New York: Norton.

Glasser, W. (1998). *Choice theory: A new psychology of personal freedom*. New York: Harper Collins.

Holcomb, T., Cheponis, G., Hazler, R., & Portner, E. (1994). *Stress busting through personal empowerment*. Muncie: Accelerated Development INC.

Holmes, T., & Rahe, R. (1967). The social readjustment rating scale. *Journal of Psychometric Research, 11*, 213–218.

HR.com-The human resources portal (2006) *Workers reveal biggest retirement concerns*. Retrieved 2/25/08 http://www.hr.com/servlets/sfs?&t = Default/gateway&i = 1116423256

Kobasa, S. (1979). Stressful life events, personality, and health: An inquiry into hardiness. *Journal of Personality and Social Psychology, 37*, 1–11.

Kail, R., & Cavanaugh, J. (2004). *Human development: A life span view* (3rd ed.). Belmont: Wadsworth

Lucas, J. (2003). *Retirement: The first year*. Alive Publishing Group. Retrieved 2/28/08 http://www.alive.com/1549a4a2.php?text_page = 2.

Maslow, A. (1970). *Motivation and personality* (2nd ed.). New York: Harper & Row

Nesbitt, J., & Aburdene, P. (1985). *Re-inventing the corporation*. New York: Warner.

Recker, N. (1996). *Laughter is really good medicine*. Retrieved 3/30/08 http://ohioline.osu.edu/hyg-fact/5000/5219.mtml

Schlossberg, N. (2004). *Retire smart retire happy*. Washington, DC: American Psychological Association

Schlossberg, N., Troll, L., & Leibowitz, Z. (1978). *Perspectives on counseling adults: Issues and skills*. Monterey: Wadsworth.

Sklody, R. (2007). *Age bias in the American workplace a "fact of life" enters its own phased retirement*. Retirement Jobs.com Research Paper

Toffler, A. (1980). *The third wave*. New York: Bantam Books.

Webster (1974). *Webster's new world dictionary* (Second College Edition) Cleveland: The World Publishing Company

Wonder, J. & Donavan, P. (1989). The Flexibility Factor: Why people who thrive on change are successful and how you can become one of them. The Doubleday Religious Publishing Group, Newyork.

Zelinski, E. (2007). *How to retire happy, wild, and free*. Berkely: Ten Speed Press.

Part III

Marriage, Family, and Sexual Life Cycle Transitions

Chapter 8

Family Transitions Following Natural and Terrorist Disaster: Hurricane Hugo and the September 11 Terrorist Attack

Disasters affect individuals, families, and entire communities. To date, the primary focus of disaster research has been on identifying the mental health consequences for individuals following natural disasters, technological disasters, and mass violence. However "...the experience (of disaster) cannot be expressed entirely in diagnoses of psychopathology" (Vlahov 2002, p. 295). An exclusive focus on individual mental health outcomes will underestimate the full psychosocial impact of a disaster for many adults, given that the consequences for adult disaster victims often unfold in the context of close relationships. The goal of this chapter is to expand the focus of disaster research by considering how disasters are related to significant family transitions. Exposure to disaster and trauma is more common than we might expect. Lifetime exposure was 22% for natural disasters (Briere and Elliott 2000) and 69% for traumatic events (e.g., combat, tragic death, automobile accident, assault; Norris 1992). Given the interdependence of married spouses (Kelley and Thibaut 1978) and the disruptive nature of disaster and trauma, we would expect these events to reverberate in people's romantic relationships.

This chapter has four goals. First, I review the literature on major stressful events and consider how they might affect family transitions. Second, I consider natural disaster and family transitions and review our study of marriage, birth, and divorce rates in South Carolina following Hurricane Hugo in 1989 (Cohan and Cole 2002). Third, I consider terrorist disaster and divorce and review our study of how the terrorist disaster of September 11, 2001 affected divorce rates in New York City (NYC) and beyond (Cohan et al. in press). (Please see the published reports for complete details.) Fourth, I discuss divorce as a function of the type of disaster.

From: *Handbook of Stressful Transitions Across the Lifespan,*
Edited by: T.W. Miller, DOI 10.1007/978-1-4419-0748-6_8,
© Springer Science+Business Media, LLC 2010

Literature Review: Stressful Events and Family Transitions

Stressful Circumstances and Marital Disruption

Research on stress and marriage shows that there are dynamic associations among stress, individual functioning, and marital functioning. The rationale for examining the stress process in marriage is derived from research indicating that in stressful times spouses are the primary sources of support and support from others does not compensate for support missing from a spouse (Brown and Harris 1978; Stroebe et al. 1996). Stress affects individual as well as interpersonal functioning. There is evidence that stress leads to negative consequences for spouses' mood, perceptions of the relationship, and relationship functioning. For example, Tesser and Beach (1998) showed that when partners reported more negative life events, they reported more depressive symptoms and lower marital satisfaction 6 months later. Three routes through which disaster might affect couples are mental health problems, marital functioning, and economic problems.

Stress and Mental Health

There is robust evidence that community-wide disasters lead to mental health problems. Mental health problems are more likely when the disaster involves more injury and death, wide-spread destruction or loss of property, disrupted social support systems, and malicious intent (Norris et al. 2001). The time course for mental health problems following a disaster is generally 1–3 years (Adams and Adams 1984; Freedy et al. 1993; Norris and Kaniasty 1996; Shore et al. 1986). In a meta-analysis of 52 studies examining the mental health consequences of natural and technological disasters, Rubonis and Bickman (1991) found that rates of psychopathology increased by 17% following a disaster compared to predisaster or control-group levels. The most common problems were anxiety, somatic complaints, alcohol problems, phobic reactions, and depression. One particular anxiety problem, posttraumatic stress disorder (PTSD), increases following natural disasters (Ironson et al. 1997; Norris 1992; Shore et al. 1986). PTSD symptoms like estrangement from others, irritability, and restricted range of affect are relevant to interpersonal functioning, because they may impede constructive communication and contribute to increased conflict.

Stress and Family Functioning

Spouses' communication behavior (i.e., resolution of marital problems, support exchanges) is the most commonly studied interpersonal process to explain the life events – marriage link. Life events may exacerbate preexisting marital conflicts or generate new ones (Christensen and Pasch 1993). Spouses' abilities to resolve a problem in their marriage have been shown to moderate the association between stress and marital adjustment such that adaptive problem-solving skills can mitigate and poorer skills can exacerbate marital distress and spouses' depressive symptoms (Cohan and Bradbury 1997; Conger et al. 1999). Stress can also interfere with the exchange of social support. When a disaster affects an entire community, support networks get disrupted. Support providers have few emotional reserves for helping others when they are trying to manage their own negative emotions. For example, spouses were less effective at soliciting and providing support to their partners when they reported more negative events (Cohan et al. 1998). Further, support providers give less help to those who express more distress (Bolger et al. 1996; Silver et al. 1990). Thus, a disaster may impair spouses' ability to get the support they need, which, in turn, may engender dissatisfaction with the relationship or conflict about the lack of support.

The limited information specific to disasters and marital functioning also shows deleterious consequences. For example, the Mount St. Helens volcano eruption was followed by increased domestic violence (Adams and Adams 1984). After Hurricane Hugo, greater injury, life threat, and financial loss predicted increased marital stress. In turn, more marital stress was related to more depressive symptoms, anxiety, and hostility (Norris and Uhl 1993), suggesting bidirectional associations between intra- and interpersonal functioning following a disaster. If we integrate the research on stress and mental health problems and marital functioning, one possible series of events linking disaster to marital outcomes is the following: a disaster can lead to a spouse feeling depressed and anxious; anxiety and depression are associated with more negative perceptions of the marriage (McLeod 1994) and deficits in marital communication (Biglan et al. 1985; Davila et al. 1997); and poorer marital quality and poorer problem-solving and social support skills are then associated with divorce (for a review, see Karney and Bradbury 1995; Pasch and Bradbury 1998).

Economic Strain and Marriage

Disasters may also affect family outcomes via economic strain. Economic strain has been shown to delay the initiation of families and hasten the breakdown of established ones. First, a dominant perspective in the sociological literature is that marriage rates shift as a function of men's employment opportunities (e.g., Easterlin 1978; Oppenheimer 1988) such that economic security facilitates the initiation of a household. When men's employment opportunities or real wages decline, they are less attractive as marriage partners, and marriage rates decline. Empirical research supports this pattern (for a review, see White and Rogers 2000). Second, fertility rates are sensitive to economic determinants similar to marriage rates. Unemployment rates and harsh economic conditions are directly related to lower fertility rates (e.g., Kelly and Cutright 1984; Rindfuss et al. 1988). Poor economic conditions can indirectly influence declines in fertility via declines in marriage rates (Kelly and Cutright 1984). Third, significant loss of income and work hours and unemployment are related to increased risk of divorce (Attewell 1999; Yeung and Hofferth 1998).

Implications for Family Transitions

Stress research indicates that marriages are vulnerable to normative and nonnormative stressors through a variety of channels. Stressful events may initiate or exacerbate processes contributing to marital instability. When spouses are taxed emotionally, marital problems increase and the quality of support exchanges decreases. Stress is associated with poorer mood and marital communication and increased domestic violence. Mood problems impede effective marital communication, and poorer marital communication and domestic violence are related to marital instability (Karney and Bradbury 1995; Pasch and Bradbury 1998; Rogge and Bradbury 1999). In addition, economic strain precedes marital instability and decreased fertility rates. Thus, stressful circumstances can be divisive and are expected to affect marriage and divorce rates in opposite directions. The literature suggests that a disaster will precipitate declines in marriage and birth rates and increases in divorce rates.

Stressful Circumstances and Marital Solidarity

On the other hand, two perspectives suggest the opposite that marital solidarity may occur after disaster. First, as the original author of attachment theory, Bowlby (1969/1982) theorized that, in response to threat, universal behavioral strategies evolved for infants to maintain proximity to their caregivers for the purpose of security, safety, and survival. Bowlby (1988) also maintained that the attachment system is active throughout the life span. Adults exhibit proximity and support seeking in response to stress that can be conceptualized as attachment behavior (Hazan and Shaver 1994). Bowlby posited that under severe threat, danger triggers efforts to be physically close to a "trusted person" (Bowlby 1969/1982, p. 207). "When sirens scream of approaching disaster, minds turn to loved ones. If they are near enough, mothers run to protect their children, and men seek their families. They huddle together and support one another through the stress…" (Hill and Hansen 1962, p. 186). In sum, attachment theory suggests that at extreme levels of danger, proximity seeking is the modal response for adults and children for physical safety and emotional comfort. Affiliation following extreme threat may translate into maintaining marital bonds by being less likely to divorce. Given the emphasis on direct threat and survival, attachment theory would predict decreases in divorces in areas directly affected by disaster and no effects for unaffected areas.

Second, terror management theory posits that reminders of mortality may increase affiliation. According to the theory, a fundamental aspect of the human condition is an existential fear of death (Pyszczynski et al. 1999; Solomon et al. 1991). In response to reminders of death, close relationships can buffer that fear through literal protection, emotional comfort, and by being symbolic of ongoing life (Mikulincer et al. 2003; Mikulincer et al. 2004). To reduce death anxiety after being primed with thoughts of death, people may be motivated to protect serious close relationships with long-term committed bonds (Mikulincer et al. 2003). Laboratory research has shown that undergraduates primed with reminders of death reported greater desire for intimacy with and greater commitment to their current partner (Florian et al. 2002; Mikulincer and Florian 2000), compromised their standards for a partner (Hirschberger et al. 2003), and sat close to others rather than alone (Wisman and Koole 2003). Similar to attachment theory, terror management theory would support the prediction that disaster would lead to an increase in marital solidarity and a decrease in divorces when the event focuses on death. However, in contrast to attachment theory, which would focus on local effects for those directly affected, terror management theory would predict affects on family transitions at large to the extent that people beyond the directly affected area are also exposed to graphic reminders of death.

A study of divorce rates and the 1995 Oklahoma City bombing provided support for the attachment and terror management perspectives applied to marriage. After the bombing, divorce rates *decreased* (1) in the 7 counties in and around Oklahoma City compared to the other 70 more geographically distant counties in Oklahoma and (2) in the 13 metropolitan Oklahoma counties compared to the nonmetropolitan ones (Nakonezny et al. 2004). The pattern of change in divorce rates showed a proximity effect as well as a metropolitan effect. Interestingly, counties geographically distant from Oklahoma City but similar in terms of metropolitan status showed a decline in divorces. This result is so striking because effects are restricted to geographic proximity with most disasters (Galea and Resnick 2005). The metropolitan effect may have occurred if residents of other metropolitan counties saw themselves as similar to those in Oklahoma City and thus felt vulnerable. In other words, though geographically distant they presumably experienced a psychological proximity to the bombing and behaved similar to people with direct exposure to the bombing.

Implications for Family Transitions

Expectations about family transitions following disaster that are derived from attachment theory and terror management theory are in the opposite direction of those from stress research. From an attachment perspective, marriage and divorce rates after disaster can be conceptualized as objective indicators of proximity seeking in response to threat, and birth rates can be viewed as an indicator of mating behavior. Considering that highly threatening circumstances should activate the attachment system and motivate people to seek or maintain proximity to an attachment figure, marriage rates should increase and divorce rates should decrease following disaster. In addition to threat, accessibility of the partner and relationship length may encourage more dating couples to transition to marriage after disaster compared to those in unaffected areas. Because dating partners are generally less accessible than married partners, disaster might motivate dating couples to marry to increase accessibility to a key attachment figure (Fraley and Shaver 1998). Increases in marriage following disaster are also likely considering that attachment-related affiliation is activated more easily when the length of the relationship is shorter, a characteristic of many dating relationships. Drawing on modern evolutionary theory (Belsky 1999; Chisolm 1993; Hazan and Zeifman 1999), birth rates following disaster should increase from premorbid levels considering that hostile environmental conditions are thought to encourage more frequent reproduction. To the extent that death and the threat of death are central to a disaster, terror management theory would also suggest that a disaster would lead to an increase in marital solidarity and a decrease in divorces.

Marriage, Birth, and Divorce Following Natural Disaster: Hurricane Hugo

Hurricane Hugo hit South Carolina on September 22, 1989 and bisected the state as it traveled northeast from the Atlantic Ocean. In the week following the class 4 storm (the maximum is 5), the 24 counties comprising the eastern half of the state received a Presidential Declaration of Disaster (Office of the Governor 1989). The economic costs were staggering. As of 1998, the Federal Emergency Management Agency ranked Hurricane Hugo fourth in natural disaster relief costs. Physical damage was estimated at over US $6 billion, approximately US $3 billion of which was unreimbursed losses. Forty percent of residences were damaged and included most of the unreimbursed losses. A year later, half of the affected counties reported lower employment compared to prestorm levels (South Carolina Governor's report 1991). The purpose of the (Cohan and Cole 2002) study was to examine how a severe stressor, Hurricane Hugo, affected three major life course transitions resulting in significant, enduring changes for individuals, couples, and families – getting married, having a baby, and getting divorced.

Sample

Using longitudinal vital statistics data across 23 years, from 1975 to 1997, we examined marriage, birth, and divorce rates for all counties in South Carolina. We compared prestorm to poststorm rates across all 46 counties collectively and between the 24 counties declared disaster sites and the 22 other counties. In the year before the hurricane (1988), there were approximately 1,900,000 citizens in the affected counties and 1,600,000 citizens in the other counties. The perspective offered by aggregate-level time series data complements other disaster research, which typically involves individual-level data gathered after the event. The prospective design provided a baseline before the hurricane against which to compare objective measures of family transitions – marriage, birth, and divorce rates – before the disaster to those after. The population data allow us to examine change in major family transitions that occur relatively infrequently in small samples.

Results and Discussion

The results showed statistically significant increases in 1990, the year following Hurricane Hugo, in all three family transitions. Moreover, these alterations were significantly more pronounced in counties directly impacted by Hugo compared to unaffected counties. During the year following Hugo, the statewide marriage rate increased by about 70 marriages per year over the baseline decline of 26 per year per 100,000 people, for a net increase of approximately 44 marriages per 100,000 people in the population ($p<0.05$). Given 1,900,00 residents in the counties declared federal disaster sites, that translates into over 800 marriages that would not have occurred in the absence of the hurricane. The predisaster decline in marriage rates resumed in 1991. Spatial dose–response analyses showed that these effects were most pronounced in the counties directly impacted by Hugo and significantly less pronounced in counties not damaged ($p<0.05$). Second, after Hurricane Hugo the predisaster downward trend in birth rates reversed to produce a significant net increase of approximately 41 births per 100,000 population members ($p<0.05$) statewide during 1990, which translates into a baby boom of approximately 780 births. Dose–response analyses examining the affected counties while controlling for birth rate changes in counties not declared disaster areas showed a significant increase in birth rates that was spatially specific to the impact of Hurricane Hugo ($p<0.01$). Thus like marriage rates, South Carolina birth rates showed a significant increase during the year following Hurricane Hugo, and the effects were significantly pronounced in all 24 counties directly affected. Third, statewide divorce rates increased significantly during the year following Hurricane Hugo ($p<0.05$). During 1990, divorce rates increased by approximately 30 per 100,000 residents before returning to basal levels in 1991. Thus roughly 570 marriages dissolved that might not have otherwise except for the hurricane. Because the processes that mediate divorce (both personal and legal) evolve over a period of months, it was interesting to find that the greatest alteration in divorce rates occurred relatively quickly, the year after the hurricane.

Dose–response analyses indicated a significantly greater increase in divorce rates among counties declared disaster areas after Hugo compared to those South Carolina counties not so declared ($p < .001$).

In sum, it appeared that a massive and destructive hurricane was the catalyst for some to take significant and relatively quick action in their personal lives that altered their life course. The increase in marriages and births supports the attachment and terror management perspectives, and the increase in divorces is consistent with the effects of mental health problems and economic strain following disasters. Another process that may capture the increase in all three outcomes is the personal growth perspective. The personal growth model of stress (Holahan and Moos 1990; Park et al. 1996) focuses on how adjustment may be *enhanced* in response to stress. According to this model, adaptive behavior enacted to cope with stressors "can create an opportunity for psychological growth" (Holahan and Moos 1990, p. 910) by stimulating coping skills, taking stock of life priorities, or enhancing personal relationships by developing problem-solving skills and exchanging support (Updegraff and Taylor 2000). Life-threatening and uncontrollable events challenge and violate the common assumption that the world is a benevolent and ordered place (Janoff-Bulman 1992). To resolve discrepancies between old assumptions that the world was safe and predictable with their new reality of danger and randomness, people are motivated to revise old schemas and establish new ones. To find meaning in the event and to establish a sense of control, survivors are motivated to reevaluate their priorities about what is important and to take action (Janoff-Bulman and Frantz 1997; Taylor 1983). Thus, the posthurricane increase in marriages and births may reflect enhanced relationship satisfaction and cohesion as a result of successful coping with a disaster. And the increase in divorce following a disaster may also reflect positive growth to the extent that the disaster crystallized one's desire to exit an abusive or dysfunctional marriage due to reevaluating one's priorities or forming new more adaptive relationships as a result of the disaster.

Divorce Following Terrorist Disaster: the September 11 Attack on New York City

The September 11 attack is a unique event in American history, similar in some ways to natural disaster and war but dissimilar in important ways. In contrast to natural disasters which have localized effects, the September 11 terrorist disaster involved the nation because it caused a large number of deaths, intimidation and fear; a threat to national security, vivid media images of death and destruction, and changes in national transportation systems. *The New York Times* (Johnson 2002) reported that most (2,654 or 88%) of the 3,025 deaths attributed to the attack were at the World Trade Center. The victims resided primarily in New York and New Jersey. Those in the family-building years between the ages of 20 and 44 were disproportionately affected.

The purpose of the (Cohan et al. in press) study was to examine how a violent man-made disaster, the September 11 terrorist attack, affected divorce rates. Our first goal was to determine if the September 11 attack had any detectable impact on divorce rates in NYC. Our second goal was to determine whether attack-related changes in divorce extended beyond NYC or whether they showed a spatial gradient that was most pronounced in the immediate vicinity of "ground zero." Our final goal was to determine whether any gradient in dissolution rates was driven primarily by spatial proximity (i.e., direct disruption of social or economic life) or by psychological proximity (i.e., perceived sense of threat). We assessed these questions by comparing pre- and post-disaster divorce rates using longitudinal population-level data in multiple counties that varied in geographic and psychological distance from NYC.

Rates of divorce can be affected by major social, political, and economic events. Major sociopolitical events such as World War II and the Vietnam War preceded an increase in divorce rates (Lipman-Blumen 1975; South 1985). Post-September 11 research has shown negative mental health consequences in NYC and across the country. One to two months after the attack, rates of probable PTSD were higher than normal in NYC (Galea et al. 2002; Schlenger et al. 2002). Depression was two times the normative rate (Galea et al. 2002), and substance use increased significantly in NYC (Vlahov et al. 2002). The prevalence of a probable PTSD diagnosis was markedly elevated in NYC but was within normal limits in other major metropolitan areas (Schlenger et al. 2002). The elevated mental health problems in NYC may have translated into increased marital distress and consequently increased marital disruption and divorce. Three national surveys conducted within weeks of September 11 showed Americans across the country felt distressed after the attack (Schlenger et al. 2002; Schuster et al. 2001; Silver et al. 2002). Consistent with the disaster literature, the three post-September 11 national surveys showed that distress increased with proximity to NYC and degree of loss. More hours of television viewing about the attacks were related to distress, suggesting that the vicarious exposure to the disaster was also potent. Although the elevated distress among Americans across the United States after September 11 did not reach clinical levels on average, it could still have an important effect on daily activities, such as decreased work productivity, avoidance of public places, and strained social relationships (Stein et al. 2004). Furthermore, considering that poor economic circumstances can hasten the breakdown of marriages, the post-September 11 job losses in NYC (Woodberry 2002) and the worst unemployment in recent times (Dillon and Schoolman 2002) could translate into post-disaster increases in divorce.

Divorce as a Function of Proximity to Disaster

Where we observe change in divorce rates and the *direction* of that change are two aspects of the spatial time series analysis that can provide insight into how the September 11 disaster affected people and their marriages. Proximity effects are the norm for natural and technological disasters such that those directly affected suffer negative consequences but those beyond do not (Galea and Resnick 2005). A disaster elsewhere is "…too far away to be tragic in any personal sense" (Bryson 1989, p. 262). But the mass violence of the September 11 attack was personal for those beyond "ground zero." That there were detectable (albeit subclinical) elevations in distress far from the site of the September 11 attack (Schlenger et al. 2002; Schuster et al. 2001; Silver et al. 2002) is remarkable in terms of disaster research and lends credence to the possibility that marriages across the country far from the direct exposure of the attacks may have been affected as well. Studies of mental health reactions to September 11 and the Oklahoma City bombing divorce study (Nakonezny et al. 2004) suggest that responses to terrorist disasters are affected by two kinds of proximity – spatial proximity and psychological proximity. Observed change may occur according to a spatially-ordered process like exposure to trauma in which there are changes in close physical proximity to the affected areas but not elsewhere, as with natural disasters. For example, mental health problems occur as a result of direct exposure and related social and economic disruptions and dissipate as one goes farther from the disaster site (Galea et al. 2002; Hanson et al. 1995).

The notion of relative risk appraisal helps to explain how psychological proximity may occur. Marshall et al. (2007) posited that relative risk appraisal may have mediated the September 11 disaster and responses to it, especially for those with indirect exposure. People tend to overestimate their risk of personal harm from rare, novel, and frightening events – characteristics of terrorism. Indirect exposure, such as through visual images of the disaster, can generate appraisals of higher risk and greater distress (Marshall et al. 2007). Perceived risk may be increased by relative proximity, perceived similarity, or a unique threat. Citizens of Los Angeles, who felt "a dark shiver of vulnerability," had a particular reason to feel at greater risk (Ness et al. 2001, p. A24). Three of the four hijacked airplanes were bound for Los Angeles. People in other urban areas with high-profile landmarks, such as the Sears Tower in Chicago, also feared attack (Yednak and Mellen 2001). Those with indirect exposure who perceive a high risk for terrorist attack may feel a psychological proximity to the World Trade Center attack that may result in similar responses as those with direct exposure and an actual degree of threat.

Sample and Hypotheses

To examine whether the September 11 terrorist attack had a significant effect on marital stability, we used a prospective longitudinal design to examine population-level vital statistics divorce data by county. We examined counties with varying degrees of spatial proximity from NYC. We examined county data for NYC, Bergen County NJ (a commuter county across from NYC), and three major counties across the country [Cook (Chicago), Los Angeles, Philadelphia]. Two records of literature suggest that the September 11 disaster will affect divorce in different directions and with different patterns. The natural disaster literature suggests that divorces will *increase* following September 11 in a pattern characterized by geographic proximity. If direct exposure explains the results, we would expect the most pronounced increases in the divorce rate in NYC, where the losses and damage were most severe, perhaps increases in Bergen County NJ, where there were less loss and damage than in NYC, and no changes in divorce rates in urban counties at greater distances that were not directly affected. On the other hand, the attachment and terrorist management theory literatures suggest that following a terrorist disaster divorces will *decrease* locally or at large, respectively. Furthermore, behavioral responses to the September 11 attack may be mediated by psychological proximity and relative risk appraisals (Marshall et al. 2007). If so, we would expect to find changes in divorce rates in locales with greater perceived risks. In this respect, Los Angeles serves as a theoretically discriminating case. Because three of the four hijacked airplanes were going to Los Angeles, the perceived risk among citizens of Los Angeles may have been greater than among those of other large urban areas that were geographically closer to the attacks, like Chicago. Put another way, the impact of September 11 on divorce rates in Los Angeles has the potential to distinguish the effects of spatial versus psychological distance on marital dissolution because those two distances are dissociated for Los Angeles but overlap for NYC and Bergen County NJ. A psychological proximity effect would be evidenced by observed changes in Los Angeles, which was indirectly involved in the attack, but not in Chicago, which was not.

Results and Discussion

Divorce rates were analyzed as in a previous study of disaster-induced changes in marital outcomes using Autoregressive Integrated Moving Average (ARIMA) time series analyses that incorporate spatial dose–response profiles (Cohan and Cole 2002). ARIMA regression models analyze the association between an outcome sequence (e.g., divorce rates over time) and a sequence of explanatory variables (e.g., the occurrence of a terrorist attack). The results are consistent with the observation that "...a disaster is more than an individual-level event, but it is also a community-level event with potential psychological consequences even for those persons who experience no direct losses (Norris 2002, p. 310)." In NYC there was a significant decrease in the rate of divorces filed in September 2001. Similarly, there was a significant decrease in divorces filed in September 2001 in Bergen, Philadelphia, and Los Angeles Counties (all $p<0.05$). There were no significant changes in divorce rates after September 2001. There were also no changes at all in Cook County (Chicago). Similar to a study of divorce following the 1995 Oklahoma City bombing, people with geographic and psychological proximity to the September 11 attack, who would have filed for divorce in September 2001 had the disaster not occurred, decided to postpone or forego a divorce. The consistency across locales in the timing and direction of the change in divorces filed lends credence to the robustness of the effect.

The effect of mass violence can move people to alter their behavior, even through indirect exposure to the disaster. The significant declines in divorce rates in NYC, Bergen County NJ, and Philadelphia are consistent with a geographic proximity effect. The significant result for Philadelphia together with the non-significant result for Chicago suggests that the impact of September 11 on divorce dissipated with spatial distance. Moreover, the non-significant result for Chicago coupled with the significant change in Los Angeles suggests there was a psychological proximity effect and that it was more nuanced than simply a metropolitan effect. The decline in divorces filed in Los Angeles County in September 2001, on the opposite side of the country from NYC, was a marked exception to a strict geographic proximity effect found with most disasters. The results suggest that a mass violence disaster can affect behavior when the exposure is vicarious and the proximity is psychological (Galea and Resnick 2005). Because three of the hijacked airplanes were going to Los Angeles, the threat of death was presumably higher for that county than a geographically closer county like Chicago. The pattern of results in the current study of mass violence corroborates an earlier study on divorce following the Oklahoma City bombing (Nakonezny et al. 2004) such that when there was specific intent to kill large numbers of people, divorces declined in areas geographically proximal as well as areas that were geographically distant but psychologically proximal. Thus vulnerability to mass violence deaths, with or without accompanying infrastructure destruction, was associated with a decrease in divorces filed, divorces that would have been filed had the September 11 attack not occurred.

Examination of monthly rates of divorces filed in the current study yielded greater precision compared to two previous studies of disaster and divorce that examined annual rates of divorces completed, with implications for refining theory (Cohan and Cole 2002; Nakonezny et al. 2004). We found a significant 1-month decline in divorces. The decline in NYC at the height of the trauma is consistent with an attachment theory interpretation. Our pattern of results is similar to Bowlby's observation that family members will stay in close proximity for "days or weeks" following a disaster because affiliation is comforting during disaster (Bowlby 1973, p. 167). Marital preservation appears to be an immediate response to mortal threat, but relaxes once the threat is less acute. Under conditions of extreme stress, uncertainty, and threat people maintain the status quo and refrain from making a major life change. Intentionally or unintentionally, humans may take quick measures to conserve resources following a severe life-threatening exogenous shock. The study also points to the power of deteriorated marriages. As massive as the September 11 disaster was, the power to preserve marriages was short-lived as it did not damp down divorces after the initial shock.

The decline in divorces in Philadelphia and Los Angeles was consistent with the terror management theory position that reminders of death can lead to actions to counter the existential fear of death. Increased commitment to a romantic partner may be one way to mitigate those fears. However, the relatively short significant decline appears more like the attachment theory idea of maintaining security and stability during the height of a crisis rather than the terror management theory idea of increased commitment, which implies a longer effect. Furthermore, the nonsignificant effect for Chicago, which was also exposed to September 11-related images of death, runs counter to the terror management theory idea that reminders of death should bolster marriages at large. It suggests that an additional dose of perceived risk was required for change in divorce behavior in locales without direct exposure. For example, Los Angeles was the destination location for three of the four airplanes and Philadelphia is relatively close to NYC and the crash of United flight 93.

Certainly, a number of important questions remain. First, it is difficult to tell from the population-level data how long the September 11 effect on divorce persisted for the people who did not file for divorce in September 2001 and whether they decided to forego divorce permanently or temporarily. Second, individual-level data are necessary to test whether the processes we posited were the mechanisms for the observed population-level declines in divorce. Alternative explanations could include urban chaos or downward social comparison (Buunk 2006; Taylor et al. 1992), such as perceiving one's distressed marriage as better than nothing compared to the young, happy families that were devastated by the disaster. Third, we conducted a number of analyses to show the results were a consequence of the September 11 terrorist attack rather than extraneous factors. However, the possibility remains with correlational data that an unexamined variable caused the results.

Divorce as a Function of the Type of Disaster

When spouses vow to stay together "for better and for worse" they are probably not anticipating that "worse" might mean the experience of a disaster. The nature of the disaster appears to contribute to whether marriages unravel. The decline in divorces following terrorist disaster (Cohan et al. in press; Nakonezny et al. 2004) contrasts the increase in divorces following natural disaster (Cohan and Cole 2002). The opposite direction of results suggests there were different dynamics for marital stability with respect to the type of disaster. Hurricane Hugo involved massive physical damage but minimal loss of human life, because the storm was predicted and people were evacuated (32 deaths in South Carolina; South Carolina Governor's 1991). When the context of the disaster involved massive destruction and the grinding stress of rebuilding, marriages were more likely to unravel. In contrast, the September 11 disaster killed approximately 3,000 people without warning by a malicious human agent. When the context of the disaster centered on death, people responded by not filing for divorce. It appears that "Goals, during crisis periods, are easily rank ordered and commonly focused upon survival or sustenance of the social system and/or individuals within it" (Lipman-Blumen 1975, p. 891). Future studies with individual-level data are necessary to identify definitively the individual or interpersonal processes that affect family transitions following disaster.

Acknowledgments: This research was supported by a grant from the National Institutes of Health (R03 HD044694-01).

References

Adams, P. R., & Adams, G. R. (1984). Mount St. Helen's ashfall: Evidence for a disaster stress reaction. *American Psychologist, 39*, 252–260.

Attewell, P. (1999). The impact of family on job displacement and recovery. *Annals of the American Academy of Political and Social Science, 562*, 66–82.

Belsky, J. (1999). Modern evolutionary theory and patterns of attachment. In J. Cassidy & P. R. Shaver (Eds.), *Handbook of attachment: Theory, research, and clinical applications* (pp. 141–161). New York: Guilford.

Biglan, A., Hops, H., Sherman, L., Friedman, L. S., Arthur, J., & Osteen, V. (1985). Problem-solving interactions of depressed women and their husbands. *Behavior Therapy, 16*, 431–451.

Bolger, N., Foster, M., Vinokur, A. D., & Ng, R. (1996). Close relationships and adjustment to a life crisis: The case of breast cancer. *Journal of Personality and Social Psychology, 70*, 283–294.

Bowlby, J. (1969/1982). *Attachment and loss: Volume 1. Attachment.* New York: Basic Books.

Bowlby, J. (1973). *Attachment and loss: Volume 2. Separation: Anxiety and anger.* New York: Basic Books.

Bowlby, J. (1988). *A secure base: Clinical applications of attachment theory.* London: Routledge.

Briere, J., & Elliott, D. (2000). Prevalence, characteristics, and long-term sequelae of natural disaster exposure in the general population. *Journal of Traumatic Stress, 13*, 661–679.

Brown, G. W., & Harris, T. (1978). *Social origins of depression*. New York: Free Press.

Bryson, B. (1989). *The lost continent: Travels in small town America*. New York: Harper & Row.

Buunk, A. P. (2006). Responses to a happily married other: The role of relationship satisfaction and social comparison orientation. *Personal Relationships, 13*, 397–409.

Chisolm, J. S. (1993). Death, hope, and sex: Life history theory and the development of reproductive strategies. *Current Anthropology, 34*, 1–24.

Christensen, A., & Pasch, L. (1993). The sequence of marital conflict: An analysis of seven phases of marital conflict in distressed and nondistressed couples. *Clinical Psychology Review, 13*, 3–14.

Cohan, C. L., & Bradbury, T. N. (1997). Negative life events, marital interaction, and the longitudinal course of newlywed marriage. *Journal of Personality and Social Psychology, 73*, 114–128.

Cohan, C. L., & Cole, S. (2002). Life course transitions and natural disaster: Marriage, birth, and divorce following Hurricane Hugo. *Journal of Family Psychology, 16*, 14–25.

Cohan, C. L., Pasch, L., & Bradbury, T. N. (1998, June). *The social support dilemma among married couples*. Poster presented at the International Conference on Personal Relationships, Saratoga Springs, NY

Cohan, C. L., Cole, S., & Schoen, R. (2009). Divorce following the September 11 terrorist attack. *Journal of Social and Personal Relationships*, 26.

Conger, R. D., Rueter, M. A., & Elder, G. H. (1999). Couple resilience to economic pressure. *Journal of Personality and Social Psychology, 76*, 54–71.

Davila, J., Bradury, T. N., Cohan, C. L., & Tochluk, S. (1997). Marital functioning and depressive symptoms: Evidence for a stress generation model. *Journal of Personality and Social Psychology, 73*, 849–861.

Dillon, N., & Schoolman, J. (2002, April 22). City can expect job losses to grow. *Daily News*, 30

Easterlin, R. A. (1978). What will 1984 be like? *Demography, 15*, 397–421.

Florian, V., Mikulincer, M., & Hirschberger, G. (2002). The anxiety-buffering function of close relationships: Evidence that relationship commitment acts as a terror management mechanism. *Journal of Personality and Social Psychology, 82*, 527–542.

Fraley, R. C., & Shaver, P. R. (1998). Airport separations: A naturalistic study of adult attachment dynamics in separating couples. *Journal of Personality and Social Psychology, 75*, 1198–1212.

Freedy, J. R., Kilpatrick, D. G., & Resnick, H. S. (1993). Natural disasters and mental health: Theory, assessment, and intervention. *Journal of Social Behavior and Personality, 8*(5), 49–103.

Galea, S., & Resnick, H. (2005). Posttraumatic stress disorder in the general population after mass terrorist incidents: Considerations about the nature of exposure. *CNS Spectrums, 10*, 107–115.

Galea, S., Ahern, J., Resnick, H., Kilpatrick, D., Bucuvalas, M., Gold, J., et al. (2002). Psychological sequelae of the September 11 terrorist attacks in New York City. *New England Journal of Medicine, 346*, 982–987.

Hanson, R. F., Kilpatrick, D. G., Freedy, J. R., & Saunders, B. E. (1995). Los Angeles County after the 1992 civil disturbances: Degree of exposure and impact on mental health. *Journal of Consulting and Clinical Psychology, 63*, 987–996.

Hazan, C., & Shaver, P. R. (1994). Attachment as an organizational framework for research on close relationships. *Psychological Inquiry, 5*, 1–22.

Hazan, C., & Zeifman, D. (1999). Pair bonds as attachments: Evaluating the evidence. In J. Cassidy & P. R. Shaver (Eds.), *Handbook of attachment: Theory, research, and clinical applications* (pp. 336–354). New York: Guilford.

Hill, R., & Hansen, D. A. (1962). Families in disaster. In G. W. Baker & D. W. Chapman (Eds.), *Man and society in disaster* (pp. 185–221). New York: Basic Books.

Hirschberger, G., Florian, V., & Mikulincer, M. (2003). Strivings for romantic intimacy following partner complaint or partner criticism: A terror management perspective. *Journal of Social and Personal Relationships, 20*, 675–687.

Holahan, C. J., & Moos, R. H. (1990). Life stressors, resistance factors, and improved psychological functioning: An extension of the stress resistance paradigm. *Journal of Personality and Social Psychology, 58*, 909–917.

Ironson, G., Wynings, C., Schneiderman, N., Baum, A., Rodriguez, M., Greenwood, D., et al. (1997). Posttraumatic stress symptoms, intrusive thoughts, loss, and immune function after Hurricane Andrew. *Psychosomatic Medicine, 59*, 128–141.

Janoff-Bulman, R. (1992). *Shattered assumptions*. New York: Free Press.

Janoff-Bulman, R., & Frantz, C. M. (1997). The impact of trauma on meaning: From meaningless world to meaningful life. In M. Power & C. R. Brewin (Eds.), *The transformation of meaning in psychological therapies* (pp. 91–106). New York: Wiley.

Johnson, K. (2002, September 8). Threats and responses: The families; in bereavement, pioneers on a lonely trail. *The New York Times*, pp. A1, A20, A21.

Karney, B. R., & Bradbury, T. N. (1995). The longitudinal course of marital quality and stability: A review of theory, method, and research. *Psychological Bulletin, 118*, 3–34.

Kelley, H. H., & Thibaut, J. W. (1978). *Interpersonal relations: A theory of interdependence*. New York: Wiley.

Kelly, W. R., & Cutright, P. (1984). Economic and other determinants of annual change in U.S. fertility: 1917 to 1976. *Social Science Research, 13*, 250–267.

Lipman-Blumen, J. (1975). A crisis framework applied to macrosociological family changes: Marriage, divorce, and occupational trends associated with World War II. *Journal of Marriage and the Family, 37*, 889–902.

Marshall, R. D., Bryant, R. A., Amsel, L., Suh, E. J., Cook, J. M., & Neria, Y. (2007). The psychology of ongoing threat: Relative risk appraisal, the September 11 attacks, and terrorism-related fears. *American Psychologist, 62*, 304–316.

McLeod, J. D. (1994). Anxiety disorders and marital quality. *Journal of Abnormal Psychology, 103*, 767–776.

Mikulincer, M., & Florian, V. (2000). Exploring individual differences in reactions to mortality salience: Does attachment style regulate terror management mechanisms? *Journal of Personality and Social Psychology, 79*, 260–273.

Mikulincer, M., Florian, V., & Hirschberger, G. (2003). The existential function of close relationships: Introducing death into the science of love. *Personality and Social Psychology Review, 7*, 20–40.

Mikulincer, M., Florian, V., & Hirschberger, G. (2004). The terror of death and the quest for love: An existential perspective on close relationships. In J. Greenberg, S. L. Koole & T. Pyszczynski (Eds.), *Handbook of experimental existential psychology* (pp. 287–304). New York: Guilford.

Nakonezny, P. A., Reddick, R., & Rodgers, J. L. (2004). Did divorces decline after the Oklahoma City bombing? *Journal of Marriage and Family, 66*, 90–100.

Ness, C., Schevitz, T., & Aguila, J. (2001, September 12). L.A. in shock—3 of the 4 crashed planes were bound for LAX. *San Francisco Chronicle*, p. A24.

Norris, F. H. (1992). Epidemiology of trauma: Frequency and impact of different potentially traumatic events on different demographic groups. *Journal of Consulting and Clinical Psychology, 60*, 409–418.

Norris, F. H. (2002). Disasters in urban context. *Journal of Urban Health, 79*, 308–314.

Norris, F. H., & Kaniasty, K. (1996). Received and perceived social support in times of stress: A test of the social support deterioration deterrence model. *Journal of Personality and Social Psychology, 71*, 498–511.

Norris, F. H., & Uhl, G. A. (1993). Chronic stress as a mediator of acute stress: The case of Hurricane Hugo. *Journal of Applied Social Psychology, 23*, 1263–1284.

Norris, F. H., Byrne, C. M., Diaz, E., & Kaniasty, K. (2001). *The range, magnitude, and duration of effects of natural and human-caused disasters: A review of the empirical literature.* Boston, MA: National Center for PTSD. Retrieved January 2, 2003 from http://www.ncptsd.org/facts/disasters

Office of the Governor. (1989). *Hurricane Hugo after action report chronology.* Columbia, SC: South Carolina Emergency Preparedness Division.

Oppenheimer, V. K. (1988). A theory of marriage timing. *American Journal of Sociology, 94,* 563–591.

Park, C. L., Cohen, L. H., & Murch, R. L. (1996). Assessment and prediction of stress-related growth. *Journal of Personality, 64,* 71–105.

Pasch, L. A., & Bradbury, T. N. (1998). Social support, conflict, and the development of marital dysfunction. *Journal of Consulting and Clinical Psychology, 66,* 219–230.

Pyszczynski, T., Greenberg, J., & Solomon, S. (1999). A dual process model of defense against conscious and unconscious death-related thoughts: An extension of terror management theory. *Psychological Review, 106,* 835–845.

Rindfuss, R. R., Morgan, S. P., & Swicegood, G. (1988). *First births in America: Changes in the timing of parenthood.* Berkeley, CA: University of California Press.

Rogge, R. D., & Bradbury, T. N. (1999). Till violence does us part: The differing roles of communication and aggression in predicting adverse marital outcomes. *Journal of Consulting and Clinical Psychology, 67,* 340–351.

Rubonis, A. V., & Bickman, L. (1991). Psychological impairment in the wake of disaster: The disaster-psychopathology relationship. *Psychological Bulletin, 109,* 384–399.

Schlenger, W. E., Caddell, J. M., Ebert, L., Jordan, B. K., Rourke, K. M., Wilson, D., et al. (2002). Psychological reactions to terrorist attacks: Findings from the National Study of Americans' Reactions to September 11. *Journal of the American Medical Association, 288,* 581–588.

Schuster, M. A., Stein, B. D., Jaycox, L. H., Collins, R. L., Marshall, G. N., Elliott, M. N., et al. (2001). A national survey of stress reactions after the September 11, 2001, terrorist attacks. *New England Journal of Medicine, 345,* 1507–1512.

Shore, J. H., Tatum, E. L., & Vollmer, W. M. (1986). Psychiatric reactions to disaster: The Mount St. Helen's experience. *American Journal of Psychiatry, 143,* 590–595.

Silver, R. C., Wortman, C. B., & Crofton, C. (1990). The role of coping in support provision: The self-presentational dilemma of victims of life crises. In B. S. Sarason, I. G. Sarason & G. R. Pierce (Eds.), *Social support: An interactional view* (pp. 397–426). New York: Wiley.

Silver, R. C., Holman, E. A., McIntosh, D. N., Poulin, M., & Gil-Rivas, V. (2002). Nationwide longitudinal study of psychological responses to September 11. *Journal of the American Medical Association, 288,* 1235–1244.

Solomon, S., Greenberg, J., & Pyszcynski, T. (1991). A terror management theory of social behavior: The psychological functions of self esteem and cultural worldviews. In L. Berkowitz (Ed.), *Advances in experimental social psychology* (Vol. 24, pp. 93–159). New York: Academic.

South, S. J. (1985). Economic conditions and the divorce rate: A time-series analysis of the postwar United States. *Journal of Marriage and the Family, 47,* 31–41.

South Carolina Governor's Office (1991). *An analysis of the damage and effects of Hurricane Hugo and status of recovery one year later.* Division of Intergovernmental Relations.

Stein, B. D., Elliott, M. N., Jaycox, L. H., Collins, R. L., Berry, S. H., Klein, D. J., et al. (2004). A national longitudinal study of the psychological consequences of the September 11, 2001 terrorist attacks: Reactions, impairment, and help-seeking. *Psychiatry, 67,* 105–117.

Stroebe, W., Stroebe, M., Abakoumkin, G., & Schut, H. (1996). The role of loneliness and social support in adjustment to loss: A test of attachment versus stress theory. *Journal of Personality and Social Psychology, 70,* 1241–1249.

Taylor, S. E. (1983). Adjustment to threatening events: A theory of cognitive adaptation. *American Psychologist, 38,* 1161–1173.

Taylor, S. E., Buunk, B. P., Collins, R. L., & Reed, G. M. (1992). Social comparison and affiliation under threat. In L. Montada, S. Filipp & M. J. Lerner (Eds.), *Life crises and experiences of loss in adulthood* (pp. 213–227). Hillsdale, NJ: Lawrence Erlbaum.

Tesser, A., & Beach, S. R. H. (1998). Life events, relationship quality, and depression: An investigation of judgment discontinuity in vivo. *Journal of Personality and Social Psychology, 74,* 36–52.

Updegraff, J. A., & Taylor, S. E. (2000). From vulnerability to growth: Positive and negative effects of stressful life events. In J. H. Harvey & E. D. Miller (Eds.), *Loss and trauma: General and close relationship perspectives* (pp. 3–28). Philadelphia, PA: Brunner-Routledge.

Vlahov, D. (2002). Urban disaster: A population perspective. *Journal of Urban Health, 79,* 295.

Vlahov, D., Galea, S., Resnick, H., Ahern, J., Boscarino, J. A., Bucuvalas, M., et al. (2002). Increased use of cigarettes, alcohol, and marijuana among Manhattan, New York, residents after the September 11th terrorist attacks. *American Journal of Epidemiology, 155,* 988–996.

White, L., & Rogers, S. J. (2000). Economic circumstances and family outcomes: A review of the 1990s. *Journal of Marriage and the Family, 62,* 1035–1051.

Wisman, A., & Koole, S. L. (2003). Hiding in the crowd: Can mortality salience promote affiliation with other who oppose one's worldviews? *Journal of Personality and Social Psychology, 84,* 511–526.

Woodberry, W. (2002, April 25). No 9/11 aid for 9,000 who lost aviation jobs. *Daily News,* 6.

Yednak, C., & Mellen, K. (2001, September 12). Chicago's high-rise landmarks take security precautions, *Chicago Tribune,* 14.

Yeung, W. J., & Hofferth, S. L. (1998). Family adaptations to income and job loss in the U.S. *Journal of Family and Economic Issues, 19,* 255–283.

Chapter 9

The Transition to Adoptive Parenthood[*]

Abbie E. Goldberg

The Transition to Adoptive Parenthood as a Stressful Life Event

The Transition to Parenthood as a Stressful Life Event

The transition to parenthood is generally regarded as a major life event that necessitates change and readjustment on the part of individuals and couples in order to negotiate a successful transition (Belsky et al. 1985). Specifically, the dyadic (couple) unit must evolve from a two-person to a three-person system; in turn, partners must expand their repertoire of roles to include that of a parent. New parents experience change and reorganization in many aspects of their lives, which can produce both rewards and stresses. While parenthood is experienced as a valued and desirable role by many (Landridge et al. 2000), the transition to parenthood is often associated with emotional and physical fatigue, increased strain between work and family responsibilities, and compromised well-being (Ballard et al. 1994; Costigan et al. 2003; and Schulz et al. 2004). The addition of a child can also result in at least temporary declines in marital intimacy and communication, which arise from the drains on couples' psychological, emotional, physical, and material resources that accompany this transition (Demo and Cox 2000; Pacey 2004). Indeed, studies of both heterosexual (Belsky and Rovine 1990) and lesbian (Goldberg and Sayer 2006) couples during the transition to parenthood have documented declines in relationship quality and increases in relationship conflict. While not all couples experience deterioration in their relationship quality (Belsky and Rovine 1990) and some couples recover relatively quickly, others experience persistent relationship instability, which in turn poses risk to child and family adjustment (Pacey 2004).

There are a number of factors that may mitigate the stress associated with the transition to parenthood. For example, possession of psychological resources

---

[*] In this chapter, the term "couples" is used, given that much of the transition to parenthood literature focuses on couples, specifically. However, much of what is discussed also applies to *individuals* who adopt children (i.e., in the absence of a partner).

From: *Handbook of Stressful Transitions Across the Lifespan,*
Edited by: T.W. Miller, DOI 10.1007/978-1-4419-0748-6_9,
© Springer Science+Business Media, LLC 2010

(such as positive well-being and high self-esteem prior to parenthood) can help to buffer the stress associated with this significant life change (Beck 2001; Hyde et al. 1995). Many studies have also established that the availability of social resources (e.g., support from friends and family) can play a key role in minimizing the stress associated with this transition (Beck 2001; Semyr et al. 2004). In particular, the role of supportive and stable intimate relationships has been emphasized as a protective guard against declines in well-being (Marks et al. 1996; Semyr et al. 2004).

The Transition to Adoptive Parenthood

The transition to parenthood literature has often focused on middle-class heterosexual couples (e.g., Belsky and Pensky 1988; Cowan and Cowan 1988). Further, the vast majority of this literature is concerned with the transition to *biological* parenthood. Thus, the current chapter focuses on aspects of the transition to parenthood for *adoptive* couples.[1] The process of becoming adoptive parents is in many ways far more multidimensional and complex than is the transition to biological parenthood (Weir 2003). Couples who seek to adopt face additional, unique challenges and stresses that may have implications for their transition to parenthood and for family functioning and adjustment over time. And yet, despite theoretical awareness of the unique concerns of adopting couples, little empirical work has explored aspects of their transition to parenthood (although notably, a reasonably large literature on adoptive parent families in general exists: e.g., Brodzinsky 1987; Miller et al. 2000).

Adoptive couples' trajectory to parenthood differs in important ways from that of biological parents. First, couples often arrive at adoption after spending months and even years trying to conceive. Further, upon deciding to adopt, couples must engage in complex decision-making about a range of factors, including what type of adoption they wish to pursue, how much money they are willing to spend, and their willingness to adopt a child of a different race and/or with special needs. Then, after a period of intensive scrutiny via the "home study" (an in-depth examination of the adoptive parents and the home environment that is required of all adoptive parents), hopeful parents may wait for months or even years before adopting. In contrast to the expectancy phase for biological parents-to-be (i.e., pregnancy), the waiting period is not culturally recognized, resulting in isolation for many adoptive parents (Daly 1989a, b). Adoption, in general, is not widely understood; thus, pre-adoptive and adoptive parents often must educate friends, family, acquaintances, and strangers about the adoption process and adoption-related issues both before and after they adopt. Finally, lesbian and gay couples, as well as couples who adopt transracially, often encounter additional unique challenges in the pre-adoptive phase and beyond. Specifically, same-sex couples must contend with societal heterosexism (in the form of legal barriers and agency unwillingness to work with lesbian, gay, bisexual, and transgendered clients), and couples that adopt transracially often encounter racism in their families and communities as they "step out" as multiracial families.

Next, the unique aspects that characterize the transition to adoptive parenthood will be discussed (e.g., conception-related difficulties; the complex decision-making process regarding adoption). Of note is that in this chapter, special effort is made to address the unique experiences and concerns of lesbian, gay, and bisexual adoptive parents. The number of children being raised by one or more gay parents has steadily risen, and it is estimated that a quarter-million children are currently living in households headed by the same-sex couples. Further, of these, 4.2% are either adopted or foster children, almost double the figure for heterosexual couples (Gates and Ost 2004). Gay parent adoption serves an important role in society in that it reduces the number of children without homes and provides lesbians and gay men with an opportunity to become parents (Brooks and Goldberg 2001). Recognizing this, adoption agencies and services are increasingly accepting and inclusive of gay/lesbian adopters (Brooks et al. 2005). And yet, despite these trends, only a small body of research has explored the experiences of gay and lesbian adoptive parents (Kindle and Erich 2005; Matthews and Cramer 2006; Shelley-Sireci and Ciano-Boyce 2002) and *no* research known to date has explored sexual minorities' transition to adoptive parenthood.

Infertility and Conception-Related Problems

Most (heterosexual) couples ultimately adopt because of a history of conception-related difficulties (Bausch 2006; Cudmore 2005). Infertility is linked to increased stress, decreased self-efficacy, decreased life satisfaction, compromised self-esteem, increased marital conflict, and negative perceptions of marital communication and intimacy, particularly among women (Abbey et al. 1991, 1992; Andrews et al. 1992; Brodzinsky and Huffman 1988; Daniluk and Hurtig-Mitchell 2003). Infertile individuals often report feeling inadequate and damaged, and the infertility problem has a negative influence on men's and women's sense of their own masculinity and femininity, respectively: Women feel "hollow" and men feel as though they are "shooting blanks" (Abbey et al. 1991). In turn, diminished self-esteem, feelings of inadequacy, and poor body image can have a negative impact on marital communication and intimacy (Abbey et al. 1991). Further, repeated and ongoing participation in medical procedures designed to identify the cause of or to treat infertility may cause distress (Daniluk 2001), and the hormonal medications commonly prescribed to stimulate ovulation often exacerbate mood instability (Daniluk and Fluker 1995). There is evidence that experience with assisted reproduction and fertility treatment is not limited to heterosexual couples. For example, Shelley-Sireci and Ciano-Boyce (2002) compared lesbian and heterosexual adoptive parents on basic family characteristics and found that regardless of sexual orientation, about 65% of parents had attempted the use of assisted reproduction at some point. Further, clinical and anecdotal evidence suggests that lesbians who are unsuccessful in conceiving may experience feelings of loss and grief that are similar to those experienced by heterosexual couples, and, in particular, heterosexual women (e.g., Jacob 1997). Indeed, the grief of not being able to produce a child tends to be shared by both men and women in heterosexual couples but is often more intense for women (Daniluk and Hurtig-Mitchell 2003).

Couples who are unable to conceive are strongly encouraged to engage in a period of mourning prior to pursuing adoption actively. However, there is evidence that many couples who seek to adopt are still in crisis at the time of their application (Cudmore 2005; Santona and Zavattini 2005). The feelings of helplessness and hopelessness associated with infertility may be alleviated somewhat, as couples cease what can seem to be a fruitless process and instead begin a journey that apparently holds greater promise in bringing them closer to parenthood. At the same time, arriving at the decision to pursue adoptive parenthood can be challenging too, as couples work to relinquish fully their long-time wish of a biological child. Additionally, once couples have begun the adoption process, they may find that it does not always proceed as easily and smoothly as imagined. Couples may find that adoption agencies, like medical professionals, usually cannot provide the easy answers or speedy solutions for which they long. Like the process of trying to conceive, the adoption process is filled with uncertainties and can seem to stretch on forever (Daly 1989a, b). In turn, both adoption and infertility can engender feelings of powerlessness and lack of control in couples (Daly 1989a; Daniluk and Hurtig-Mitchell 2003). Furthermore, the experience of being "pregnant without a due date" (Sandelowski et al. 1991) can be isolating and frustrating: Prospective adoptive couples prepare to become parents without the social recognition and validation that pregnant couples receive. They may feel isolated and estranged from their peer group, in that many of their friends may have already had biological children (Daly 1989a; Weir 2003) and may feel hesitant about sharing their worries specific to parenting an adoptive child, such as fears about bonding, fears about their ability to love a biologically unrelated child, and concerns about being judged and/or on display as an adoptive parent (Farber et al. 2003).

Complex Decision-Making

Choosing an Adoption Path

After working through the grief and loss associated with infertility and coming to terms with the fact that they may never have a biological child, couples that ultimately seek to adopt must engage in a series of complex decisions. These decisions appear in Table 9-1, which summarizes pre-parenthood and post-parenthood "tasks" for biological parent, adoptive parent, transracial adoptive parent, and gay/lesbian adoptive parent families. One of the first major decisions that couples face is what *type of adoption* to pursue. Couples must weigh their goal of becoming a parent quickly and easily with the need to be realistic about the level and type of child-related problems that they are willing and able to take on. Additionally, they may consider financial constraints: For example, many couples have exhausted significant financial resources in their attempts to become pregnant and therefore, arrive at adoption with very little money to spare. Thus, a variety of factors may be influential in couples' decision-making about what type of adoption to choose.

The major types of adoption are international adoption, public domestic adoption (through the foster care or child welfare system), and private domestic adoption (e.g., through a lawyer or agency). Private domestic adoptions, in turn, may be either "open" or "closed." Open adoption (which is increasingly common in U.S. private domestic adoptions and now represents the norm rather than the exception) refers to a continuum of openness that allows birth parents and adoptive parents to have information about and to communicate with each other before and/or after placement of the child. Contact may vary in form (e.g., information, pictures, phone calls, letters, in-person visits) as well as in frequency and duration (Brooks et al. 2005). In open adoptions, the birth mother or birth parent often chooses the adoptive parents. In all cases, the birth parents legally relinquish all parental rights to the child, and the adoptive parents are the child's legal parents. Closed adoptions, on the other hand, refer to arrangements in which the birth parents and adoptive parents do not exchange

Table 9-1. The transition to parenthood: tasks for biological, adoptive, transracial adoptive, and gay/lesbian adoptive parents.

	Biological parents	Adoptive parents	Transracial adoptive parents	Gay/lesbian adoptive parents
Pre-parenthood tasks	Attend prenatal appointments	Mourn infertility; turn towards adoption	Mourn infertility; turn towards adoption	(Mourn infertility); turn towards adoption
	Make birth plan	Choose adoption path	Choose adoption path	Choose adoption path, *weighing implications of being "out" for each one*
		Choose adoption agency	Choose adoption agency	Choose adoption agency, *with eye towards evidence of comfort w/GL adopters*
		Complete home study	Complete home study	Complete home study, *possibly as single heterosexual parent*
		Attend pre-adoption classes and trainings	Attend pre-adoption classes + trainings, *attend trainings and read materials on TRA*	Attend pre-adoption classes + trainings
		Make decisions about preferred child characteristics	Make decisions about preferred child characteristics; *talk to family/ friends about TRA*	Make decisions about preferred child characteristics
		Negotiate feelings/preferences about birth parent contact (if open)	Negotiate feelings/preferences about birth parent contact (if open)	Negotiate feelings/preferences about birth parent contact (if open)
Transitional tasks	Physical recovery	Travel (for international and some domestic)	Travel (for international and some domestic)	Travel (for international and some domestic)
	Breastfeeding	Negotiate relationship with birth parent(s), if open	Negotiate relationship with birth parent(s), if open	Negotiate relationship with birth parent(s), if open
	Bonding	Bonding, *sensitive to how child risk factors might impact bonding*	Bonding, *sensitive to how child risk factors might impact bonding*	Bonding, *sensitive to how child risk factors might impact bonding*
	Fatigue	Fatigue	Fatigue	Fatigue
	Financial concerns	Financial concerns	Financial concerns	Financial concerns
	Child care planning	Child care planning	Child care planning	Child care planning
	Balance work and family	Balance work and family	Balance work and family	Balance work and family
	Maintain communication w/partner	Maintain communication w/partner	Maintain communication w/partner	Maintain communication w/partner
	Meet personal needs	Meet personal needs	Meet personal needs	Meet personal needs
		Finalize adoption	Finalize adoption	Finalize adoption; *Complete legal paperwork to protect second parent if did not coadopt*
		Educate family/friends about adoption	Educate family/friends about adoption, *with attention to race/culture*	Educate family/friends about adoption

TRA = transracial adoption

identifying information and there is no contact whatsoever between the birth parents and the adoptive parents or the child.

Couples may choose private domestic open adoption because they are attracted to the possibility of maintaining contact with birth parents and/or being able to provide their child with information (possibly ongoing) about their birth parent(s) (Goldberg et al. 2007; Haugaard et al. 2000; Siegel 1993). They may also be drawn to open adoption because of the greater likelihood of adopting an infant compared to international or public domestic adoption (Goldberg et al. 2007). Further, there is some evidence that lesbians and gay men may be drawn to open adoption specifically, because the philosophy of open adoption fits with their desire to be "out" and honest about their sexual orientation and relationship status during the adoption process. That is, they choose open adoption because they do not wish to closet themselves and pose as single (heterosexual) parents, which is necessary to adopt internationally (Goldberg et al. 2007).

Many prospective adoptive parents select international adoption to avoid the long wait associated with domestic private adoptions of healthy infants (Grotevant et al. 2000; Hollingsworth and Ruffin 2002). Some gay and lesbian prospective parents are particularly drawn to international adoption for this reason: Indeed, they suspect that birth mothers are unlikely to choose a gay couple and therefore, they will end up waiting "forever" (Goldberg et al. 2007). Such concerns are not unrealistic. Research suggests that birth parents may specifically protest the placement of their child with gay/lesbian parents (Downs and James 2006). On a more general level, some couples are drawn to adoption because of their desire for a confidential adoption. They do not wish to have contact with the birth parents and may wish to raise the child as if they had been born to them biologically (Hollingsworth and Ruffin 2002). Relatedly, couples may choose international adoption because of concerns about negotiating birth parent relationships (e.g., they harbor fears that birth parents will try to "steal" their children back) and/or they worry that birth parent relationships will create confusion for their children (Daly 1988; Haugaard et al. 2000; and Siegel 1993). Also, some men and women report choosing international adoption because of a special relationship with a country: For example, some couples seek to adopt from a particular country because they have family members that are from that country and/or they have personally lived in that country (Goldberg 2009).

Couples who adopt through the public welfare system are often, in part, motivated by finances. Barth et al. (1995), for example, found that parents who adopted children through public agencies tended to have lower incomes than parents who adopted through private agencies. Indeed, adoptions through the public sector typically range from $0 to $2,500, whereas the cost of private domestic adoptions ranges from $5,000 to $40,000 and the cost of international (intercountry) adoption ranges from approximately $7,000 to $30,000 (Child Welfare Information 2004). Also, some men and women pursue public adoption out of social or community concerns: They are concerned about the number of children without permanent homes and wish to give a child a permanent family (Cole 2005). Such altruistic motivations are also common among people who seek to foster but not necessarily adopt (Cole 2005; Rodger et al. 2006). Finally, some men and women that pursue public adoption do so out of a desire to adopt an older child, specifically.

Path-Specific Stresses

There are a number of unique stresses that characterize each of these paths to adoption. Couples who pursue open adoption may experience strong feelings of helplessness and fears of rejection, insofar as they must wait for a birth mother to choose them (Sandelowski et al. 1991). For example, birth mothers are often cast as even more powerful than adoption agencies in determining waiting couples' "fate" (Goldberg et al. 2007; Sandelowski et al. 1991). Couples who pursue open adoption also may experience intermittent or ongoing anxieties about negotiating the level of openness that will characterize their future interactions with birth parents (Mendenhall et al. 1996). They may also meet resistance from family members, friends, and coworkers regarding their choice to seek an open adoption. Open adoption is a relatively new phenomenon and one which is not broadly understood. For example, one study of community attitudes regarding open adoption found that many people believe that adoption will create conflict between two sets of parents and will confuse the adopted child (Miall 1998).

In some ways, international adoption is characterized by a more clear and certain path, in that families participate in a home study and then, after a period of waiting, receive a referral for a child. At this point, many families travel overseas to visit with the child that they will adopt before the actual adoption (which can occur after several or many months). However, the waiting period can be equally as indeterminate, and feelings of helplessness and lack of control may be compounded by the fact that the ease of adoption proceedings are, in part, determined by the (changing) laws and policies of other countries' governments. Specifically, couples who seek to adopt internationally must consider the possibility that political unrest, national or governmental crises, and/or governmental policy changes might interfere with their adoption plans.

Finally, couples and individuals who adopt through the public sector encounter other unique challenges and concerns. For example, they may experience frustration with what they perceive as disorganized, inefficient, or slow social service agencies. Additionally, they may worry about the possibility of adopting a child whose emotional/behavioral problems are too severe for them to handle, and they may experience (realistic) concerns about attachment-related challenges. Alternatively, they may hold (unrealistic) expectations about their future child's adjustment, believing that "if we just love him/her enough, everything will be fine." Violation of idealized expectations can have negative consequences for family stability and may result in disruption of the adoptive placement (Brodzinsky and Pinderhughes 2002).

Choosing an Agency/Lawyer

Upon settling on a route to parenthood, couples must then choose an *agency*. While this process is somewhat straightforward for heterosexual couples, it can be challenging and time-consuming for gay/lesbian couples. Because of their vulnerability in the adoption process, it is not surprising that many lesbians and gay men expend significant time and effort researching potential adoption agencies (Goldberg et al. 2007). In selecting an agency, a primary consideration for many lesbians and gay men is the perceived gay-friendliness of the agency. That is, does the agency's materials (website, offices, printed materials) contain images of the same-sex couples? Does the agency explicitly state their openness to working with lesbians and gay men (i.e., in their materials, on their website, in their mission statement)? Are staff members friendly and respectful in initial in-person and telephone interactions? Does the agency have specialized support groups or services for gay/lesbian adoptive parents and prospective parents? Does the agency actively engage with and recruit from the gay/lesbian community? Agencies that receive high marks in these categories are perceived as gay-friendly and thus more likely to be selected by lesbians and gay men (Goldberg et al. 2007).

Sometimes gay/lesbian couples choose agencies that they believe will be accepting and affirming, but ultimately face (often subtle) forms of heterosexism further into the process. For example, gay and lesbian couples often encounter forms, materials, and support groups that seem to focus on heterosexual couples only (e.g., they presume infertility) (Goldberg 2009; Matthews and Cramer 2006). They may also confront specific adoption workers who seem to hold discriminatory stereotypes and attitudes towards gay men and lesbians (e.g., workers who seem to presume that lesbians are "anti-men": Hicks 2000). Although such treatment can be upsetting, gay and lesbian couples may choose to stay silent about their feelings so as not to "make waves" in that their goal is often to adopt as quickly and easily as possible.

Of course, some lesbians and gay men are limited by financial resources and geographic location, such that they have few choices with regard to adoption agencies. Indeed, in many states, gay/lesbian couples are *not* allowed to jointly legally adopt (a fact which will be returned to later). Thus, they may remain closeted throughout the adoption process (e.g., one partner poses as a single heterosexual adopter) for fear of jeopardizing their chances of adopting (Downs and James 2006; Mallon 2004). At times, this is in response to an informal "don't ask, don't tell" policy that appears to be operating at the agency level (Downs and James 2006; Goldberg et al. 2007; Matthews and Cramer 2006). While the hiding of one's sexual orientation may be experienced as a necessary and possibly successful coping strategy, it is not ideal. For example, closeting may contribute to poor psychological and physical health (Cole 2006), and it inhibits the development of a meaningful and supportive relationship between the adoptive parents and the agency.

Deciding on Child-Related Characteristics

Prospective adoptive parents must think carefully about the *child-related characteristics* that they feel capable of and willing to take on as an adoptive parent. Issues concerning the health of the child warrant serious consideration. For example, prospective adoptive parents are asked to consider the level of risk that they are willing to consider with respect to prenatal drug and alcohol exposure. Additionally, for individuals and couples who are adopting older children either domestically or internationally, applicants must consider whether they are open to adopting a child with known emotional or physical handicaps, and, if so, what level and types of difficulties they feel that they can manage. Prospective parents who are unrealistic about the demands of parenting a child with special needs (e.g., an older child; a child with a significant abuse history) are vulnerable to poorer adjustment and greater stress in the post-adoption phase; thus, realistic inventory of one's strengths and limitations is important (Brooks et al. 2005). Importantly, gay and lesbian prospective adopters sometimes report feeling that they are *expected* to be more open to special needs or hard-to-place children (e.g., children with emotional/behavioral problems; older children; sibling groups) and may wonder whether agencies that push high-risk children on them are engaging in a practice of attempting to match the *least desirable* applicants with the *least desirable* children (Goldberg et al. 2007; Matthews and Cramer 2006). Should gay prospective adopters give in to real or perceived pressures to adopt a child whose characteristics lie outside of their comfort zone, they may be placing themselves, and the adoption, at risk.

Additionally, couples must think critically about the *race* of the child whom they are willing to adopt. There is some evidence that the same-sex couples are more likely to adopt transracially than heterosexual couples, at least with regard to international adoption (Gates et al. 2007; Shelley-Sireci and Ciano-Boyce 2002). In a study of lesbian and heterosexual pre-adoptive couples, Goldberg (2009) explored: (1) whether there were different rates of willingness to adopt transracially in the two groups; and (2) couples' explanations for why they were willing or unwilling to adopt transracially. Lesbians were significantly more likely to be willing to adopt transracially than heterosexual couples. Lesbian and heterosexual couples cited the following reasons for being open: they lived in a racially diverse community (and therefore, they felt that they could provide an environment that supported and reflected their child's race/ethnicity); their families and/or friendship networks were racially diverse; and they perceived their family members as supportive (i.e., not racist) and were confident that their families would accept and love a family member that was racially different. Some lesbian partners also felt that it would not be fair to discriminate against a child on the basis of race in the light of their own experiences of discrimination. Reasons for being unwilling to adopt transracially included: a lack of racial/ethnic diversity in their communities; racism/lack of support from family; personal "internalized" racism; and the sense (from lesbians) that having gay parents, being adopted, and being racially different from one's parents was simply too much for a child to handle. Of note is that both heterosexual and lesbian prospective adopters noted particular concerns about adopting Black children, specifically. They stated that racism against Black people in their communities would make it difficult to raise their children in a supportive and affirming environment (Riley and Goldberg 2007).

Transitioning to Parenthood: Protective and Risk Factors

Given the complex nexus of factors that are unique to prospective adoptive couples, their transition to adoptive parenthood may be quite different from couples who transition to biological parenthood in certain ways. For example, unresolved grief associated with infertility, financial worries, challenges related to the characteristics of the adopted child (such as behavioral and emotional problems, and attachment difficulties), and legal issues (i.e., for the same-sex couples) may all complicate adoptive couples' transition to parenthood. In the light of such potential stresses, attention to the protective factors that might buffer the strains associated with the transition to adoptive parenthood is important.

Social Resources

Social support is an important resource to all couples during the transition to parenthood. Social support has been shown to reduce parenting stress, marital strain, and depression/anxiety during the transition (Bird et al. 2002; Budd et al. 2006), and intimate partner support, specifically, is related to mental health during the transition to parenthood (Semyr et al. 2004). Interestingly, in one of the few studies of the transition to adoptive parenthood, Levy-Shiff et al. (1991) found that heterosexual couples ultimately experienced greater support from family members than they initially expected. Furthermore, they found that adoptive parents were more satisfied with their families' support than biological parents. They also observed that social support, measured preadoption, was an important predictor of later family adjustment for adoptive parents. Cross-sectional research on adoptive parents has also found that higher levels of social support are related to less parenting stress (Bird et al. 2002).

Of note is that lesbian and gay adoptive couples may be at risk for compromised social support during this critical life transition. Sexual minorities, in general, tend to perceive less support from their families of origin compared to heterosexual men and women (Kurdek 2001; Kurdek and Schmitt 1987). Further, Goldberg and Smith (2008) examined lesbian and heterosexual preadoptive parents and found that lesbians reported less support from family members but similar levels of support from friends and that low levels of perceived support from family was associated with increased depression among both types of couples. Similarly, Kindle and Erich (2005) found that lesbian and gay adoptive parents relied much less on their families of origin than heterosexual adoptive parents, although there were no differences in overall levels of support.

Couples who adopt transracially (either through domestic adoption or international adoption) may also be at risk for compromised support from family members, who may struggle with their own racism and express uncertainty that they will be able to love a child that is racially different from themselves (de Haymes and Simon 2003; Goldberg 2009; Johnson and O'Connor 2002). In the absence of unqualified support from family members, adoptive parents may be at risk for feelings of isolation and frustration, particularly if they lack alternative sources of support. Sometimes, however, family members do become less resistant and more accepting of the adopted child over time (Bennett 2003; de Haymes and Simon 2003). Alternatively, couples who anticipate extreme resistance from their family members are less likely to adopt transracially (Goldberg 2009).

Psychological Resources

The psychological resources (e.g., self-esteem, mental health) that adoptive parents possess also may have implications for their ability to navigate through the changes and challenges associated with parenting. Most couples who suffer from conception-related difficulties experience some impairment in their relationships and sense of self; however, it is possible that such impairments may be short-lived and/or may not negatively affect their transition to (adoptive) parenthood. For example, it is possible that after a lengthy period of longing to be a parent, adoptive parents may be more appreciative of the *rewards* of parenthood and may be less unsettled by its challenging aspects (Brodzinsky and Huffman 1988). Some research with previously infertile couples (who ultimately succeeded in conceiving) suggests exactly this outcome – at least for women. Abbey et al. (1994) conducted a study in which they compared fertile and previously infertile couples (who ultimately conceived) and found that previously infertile women experienced the greatest benefits of parenthood: In contrast to other participants, they experienced significantly less stress and increased personal control after becoming a parent. However, previously infertile women and their spouses also reported less intimacy in their marriages compared to fertile parents, suggesting a prolonged impact of infertility treatments on intimacy (additionally, these couples may not have been prepared for the impact of fatigue and childcare responsibilities on their sex lives).

Levy-Shiff et al. (1991) interviewed adoptive parents and biological parents before the placement/birth of their child and found that adoptive parents actually expressed more positive expectations about parenthood than biological parents. Having yearned for a child for so long, these couples were highly optimistic about parenthood. Further, in their 4-month post-placement/birth followup, they found that for both adoptive and biological parents, pre-parenthood expectations largely matched post-birth experiences, suggesting the potentially powerful role of optimism. These findings counter concerns that conception-related difficulties necessarily have long-term implications and suggest that adoptive couples may, in fact, possess enhanced coping resources in certain areas. Indeed, their positive adjustment may be related to the fact that adoptive parents on the whole tend to be older, to have been married longer, and to have more financial resources compared to biological parents; such factors may facilitate the development of a wide array of coping strategies that protect against maladjustment (Brodzinsky and Huffman 1988). However, the short-term nature of the assessment period in Levy-Shiff et al.'s study leaves many questions unanswered. For example, it is possible that as the initial "honeymoon" phase wears off, adoptive parents experience greater stress. Further, some adoptive parents' idealized expectations may not be belied in the immediate post-placement phase, but later on, if and when their children manifest more challenging and perhaps atypical behaviors. Reasonable expectations are a critical component of successful adoptions (Brodzinsky et al. 1998), and unmet or unrealistic parental expectations of their adopted children are associated with problems in family functioning (Brodzinsky and Pinderhughes 2002; Brooks et al. 2005). Additionally, it is possible that adoptive parents who have unresolved feelings regarding infertility (e.g., they have not yet fully mourned the biological child they cannot have) and/or adoptive parents who are placed with a child on short notice may experience a more difficult adjustment: They may be emotionally unprepared and/or may experience ambivalent feelings towards their adopted child, which they may (inadvertently) communicate (Brinich 1995).

Compared to couples with a long history of conception-related difficulties, preferential adopters – that is, adoptive couples who turn to adoption first, as opposed to as a "last resort" (i.e., because they are unable to conceive) – may theoretically possess greater psychological resources at the time of adopting. Preferential adopters may represent couples who choose to adopt for altruistic reasons, health reasons (e.g., prior illnesses such as childhood cancer that prevent conception), or age-related reasons (some couples delay the decision to pursue parenthood past the childbearing years and find themselves with little choice but to pursue adoption) (Hollingsworth 2000). Lesbians, who lack a partner with whom to conceive, are more likely to be preferential adopters than heterosexual couples (Goldberg and Smith 2008; Matthews and Cramer 2006; and Tyebjee 2003). Lesbian couples typically choose between pursuing alternative insemination (which would allow one partner to carry and bear the child) and adoption. Faced with this decision, many lesbians choose adoption, perhaps in part because of a broader definition of family that is based less on biological ties and more on affective ties (Oswald 2002). Lesbians (and gay men, for that matter) may, therefore, experience the road to adoption as less painful than heterosexual couples and may arrive at adoption with greater psychological resources. On the other hand, lesbians and gay men are vulnerable to heterosexism as well as extreme scrutiny in their quest to become parents (e.g., adoption workers may hold them to higher standards than heterosexual couples: Hicks 2000), which may serve deplete their psychological resources. However, at least one study of lesbian and heterosexual pre-adoptive parents found *no* differences in well-being as a function of sexual orientation (Goldberg and Smith 2008).

Although most heterosexual couples who pursue adoption do so because they were not successful at conceiving a biological child (and therefore, there may be fewer heterosexual preferential adopters than lesbian/gay preferential adopters), there is variability among heterosexual couples in terms of how far they will go to conceive – that is, their willingness to seek increasingly expensive and sophisticated medical solutions to their problem (Daniluk 2001). Some couples undergo extensive medical testing and interventions, which are time-consuming, costly, and painful, while others do not. It is possible that couples who resist medical intervention and turn to adoption sooner might retain greater psychological resources, which in turn might buffer the stresses of transitioning to adoptive parenthood. Consistent with this notion, Goldberg and Smith (2008) studied heterosexual and lesbian couples in the pre-adoptive phase and found that couples who had previously pursued in vitro fertilization (IVF) (a high-tech, invasive, and expensive intervention) and failed reported higher depression levels. However, it is unknown whether IVF experiences continue to impact couples' well-being beyond the pre-adoptive phase. Further, although this study did not investigate whether extensive experience with medical interventions was associated with compromised relationship quality and intimacy, prior research with infertile (but not pre-adoptive) couples suggests that it is (e.g., Abbey et al. 1992; Benazon et al. 1992; and Daniluk 2001). In turn, it is possible that such experiences continue to exacerbate intimacy problems during the transition to adoptive parenthood. Longitudinal research in this area is obviously needed.

Characteristics of the Adoption and the Child

Characteristics of the child and of the adoption may also influence parents', children's, and families' adjustment. For example, there is evidence that as the child's age at adoption increases, the likelihood of poorer child and family outcomes increases (Brooks et al. 2005). A history of neglect or abuse prior to placement, a greater number of prior placements, and prenatal drug exposure are also associated with poorer child, parent, and family outcomes (Brooks et al. 2005; Feigelman and Silverman 1983; and Simmel et al. 2001), although importantly, the number of risk factors present may be the most significant predictor of family adjustment to adoption, more so than any individual risk factor (McDonald et al. 2001). Of note is that for some families, adjustment outcomes may improve over time, particularly when children are adopted at an early age. For example, McCarty et al. (1999) studied parents of adopted children with prenatal substance exposure and found that parents perceived better circumstances when their children were 13–15 months compared to when they were 3–5 months, including better attachment, less stress, and less concern over prenatal substance exposure.

Children adopted through the public sector (e.g., via foster care) are most likely to have the above "risk factors": that is, to be older, to have experienced multiple placements, to have prenatal drug exposure, and to have been abused. Likewise, some research suggests that families that adopt children via foster care experience a more challenging adjustment than families who adopt children via private domestic or international adoption. Howard et al. (2004) conducted a large study of child welfare adoptions, domestic infant adoptions, international adoptions, and birth families. Parents provided information on their families and their adopted children, who ranged in age from 6 to 18. They found that child welfare and internationally adopted children were the most likely to have suffered early adverse experiences. Children adopted from the child welfare system experienced the highest level of behavioral problems, followed by children who were adopted internationally, according to their parents. Most parents were satisfied with their adoption experiences, although child welfare adopters were less satisfied than other types of families. While this study focused primarily on child outcomes (as opposed to parent/family outcomes) and did not capture the early adjustment phase, the findings are important in that they suggest that families' needs and experiences may differ as a function of adoption type. Future longitudinal research is needed that explores how family outcomes and adjustment processes unfold over time, beginning in the pre-adoptive or early post-adoptive phase.

Families who adopt transracially encounter unique challenges and concerns in the early months and years of parenthood. They may need to educate themselves about the racial and cultural needs of their children, including how to help their children develop a sense of pride in themselves, as well as more pragmatic issues such as how to address health, hair, and/or skin needs that may differ from their own (Lev 2004). Additionally, their decision to adopt a child that is racially/ethnically/culturally different may be met with discomfort or lack of support from family members, friends, neighbors, and the community at large (de Haymes and Simon 2003; Johnson and O'Connor 2002). In general, children who are transracially adopted experience a lack of privacy because of the inability to keep the fact of their adoption from others (Brodzinsky and Pinderhughes 2002; de Haymes and Simon 2003); thus, these children and their families may be faced with more intensive scrutiny (e.g., questions and stares) than families with inracially adopted children who may "pass" as biogenetically related. Of note is that gay and lesbian parent families are also more visible than heterosexual parent families in that they do not conform to the stereotypical nuclear family model. Thus, gay/lesbian parent families who adopt transracially may experience a "double visibility," a phenomenon that has not been investigated to date.

Ideally, parents who adopt a child of a different or minority race seek to create a new multiracial, multicultural identity for the family and to learn about their child's racial and ethnic heritage so that they can help to foster a healthy self-image and secure racial identity in their child (Park and Green 2000). However, research by Johnson et al. (1987) and Shireman and Johnson (1986) found that three-quarters of White families who adopted children of color lived in white neighborhoods and sent the children to predominantly White schools. Though parents acknowledged the need for greater contact with people of color they did not change their lifestyles and tended to minimize the importance of race and to downplay incidents of discrimination. Furthermore, the creation of racially integrated environments may have important implications for child and family adjustment. Feigelman (2000) found that when adoptive families lived in racially heterogeneous settings, parents were less likely to report that their children experienced discomfort about their appearance.

Legal Issues

Another set of variables that can complicate gay and lesbian couples' transition to adoptive parenthood are the laws and practices regarding gay adoption in the states in which couples live. Indeed, couples who adopt in states that do not equally recognize both partners' parental statuses may be at risk for negative outcomes. Ideally, gay and lesbian couples can pursue a *co-parent adoption*, which allows both partners to adopt their child together, at the same time, ensuring legal recognition of both parents. Couples who live in states that do not allow co-parent adoptions, then, must choose one partner to officially adopt as the legal parent. The non-legal partner can then in some states seek out a *second parent adoption*, which allows them to adopt their partner's child after the primary parent has adopted. Similarly, couples that pursue international adoption (which requires that only one partner can officially adopt, as a single parent) may then later, in their home state, pursue a second parent adoption for the non-legal parent (HRC 2000). Couples who live in states with unfavorable rulings concerning second parent adoption, of course, are resigned to a situation in which their child has only one legal parent. This may lead to feelings of insecurity and/or invisibility on the part of parents and children (e.g., Connolly 2002; Goldberg et al. 2007). Further, when only one parent is legally recognized as the parent, the other parent has to go out of their way to assert his or her parental role, which can be stressful to both members of the couple (Mallon 2004).

Conclusions: The Transition to Adoptive Parenthood

Despite a relatively large literature on adoption, we know relatively little about the transition to adoptive parenthood and about couples', children's, and families' adjustment experiences during this transitional phase. The extant research in this area suggests that this period is challenging, but it may not really have the negative and long-term impact as might be expected. Despite the potentially painful road that may lead couples to pursue adoption and the challenges associated with the adoption process, many couples do appear to transition to parenthood relatively smoothly. More research is, of course, needed that follows couples over time, in order to gain a better long-term perspective on couple and family adjustment, as well as the factors (particularly those that are present in the pre-adoptive stage) that are associated with enhanced (or compromised) functioning. Further, research on the transition to adoptive parenthood among couples who adopt transracially and transculturally is needed in order to identify the sorts of unique challenges that these couples are faced with in the early transitional phase. Additionally, examination of how different types of couples (i.e., heterosexual, lesbian, and gay parent couples) negotiate the stresses and joys of adoptive parenthood is of interest. Some risk and protective factors may be more salient for certain groups than others.

Suggestions for Practitioners

Based on the literature, I offer several recommendations for professionals that work with couples at various phases of the adoption process (e.g., social workers, adoption agency personnel, lawyers, other adoption professionals). First, gay and lesbian couples that seek to adopt but who closet their relationships (e.g., because they feel that they have no other choice but to do so) may receive inadequate pre-adoptive preparation. Adoption professionals who believe that they are working with a single parent, for example, will emphasize certain key factors (and ignore others) in the preparation and placement stages. Further, they will be unaware of, and therefore unable to draw on, particular strengths that both partners bring to parenthood. They will also be unable to address and respond to the unique concerns of gay and lesbian couples (e.g., legal concerns; concerns about negotiating both racism and heterosexism). Adoption professionals who are open to working with gay/lesbian couples are, therefore, strongly encouraged to be demonstratively affirming in their materials in order to encourage openness in prospective clients (Goldberg et al. 2007). Social workers who conduct home studies should be especially careful to clearly communicate – in their language, affect, and overall demeanor – that they are open and accepting of lesbians and gay men, starting in their very first encounters with couples and individuals (Mallon 2007). Indeed, in that applicants may not be "out" in the first interview, it is important for social workers not to assume that, for example, a single man is necessarily heterosexual.

Second, adoption and healthcare professionals who work with adoptive couples in the pre- and post-adoptive phases are encouraged to maintain a long-range view of couples' experience. Specifically, adoption professionals who work with couples in the pre-adoptive stage are encouraged to elicit details about clients' specific parenthood trajectories, including their infertility history (if applicable), the factors that led them to adopt, and their expectations, hopes, and fears about parenthood in general and adoptive parenthood, in particular. Professionals should be cognizant of the fact that unrealistic expectations regarding parenting are linked to poor parental adjustment and should therefore aim to provide a comprehensive pre-adoptive training to prospective adopters, placing special emphasis on the challenges of parenting children with special needs (Brooks et al. 2005). In the post-adoptive stage, it is important to assess the degree to which parents' expectations have been met in the short-term as well as the long-term (Levy-Shiff et al. 1991) and to provide needed support in areas that were unanticipated (e.g., adopting a different-race child). Further, ongoing support and services may be needed, particularly for couples who adopt via foster care and/or who adopt transracially (de Haymes and Simon 2003).

Research suggests that couples who are not willing to adopt transracially often cite family unsupportiveness and lack of community diversity as reasons (Goldberg 2009). For some couples, these reasons may function as excuses (e.g., couples may be ashamed of to admit their own discomfort with adopting outside of their own race). However, for others, these represent true, genuine concerns. Adoption workers should encourage clients to engage in open and frank dialogue about their individual and couple-level beliefs and concerns regarding transracial adoption. In this way, adoption professionals can differentiate between (and appropriately serve) clients who might be willing to adopt transracially but are concerned about the lack of diversity in their school system, for example, and clients who are personally uncomfortable with the idea of adopting transracially but who claim concern for school diversity as the reason for their unwillingness.

School personnel, child care workers, pediatricians, and other child/family practitioners should be familiar with the varied ways in which families are created. Specifically, they should have a basic understanding of both biological and adoptive family formation, and they should be aware of both the unique and common factors of biological and adoptive couples' transition to parenthood (see Table 9-1). Further, as this review illustrates, adoptive families are not a monolithic group but are complex, diverse, and multifaceted. Practitioners should, therefore, acknowledge the many sources of diversity in adoptive families (e.g., type of adoption, racial makeup, parental sexual orientation) and attend carefully to the ways in which they can shape the experiences of parents, children, and families.

References

Abbey, A., Andrews, F. M., & Halman, L. J. (1991). Gender's role in responses to infertility. *Psychology of Women Quarterly, 15*, 205–316.

Abbey, A., Andrews, F. M., & Halman, L. J. (1992). Infertility and subjective well-being: The mediating roles of self-esteem, internal control, and interpersonal conflict. *Journal of Marriage and the Family, 54*, 408–417.

Abbey, A., Andrews, F. M., & Halman, L. J. (1994). Infertility and parenthood: Does becoming a parent increase well-being? *Journal of Consulting and Clinical Psychology, 62*, 398–403.

Andrews, F. M., Abbey, A., & Halman, L. J. (1992). Is fertility-problem stress different? The dynamics of stress in fertile and infertile couples. *Fertility and Sterility, 57*, 1247–1253.

Ballard, C. G., Davis, R., Cullen, P. C., Mohan, R. N., & Dean, C. (1994). Postnatal depression in mothers and fathers. *British Journal of Psychiatry, 164*, 782–788.

Barth, R., Brooks, D., & Iyer, S. (1995). *California adoptions: Current demographic profiles and projections through the end of the century*. Berkeley, CA: University of California, Child Welfare Research Center.

Bausch, R. S. (2006). Predicting willingness to adopt a child: A consideration of demographic and attitudinal factors. *Sociological Perspectives, 49*, 47–65.

Beck, C. (2001). Predictors of postpartum depression: An update. *Nursing Research, 50*, 275–285.

Belsky, J., Lang, M., & Rovine, M. (1985). Stability and change in marriage across the transition to parenthood: A second study. *Journal of Marriage and the Family, 47*, 855–866.

Belsky, J., & Pensky, E. (1988). Marital change across the transition to parenthood. *Marriage and Family Review, 12*, 133–156.

Belsky, J., & Rovine, M. (1990). Patterns of marital change across the transition to parenthood: Pregnancy to three years postpartum. *Journal of Marriage and the Family, 52*, 5–19.

Benazon, N., Wright, J., & Sabourin, S. (1992). Stress, sexual satisfaction, and marital adjustment in infertile couples. *Journal of Sex and Marital Therapy, 18*, 273–284.

Bennett, S. (2003). International adoptive lesbian families: Parental perceptions of the influence of diversity on family relationships in early childhood. *Smith College Studies in Social Work, 74*, 73–91.

Bird, G. W., Peterson, R., & Miller, S. H. (2002). Factors associated with distress among support-seeking adoptive parents. *Family Relations, 51*, 215–220.

Brinich, P. M. (1995). Psychoanalytic perspectives on adoption and ambivalence. *Psychoanalytic Psychology, 12*, 181–199.

Brodzinsky, D. M. (1987). Adjustment to adoption: A psychosocial perspective. *Clinical Psychology Review, 7*, 25–47.

Brodzinsky, D. M., & Huffman, L. (1988). Transition to adoptive parenthood. *Marriage & Family Review, 12*, 267–286.

Brodzinsky, D. M., & Pinderhughes, E. (2002). Parenting and child development in adoptive families. In M. H. Bornstein (Ed.), *Handbook of parenting: Vol. 1: Children and parenting* (2nd ed., pp. 279–311). Mahwah, NJ: Erlbaum.

Brodzinsky, D. M., Smith, D. W., & Brodzinsky, A. B. (1998). *Children's adjustment to adoption*. Thousand Oaks, CA: Sage.

Brooks, D., & Goldberg, S. (2001). Gay and lesbian adoptive and foster care placements: Can they meet the needs of waiting children? *Social Work Journal, 46*, 147–157.

Brooks, D., Simmel, C., Wind, L., & Barth, R. P. (2005). Contemporary adoption in the United States: Implications for the next wave of adoption theory, research, and practice. In D. M. Brodzinsky & J. Palacios (Eds.), *Psychological issues in adoption: Research and practice* (pp. 1–25). Westport, CT: Praeger.

Budd, K. S., Holdswirth, M. J., & HoganBruen, K. D. (2006). Antecedents and concomitants of parenting stress in adolescent mothers in foster care. *Child Abuse & Neglect, 30*, 557–574.

Child Welfare Information Gateway (2004). *Costs of adopting: Factsheet for families.* Retrieved on June 18, 2007 from http://www.childwelfare.gov/pubs/s_cost/s_costb.cfm.

Connolly, C. (2002). The voice of the petitioner: The experiences of gay and lesbian parents in successful second-parent adoption proceedings. *Law & Society Review, 36*, 325–346.

Cole, S. A. (2005). Foster caregiver motivation and infant attachment: How do reasons for fostering affect relationships? *Child and Adolescent Social Work Journal, 22*, 441–457.

Cole, S. W. (2006). Social threat, personal identity, and physical health in closeted gay men. In A. M. Omoto & H. S. Kurtzman (Eds.), *Sexual orientation and mental health: Examining identity and development in lesbian, gay, and bisexual people* (pp. 245–267). Washington, DC: American Psychological Association.

Costigan, C. L., Cox, M. J., & Cauce, A. M. (2003). Work-parenting linkages among dual-earner couples at the transition to parenthood. *Journal of Family Psychology, 17*, 397–408.

Cowan, C. P., & Cowan, P. A. (1988). Who does what when partners become parents: Implications for men, women, and marriage. In C. P. Cowan & P. A. Cowan (Eds.), *Transitions to parenthood* (pp. 105–131). New York: Haworth.

Cudmore, L. (2005). Becoming parents in the context of loss. *Sexual and Relationship Therapy, 20*(3), 299–308.

Daly, K. (1988). Reshaped parenthood identity: The transition to adoptive parenthood. *Journal of Contemporary Ethnography, 17*, 40–66.

Daly, K. (1989a). Preparation needs of infertile couples who seek to adopt. *Canadian Journal of Community Mental Health, 8*, 111–121.

Daly, K. (1989b). Anger among prospective adoptive parents: Structural determinants and management strategies. *Clinical Sociology Review, 7*, 80–96.

Daniluk, J. C. (2001). "If we had it to do over again…": Couples' reflections on their experiences of infertility treatments. *Family Journal, 9*, 122–133.

Daniluk, J. C., & Fluker, M. (1995). Fertility drugs and the reproductive imperative: Assisting the infertile woman. *Women & Therapy, 16*, 31–47.

Daniluk, J. C., & Hurtig-Mitchell, J. (2003). Themes of hope and healing: Infertile couples' experiences of adoption. *Journal of Counseling & Development, 81*, 389–399.

de Haymes, M. V., & Simon, S. (2003). Transracial adoption: Families identify issues and needed support services. *Child Welfare Journal, 82*, 251–272.

Demo, D., & Cox, M. (2000). Families with young children: A review of research in the 1990s. *Journal of Marriage and the Family, 62*, 876–895.

Downs, C. A., & James, S. E. (2006). Gay, lesbian, and bisexual foster parents: Strengths and challenges for the child welfare system. *Child Welfare, 85*, 281–298.

Farber, M. L. Z., Timberlake, E., Mudd, H. P., & Cullen, L. (2003). Preparing parents for adoption: An agency perspective. *Child and Adolescent Social Work Journal, 20*, 175–196.

Feigelman, W. (2000). Adjustments of transracially and inracially adopted children. *Journal of Child and Adolescent Social Work, 17*, 165–184.

Feigelman, W., & Silverman, A. R. (1983). *Chosen children: New patterns of adoptive relationships*. New York: Praeger.

Gates, G., & Ost, J. (2004). *The gay and lesbian atlas*. Washington, DC: Urban Institute Press.

Gates, G., Badgett, M. V. L., Macomber, J. E., & Chambers, K. (2007). *Adoption and foster care by gay and lesbian parents in the United States*. Washington, DC: The Urban Institute.

Goldberg, A. E. (2009). Lesbian and heterosexual preadoptive couples' openness to transracial adoption. *American Journal of Orthopsychiatry, 79*, 103–117.

Goldberg, A. E., Downing, J. B., & Sauck, C. C. (2007). Choices, challenges, and tensions: Perspectives of prospective lesbian adoptive parents. *Adoption Quarterly, 10*, 33–64.

Goldberg, A. E., & Sayer, A. (2006). Lesbian couples' relationship quality across the transition to parenthood. *Journal of Marriage and Family, 68*, 87–100.

Goldberg, A. E., & Smith J. Z. (2008). Social support and well-being in lesbian and heterosexual preadoptive parents. *Family Relations, 57*, 281–294.

Grotevant, H. D., Dunbar, N., Kohler, J. K., & Esau, A. M. (2000). Adoptive identity: How contexts within and beyond the family shape developmental pathways. *Family Relations, 45*, 309–317.

Haugaard, J. J., West, N. M., & Moed, A. M. (2000). Open adoption: Attitudes and experiences. *Adoption Quarterly, 4*, 889–899.

Hicks, S. (2000). 'Good lesbian, bad lesbian…': Regulating heterosexuality in fostering and adoption assessments. *Child & Family Social Work, 5*, 157–168.

Hollingsworth, L. D. (2000). Who seeks to adopt a child? Findings from the National Survey of Family Growth (1995). *Adoption Quarterly, 3*, 1–23.

Hollingsworth, L., & Ruffin, V. M. (2002). Why are so many U. S. families adopting internationally? A social exchange perspective. *Journal of Human Behavior in the Social Environment, 6*, 81–97.

Howard, J. A., Smith, S. L., & Ryan, S. D. (2004). A comparative study of child welfare adoptions with other types of adopted children and birth children. *Adoption Quarterly, 7*, 1–30.

Human Rights Campaign Foundation. (2002). *The state of the family*. Washington DC: Human Rights Campaign.

Hyde, J., Klein, M., Essex, M., & Clark, R. (1995). Maternity leave and women's mental health. *Psychology of Women Quarterly, 19*, 257–285.

Jacob, M. C. (1997). Concerns of single women and lesbian couples considering conception through assisted reproduction. In S. R. Leiblum (Ed.), *Infertility: Psychological issues and counseling strategies* (pp. 189–206). Oxford, England: Wiley.

Johnson, P. R., Shireman, J. F., & Watson, K. W. (1987). Transracial adoption and the development of black identity at age eight. *Child Welfare, 66*, 45–55.

Johnson, S. M., & O'Connor, E. (2002). *The gay baby boom: The psychology of gay parenthood*. New York: New York University Press.

Kindle, P. A., & Erich, S. (2005). Perceptions of social support among heterosexual and homosexual adopters. *Families in Society, 86*, 541–546.

Kurdek, L. (2001). Differences between heterosexual-nonparent couples and gay, lesbian, and heterosexual-parent couples. *Journal of Family Issues, 22*, 727–754.

Kurdek, L., & Schmitt, J. P. (1987). Perceived emotional support from family and friends in members of homosexual, married, and heterosexual cohabiting couples. *Journal of Homosexuality, 14*, 57–68.

Landridge, D., Connolly, K., & Sheeran, P. (2000). Reasons for wanting a child: A network analytic study. *Journal of Reproductive and Infant Psychology, 18*, 321–338.

Lev, A. I. (2004). *The complete lesbian and gay parenting guide.* New York: Penguin.

Levy-Shiff, R., Goldschmidt, I., & Har-Even, D. (1991). Transition to parenthood in adoptive parents. *Developmental Psychology, 27*, 131–140.

Mallon, G. P. (2004). *Gay men choosing parenthood.* New York: Columbia University Press.

Mallon, G. P. (2007). Assessing lesbian and gay prospective foster and adoptive families: A focus on the home study process. *Child Welfare, 86*, 67–86.

Marks, M. N., Wieck, A., Checkley, S. A., & Kumar, R. (1996). How does marriage protect women with histories of affective disorder from post-partum relapse? *British Journal of Medical Psychology, 69*, 329–342.

Matthews, J. D., & Cramer, E. P. (2006). Envisaging the adoption process to strengthen gay- and lesbian-headed families: Recommendations for adoption professionals. *Child Welfare, 85*, 317–340.

McCarty, C. J., Waterman, J. D., Burge, D., & Edelstein, S. B. (1999). Experiences, concerns and service needs for families adopting children with prenatal drug exposure: A summary and recommendations. *Child Welfare, 78*, 561–577.

McDonald, T., Propp, J., & Murphy, K. (2001). The postadoption experience: Child, parent, family predictors of family adjustment to adoption. *Child Welfare, 80*, 71–94.

Mendenhall, T. J., Grotevant, H. D., & McRoy, R. G. (1996). Adoptive couples: Communication and changes made in openness levels. *Family Relations, 45*, 223–229.

Miall, C. E. (1998). Community assessments of adoption issues: Open adoption, birth reunions, and the disclosure of confidential information. *Journal of Family Issues, 19*, 556–577.

Miller, B. C., Fan, X., Christensen, M., Grotevant, H. D., & van Dulmen, M. (2000). Comparisons of adopted and nonadopted adolescents in a large nationally representative sample. *Child Development, 71*, 1458–1473.

Oswald, R. (2002). Resilience within the family networks of lesbians and gay men: Intentionality and redefinition. *Journal of Marriage and Family, 64*, 374–383.

Pacey, S. (2004). Couples and the first baby: Responding to new parents' sexual and relationship problems. *Sexual and Relationship Therapy, 19*, 223–246.

Park, S. M., & Green, C. E. (2000). Is transracial adoption in the best interests of ethnic minority children?: Questions concerning legal and scientific interpretations of a child's best interests. *Adoption Quarterly, 3*, 5–34.

Riley, A., & Goldberg, A. E. (2007). *Preferences and attitudes towards race in adoptive parenthood.* Poster presented at the American Psychological Association annual conference, San Francisco, CA.

Rodger, S., Cummings, A., & Leschied, A. W. (2006). Who is caring for our most vulnerable children? The motivation to foster in child welfare. *Child Abuse & Neglect, 30*, 1129–1142.

Sandelowski, M., Harris, B. G., & Holditch-Davis, D. (1991). "The clock has been ticking, the calendar pages turning, and we are still waiting": Infertile couples' encounter with time in the adoption waiting period. *Qualitative Sociology, 14*, 147–173.

Santona, A., & Zavattini, G. (2005). Partnering and parenting expectations in adoptive couples. *Sexual & Relationship Therapy, 205*, 302–322.

Schulz, M. S., Cowan, P. A., Cowan, C. P., & Brennan, R. T. (2004). Coming home upset: Gender, marital satisfaction, and the daily spillover of workday experience into couple interactions. *Journal of Family Psychology, 18*, 250–263.

Semyr, L., Edhborg, M., Lundh, W., & Sjogren, B. (2004). In the shadow of maternal depressed mood: Experiences of parenthood during the first year after childbirth. *Journal of Psychosomatic Obstetrics and Gynecology, 25*, 23–34.

Shelley-Sireci, L., & Ciano-Boyce, C. (2002). Becoming lesbian adoptive parents: An exploratory study of lesbian adoptive, lesbian birth, and heterosexual adoptive parents. *Adoption Quarterly, 6*, 33–43.

Shireman, J. F., & Johnson, P. R. (1986). A longitudinal study of Black adoptions: Single parent, transracial, and traditional. *Social Work, 31*, 172–176.

Siegel, D. H. (1993). Open adoption of infants: Adoptive parents' perceptions of advantages and disadvantages. *Social Work, 38*, 15–23.

Simmel, C., Brooks, D., Barth, R. P., & Hinshaw, S. P. (2001). Externalizing symptomatology among adoptive youth: Prevalence and preadoption risk factors. *Journal of Abnormal Child Psychology, 29*, 57–69.

Tyebjee, T. (2003). Attitude, interest, and motivation for adoption and foster care. *Child Welfare, 82*, 685–706.

Weir, K. N. (2003). Adoptive family leap-frogging patterns. *Adoption Quarterly, 7*, 27–41.

Chapter 10

Transitioning the Impact of Divorce on Children Throughout the Life Cycle

Brian Barczak, Thomas W. Miller, Lane J. Veltkamp, Sarah Barczak, Clay Hall, and Robert Kraus

Introduction

It is unfortunate that despite an alarming, worldwide increase in the rate of divorce in recent decades, there has been a general paucity of mental health literature written with the express purpose of focusing on and discussing the many and varied deleterious effects of parental divorce on child and adolescent populations in society at large. In addition to this dearth of available literature, there have been even fewer publications written to address potential treatment protocols and clinical "pearls," which may be useful to mental health professionals working with affected youth from these disrupted home environments resulting from parental divorce.

In response to the relative lack of valuable literature, this chapter will first comprehensively review and summarize the most up-to-date literature available, addressing the ever-increasing problem of parental divorce in the lives of today's youth. This chapter will then highlight the clinical principles presented in the literature review through an in-depth discussion of details of a pertinent case history, in which an individual family's experiences throughout the divorce process are described in detail. Finally, this case history will be used to demonstrate a variety of clinically salient facts, observations, and treatment options for youth struggling with the negative effects of parental divorce throughout their lives. The most clinically relevant information will be compiled as a separate section of take-home points at the end of this chapter in order to facilitate future reference to the clinical materials discussed herein.

Conceptual Framework

The impact of the stressful transitions required during family dissolution and divorce has been the focus of clinicians and researchers. Wallerstein et al. (2001) studied this phenomenon in one of the most recognized longitudinal studies spanning almost three decades and concluded from their research of some 45 cases involving divorced families that divorce causes lasting damage to the children involved in divorces. These clinician-researchers attribute

From: *Handbook of Stressful Transitions Across the Lifespan,*
Edited by: T.W. Miller, DOI 10.1007/978-1-4419-0748-6_10,
© Springer Science+Business Media, LLC 2010

the subsequent psychological problems in the children to the divorce itself as opposed to the psychopathology of the parents, the trauma of their parenting, and their conflicted marriage. Other researchers have found that just after divorce, children have more symptoms than those in high-conflict, nondivorced families but that as children adapt to the new situation, the pattern of differences reverses. When divorce is associated with children moving into a less stressful situation, children from divorced families have similar adjustment to those from normal intact families. Wallerstein began her research in the early 1970s with 131 children of divorce. She interviewed at length both the children and their parents. She has continued to follow those same families as the children have matured into adulthood and begun families of their own, continuing periodic interviews and checking their progress through life. Wallerstein's research is different from its predecessors because it continued for so long after the actual divorce. Her research is the product of hundreds of hours of interviews with children of divorce and their parents. It is an extraordinary gift, and she deserves our deepest thanks and praise for her monumental efforts.

Most significant among Wallerstein's conclusions (by far) is the realization that the effects of divorce on children are *not* short-term and transient. They are long-lasting, profound, and cumulative. The children in Wallerstein's study view their parents differently, and they have lingering fears about their ability to commit to relationships, which affect their own marriages. Children experience divorce differently from their parents, and on different schedules. By and large, divorcing spouses go through a period of high conflict and intense emotional suffering during the divorce process. The pain experienced in divorce continues for years after divorce, but healing is usually more or less complete within 3 years after divorce. Wallerstein's research indicates that the effects of the divorce for children may continue for decades. Wallerstein notes that the children studied complained bitterly about being forced to disrupt their lives to spend time with the noncustodial parent. There was consistently a desire to see the other parent but they felt that all the arrangements were made for their parents' convenience and not theirs. Furthermore, the children Wallerstein studied were more likely to have a history of problems with drugs, alcohol, and adult sexuality. As many as 50% of the children she studied were involved in serious abuse of alcohol and drugs, some as early as age 14. When this occurred, these children, more often girls, showed a tendency to be sexually active earlier than usual.

In her book, *The Unexpected Legacy of Divorce*: *A 25 Year Landmark Study*, Wallerstein et al. (2001) examine how seven of these children have fared as adults. This group showed consistent clinical patterns marked by delayed adolescence. Thus, divorce is not a temporary crisis, as children often fear being married or becoming parents themselves. In addition, children of divorce and children from intact families experience childhood differently. *The take-home messages included the realization that parents in the midst of a divorce become more conscious of the needs for children's playtime, by focusing first on the needs of the child, even if mediators and lawyers encourage them to do otherwise.* Furthermore, it is important to share marital history, perhaps during the teen years, gives children a reference to use when navigating the terrain of their own, hopefully better relationships. And finally, Wallerstein argued that strengthening the relationship between grandparents and grandchildren during the divorce and the years that follow, provides critical relationship in aiding children and their ability to cope with the divorce experience.

Review of the Current Literature

General Effects of Divorce on Children and Adolescents

Many studies have focused on the general effects of divorce on child and adolescent populations, the outcomes of which are quite varied. For example, Wilcox Doyle et al. (2003) confirmed their hypothesis that positive events are indeed protective for children and adolescents experiencing frequent negative events during significant family transitions, including marital disruption and divorce. Conversely, Single-Rushton et al. (2005) examined both the short-term and long-term negative effects of divorce on youth from different-aged cohorts and discovered very little evidence of any change in the impact of negative effects of divorce on children, despite the fact that divorce rates continue to climb on a worldwide scale.

In their study of genetic and environmental risk factors among parents contributing to subsequent maladjustment in their offspring, D'Onofrio et al. (2007) demonstrated that when controlling for these variables (as well as for measured characteristics of both parents of the child), a specific causal connection exists between parental divorce and eventual substance use problems in these parents' offspring. Additionally, the genetic liability shared between divorced parents and their offspring was shown to better account for the increased risk of internalizing problems in the offspring as they matured throughout their adult years. Ultimately, this study demonstrates that selection versus causal mechanisms may function quite differently when determining the future risk of both substance abuse and internalizing problems in the offspring of divorced parents.

Psychosocial Effects of Divorce on Children

In an effort to focus more specifically on the psychosocial effects of divorce on child populations, excluding adolescents, Wood et al. (2004) conducted a chronological study of fourth-grade students born into middle class, divorced, single-mother families. Results of this study complemented those of D'Onofrio et al. (2007), demonstrating that the association between divorce and child internalizing behavior was partially mediated by depressive/withdrawn parenting style when the children were in the fourth and fifth (but not in later) grades.

Lansford et al. (2006) studied the trajectories of internalizing and externalizing behaviors, as well as school grades in cohorts of children from both divorced parents and intact families. Internalizing behaviors include symptoms consistent with the presentation of mood, anxiety, and/or neurotic mental disorders, while externalizing behaviors include symptoms consistent with disruptive behavior diagnoses (for example, ADHD, ODD, Conduct Disorder, etc.) and/or out-of-control clinical presentations (for example, those potentially related to prominent Axis II [oftentimes Cluster B] traits). The results of this study demonstrated that *early* parental divorce or separation appears to be more negatively related to the trajectories of both internalizing and externalizing behaviors and that children may therefore benefit most from psychosocial interventions focusing on the prevention of these behaviors. In contrast to this aforementioned trend among families with early parental divorce or separation, *later* parental divorce or separation was found to be more specifically and negatively related to the trajectories of academic grades, suggesting that these children may benefit most from social, environmental, and educational interventions aimed at promoting academic achievement in school.

Nair and Murray (2005) examined numerous mother–child dyads in an attempt to predict the impact of parental divorce on attachment security in preschool children. Demographic variables between two cohorts within this study were markedly different, as mothers from divorced families were found to be typically younger, had lower income, were less educated, and had significantly higher reported levels of stress, depression, conflict with their spouses, as well as increased need for social support. In addition to these characteristic differences, mothers from intact families tended to utilize a generally more positive and authoritative parenting style. Children in the divorced group reported a lower sense of security on assessment instruments than children from intact families. Ultimately, this study demonstrated that maternal parenting style and parental temperament are the major factors in mediating the relationship of parental divorce to preschoolers' sense of attachment security.

In a recent study, Ahrons (2007) utilized data from a previous longitudinal "Binuclear Family Study" (in which children were interviewed as adults 20 years after their parents' previous divorce(s)), to illustrate that the parental subsystem continues to impact the binuclear family in a long-term manner. This influence seems to be directly exerted by the parental subsystem on the quality of the children's own numerous relationships within the nuclear and extended family systems. These findings are supported by the fact(s) that: (1) While most children experience the remarriage of one or both parents after a divorce, as many as one-third of children remember the remarriage as being more stressful than the initial divorce; (2) Children who experienced remarriage of both of their parents reported that their father's remarriage was more stressful than their mother's remarriage; and finally, (3) Children whose relationships with their fathers deteriorated after a divorce were found to lack meaningful relationships with their paternal relatives.

Finally, Kelly (2007) both highlighted historical determinants of child custody arrangements following parental separation and divorce, as well as reviewed empirical and clinical research relevant to shaping children's living arrangements after parental marital disruption. Kelly's study notes that the traditional visitation patterns and guidelines seem to be outdated, unnecessarily rigid, restrictive, and fail to address the best interests of the majority of children from divorced families, from both short- and long-term perspectives. Currently, the more modern research-based parenting plan models appear to most appropriately serve the developmental and psychological needs of children from divorced families.

Psychosocial Effects of Divorce on Adolescents

Focusing more heavily on the psychosocial effects of divorce on adolescents, Roustit et al. (2007) utilized data from the previous "Social and Health Survey of Children and Adolescents (in Quebec, Montreal, Canada)" to more closely examine the associations between family dissolution and adolescents' subsequent maladjustment, that is, the adolescents' risk of eventual development of internalizing disorders, externalizing disorders, (non-alcoholic) substance use, and/or alcohol consumption. This study's results complemented those of both

D'Onofrio et al. and Wood et al., in that, all four of the aforementioned indicators of adolescents' subsequent psychosocial maladjustment were significantly associated with family breakup. Internalizing disorders were specifically mediated by both parental psychological distress and low parental emotional support. An independent association was also noted between adolescents' development of internalizing disorders and the witnessing of interparental violence at some point in the adolescent's past. Both family breakup and family-functioning variables had independent effects on mediating the adolescents' risk of developing the latter three indicators of psychosocial maladjustment, Thus, family-based interventions and social approaches are viewed to be complementary support modalities for adolescents who have experienced or are currently experiencing family disruptions.

A pair of Norwegian studies by Størsken et al. (2005, 2006) yielded the following clinically significant findings: (1) Parental divorce was determined to be prospectively associated with relative changes in the frequency of adolescent anxiety and depressive symptoms, as well as in adolescents' sense of subjective well-being, self-esteem, and school problems (more specifically, parental divorce was prospectively associated only with school problems in adolescent males, while it was associated with all of the aforementioned variables studied, especially long-term depressive and anxiety symptoms, among adolescent females); and (2) Both parental divorce and parental distress contributed independently to adolescents' subsequent distress. The authors found that the general prevalence of substantial symptoms of psychological distress (examples, as above, included anxiety, depression, etc.) was more than doubled (~30% vs. ~14%) among adolescents from divorced and distressed parents (when compared to same-aged peers from families with non-divorced and non-distressed parents).

In examining the long-term psychosocial effects of parental divorce on youth from adolescence to adulthood, Huurre et al. (2006) found that females from divorced families reported more psychological and interpersonal problems than both their male counterparts from divorced families, as well as their same-aged female peers from non-divorced families. In actuality, when compared to peers from non-divorced families, subjects of both genders with a background of parental divorce reported a higher frequency of various future psychosocial problems throughout their lives, including shorter education, unemployment, divorce, negative life events, and more unhealthy, risk-taking behaviors. Thus, parental divorce appears to be an indicator of significant stress in childhood and adolescence, due to the fact that its various long-term negative effects persist well into adulthood.

Peris and Emery (2004) examined: (1) The consequences of marital disruption on adolescents' adjustment; (2) The extent to which pre-disruption family dynamics accounted for both pre- and post-disruption group differences in overall youth functioning; as well as (3) The interaction between the level of marital discord and subsequent marital disruption. Group differences appeared to emerge in adolescents' adjustment during both pre-and post- marital disruption. Ultimately, these differences were felt to be better accounted for by family-level variables than by actual parental marital disruption.

Silverberg Koerner et al. (2004) found that, despite the fact that the majority of adolescents experience some level of maternal disclosure after parental divorce, neither the frequency nor detail of maternal disclosure differed as a function of the adolescents' gender, yet most detailed disclosures were significantly associated with at least some degree of adjustment difficulties during adolescence, especially in the form of symptoms of psychological distress. It is important to note that, additionally, the way in which these disclosures are actually made by the parent(s) may be the ultimate mediator of potential gender differences in adolescents' specific reactions to these sensitive disclosures after they have experienced parental divorce.

Lazar and Guttmann (2004) examined the relationships between adolescents' experience of parental divorce, their perception of their parents' characteristics, and their perceptions of their future ideal mate's characteristics. No significant differences were found between adolescents included in this study (i.e., from both intact and non-intact [divorced] families) in the independence of their characterizations of an ideal mate from those of their parents.

In a later study, Reese-Weber and Kahn (2005) examined whether predictors of romantic-partner conflict vary as a function of family structure. The investigators found that for both positive and negative behaviors among all adolescents in the study, mother-adolescent and father-adolescent conflict resolutions behaviors mediated the relationships between interparental and sibling conflict resolution. Additionally, mother-adolescent and sibling conflict resolution behaviors mediated the relationship between interparental and romantic-partner conflict resolution behaviors. These results support the fact that the vast majority of clinical conflict resolution behaviors within an adolescent's family appear to spill over into romantic relationships for these adolescents outside of their family, regardless of whether the adolescent lives in either an intact or a divorced (non-intact) household.

Lastly, a study by Ge et al. (2006) examined the trajectories of depressive symptoms among a cohort of over 500 male and female Midwestern adolescents from both intact and non-intact (divorced) families. Clinically significant findings of this study included: (1) Depressive symptoms appeared to increase during early to mid-adolescence, especially among females, and then subsequently declined as subjects approached late adolescence and young adulthood; (2) Female subjects experienced a greater number of ongoing depressive symptoms in adolescence and early adulthood when compared to their male counterparts; (3) Adolescents who experienced parental divorce by age 15 displayed a sharper increase in the number of depressive symptoms experienced when compared to peers from intact families; (4) Stressful life events experienced shortly after parental marital disruption and divorce mediated the actual effects of parental divorce on the adolescents' depressive symptoms; and finally, (5) Time-variable stressors, such as those related to either personal losses or relationship losses, were significantly associated with the present and future trajectories of depressive symptomatology in adolescents.

Biological Effects of Divorce on the Physical Health of Children and Adolescents

Examining more closely the potential myriad short- and long-term physical health implications and sequelae of divorce in both child and adolescent populations, Troxel and Matthew (2004) studied whether parental marital conflict and subsequent dissolution influence the risk trajectory of children's eventual physical health risk. This study demonstrated that because of stressors associated with marital conflict and subsequent disruption, parenting practices in these situations are often compromised. As a result, the offspring of divorced parents experience deficits in affective, behavioral, and cognitive domains, which eventually increase the overall physical health risk in these individuals by contributing to poor health behaviors, as well as by altering and compromising innate physiological stress-response systems (including cardiovascular, neuroendocrine, and neurotransmitter functioning).

Examining data collected from participants in the previous "US Terman Life Cycle Study," Martin et al. (2005) determined that the stress of parental divorce during childhood does not necessarily lead to later negative outcomes throughout the lives of the divorced parents' offspring. Though the investigators found that mediating and moderating variables of socioeconomic status (SES) and family psychosocial environment were related to eventual parental divorce, these variables neither fully nor adequately explained the short- and long-term effects of parental divorce on the health and vitality of the children from these families. In addition, the study's investigators found that a higher mortality risk in the offspring of divorced parents was decreased among the children (especially in males) who had achieved a sense of personal satisfaction with their lives by their mid-life years. Of note, from a behavioral standpoint, smoking in these divorced parents' offspring was the strongest mediator of the link between parental divorce and subsequent offspring mortality.

Fabricius and Luecken (2007) examined and tested a biopsychosocial model in which both young adults' long-term paternal relationships, as well as their ongoing distress caused by their parents' divorce(s) mediated the relationship between the disrupted parenting within their families of origin and various eventual indicators of the young adults' own physical health. The authors found that the more time children lived with their fathers, the better their current paternal relationships were, regardless of the presence of divorce-related parental conflict in the past. In contrast to this finding, however, was the fact that the more parental conflict witnessed by the children both throughout and after their parents' divorce proceedings, the worse their relationships were with their fathers in general, and the more distress they felt about their parents' divorce, regardless of the amount of time spent living with their fathers. In addition to these findings, poor-quality father–child relationships and more distress experienced by the children predicted poorer future overall health status in these offspring as they matured throughout their teenage and young adult years. Thus, this study highlights the impact of the quality of both the maternal–child relationship *and* the paternal–child relationship on the potential for both positive and negative, short- and long-term health effects in children and adolescents who struggle in the disruptive wake of their parents' divorce.

Lastly, in an effort to illustrate the effects of parental divorce on specific medical condition(s) in these parents' offspring, Bockelbrink et al. (2006) utilized responses from parent participants in an ongoing German survey study in order to examine the lifetime prevalence of Atopic Eczema [AE] in the children of parents who reported that significant stressful life events had occurred within their families, including parental divorce. The authors found that prevalence of Atopic Eczema [AE] among the offspring of the all of the parents included in this study was approximately 21.4% until the age of 4 years. The incidence of reported parental divorce/separation within the sample of parental participants studied was 3.4%. Parental divorce/separation was determined to be associated with a significantly increased odds ratio (OR) of 3.59 for the development of AE in these children's cases (that is, revealing that a significantly higher potential development of AE in the offspring of these divorced parents existed during the children's subsequent years of life). Thus, parental divorce/separation was found to significantly influence the risk of these divorced parents' offspring developing eventually later-life medical comorbidities, including Atopic Eczema [AE].

Case History

In order to illustrate the pertinent clinical concepts discussed above, this chapter will focus on the case history of one specific family separated by divorce. The Jones family is a Midwestern family comprising a group of eight people with which the authors of this chapter were familiar a number of years ago because of the family's collective requests for psychological evaluation and psychotherapeutic treatment through the local outpatient mental health clinic following the start of the divorce proceedings between Mr. and Ms. Jones. In fact, the family's first visit to clinic occurred within weeks of the divorce papers being jointly filed by Mr. and Ms. Jones in January, 1997.

The Parents

The father of the family, Mr. Jones, was a 45-year-old Caucasian male physician who during the initial interview readily identified the fact that he felt he was "a good father." As a working man, Mr. Jones had been relatively successful throughout his career in medicine – to illustrate this point, prior to the divorce proceedings Mr. Jones had worked as the sole consulting practitioner in his particular medical specialty for four separate hospitals simultaneously and his sense of self-esteem seemed to, in large part, hinge upon, and appeared to be most closely related to, his self-perception as "a good father," the "head of the household," a "hard worker" and the primary provider or "breadwinner" of the family. Throughout the evaluation process, Mr. Jones appeared to be an individual who was quite rigid and very uncompromising in his beliefs and attitudes toward his family, peers, and patients. For example, he identified himself as a "traditional Roman Catholic" and viewed himself as an individual with most of the power and "say-so" in the daily goings-on within the household because of his financial support of the rest of the family, as well as his status as "the man of the house."

Ms. Jones was a 41-year-old Caucasian female physician who worked primarily as a college professor of basic sciences, despite the fact that she herself had also graduated from medical school. In fact, Ms. Jones had taken classes alongside Mr. Jones at the same academic medical institution where they had matriculated together – there they had met and were married 3 years later, all of this occurring during their medical school training experience together. Over the years, because of the enormous responsibilities of rearing the couples' six children, however, Mr. Jones had allegedly decided (and Ms. Jones had initially albeit reluctantly agreed) that it would be best for her to remain at home to be with and care for the children each day. Because of Mr. Jones' traditional belief system, the decision was also made to home-school all six children in the family until they reached their high school years (at which time, each of the children could choose to continue being home-schooled or go to either a public or a private high school), a super-human task which largely appeared to rest primarily on the shoulders of Ms. Jones, due to her homemaker and housewife status. Ms. Jones frequently mentioned that her occupation was one which she felt allowed Mr. Jones to "go out and be the breadwinner of the family" as previously mentioned. Despite the fact she herself had suffered clinically significant depression (which had been intermittently treated with SSRI medications over the years) throughout her marriage to Mr. Jones, Ms. Jones appeared to view herself as the more giving, nurturing parent for the six children in the family, as she had clearly had more opportunities to spend time with and interact with them each day. Because of this dynamic and accompanying self-perception, Ms. Jones also readily concluded on several occasions that, from her own perspective, Mr. Jones was, in fact, generally more "out of touch" and "aloof" than she with respect to knowledge of "what was actually going on with the kids" within their family.

The Children

Clark Jones was a 16-year-old Caucasian male who was a senior at a local high school at the time of his family's initial presentation to clinic. Clark appeared to be precociously mature for his age and seemed to be able to relate more easily to adults than either to his younger siblings or, for that matter, to his same-aged peers. The apparent downside or trade-off related to Clark's precocious sense of maturity was his apparent development of an excessively anxious and obsessive–compulsive personality type. Psychological testing of Clark and his siblings as a part of the evaluation process revealed that Clark was one of two family members who appeared to have "Superior Intelligence." This high level of cognitive functioning and his accompanying history of high academic achievements to-date seemed to be related to the way in which Clark interpersonally appeared to be driven by a perceived parental pressure to try and excel at any task set before him. In doing so, his parents felt that he would be able to "set a good example" for his younger siblings on a routine basis. To this perceived external stressor from his parents, Clark added his own internal perception that the divorce between his parents was his own "fault" for a variety of reasons. Clark cited numerous examples of how his general and routine alignment with his father's point of view on most major family issues and decisions, as well as his corresponding strained relationship with his mother over the same situations, had in his mind contributed to the growing sense of animosity among and, ultimately, the decision to divorce between his parents. Thus, Clark seemingly took it upon himself (or at least allowed himself) to be labeled as the family's *voluntary scapegoat* of sorts – in essence, he willingly became the family's so-called *symptom-bearer*, a role so often seen in at least one individual member of troubled families presenting together for mental health treatment.

Sally Jones, the next-oldest child in the family's birth order, was a 12-year-old Caucasian female who was an eighth-grade student at the time of her family's presentation to clinic. Sally also appeared to be precociously mature for her age and psychological testing of her and her siblings' intellectual prowess revealed that she (like Clark) was the other family member who appeared to have been blessed with "Superior Intelligence." This innate gift, however, was likewise not without its own accompanying trials and tribulations in her case. The apparent downside to Sally's precocious sense of maturity and her superior intellect was her tendency to constantly find new and creative ways to rebel against anything and everything in her desperate efforts to cope with her own life's seemingly out-of-control stressors. Sally responded quite flippantly to the perceived pressure from her parents to excel at any task set before her, and she seemed to almost enjoy at times utilizing her intellectual capabilities to show others in the family, especially her parents, why her point of view was more "right" or correct than theirs – in essence, showing them how she would not allow anyone to command, coerce, or force her to do anything she did not feel like doing herself. On the surface, Sally did not overtly share Clark's burden of the autonomous perception that the divorce between her parents was indeed her fault in some way. Sally also did not openly display any explicit allegiance to either her mother's or her father's perspectives regarding their divorce. However, when the divorce papers were filed and a restraining order was issued on Ms. Jones' behalf against Mr. Jones, Sally (like her older brother Clark) determined that the best short-term placement for her at that time was in her father's household. Thus, during the divorce proceedings, while the younger four children remained with Ms. Jones in the family's original home, Mr. Jones and Clark moved to a new apartment along with Sally, who accompanied her father to his new living quarters in an almost dutiful manner.

Jenifer Jones was an 11-year-old Caucasian female who was a fifth-grade student at the time of her family's presentation to clinic. Unlike her older two siblings, Jenifer did not appear to be precociously mature for her age – in fact, Jenifer rather enjoyed her status as the family's most carefree and (in her own words) "happy-go-lucky" individual. Due to the progression of the family's birth order and the relative lack of significant age difference(s) among the youngest members of the family, Jenifer related much more easily to her younger three siblings than did either Clark or Sally. Jenifer took great pride in identifying herself as the true "middle child" of the family, both through her own verbalizations of this status, as well as through intermittent external reminders and reinforcing statements of this fact made by other members of the family. Because of her rank in the birth order, Jenifer best utilized her "middle child" status to acquire the attention of others, especially her parents, by reminding them that she didn't "get treated the same" as her two older siblings, nor did she "get everything" that she might have wanted "like the little kids" (the youngest three siblings) in the family did. As with her sister Sally's case, superficially, Jenifer did not perceive that the divorce between her parents was any fault of her own. Finally, despite her living arrangement in her mother's household and her own routine alignment with her mother's point of view on most major family issues and decisions, Jenifer was the one child among all six siblings in this family who steadfastly remained the most open to wanting to maintain an active relationship with both of her parents. Jenifer appeared consistently to be the most emotional member of the family and would often make statements to her parents both before and after the divorce such as "…When you go away, my heart just hurts."

Gerald Jones was an 8-year-old Caucasian male who was a second-grade student at the time of his family's presentation to clinic. Gerald was an extremely likeable and humorous young man, and he quickly appeared to stand out from among his siblings as the family's self-labeled "clown" and "the life of the party" (in his own estimation, as well as according to his parents' and siblings' perspectives). In fact, Gerald's capacity to turn any situation into a joke for the pure pleasure of creating some comic relief for those around him was one of the most noticeable and attractive aspects of his personality. As in the case of his elder sister, Jenifer, Gerald seemed to be able to more easily relate to his younger siblings – in fact, the age and maturity differences between Clark, Sally, and Gerald appeared to contribute to intermittent personality clashes and squabbling between these three particular siblings. Gerald's outgoing personality and uncanny capacity for socialization with nearly anyone he met unfortunately appeared to be offset by a very poor sense of self-esteem. To illustrate this point, Gerald historically had had difficulties with toilet training as a child and he continued to experience episodes of enuresis until he was approximately the age of six. The teasing by his siblings over this fact, coupled with a variety of instances in which Gerald had been severely disciplined by his parents for various age-related defiant behaviors (including multiple spankings with a belt, as well as reportedly with a two-by-four board on at least one occasion) all seemed to have scarred Gerald's sense of self-esteem in a very deep and profound way. Thus, his most obvious and apparent defense against these feelings of inadequacy and perceived extremely low self-worth was his effort to make himself likeable to anyone and everyone around him in his life.

Katie Jones was a 6-year-old Caucasian female who was a first-grade student at the time of her family's presentation to clinic. Katie appeared to be more endearing and attractive than the majority of her siblings, and she also displayed evidence of the fact that she was also quite precociously mature for her age (in a manner which was more similar to either Clark or Sally's persona than it was to either Jenifer or Gerald's personalities). She seemed to be more capable of and more comfortable with relating easily to her older siblings and adults than she was able to relate to her youngest brother. Unlike her two oldest siblings, Clark and Sally, however, Katie seemed to have no trouble whatsoever relating to her same-aged peers. Because of her position in the birth order, Katie often seemed to become involved in sibling rivalries and fighting with the two siblings closest to her own age in the family, her elder brother Gerald and her younger brother Jackson. Throughout the evaluation process, Katie did not openly admit to any perception on her part that the divorce between her parents was her fault in any way, shape, or form. She also seemed to be the sibling who was least capable of understanding why her parents could not simply put aside their differences and "get along," "live together," and "stay married." Aside from this innate and innocent sense of naivete, Katie was felt to be an extremely bright young woman by the clinical examiners involved in the case, in fact, their conclusion was that Katie was a true "people person" and the one family member who would most definitely be able to be successful in whatever she chose to do with her life.

Lastly, Jackson Jones was a 4-year-old Caucasian male who was not yet in preschool at the time of his family's presentation to clinic. Upon meeting him for the first time, the clinical examiners involved in the family's case felt that Jackson appeared to be "by far and away the most genuine and resilient member of the family" – he was the most innately happy and also the most unconditionally accepting of all of the other family members, including both of his quarreling parents. Jackson appeared to not even have to try to like others or be liked by them – he was a naturally charismatic young man with a uniquely mature personality despite his extremely young age. Jackson was most definitely the one member of the family who was able to seamlessly relate to everyone around him, including adults, all of his older siblings, as well as his own same-aged peers. During the evaluation process, Jackson displayed no evidence of any negative self-perception that the divorce between his parents was his fault for any reason whatsoever. Finally, Jackson seemed to be the one child who was able to enjoy himself at all times in the presence of either or both of his parents throughout the divorce process. To illustrate this last fact, despite his primary living arrangement with his three immediate elder siblings in his mother's household, Jackson seemed to be equally comfortable at his father's apartment throughout all of the divorce proceedings, including during any and all visitation sessions with his father and seemingly estranged elder siblings, Clark and Sally.

Summary of the Family Dynamics

Mr. and Ms. Jones had been married for over 17 years at the time of their initial marital separation in January, 1997. When the divorce proceedings began and tensions between Mr. and Ms. Jones rose, the family began to splinter, as all eight individuals in the family were no longer able to live together under one roof. As mentioned above, after the divorce papers were mutually signed by their father and mother, the children were all gathered together in the basement of the house by their parents and immediately given a choice as to where they preferred to live – "with mom, or with dad." As previously mentioned, the four younger children remained with their mother in the family's original house, while their father and the two older children, Clark and Sally, moved first to a hotel, where they lived for approximately 2 months prior to Mr. Jones finding a new apartment in town to which they were finally able to move into in March, 1997.

When news of their parents' decision to divorce reached them, the six Jones children all seemed to band together at first in expressing their mutual shell-shocked feelings generated by this situation, including disappointment, frustration, and anger at both Mr. and Ms. Jones for deciding to end their marriage. With time, however, old sibling rivalries grew to new heights while new rivalries quickly began; new and old alliances among these six children were dissolved and created, respectively, based in large part by the children's' proximities to either parent. For example, the children quickly developed a system of relating to one another which directly reflected the details of their living situation – the two older children seemed to be pitted against the younger four children during their visitations and various other interactions together. This phenomenon was apparently related to the fact that the two older children had been labeled as choosing "to live with dad instead of mom," a fact which unfortunately seemed to engender significant animosity on both sides of this issue. As an example to illustrate this last point, the two older children viewed themselves as involuntary outcasts who had had little choice but to go and live with their father throughout this tumultuous period. Clark and Sally quickly identified the fact that they "felt sorry for" their father and "didn't want him to be alone" during this incredibly stressful time in the family's history.

Because of their aforementioned dedication to their father, the two older children viewed their four younger siblings as "traitors" who had seemingly abandoned their father by choosing to live with their mother throughout the divorce process. In a very similar manner, the younger four children viewed the departure of their two older siblings as a betrayal of their mother, who they viewed as particularly fragile and victimized throughout the divorce proceedings. This trend was definitely most noticeable in Gerald's case, as Gerald often quickly grew quite angry and volatile when he was visiting with his older siblings at his father's apartment. Verbal arguments rapidly escalated on a frequent basis between Gerald and both Clark and Sally over the fact that they had, in his perception, left their mother "all by herself" by choosing to live with their father throughout this extremely nerve-racking situation.

The children in the family, however, were not the only people involved in controversy and troubled feelings of distrust. As might be expected, the parents' animosity in this case toward each other grew exponentially once divorce papers were filed and their divorce proceedings officially began. However, in varying degrees all six of the children appeared to feel on some level that they were frequently being used by their parents as "battering rams" so that their father and mother could "get back at each other" because of their respective angry and resentful feelings generated by the divorce process. Examples of this "battering ram" phenomenon included Mr. and Ms. Jones' efforts to win sole custody over all six children, which included two separate custody evaluations and a special hearing between all six children and the judge presiding over the case (which was held outside of the courtroom in the judge's quarters). A deposition of Clark by his mother's attorney soon followed – this legal proceeding was allegedly planned to try and elicit information from Clark which might implicate his father as the supposed mastermind behind manipulating all of the children, including Clark, to turn against their mother during the days and months immediately preceding the filing of the divorce papers.

Wallerstein's groundbreaking research on the long-term outcome of divorce highlights the fact that *the quality of the parental pre- and post-divorce relationship is the absolute most important overall factor in determining whether or not subsequent delayed effects of divorce on children and adolescents will occur and be manifested clinically.* If one therefore accepts the classic research findings by Wallerstein and Blakeslee (1989) as accurate, valid, and reliable, then the Jones family was a living, breathing example of how parental feelings of animosity and disdain contribute to generally poor long-term divorce outcomes throughout their childrens' lives. The Jones' divorce case was dragged through the local court system for nearly 3 years – finally, in the late Fall of 1999, a settlement between Mr. and Ms. Jones was reached and the paperwork was finalized. An annulment followed shortly thereafter in the following Spring of 2000 at the request of Mr. Jones.

The Outcome

Thus, while the steps of the divorce proceedings appeared to be finalized on a superficial level, the resultant long-term, generally negative behavioral effects and personality structure defects in the cases of the six Jones children (all of which manifested themselves in the years following the conclusion of their parents' divorce process) became lasting testaments to how truly indelible and life-altering the traumatic experience of parental divorce is on the impressionable minds of youth who are caught up in the metaphorical crossfire and animosity amidst the seemingly titanic struggles between all-too-human, bickering parents entangled in divorce proceedings. Specific examples of these negative behavioral effects and personality structure defects, which occurred in the cases of each of the Jones children are detailed below.

Clark became a self-labeled "workaholic" and completed a 4-year basic medical sciences program at a prestigious Midwestern university before being accepted into medical school. Clark's parents attempted to dissuade him from pursuing a career in medicine, each of them citing various examples of how medicine had, in their opinions, dramatically "changed (for the worse)" since they both had attended medical school. Despite this lack of parental support, Clark nonetheless pursued his dream to become a doctor in order to try and "help other kids from divorced families get the help and support" that he felt he and the rest of his siblings had never received (both during and after his own parents' marital disruption). At his 10-year follow-up appointment in the mental health clinic where Clark and his family had initially received treatment, Clark informed staff that he had eventually married in his mid-1920s, that he had been treated for clinical depression (with both therapy and medication interventions) for a number of years, and that he and his wife routinely struggled with his perception that she would leave him and file for divorce if he upset her in any way. Thus, Clark's motivated, driven persona served primarily to mask the feelings of inadequacy and insecurity throughout his life, which had been direct consequences of his own parents' divorce many years prior.

Sally became a talented artist who worked in a variety of media after receiving both her Bachelor's and Master's degrees in art from schools well known throughout the country. She quickly married a boyfriend whom she had met during her undergraduate training at a southern art school. Within a year, however, they were themselves divorced for a variety of interpersonal reasons. At her 10-year follow-up appointment in the mental health clinic where she and her family had initially received treatment, Sally informed staff that she had eventually moved to the West Coast where she remarried and had had her first child while working as an artist in the Bay Area. Sally was very reluctant to discuss her parents' divorce (much less her own divorce experience) during the aforementioned follow-up appointment in clinic. Despite her lack of verbalization of her feelings, she seemed to be very angry and frustrated with both of her parents because of their marital split, regardless of the number of years which now separated her from the timeframe of her parents' separation. Sally also eventually admitted that she had intermittently begun consuming alcohol on a relatively heavy basis and had likewise turned to recreational use of illicit substances at various times during her teenage and young adult years as a means of trying to distance herself from the stress generated by her negative feelings surrounding her parents' divorce. In a similar manner, Sally's attempts to distance herself from her family physically throughout her teenage years and young adult life (for example, settling down to live on the West Coast) were yet another direct reflection of the ever-present emotional distance that she felt toward both her parents and many of her siblings in the years following her parents' divorce.

Jenifer became a perpetual part-time student of sorts in the years following her parents' separation. Her lack of self-reliance and self-assuredness led her to initially experience difficulties in maintaining long-term, committed romantic relationships; she also frequently had trouble keeping jobs for longer than a few months at a time while she was in school. In a similar manner, she frequently changed not only the universities that she attended, but she just as quickly seemed to change her college majors and courses of study (for example, from Law, to Psychology, to Interior Design, etc.). Overall, Jenifer appeared to be one of the least satisfied and most restless siblings in this family. At her 10-year follow-up appointment in the mental health clinic where she and her family had initially received treatment, Jenifer admitted that after her parents' divorce, she had eventually begun to suffer intermittent symptoms of panic attacks, had (like her elder sister, Sally) occasionally turned to alcohol and recreational substance use as a means of stress relief in her daily life, and that she had ultimately become preoccupied with the eventual demise of both of her aging parents. Because of this preoccupation, she planned to be "the one person out of all the kids to stay in the area" around which her parents lived so that "somebody would be there to take care of them, if need be." In addition to these feelings of chronic anxiety about her parents' health and well-being, Jenifer also admitted to feelings of inadequacy when compared to her other siblings who had left the geographical area to attend various colleges throughout the country. In Jenifer's own words "they (her other siblings) probably think that I'm a loser because I stay around."

Gerald became a very dark, mysterious, and brooding young man who was preoccupied with the nihilistic side of life in the years following his parents' marital split. At his 10-year follow-up appointment in the mental health clinic (which had been scheduled in a manner similar to the appointments for his aforementioned elder siblings), Gerald informed staff that he too had moved to the Bay Area of the West Coast and was attending a local film school in his attempts to receive an undergraduate degree in videography. Gerald reluctantly admitted to staff that he had also suffered symptoms of clinical depression, that he had had difficulties in maintaining stability in his interpersonal relationships with others (for example, Gerald had recently become involved in a serious dating relationship with an older, married woman), and that he had been on at least one occasion involuntarily kept overnight in a local Psychiatric Emergency Department on suicide watch at the behest of not only his family but also concerned law enforcement authorities because of the intermittent worsening of his baseline depression. This event was reportedly precipitated by the fact that Gerald had made a variety of statements concerning his own suicidal plans to various family members via telephone shortly after moving out to the West Coast. While Gerald continued to remain very likeable and socially appealing to those in his immediate environment, it was obvious that he had become a mere shadow of his former self. All of the characteristic mirth, joy, and childlike innocence behind his developmentally appropriate mischievousness had gradually vanished completely following his parents' divorce. It became obvious at his 10-year follow-up appointment that in his efforts to battle his longstanding personal struggles with poor self-esteem, Gerald had developed what appeared to be the beginnings of an arrogant and malignantly narcissistic personality. At one point during the follow-up interview, Gerald stated very haughtily that he had "cut ties" with various members of his family in recent years because they "were of no further use to me (him) in my (his) life right now."

Katie became interested in the performing arts in the years following her parents' divorce. At her own individual 10-year follow-up appointment in the mental health clinic where she and her other siblings had been treated over the years, Katie informed staff that she had recently begun attending undergraduate classes at a smaller Midwestern university where she could focus her time and efforts on completing her performing arts degree. Katie seemed to be relatively disinterested during her follow-up appointment in discussing both the current and long-term effects of her parents' marital separation on her self-esteem and her personality. It appeared that Katie's most successful defense against the overwhelming disappointment and negative feelings generated by her parents' divorce was her ability to minimize the impact of the event on all the various aspects of her life, including her own rare alcohol and recreational substance use (which she minimized when comparing her habits to those of her elder sisters, Sally and Jenifer, by stating "…at least I don't drink or smoke as much as they [Sally and Jenifer] do…"). Katie generally seemed to be the most flippant sibling in this family who was interviewed at her individual follow-up appointment. However, her tough outward appearance merely highlighted (rather than masked) the obvious distress and ego-dystonic emotions she felt but was unwilling to express verbally to pertinent clinic staff members familiar with the family's case.

Even as a high school student, Jackson had become a very talented artist who also worked in a variety of media in the years following his parents' marital separation. At his own 10-year follow-up appointment in the same mental health clinic where he and his family members had received treatment, Jackson displayed some of his latest art projects when speaking with the clinic staff. The vast majority of his artwork seemed relatively dark and disturbing, as it frequently showcased his apparent inner feelings of conflict and pain, none of which had never been fully dealt with or adequately verbalized since his parents' marital split. At this same follow-up appointment, however, Jackson did appear to have maintained and nurtured his innate talent of relating interpersonally to everyone around him in his immediate environment in a seamless fashion (in a manner which was truly contrary to the vast majority of his elder siblings). In addition, Jackson was obviously the one family member who had truly remained a child at heart. He continually displayed his unique abilities from among his elder five siblings to enjoy himself at all times, to be unconditionally accepting of all of the other members of his family, and to be equally comfortable in the presence of either or both of his parents. Jackson attributed this last attractive character trait to his mere acceptance of the fact that he "couldn't change what happened between mom and dad," so he felt that he had eventually "just grown to learn to live with it."

To reiterate a previous point, while divorce proceedings between parents may eventually end, the rift that they cause in the structure and dynamics of the average modern family frequently leaves lasting, painful scars on the psyches of both parents who are involved in the seemingly herculean struggle often inherent in contested divorce proceedings. In addition to the injuries to the parents' own psyches, the divorce process itself seems to even more permanently damage the ego structures of the "innocent bystanders" – the children and adolescent victims of this all-too-common and truly traumatic, life-changing event. A more detailed discussion of this phenomenon, various useful treatment options and therapeutic techniques available to clinicians working with youth from divorced families, as well as the most clinically relevant take-home points will be reviewed in the subsequent sections of this chapter.

Discussion of the Clinical Impact of Divorce on Children and Adolescents

While there are myriad potential biopsychosocial developmental theories that could be called upon to further explain the short- and long-term, lasting negative effects on children and adolescents from divorced families, to find a satisfactory and clinically relevant explanation of why these children and adolescents develop so differently (when compared to their same-aged peers from non-divorced [intact] families), one actually does not need to look much farther beyond classic psychodynamic principles, such as Freud's own revolutionary theories on the Stages of Psychosexual Development in youth and young adults, as well as Erikson's innovative theories of the Epigenetic principle and his accompanying proposed Stages of the Life Cycle (Sadock and Sadock 2005).

Utilizing the Jones family's clinical case history presented above regarding their individual and collective experiences during and after the dissolution of Mr. and Ms. Jones' marriage, both the principles of the Freudian Psychosexual Developmental Stages and Eriksonian Epigenetic/Life Cycle Stage principles, as well as results of pertinent clinical studies from the aforementioned *Review of the Current Literature* section above will be utilized here to further elucidate (theoretically) how and why the Jones children grew and matured as they did over the years following their parents' marital disruption.

One fundamentally simple, yet undeniably important, clinical principle that the reader should keep in mind when reviewing the clinical material below is the following: *children and adolescents in different developmental stages will necessarily react quite differently (in both short-term and long-term settings) to the phenomenon of parental divorce*. This statement has a number of far-reaching interpersonal implications within and outside the home environment(s) of these afflicted families, as well as in the midst of the clinical setting (from both diagnostic and treatment perspectives), a fact which is readily identifiable and known all-too-well by mental health practitioners with experience in working with members of divorced families.

Clark

From a Freudian Psychosexual Developmental Stage perspective, Clark at 16 years of age was in the midst of his "Genital" stage of development at the time of his parents' divorce. Because of the significant distress related to his parents' marital difficulties, Clark appeared to have become at least partially arrested in this stage of development and subsequently struggled to successfully meet the goals of this psychosexual stage for a number of years (i.e., the goals of separating from one's parents, as well as developing not only mature object relations but also a more secure sense of identity and traditional adult roles). Clark also seemed to suffer intensely from the pathology associated with this psychosexual developmental stage, in that he struggled with the reopening of previous conflicts from earlier developmental stages, as well as with the predictable subsequent regression in one's personality organization that often accompanies the reopening of these previous developmental conflicts.

From an Eriksonian perspective, Clark was in the midst of his own "Identity vs. Role Confusion" life cycle stage when news of his parents' divorce upended the established order in his family. While Clark eventually became a "workaholic," he continued to struggle with ongoing difficulties with any major change(s) in his life in general, as well as with more specific changes in his everyday routine, such as transitioning into new roles and learning new skills associated with occupational prototypes. Because of the fact that Clark seemed to suffer from an unresolved identity crisis in the wake of his parents' divorce, his identity became diffused and his role(s) both within and outside of his nuclear family became confused. This may in fact be the most appropriate explanation as to why Clark became his family's *voluntary scapegoat* or primary *symptom bearer* with respect to his parents' divorce. In essence, Clark attempted to voluntarily blame himself for the relationship problems between his parents, because it was easier to displace his anger and turn his frustration at the situation inward on himself (in an almost quasi-masochistic manner) rather than confront his parents openly about his feelings of disappointment and regret caused by their marital difficulties. Theoretically speaking, divorced families will oftentimes contain not only a *voluntary scapegoat* (who blame themselves for their parents' marital struggles, as in Clark's case in this particular family), but also one or more *involuntary scapegoat(s)* or other *symptom-bearer(s)* who are blamed by others (including the parents and/or their siblings) for the parents' relationship difficulties and subsequent marital disruption.

Clark's pattern of behavior and development over the years following his parents' divorce coincides with the findings of D'Onofrio et al. (2007). Clark's increased risk of experiencing depressive symptoms in the wake of his parents' divorce could be partially explained by D'Onofrio's assertion that shared genetic liability found in divorced parents and their offspring seems to better account for the increased risk of internalizing problems in the offspring. Specifically, Clark's mood symptoms can be related to those of his mother which she had previously experienced during her own history of clinical depression.

Clark also displayed behaviors which supported the findings of Lansford et al. (2006), in that, as an adolescent from a divorced family, he would have most likely benefitted from social/environmental and educational interventions focusing on promoting academic achievement in school, since academic achievement was such an important determinant of his self-esteem and his personal sense of accomplishment following the dissolution of his parents' marriage. As was true in the case of his five younger siblings, Clark manifested behaviors which were consistent with the clinical findings of Silverberg Koerner et al. (2004) – specifically, Clark and his siblings were exposed to frequent and detailed maternal and paternal disclosures about their parents' divorce, all of which seemed to be associated with eventual adjustment difficulties during the years following the marital disruption. In fact, the way in which these parental disclosures were made to Clark and his siblings became (1) the ultimate mediator of both interpersonal differences in the various Jones children's overt reactions to these sensitive parental disclosures, as well as (2) the primary determinant of the frequency and severity of the baseline psychopathological symptoms indicative of the aforementioned varying levels of biopsychosocial maladjustment throughout the lives of each and every one of the Jones children.

Clark's insecurity in his interpersonal relationships with others, including his romantic relationship with his wife, coincides with the findings of Reese-Weber and Kahn (2005) – that is, clinical resolution behaviors within an adolescent's family appear to spill over into romantic relationships for these adolescents outside of their family, regardless of whether the adolescent lives in either an intact or a non-intact household. Ultimately, Clark's case is also an example consistent with the sample of subjects included in the study by Martin et al. (2005). Specifically, one might expect that the higher mortality risk in the offspring of divorced parents may actually be decreased in Clark's case, as he was a male from a divorced family who had not only achieved some semblance of personal satisfaction via his academic achievement(s) prior to his mid-life years, but he had also managed to avoid adopting unhealthy behaviors such as smoking and other recreational substance use which might have otherwise affected his mortality risk. In essence, from a strictly biological or physical health perspective, the stress of parental divorce during Clark's youth did not necessarily lead to strictly negative future outcomes by his 10-year follow-up appointment.

Sally

According to Freud's Psychosexual Developmental Stage theories, Sally at 12 years of age was in the midst of her "Latency" stage of development at the time of her parents' divorce. Because of the significant distress related to her parents' marital difficulties, at her 10-year follow-up appointment in clinic, Sally admitted to having what seemed to be at least superficial difficulties in the years following her parents' divorce in integrating her oedipal identifications between both of her parents, as well as experiencing inherent difficulties in consolidating her expected gender role(s) and identity. Sally also seemed to suffer moderately from the pathology associated with this particular psychosexual developmental stage, in that she struggled with developing meaningful internal controls and coping skills. In fact, Sally seemed to have developed these internal controls only very minimally; because of this fact, Sally (unlike her older brother) had turned to numerous romantic relationships and recreational substance use as potential external sources of control over primarily depressive symptoms (potentially in an attempt to compensate for her previously mentioned underdeveloped internal controls).

Erikson would have most likely classified Sally as being in the midst of her own "Industry vs. Inferiority" life cycle stage when her parents' divorce occurred. Because the significant trauma of her parents' divorce contributed to Sally's feelings of being (as she put it) "frozen in time" at this particular developmental stage for a number of years, she appeared to experience predictable deficits in her ability to quickly and easily learn new skills necessary for imagining and realizing future roles. In addition to this, Sally demonstrated frequent procrastinating and poor planning behaviors as a result of her arrest at this developmental stage; these negative behaviors seemed to directly result in frequent feelings of inferiority and inadequacy when Sally compared herself to others (a phenomenon which also may have led Sally to turn to recreational substance use to try and suppress and/ or mitigate these negative, self-loathing feelings).

Sally's interpersonal behaviors and developmental arrest(s) in the years following her parents' divorce reflect to the premise put forth by D'Onofrio et al. (2007) that a robust association exists between parental divorce and subsequent substance use problems in these parents' offspring, since this was most certainly true in Sally's life during the years following her parents' marital disruption.

In addition, Sally displayed numerous behaviors which supported the findings of Roustit et al. (2007), namely, numerous indicators of psychosocial maladjustment in adolescents are significantly associated with family dissolution. As was true in the case of both her older brother and her four younger siblings, Sally also manifested behaviors which were consistent with the clinical findings of Silverberg Koerner et al. (2004), in that, she and her siblings were exposed to frequent and detailed maternal and paternal disclosures about their parents' divorce, all of which seemed to be associated with her eventual adjustment difficulties during the years following her parents' marital dissolution.

Sally's case seemed to also coincide with conclusions of Størsken et al. (2005, 2006), due to the fact that, as an adolescent, she seemed to intermittently experience anxiety and depressive symptoms, with depressive symptoms being more frequent and prominent throughout her teenage and young adult years. Sally also suffered from a lowered sense of subjective well-being, self-esteem, and school problems in the wake of her parents' divorce. In fact, as a general rule, anxiety and long-term depressive symptomatology appeared to be much more common among the female siblings in the Jones family when compared to their male sibling counterparts. Likewise, the work of Huurre et al. (2006) appears to be particularly relevant in Sally's case, as her parents' divorce appeared to be an incredibly significant a stressor throughout her childhood and adolescence, so much so that its various long-term negative effects persisted well into her adulthood years.

Finally, Sally's conflict resolution behaviors within her family appeared to infiltrate and negatively impact her future romantic relationships, a trend which is consistent with the findings of the Reese-Weber and Kahn (2005) study. Specific, time-variable stressful events throughout her life in the years following her parents' divorce also relate to the work of Ge et al. (2006) and are particularly relevant in Sally's case, as they were significantly associated with the variable trajectory of the depressive symptoms which she experienced intermittently as she moved through her adolescent years into her young adult life.

Jenifer

Jenifer's developmental trajectory quite remarkably mirrored Sally's own developmental experiences from both a Freudian and Eriksonian perspective. Like her elder sister, Jenifer at 11 years of age was in the midst of her Freudian "Latency" psychosexual developmental stage. Once again, on account of the significant distress related to her parents' marital difficulties, at her 10-year follow-up appointment in clinic, Jenifer (like Sally) also reported having at least superficial difficulties in the years following her parents' divorce in integrating her oedipal identifications between both of her parents, as well as experiencing inherent difficulties in consolidating her expected gender role(s) and identity. In addition to these aforementioned difficulties, Jenifer also seemed to suffer moderately from the pathology associated with this particular psychosexual developmental stage, in that she struggled with developing meaningful internal controls and coping skills. In fact, Jenifer seemed to have developed these internal controls only very minimally; because of this fact she (unlike her older brother and sister) had turned to numerous romantic relationships and recreational substance use as potential external sources of control in the wake of numerous anxiety (specifically, panic attack) symptoms (once again [as has been true in Sally's case], potentially in an attempt to compensate for her aforementioned underdeveloped internal controls).

From an Eriksonian Epigenetic/Stages of the Life Cycle point of view, Jenifer would also be identified as being in the midst of her own "Industry vs. Inferiority" life cycle stage when her parents' divorce occurred. Because of her obvious developmental arrest in this particular developmental stage for a number of years, Jenifer (like Sally) also appeared to experience predictable deficits in her ability to easily and quickly learn new skills necessary for imagining and realizing future roles. In addition to these difficulties, Jenifer demonstrated frequent procrastinating and poor planning behaviors; these negative behaviors may have directly resulted in not only Jenifer's pattern of indecisiveness (in changing job plans, educational plans, relationship plans in an almost routine manner), but also to her nagging feelings of inferiority and inadequacy when Jenifer compared herself to others, especially her five siblings.

As in the case of her two elder siblings, Jenifer's interpersonal behaviors and developmental struggles during the years following her parents' divorce correspond closely with the conclusions of D'Onofrio et al. (2007). Jenifer's substance-use behaviors, much like Sally's, during the years following her parents' marital disruption clearly illustrate the relationship between parental divorce and subsequent substance-use problems in divorced parents' offspring.

Jenifer, like Sally, also displayed numerous behaviors which supported the premise that indicators of psychosocial maladjustment in adolescents are significantly associated with family breakup, as described by Roustit et al. (2007). Jenifer also manifested behaviors which were consistent with the clinical findings of Silverberg Koerner et al. (2004), in that, she and her siblings were exposed to frequent and detailed maternal and paternal disclosures about their parents' divorce, all of which appear to be linked with the adjustment difficulties she faced subsequently during her adolescent and young adult years.

The findings of Størsken et al. (2005, 2006) are evident in Jenifer's case as well. As an adolescent female from a divorced family, Jenifer seemed to intermittently experience anxiety and depressive symptoms (with anxiety symptoms being more prominent, frequent, and severe in her case than were overt depressive symptoms), as well as a lowered sense of subjective well-being, self-esteem, and school problems, all of which occurred in the wake of her parents' divorce. In fact, in light of the long-term effects of her parents' divorce, Jenifer's case is also an example of the findings of Huurre et al. (2006). Her parents' divorce was clearly a significant stressor during her childhood and adolescence, and is evidenced by the chronic negative effects which persisted well into her adult years.

Again, like Sally, Jenifer also seemed to exhibit behaviors consistent with the findings of Reese-Weber and Kahn (2005), because of the fact that her conflict resolution behaviors within the family were carried over into the frequent and superficial romantic relationships which occurred during her adolescent, teenage, and young adult years. The work of Ge et al. (2006) could be used to assert that time-variable stressful events throughout the years following Jenifer's parents' divorce were significantly associated with the unpredictable course of her anxiety and depressive symptoms, the majority of which she experienced rather frequently throughout her maturation during her adolescent and young adult years.

Gerald

While technically Gerald's developmental trajectory overlapped those of his two elder sisters from both Freudian and Eriksonian developmental stage perspectives, Gerald's baseline symptomatology throughout his adolescence and his early adult years was actually quite different than the symptoms observed in the aforementioned cases of Sally and Jenifer. Like his elder sisters, Gerald at 8 years of age was in (albeit the earlier portion of) his Freudian psychosexual developmental ("Latency") stage. Unlike his elder sisters, Gerald did not display prominent difficulties in integrating oedipal identifications and/or consolidating his expected gender role(s) and identity. In fact, Gerald's internal controls appeared to be much more highly developed when compared to those exhibited by his elder sisters – in Gerald's case, these controls may very well have been overdeveloped, as Gerald intermittently displayed characteristics consistent with an obsessive–compulsive and generally quite controlling personality as he matured throughout his teenage and young adult years.

Epigenetically speaking, Gerald was in the midst of his own "Industry vs. Inferiority" life cycle stage when the news of his parents' divorce was revealed to him. While Gerald did not display an obvious developmental arrest in this particular developmental stage (as had both Jenifer and Sally, as mentioned above), the trauma of his parents' divorce most definitely contributed to a lack of reliable and secure parental role models for Gerald to rely upon and look up to in his everyday life. Because of this baseline insecurity, Gerald became more and more introverted as he relied more and more heavily on himself for his own self-actualization and self-soothing needs. By his mid-teens, Gerald had gradually developed the underlying malignantly narcissistic personality which eventually manifested itself at his 10-year follow-up appointment in clinic, at which, he made it perfectly clear that he no longer needed other for "anything" – in fact, he planned on caring for himself and only himself, because, as he perceived it, no one had ever cared enough about him to focus on his needs in the devastating time period of (both during and after) his parents' divorce. In his quest for individuation, Gerald appeared to have taken the concept of self-reliance to an extreme and subsequently asserted (in a pathologically defensive manner) that he did not "need anyone" in his life at all.

Gerald's unique interpersonal struggles and developmental challenges during the years following his parents' divorce lend credence to the findings of both Wood et al. (2004) and Nair and Murray (2005). Wood et al. (2004) asserted that the association between divorce and child internalizing behavior was partially mediated by depressive/withdrawn parenting style when the children are younger, while Nair and Murray (2005) explored how parenting style made a direct and independent contribution to the sense of attachment security in younger children. Parental temperament also appeared to be directly related to Gerald's extremely poor/low level of attachment security.

Since Gerald prominently manifested both internalizing and externalizing behaviors at differing times throughout the years following his parents' divorce, he would likely have benefitted from various psychosocial interventions focusing on the prevention of these negative behaviors, as suggested by Lansford et al. (2006). As was true in the cases of all three of his elder siblings, Gerald, was exposed to repeated and in-depth disclosures by his parents about their divorce. Thus, Gerald's eventual adjustment difficulties in the years following his parents' marital disruption also draw a parallel to the findings of Silverberg Koerner et al. (2004).

Katie

Katie's developmental trajectory was also quite remarkably different from those of either of her two elder sisters, despite the fact that she herself was technically in the midst of the same Freudian and Eriksonian developmental stages as her three immediate elder siblings. Unlike her elder sisters, Katie at 6 years of age was merely at the beginning of her Freudian "Latency" psychosexual developmental stage. This developmental difference between the maturity levels of Katie and her elder sisters at the time of their parents' divorce may account for the fact that Katie did not seem to suffer from either difficulties in integrating her oedipal identifications between both of her parents, nor did she seem to overtly experience inherent difficulties in consolidating her expected gender role(s) and identity. In addition to the lack of these aforementioned difficulties, Katie did not appear to struggle greatly with the development of meaningful internal controls and coping skills. In fact, despite Katie's outwardly flippant and disinterested demeanor as an adult, she did genuinely seem to be generally better adjusted than either of her two elder sisters, due to the fact that she had seemingly developed her own internal controls to a much higher degree than had either Sally or Jenifer throughout their respective teenage or young adult years.

According to Erikson's theories regarding the Epigenetic principle and accompanying Stages of the Life Cycle, Katie would have been beginning her own "Industry vs. Inferiority" life cycle stage at the time of her parents' divorce. Once again, due to Katie's young age at the time of her parents' marital disruption, unlike her two elder sisters, Katie appeared to have managed to avoid developing significant pathology with respect to experiencing prominent, frequent feelings of inferiority and inadequacy which are typically associated with maldevelopment during this particular life cycle stage. In addition to this developmental difference, when compared to her two elder sisters, Katie also appeared to be more able to readily embrace daily changes in her life; she was notably quite capable of acquiring and developing new skills for the purposes of realizing potential future roles throughout her lifetime.

As previously discussed in the cases of her two elder sisters, Katie's case illustrates the relationship found by D'Onofrio et al. (2007) to exist between parental divorce and subsequent substance-use problems in the offspring of these parents. During the years following her parents' marital disruption, Katie, too, occasionally experimented with drugs and alcohol. However, in her particular case, Katie tried to minimize her substance-use behaviors by comparing them with the personal habits of her elder sisters, Sally and Jenifer.

Katie also manifested behaviors reflective of the findings of Silverberg Koerner et al. (2004). As Katie was not excused from the recurrent, detailed disclosures by her parents regarding their divorce, she too experienced unique maladjustment difficulties in the years following her parents' marital disruption. However, like her elder brother Clark, Katie's developmental experiences in the wake of her parents' divorce support the findings of Martin et al. (2005), as the childhood stresses she experienced following her parent's divorce did not necessarily exclusively lead to later negative outcomes in her young adult years.

Jackson

Due to the fact that he was a mere 4 years of age at the time of the announcement of his parents' impending divorce, Jackson's developmental trajectory was quite unique and remarkably different from those of all five of his elder siblings. Unlike his elder siblings, Jackson was at the midpoint of his Freudian "Phallic" psychosexual developmental stage. This developmental difference between Jackson and his siblings may very well explain why Jackson himself eventually became the most well-adjusted member of the sibling group in the Jones family. Specifically, Jackson appeared to be able to master his oedipal complex feelings and readily mastered his internal impulses by allowing his superego to develop appropriately and help him channel his negative feelings surround his parents' divorce into productive activities, such as creating complex, visually stimulating, and generally haunting artwork.

From an Eriksonian point of view, Jackson was also at the midway point of experiencing his own "Initiative vs. Guilt" life cycle stage at the time of his parents' divorce. As his locomotion and language skills improved throughout this developmental stage, Jackson successfully appeared to become more active and was able to participate more fully in the daily goings-on at both his mother's and his father's home(s). Unlike his siblings, Jackson seemed to be more ready and willing to accept the status quo of the new family living arrangements in the wake of his parents' marital disruption (as his frame of reference was obviously different from his elder siblings, all of whom had known only a two-parent household lifestyle throughout their developmental years). Once again, as had been true in his elder sister Katie's case, Jackson's young age at the time of his parents' marital disruption appeared to have shielded him from developing significant pathology (such as conversion disorder symptoms, general inhibition, and specific phobias) typically associated with maldevelopment during his particular life cycle stage.

Jackson's case echoes the findings by Wilcox Doyle et al. (2003), in that, positive events appear to be protective for children and adolescents experiencing high levels of negative events during significant family transitions. It appears that Jackson's generally positive attitude and outlook on life facilitated the remarkable frequency of his positive life experiences, despite the fact that the majority of his life occurred within a post-divorce home environment. Jackson, along with his five elder siblings, also manifested behaviors similar to those discussed by Silverberg Koerner et al. (2004). The frequent nature his parent's disclosures regarding their divorce were predictors of the inimitable adjustment difficulties Jackson would face in the years following his parents' marital disruption. Finally, Jackson's developmental experiences mirror the findings of Martin et al. (2005), as the strain caused by his parent's divorce did not necessarily lead to negative outcomes thus far throughout his young life (that is, throughout his teenage years to date).

Therapeutic Treatment Options and Strategies for Children and Adolescent Victims of Parental Divorce

Within the continuum of appropriate treatment interventions for members of divorced families, a number of classic strategies have been frequently utilized to minimize family disruption and improve the psychological health and well-being of all individuals involved in various conflicts created by the phenomenon of parental divorce. These enduring strategies (whether voluntary or court-ordered) include the following:

1. *Group therapy*, which targets and treats symptoms in the cases of various members of the divorced family in differing ways:
   (a) Divorced couples' groups – promote psychoeducation and psycho-therapeutic interventions among divorcing parents (sessions may be attended within a therapeutic group setting either individually or jointly).
   (b) Groups for preschool/latency-aged children – promote psychoeducation and sharing/interpersonal techniques among the youngest victims and survivors of parental divorce.
   (c) Groups for adolescents – like those conducted for children, these groups also promote psychoeducation and sharing/interpersonal techniques among teenagers and their peers in the wake of parental divorce.
2. *Mediation*, a technique which targets the conflict between the divorcing couple itself and challenges each member of this strained dyad to put aside personal differences and formulate a plan prioritizing their children's needs. In the midst of any successful mediation process, two basic yet extremely relevant clinical principles must be realized at all times:
   (a) Children and adolescents all need frequent and liberal contact with both of their parents in order to minimize family conflict and promote inter-personal healing among the numerous damaged relationships within these families.
   (b) Children and adolescents will experience significantly fewer adverse consequences throughout their lives (both short-term and long-term) if the level of interpersonal conflict between the divorcing parents is kept to a minimum.
3. *Psychotherapy for divorcing couples*, a technique which focuses on behavioral and communication characteristics and trends between divorcing parents in order to more thoroughly understand the psychodynamic interplay between the couple, as well as to minimize the short-and long-term adverse consequences of both marital dissolution and ongoing strained relationships between these individuals with each other, as well as the strained relationships between each of these individuals and their children within the now divorced family.
4. *Individual psychotherapy*, targeting children, adolescents, and parents. This technique appears to be the most beneficial strategy for addressing the individual needs of various divorced family members (for example, individual

treatments for problems related to poor interpersonal functioning, domestic violence, addictions, and residual feelings of anger/rage within any of the members affected by this familial crisis, etc.).

In addition to these more traditional treatment techniques, two recent studies focused more specifically on treatment options and strategies for children and adolescents from divorced families. Lebow and Newcomb Rekart (2007) examined an integrative family therapy approach to target high-conflict, intractable disputes over child custody and visitation issues among families in the midst of parental divorce proceedings. The authors found that the Integrative Family Therapy approach appears to successfully create a "good enough" post-divorce climate for families in order for new family structure(s) to be established in the midst of high levels of intra-family conflict. The new family structure(s) established during the course of the Integrative Family Therapy process subsequently allow(s) the involved parents to not only keep physical and emotional distance from each other, but also to help minimize conflict and triangulation within their families.

Bernstein (2007) addressed multiple themes of successful therapeutic interventions in work with complex post-divorce families. The author concluded that the following treatment recommendations are absolutely essential to positive clinical progress sought by treating mental health practitioner(s) and members of complex post-divorce families: (1) The assumed "Child of Divorce" disposition "script" must be deconstructed by the therapist, in order to prevent the restriction of possibilities and the subsequent development of negative self-fulfilling prophecies in the lives of both the children and their divorced parents; (2) The gap between possibilities and positive/negative preconceptions in both the "new extended family" and other new partnerships created by divorce must be discussed throughout the course of clinical work with divorced family members; and lastly, (3) The potential for repairing relationships (especially the relationships between divorced parents and their adult children) which have been damaged through the marital disruptions and challenging transitions inherent in the divorce process must be exclusively addressed as a part of any successful family therapy.

Take Home Messages

For the reader's ease of usage and future reference to this chapter and the clinical materials contained therein, the following list of clinically significant take-home points regarding the topic of divorce and its deleterious effects on children and adolescents has been assembled:

Clinical research on the long-term outcome of divorce highlights the fact that *the quality of the parental pre- and post-divorce relationship is the most important overall factor in determining whether or not subsequent delayed effects of divorce on children and adolescents will occur and be manifested clinically.*

Children and adolescents in different developmental stages of life will necessarily react quite differently (in both short-term and long-term settings) to the phenomenon of parental divorce.

While some may argue or assume that children and adolescents are sufficiently resilient to simply "get over" the negative effects of divorce throughout their lives, the most recent clinical research findings refute this claim.

Parents in the midst of a divorce absolutely must become more conscious of the needs of their children during this incredibly stressful life event. Parents should also realize that in order for their children to successfully adapt to the unique stresses in a divorced family, they themselves need to focus first on the needs of the child (including basic needs for parental attention and nurturance, such as playtime, etc.), even if mediators and lawyers encourage them to do otherwise.

Parenting style may make a direct and independent contribution to the sense of attachment security in young children. In addition, the parental temperament appears also to be directly related to the children's sense of attachment security; however, it does not overshadow or diminish the influence of parenting style on the children's sense of attachment security. Ultimately, the maternal parenting style is felt to be the major factor in mediating the relationship of divorce to younger children's sense of attachment security.

Based upon the available research in the current literature, it appears that the traditional parent–child visitation patterns and guidelines are outdated, unnecessarily rigid, restrictive, and fail (in both short-term and long-term timeframes) to address the best interests of the majority of children from divorced families. Research-based parenting plan models appear to more appropriately serve children from divorced families' developmental and psychological needs (than do the aforementioned traditional visitation pattern models).

An association between divorce and children's subsequent externalizing and internalizing behaviors may exist and be at least partially mediated by a depressive/withdrawn parenting style when the children are in elementary school grade(s).

Early parental divorce or separation is more negatively related to the trajectories of both children's externalizing and internalizing behaviors (when compared to later parental divorce/separation). However, later parental divorce or separation is more negatively related to trajectories of academic grades as children grow older and mature. Thus, children may benefit most from interventions focusing on preventing both internalizing and externalizing behaviors, while adolescents may benefit most from interventions focusing on promoting academic achievement in school.

Indicators of psychosocial maladjustment in adolescents (i.e., internalizing disorders, externalizing disorders, (non-alcoholic) substance use, and alcohol consumption) appear to be significantly associated with family breakup. In addition to this fact, an independent association between adolescents' development of internalizing has been noted to be strongly related to these young individuals' previous experience(s) of witnessing interparental violence at some point in their past. It appears that, ultimately, family-based interventions and social approaches are definitely complementary support modalities for adolescents who have experienced or are experiencing family disruptions.

A robust association appears to exist between parental divorce and offspring substance-use problems; while these results do not prove that a connection exists between the above variables, all the same, they are associated with a causal connection between parental divorce and offspring substance-use problems. In direct contrast to this, however, the shared genetic liability in divorced parents and their offspring seems to better account for the increased risk of internalizing problems in the offspring from these divorced families as they mature throughout their adolescent and adult years. Thus, the increased risk of internalizing problems in this population appears to be a selection artifact as a part of the clinical research process. Ultimately, unmeasured genetic and environmental selection factors must be considered when studying the effects of parental divorce on their offspring. In addition to this fact, selection versus causal mechanisms may function quite differently for substance abuse in offspring of divorced parents (a potential causal connection) and internalizing problems in these same offspring (a selection artifact).

Parental divorce was prospectively associated with relative changes in the frequency of adolescent anxiety and depressive symptoms, as well as in subjects' sense of subjective well-being, self-esteem, and school problems. In addition, parental divorce was prospectively associated only with school problems in adolescent males, while parental divorce was prospectively associated with all of the variables listed above among adolescent females.

Parental divorce is associated with higher mean levels and larger variances in adolescent problems; both divorce and parental distress appear to contribute independently to adolescents' distress. The prevalence of substantial adolescent distress symptoms has, reportedly, more than doubled among adolescents from divorced and distressed parents when compared to the prevalence of these symptoms in their same-aged peers from non-divorced and non-distressed parents. In addition, long-term effects of divorce on anxiety and depressive symptoms seem to be more overt and clinically significant among adolescent females than among their adolescent male counterparts.

Females from divorced families report more psychological problems (incl. higher scores on the Beck Depression Inventory (BDI) instrument) and more problems in their interpersonal relationships with others; however, these particular findings are not necessarily found among their male peers. Ultimately, subjects of both genders with a background of parental divorce report a higher frequency of various psychosocial problems throughout their lives (when compared to peers from non-divorced families), including shorter education, unemployment, divorce, negative life events, and more risk-taking (unhealthy) behaviors. Thus, parental divorce appears to be an indicator of sufficient stress in childhood and adolescence, due to the fact that its various long-term negative effects persist well into adulthood (perhaps with a wider scope of negative effects among females when compared to male counterparts).

Among adolescents from divorced (non-intact) families, (1) Depressive symptoms appear to change in a curvilinear pattern throughout the adolescent years (especially among the females) (depressive symptoms appeared to increase during early- to mid-adolescence and then subsequently declined as subjects approached late adolescence and young adulthood); (2) Females experience an ongoing greater number of depressive symptoms in adolescence and early adulthood when compared to their male counterparts; (3) Adolescents who experienced parental divorce by age 15 tend to display a sharper increase in the number of depressive symptoms experienced when compared to their peers from non-divorced families; (4) Stressful life events experienced shortly after parental marital disruption and divorce appear to mediate the actual effects of parental divorce on the adolescents' depressive symptoms; and finally, (5) Time-variable stressful events throughout the adolescents' lives (especially those related to either personal losses or relationship losses) are significantly associated with the trajectories of depressive symptoms in the typical adolescent member of a divorced family.

Conflict resolution behaviors within an adolescent's family appear to spill over into romantic relationships for these adolescents outside of their family, regardless of whether the adolescent lives in either an intact or a divorced (non-intact) household.

Because of stressors associated with marital conflict and subsequent disruption, parenting practices in these situations are often compromised. As a result, the offspring of these parents often experience deficits in affective, behavioral, and cognitive domains, which eventually increase the overall physical health risk in these individuals (by contributing to poor health behaviors, as well as altering and compromising innate physiological stress-response systems, including cardiovascular, neuroendocrine, and neurotransmitter functioning). On the basis of all of the above conclusions, there appears to be a definite cost of marital conflict between parents via the disruption of their children's overall physical and mental health.

A higher mortality risk in the offspring of divorced parents was decreased among the children (especially in males) who had achieved a sense of personal satisfaction with their lives by their mid-life years. From a behavioral standpoint, smoking in these divorced parents' offspring was the strongest mediator of the link between parental divorce and subsequent offspring mortality. Ultimately, the fact remains that the stress of parental divorce during childhood does not necessarily lead to later negative outcomes throughout the lives of the divorced parents' offspring.

Within the continuum of appropriate treatment interventions for members of divorced families, a number of classic strategies have been utilized to minimize family disruption and improve the psychological health and emotional well-being of all individuals involved. These enduring strategies include: group therapy, mediation, psychotherapy for divorcing couples, and individual psychotherapy for any and all members of divorced families who might require and benefit from this treatment option (including children, adolescents, and parents).

The Integrative Family Therapy approach appears to successfully create a "good enough" post-divorce climate for families with high levels of conflict throughout their divorce proceedings in order for new family structures to be established. The new family structures established during the course of the Integrative Family Therapy process allow the involved parents to not only keep physical and emotional distance from each other, but also to help minimize conflict and triangulation within their families.

In order to facilitate successful clinical work between mental health practitioners with members of complex post-divorce families, the following clinical treatment recommendations should be considered – the assumed "Child of Divorce" disposition "script" must be deconstructed by the therapist, in order to prevent the restriction of possibilities and the subsequent development of a self-fulfilling prophecy in the lives of children and their divorced parents. In addition to the deconstruction of the aforementioned disposition narrative, the gap between possibilities and (positive and negative) preconceptions in both the "new extended family" and new partnerships created by divorce must be discussed throughout the course of clinical work with divorced families. Finally, the potential for repairing relationships (especially the relationships between divorced parents and their adult children) damaged through the marital disruptions and transitions inherent in the divorce process must be exclusively addressed as a part of any successful family therapy when one is working clinically with individuals and families from this complex post-divorce population.

References

Ahrons, C. (2007). Family ties after divorce: Long-term implications for children. *Family Process, 46*(1), 53–65.

Bernstein, A. (2007). Re-visioning, restructuring, and reconciliation: Clinical practice with complex post-divorce families. *Family Process, 46*(1), 67–78.

Bockelbrink, A., Heinrich, J., Schäfer, I., Zutavern, A., Borte, M., Herbarth, O., et al. (2006). Atopic eczema in children: Another harmful sequel of divorce. *Allergy, 61*, 1397–1402.

D'Onofrio, B., Turkheimer, E., Emery, R., Maes, H., Silberg, J., & Eaves, L. (2007). A children of twins study of parental divorce and offspring psychopathology. *Journal of Child Psychology and Psychiatry, 48*(7), 667–675.

Fabricius, W., & Luecken, L. (2007). Postdivorce living arrangements, parental conflict, and long-term physical health correlates for children of divorce. *Journal of Family Psychology, 21*, 195–205.

Ge, X., Natsuaki, M., & Conger, R. (2006). Trajectories of depressive symptoms and stressful life events among male and female adolescents in divorced and non-divorced families. *Development and Psychopathology, 18*, 253–273.

Huurre, T., Junkkari, H., & Aro, H. (2006). Long-term psychosocial effects of parental divorce: A follow-up study from adolescence to adulthood. *European Archives of Psychiatry & Clinical Neuroscience, 256*, 256–263.

Kelly, J. (2007). Children's living arrangements following separation and divorce: Insights from empirical and clinical research. *Family Process, 46*(1), 35–52.

Lansford, J., Malone, P., Castellino, D., Dodge, K., Pettit, G., & Bates, J. (2006). Trajectories of internalizing, externalizing, and grades for children who have and have not experienced their parents' divorce or separation. *Journal of Family Psychology, 20*(2), 292–301.

Lazar, A., & Guttmann, J. (2004). Adolescents' perception of the ideal mate: Its relationship to parental characteristics in intact and nonintact families. *Adolescence, 39*(154), 389–396.

Lebow, J., & Newcomb Rekart, K. (2007). Integrative family therapy for high-conflict divorce with disputes over child custody and visitation. *Family Process, 46*(1), 79–91.

Martin, L., Friedman, H., Clark, K., & Tucker, J. (2005). Longevity following the experience of parental divorce. *Social Science & Medicine, 61*, 2177–2189.

Nair, H., & Murray, A. (2005). Predictors of attachment security in preschool children from intact and divorced families. *The Journal of Genetic Psychology, 166*(3), 245–263.

Peris, T., & Emery, R. (2004). A prospective study of the consequences of marital disruption for adolescents: Predisruption family dynamics and postdisruption adolescent adjustment. *Journal of Clinical Child and Adolescent Psychology, 33*(4), 694–704.

Reese-Weber, M., & Kahn, J. (2005). Familial predictors of sibling and romantic-partner conflict resolution: Comparing late adolescents from intact and divorced families. *Journal of Adolescence, 28*, 479–493.

Roustit, C., Chaix, B., & Chauvin, P. (2007). Family breakup and adolescents' psychosocial maladjustment: Public health implications of family disruptions. *Pediatrics, 120*(4), e984–e991.

Sadock, B., & Sadock, V. (2005). *Kaplan & Sadock's comprehensive textbook of psychiatry* (8th ed., Vol. 1, pp. 725–734). Philadelphia, PA: Lippincott Williams & Wilkins.

Silverberg Koerner, S., Wallace, S., Jacobs Lehman, S., Lee, S., & Escalante, K. (2004). Sensitive mother-to-adolescent disclosures after divorce: Is the experience of sons different from that of daughters? *Journal of Family Psychology, 18*(1), 46–57.

Single-Rushton, W., Hobcraft, J., & Kiernan, K. (2005). Parental divorce and subsequent disadvantage: A cross-cohort comparison. *Demography, 42*(3), 427–446.

Størsken, I., Røysamb, E., Holmen, T. L., & Tambs, K. (2006). Adolescent adjustment and well-being: Effects of parental divorce and distress. *Scandinavian Journal of Psychology, 47*, 75–84.

Størsken, I., Røysamb, E., Moum, T., & Tambs, K. (2005). Adolescents with a childhood experience of parental divorce: A longitudinal study of mental health and adjustment. *Journal of Adolescence, 28*, 725–739.

Troxel, W., & Matthew, K. (2004). What are the costs of marital conflict and dissolution to children's physical health? *Clinical Child and Family Psychology Review, 7*(1), 29–57.

Wallerstein, J., & Blakeslee, S. (1989). *Second chances: Men, women, and children a decade after divorce*. New York, NY: Ticknor & Fields.

Wallerstein, J., Lewis, J., & Blakeslee, S. (2001). *The unexpected legacy of divorce: A 25 year landmark study*. New York, NY: Hyperion.

Wilcox Doyle, K., Wolchik, S., Dawson-McClure, S., & Sandler, I. (2003). Positive events as a stress buffer for children and adolescents in families in transition. *Journal of Clinical Child and Adolescent Psychology, 32*(4), 536–545.

Wood, J., Repetti, R., & Roesch, S. (2004). Divorce and children's adjustment problems at home and school: The role of depressive/withdrawn parenting. *Child Psychiatry and Human Development, 35*(2), 121–142.

Chapter 11

Stress, Mindful Parenting, and the Transition to Adulthood

Jeanne Joseph Chadwick

In our time, families are often wound up in social, professional, and occupational pursuits that inhibit the potential for establishing secure emotional bonds (Elkind 1994; Brazelton and Greenspan 2000; and Gottman 1997). This inhibition is serious under any circumstances, but it becomes even more conspicuous and damaging at moments when members of a family face new challenges and developmental transitions (Elkind 1994; Wallerstein 2003). These transitions are prompted by a variety of stressful life events that tend to arise at different points in the family life cycle. For parents, these events may include divorce, remarriage, loss of job, relocation of job, or care-giving responsibilities for aging parents. For children, these events are often associated with developmental challenges that give rise to a new set of emotional needs. During such transitions, a nurturing social environment that the child experiences as occurring for his/her sake is the optimal context for healthy development (Elkind 1994, 2008; Garbarino 1992; and Devereux et al. 1969).

While this idea may be intuitive to parents and researchers, the kind of environment that supports families in the midst of life changes has, thus far, been difficult to articulate. The parenting literature prescribes several different approaches, including early attachment to caregivers, acceptance of children's temperamental differences, spending quality time with children or increasing parental supervision, and making available social support networks such as effective childcare outside of the family (Bowlby 1988; Karen 1994; Lerner and Lerner 1987; Rosenfeld and Wise 2001). Much of the parenting literature also cautions, however, that parenting behaviors alone are not enough. Some even suggest that regardless of the child's age, even if parents were to do all that is prescribed, under the duress of stressful life events, there is no guarantee that children would appreciate these behaviors as having occurred for their sake (Garbarino 1992; Bronfenbrenner 1979).

Ecological systems theory has held promise as a conceptual framework for describing the kind of environment that incorporates many of these prescribed behaviors for parents (Garbarino 1992; Bronfenbrenner 1979). However, as

From: *Handbook of Stressful Transitions Across the Lifespan,*
Edited by: T.W. Miller, DOI 10.1007/978-1-4419-0748-6_11,
© Springer Science+Business Media, LLC 2010

convincingly argued by Wakefield (1996), this theory is difficult to translate directly into practice and falls short of capturing the relational complexity of the parent-child bond. Of course, one cannot expect that any one theory or approach will serve this purpose. Therefore, this chapter will use a number of related theories to examine variables that, taken together, may be indicators of the kind of environment that is most suitable for effective developmental transitions within families. It will prudently borrow and translate the concepts from both humanistic psychology/phenomenology (Rogers 1959), and systemic object relations' theory (Winnicott 1971) as the theoretical basis. In addition to these theories, the concept of *mindfulness* will be borrowed from the parenting literature that is derived from an Eastern philosophical perspective (Kabat-Zinn 1997).

Mindfulness is a concept that is discussed primarily in the philosophy, behavioral medicine, and public health literature. It is an orientation or focus that results in being fully present (paying attention) to the experiences of others in addition to one's own experiences. It has been defined in the philosophy literature as a way of being *consciously present* to one's internal and external environment (Thoreau 1854).

Mindful Parenting has been defined in the philosophy/psychology literature as a skillful way of being present to children and to everyday experiences that results in greater self-awareness, clarity of purpose and accelerated human development (Kabat-Zinn 2004). Lifespan, public health and social psychology literature has also shown this skillful way of being in relationship to be associated with higher levels of moral behavior (Kohlberg 1998) and positive emotional development (Devereux et al. 1969; Chadwick 2005). It is also inherently related to the concept of "generativity" from the psychosocial development literature (Erikson 1959). Generativity is defined as a special investment in or focus on one's child. Mindful Parenting, however, takes this one step further and includes an awareness or investment in one's own physical/emotional/spiritual needs. This awareness allows one to cultivate an inner sense of stillness/quiet and control over emotional reactions. This distinction is important for parents because knowing that one is capable of being calm and responsive to situations rather than reactive to them helps parents to develop a greater sense of self-efficacy and self-competence (Segal et al. 2002). This sense of competence appears to be significant for parent-child relationships during developmental transitions. This chapter focuses specifically on the challenges of parenting children in emerging adulthood.

For our purposes, the term "emerging adult" denotes developmental status (Arnett 2000), while the terms "child," "children," "child-focused" and "mindful focus on the child" reflect the relational status of emerging adults to the extent that the child is the offspring of the parent (Kabat-Zinn and Kabat-Zinn 1997; Devereux et al. 1969).

The tendency of an individual to focus on the needs of others (in terms of parenting, this could be described as child-focused) stands in direct contrast to assuming a reactive "self-focus" that is associated with an absence of mindfulness (Chadwick 2004). The public health literature suggests that such self-focused attitudes and behaviors are not only toxic to children but *can* also lead to depression and anxiety for adults (or parents); they are more likely to occur when these adults are experiencing cumulative and protracted episodes of stressful life events (Dohrenwend 1974). A study by Chadwick (2004) shows that this process is exacerbated when the adults, under stress, are also parents of emerging adult children. This study highlighted how stress processes influence human development when the parents' stress coincides with their children's transition to adulthood.

Focusing on psychosocial risk and the transition to adulthood, Hill and Maughan (2000) have attempted to clarify how parent-child relationships in this period may well have important implications for one's overall *functioning* as an adult. Their study of the transition to adulthood suggests that changes in the early adult period can be a "window of opportunity" that supports new patterns of development. These key transitional events and changes can alter the life trajectory to the extent that significant relationships that occur within this period hold the potential to offset earlier childhood disadvantage. In general, the years of emerging adulthood are characterized by a high degree of emotional instability and are typically used for discovering identity and negotiating changes in careers, geography, and relationships (Arnett 1998; Rindfuss 1991).

In terms of identity/self-perception, emerging adults do not see themselves as adolescents, yet many of them do not see themselves as adults either. According to Arnett (2000), when asked whether they feel they have reached adulthood, the majority of people at this age answer neither 'no' nor 'yes' but the ambiguous "in some respects, 'yes' and in some, 'no.'" This suggests the subjective sense on the part of emerging adults of being in a kind of developmental "limbo." It also reflects the sense that emerging adulthood is a period that is culturally constructed, and it is not universal or inflexible. This supports the emerging adult's need for stable family relationships to negotiate this state of *uncertainty*.

The Mindful Parenting model provides a map for parents to navigate this limbo and provide the necessary stability for emerging adults to make healthy developmental transitions. It does so by focusing on four key parenting dimensions that have been shown to be important to human development.

Dimensions of Mindfulness in the Parenting Relationship

As shown in Fig. 11-1 above, the dimensions of Mindful Parenting are the emerging adults' perceptions of mattering, their perception of unconditional support (unconditional acceptance), perception of parental regard (respect),

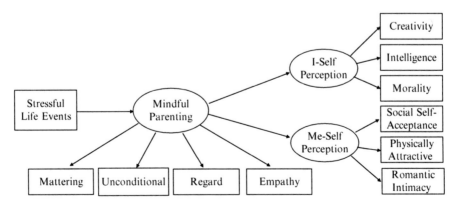

Fig. 11-1. Mindful parenting: a way of being child – focused

and their perception of parental empathy (Chadwick 2009). When these four parenting dimensions are present for emerging adults, it is theorized that Mindful Parenting is operating. Empathy is defined as the parents' response to the child that conveys an understanding of the child's needs. Unconditionality is the dimension indicating that the child experiences the parent as warm and accepting. Mattering is the overall sense of significance in the parents' lives. Studies show that mattering to parents is associated with the belief that one is also relevant in the lives of others (Taylor and Turner 2001). Regard is the child's perception that trust and respect are present in the relationship insofar as the child is seen as a unique and valued individual.

These four dimensions are discussed in the Eastern philosophical literature as representative of Mindfulness; the responsiveness to one's own needs (self-awareness) and to the needs of others (clarity of purpose/meaningful relatedness) (Kabat-Zinn and Kabat-Zinn 1997). From the clinical psychology literature, empathy and unconditionality have been shown to cultivate a sense of relatedness between individuals (Winnicott 1971; Rogers 1959; and Epstein 1997) while regard (respect for uniqueness) and mattering support autonomy (Marshall and Fleming 2001; Hauser et al., 1986; Grotevant and Cooper 1986).

Combining these four dimensions and attending to the needs of one's child in this way is thought to reflect a way of being that is "child-focused" (Devereux et al. 1969). The overarching assumption of this chapter is that when "children" are exposed to parenting dimensions and orientations that are sufficiently mindful or child-focused, they experience themselves as mattering to parents and to others. This, in turn, facilitates their healthy sense of *self* and psychosocial adjustment. By the same token, the experience is mutual given that what is gained by the parent is greater self-awareness, and a deeper sense of purpose and meaning in being a parent.

This idea that human development can occur mutually in certain kinds of relationships is suggested by the humanistic psychologist/phenomenologist, Carl Rogers. He describes a process that is similar to mindfulness in his use of the term "unconditional positive regard." While he did not refer specifically to parents and children, Rogers (1959) claims that when unconditional positive regard is generated in any significant relationship, a warm and trusting climate is likely to be present that nurtures emotional development. This sets up an experience of relatedness that Rogers describes in the following statement: " I have found it personally transforming when I can unconditionally accept another person" (Rogers 1957; p. 20). From a mindfulness perspective, Kabat-Zinn takes this idea further saying, "when I fully accept another person, especially when that person is my child, both myself and my child are transformed in that moment" (Kabat-Zinn and Kabat-Zinn 1997). When the parent is attuned and intentionally present in the moment, this sense of mutual transformation is the experience of Mindful Parenting. The practice of Mindful Parenting allows children and parents to experience an inner sense of calm and quiet. Thus, the experience of many of these moments over time is likely to lead to mutually transforming human growth and development (Chadwick 2004).

Segal et al. (2002) has described the practice of mindfulness this way: "one opens oneself up and is receptive to the flow of sense perceptions, emotions and thought processes in each given moment while attempting to hold judgment in abeyance. This is done with no other goal than to be as present as one can possibly be within each and every moment. One does this with an intimate attention that is very different from a scrutinizing, objective stance. Rather than being a distant observer of a set of experiences, one is a participant-observer, and what one observes is not only the sense impressions of the 'outside' world (i.e., stressful situations or the needs of one's child), but also one's own subjective reactions to that world" (Segall 2003, p. 79). Attending to one's child with mindfulness provides direct training in this regard. Knowing that one can be calm and responsive to situations rather than reactive to them helps parents to develop a greater sense of competence. The ability to do this for oneself reduces dependence on others and relieves emerging adult children from the burden of having to meet parents' needs as well as their own. This ability is thought to be most useful during periods of stress or transition because differences in the perception of self for emerging adults are associated with the number of stressful events that are encountered by their parents (Chadwick 2004).

The importance of addressing Mindful Parenting as a map for parents to follow is highlighted by the fact that studies on emerging adult development show that as children near the transition to adulthood the role of parents becomes less well-defined (Steinberg and Silk 2002). This uncertainty makes it difficult for parents to know how to sustain close and long-lasting relationships with emerging adults (Coleman et al. 2000). There is some evidence that these uncertainties about parenting are also driven by parents' own concerns about their transition into mid-life (Paikoff et al. 1991). These transitions for parents often involve changes of employment or career decisions, divorce, empty nest anxiety, or care-giving relationships with their own aging parents. In order to understand how these issues impact on the ability to be mindful or child-focused during the transition to emerging adulthood, it is important to examine the stressful life events pressing upon parents.

The Research on Stressful Life Events

Studies about how stressful life events in parents' lives impact older children are inconsistent. While some studies report a significant association between the levels of negative life events experienced by parents and their children's behavior problems (Furgusson et al. 1985; Holahan and Moos 1987), others do not observe a significant relationship between the two phenomena (Cohen et al. 1987; Thomson and Vaux 1986). A review of the stressful life events research suggests at least two limitations that may account for these empirical inconsistencies.

First, most studies testing the link between stressful life events experienced by parents and children's development use the parent as a single informant. When this method is used, significant prediction of life events to child outcomes appears to be likely (Furgusson et al. 1985; Holahan and Moos 1987). On the other hand, those who use one source of information to measure stressful life events and a different reporter for adolescent functioning do not find a significant stress effect (Compas et al. 1989; Cohen et al. 1987; and Thomson and Vaux 1986). Thus, it appears that parental stress is related to adolescent developmental outcomes only when the same informant is used to assess both constructs. It is the view of the Mindful Parenting framework that the reports from emerging adults about both stressors in the family and their own developmental outcomes would be more useful to researchers in eliminating this problem.

A second limitation in earlier studies of stressful life events and developmental outcomes involves the failure to take into consideration possible mediational mechanisms linking these two phenomena. Over the years, there has been a growing consensus that family processes play an important role in the etiology and maintenance of adolescent psychological distress (Downey and Coyne 1990; Rutter 1990). However, studies only vaguely describe how this occurs. For example, Rutter (1990) suggests that the relationship between negative life events for the parents and children's psychological dysfunction may be indirect and mediated by family processes. Other studies lend support to the idea that stressful life events experienced by parents amplify pathological family processes that subsequently lead to problematic child and adolescent developmental outcomes (Elder 1974; Elder et al. 1985; Patterson 1983; and Patterson et al. 1989). Building upon this research, the study by Chadwick (2004) investigated the role of Mindful Parenting as a possible mediator between stressful life events and the perception of *self*.

According to the path model diagram (Recall Fig. 11-1) stressful events experienced by parents set in motion a chain of events involving four indicators of the parents' behaviors, attitudes and emotions. This is quite consistent with studies of stress processes that have demonstrated that people exposed to a greater number of stressors experience more emotional problems and overall distress (Conger et al. 1993; Dohrenwend et al. 1978). This negative chain of events was investigated with regard to its effect on the self-perception of emerging adults. The self-perception of emerging adults is an important indicator of a healthy transition to adulthood.

The second model (Fig. 11-2 below) shows a model of aspects of the emerging adult self (Harter 1994) that were investigated using CFA (Confirmatory Factor Analysis), a type of structural equation modeling (Chadwick 2004; Baron and Kenny 1986) (Table 11-1).

As shown above, the six domains of self were highly correlated. A Varimax rotation was conducted to show how each of these domains factored into a two-factor model that would be consistent with James' (1890) conception of the self as the I-Self and the Me-Self (Harter, 94). The results of this showed that the six subscales of the measure fell into two distinct factors. From the table above we see that "intelligence" loads onto component 1 at 0.392 and higher on component 2 at 0.652. It is followed by higher loadings on the same factor for "creativity" and "morality" at 0.567 and 0.807, respectively. Thus, in an effort to specify a more precise structural model this factor/domain was separated from the three other subscales "social acceptance," "physical appearance," and "romantic intimacy," that factored into Component 1 of the matrix. The grouping of subscales that occurred through this analysis was thus, referred to as "socially independent" given that these variables appear to relate to internal processes, e.g., internal working models of self. They are the subscales for intelligence, creativity and morality. The other grouping was referred to as the "socially dependent" aspects of self given that these indicators of self-perception are thought to be dependent upon a person's particular social context. These included social acceptance, physical appearance, and the perception of romantic intimacy. These separate aspects of the self, represent

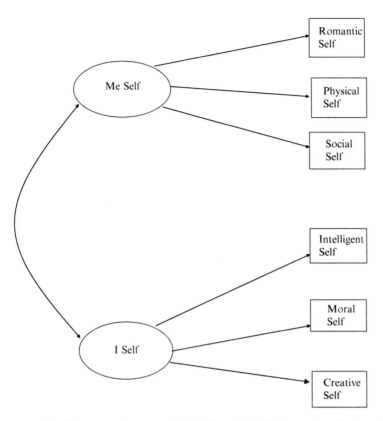

Fig. 11-2. Confirmatory factor model for Harter's Self Perception Scale with two factors

Table 11-1. Factor loadings from principle components analysis with a two-factor solution for the Self Perception Scale ($N = 580$).

Item	Factor loading		Communality
	1	2	
Intelligence	.392	**.652**	.579
Social acceptance	**.694**	.220	.530
Creativity	.358	**.567**	.449
Physical appearance	**.699**	.273	.564
Morality	.122	**.807**	.655
Romantic intimacy	**.780**	.130	.608

Note: Boldface indicates highest factor loadings

an outcome variable made up of two unobserved latent variables: the I-Self (socially independent aspects of self) and the Me-Self (socially dependent aspects of self).

One important consequence of stress-related experience is that it results in parenting behavior that may be harsh, hostile, and inconsistent, as shown in earlier studies of parents who suffer from depression (Field 1995; Berkowitz 1989; Burbach and Borduin 1986; Downey and Coyne 1990; Hammen et al. 1987;

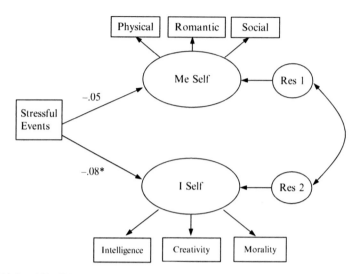

Fig. 11-3. Mindful parenting as mediator variable

and Weissman and Paykel 1974). The studies reviewed earlier from the emerging adult and stressful life event literature suggest that stressful life events give rise to more irritable parental responses toward children thus distracting them from the effort involved in skillful parenting. Using these studies as a guide, the diagram above illustrates how Mindful Parenting mediates important processes that impact the emerging adults' sense of self in the six areas that showed statistical relevance in the factor analysis (Fig. 11-3).

This test of the Mindful Parent model was designed to reveal the relationship between stressful life events (SLEs) and self-perception for emerging adults. The intention was to determine whether or not Mindful Parenting functions as a *mediating variable* in this causal pathway (Baron and Kenny 1986). According to Kenny, a given variable can be said to function as a mediator to the extent that it accounts for the relation between the predictor and the criterion. With this in mind, the paths from the predictor variable SLEs have been drawn directly to the criterion variables, I-Self (Socially Independent) and Me-Self (Socially Dependent) domains of self-perception (James 1890). According to Kenny's definition, mediators explain how external physical events (in this case, SLEs) take on internal psychological significance (the perception of self). The figure above shows how the measurement model was drawn before it was submitted to the AMOS 5.0 program.

The findings from this investigation are consistent with Kenny's theory of how mediator variables function. The study that proposed this model originally tested the full structural model that showed non-significance in the path coefficients between SLEs and self-perception when Mindfulness was included in the model. When Mindful Parenting was taken out of the model (see Chadwick 2004), the original paths were significant. This finding supported the mediator hypothesis indicating that Mindful Parenting mediated the relationship between parents' stressful life events and the emerging adults' sense of self. When the sense of self was tested as a single variable (combining the two aspects of self), it revealed the presence of a single significant pathway between SLEs and the sense of self in six domains.

When the model was tested with self-perception constructed as two separate domains (see Fig. 11-2), a new finding occurs. That is, the path from SLEs to the I-Self shows significance while the path from SLEs to the Me-Self dimension shows nonsignificance. Thus, Mindful Parenting was shown to lead to the sense of self in the domain of I-Self thereby affecting whether or not one views himself/herself as intelligent, creative and moral. It is, however, less important in the domain of socially dependent aspects of the Me-Self (i.e., physical attractiveness, romantic and social self) (Chadwick 2004) (Tables 11.2 and 11.3).

It was also thought that parent gender would operate as a second mediator within this path model. This was dealt with intuitively by separately analyzing the models by sex of parent. The conclusion is that the Mindful Parenting model, represented by four dimensions of experience, mediated the relationship between SLEs and the sense of self for emerging adults. These results are scaffolded by the synthesis of ecological and object relations' theory. These theories suggest that through mindfulness, a uniquely special environment is created. This environment is unique in that it "holds" the emerging adult through the turbulence of the developmental transition to adulthood.

The British pediatrician and psychoanalyst, D.W. Winnicott's concept of the "holding environment" and its elements are central in guiding this discussion of what it means to be Mindful or child-focused in parenthood, not just in infancy, but throughout development and specifically, during the emerging adult years and in the context of family stressors.

Winnicott's Developmental Theory of the Self

During his long career, Winnicott reportedly observed more than 60,000 children and parents (Winnicott 1956; Rudnytsky 1991). From these observations, he identified a series of behaviors and processes that he subsumed under

Table 11-2. Fit statistics for mediation model (Fig. 5-1).

Test 2 models	Df	X2	GFI	CFI	RMSR	IFI
Mediation model	12	25.07	.999	.999	.043	.999

GFI goodness-of-fit index; *CFI* comparative fit index; *RMSR* root-mean-square residual; *IFI* incremental fit index
$p < 0.01$

Table 11-3. Maximum likelihood estimates of test for mediation.

Regression weights	Estimate	Standard error	Critical ratio	Significance
ToPeri3 to Me-Self	−0.056	0.030	−1.869	
ToPeri3 to I-Self	−0.084	0.031	−2.705	***
Me-Self to Phyself2	1.000			
Me-Self to Romself2	0.863	0.117	7.347	***
Me-Self to Socself2	0.819	0.111	7.357	***
I-Self to Crease12	0.574	0.148	3.891	***
I-Self to Intself2	1.000			
I-Self to Morself2	0.365	0.099	3.690	***

*** means significance at the 0.01 probability level

the term "holding." He called the context in which these behaviors occurred as the "holding environment."

The holding environment is a concept introduced by D. W. Winnicott and his wife, Claire Britton Winnicott, while helping displaced families in the World War II Evacuation Project in London (Winnicott 1956). The couple used the term in two ways: to describe the bio-psychosocial context in which infants are sensitively tended to by their caregivers (particularly while under the duress of war); and as a metaphor for the silent, sustaining therapeutic functions (the relational matrix) of effective support efforts for those working with distressed families (Winnicott 1960).

Winnicott referred to the "holding" roles of both the parent and the therapist in virtually all of his writings (Winnicott 1956, 1960, 1965, and 1971). These references are consistent with ecological theory and also describe important aspects of Mindful (child-focused) Parenting. The key aspects are the child's perceptions in the parent-child relationship, the adaptation of the child's environment to his/her needs, and the importance of emotional support generated by the family, school or community. These holding references translate into the variables that constitute the Mindfulness framework to the extent that parents' focus of attention or orientation toward their children is likely to convey to children the existence of empathic concern, unconditional acceptance, a sense of regard, and the reassurance that they matter to parents.

While Winnicott's holding theory articulates the relationship of infants and young children to their parents, the main ideas are applicable to the parent-child relationship at any age. This chapter posits that this idea is particularly relevant to developmental issues that arise for older children at a time when they must establish their own holding environments away from the family. The holding environment theory is developmental and therefore, just as the child's needs change as he/she develops, the holding environment also changes to meet these developmental needs. In addition to holding, Winnicott suggests that through gestures and movements, parents mirror back (the process of mirroring) that they are experiencing and begin to co-construct with the child his/her psychosocial life (Winnicott 1960).

Winnicott also hypothesized that, from repeated experiences of adaptive holding and mirroring, there develops a profound mutuality between parents and children. He referred to this as "ego-relatedness" (Winnicott 1960). This term means that the child experiences an emotional bonding with parents and this allows him/her to "go-on-being" toward an integrated sense of self. This integrated self is also referred to as the "true self." This integrated true self ultimately lays the groundwork for the development of "unit status" (individuation from the parents) that is the task of older adolescents.

In a memorable meeting of the British psychoanalytic society, Winnicott (1956) declared, "There is no such thing as a baby!" (p. 39). By this, he meant that only in a facilitating holding environment that includes a partnership with an empathic caregiver is the baby able to come into existence as a whole person. Paradoxically, however, the core condition of ego-relatedness is the capacity to be alone; a capacity that he believed can only develop through repeated experiences of being alone in the presence of another (Winnicott 1971; Epstein 1997).

That which Winnicott referred to as ego-relatedness, could be viewed from the perspective of Mindful Parenting (Chadwick 2009). From this perspective, one could expect that given a non-demanding yet present caregiver, the child can enjoy periods of "un-integration" (the sense of being on one's own) without excessive anxiety. This conception may relate to the young child playing in the presence of an unintrusive, yet not-too-distant parent or to the older child/emerging adult who is physically distanced from parents yet protected by the sense that he/she still matters to them. According to this theory, the emerging adult's sense that he/she matters to parents is validating and leads him/her to a healthy sense of self (Chadwick 2004).

The emerging adult who perceives that he/she matters, begins the establishment of a reliable, comforting internal holding environment (the ability to withstand being alone) and this forms the foundation for healthy self-perception. In addition, it is perhaps, this sense of safety in one's internal holding environment that allows the emerging adult to trust others. According to Winnicott, having met these conditions (trust and the ability to be alone) the individual observes a coming together of a solidly grounded and accessible true self (Winnicott 1971).

By contrast, when development is substantially compromised, a less adaptive "false self" dominates relatedness. The development of this false self is more likely to happen by not attending to the child's needs because a parent who is constrained by stressful life events is more likely to assume a reactive self-focus. According to Winnicott, the false self is marked by social compliance, a lack of spontaneity, and a subsuming of one's own needs to those of others (Winnicott 1971). The false self is thought to suppress the expression of the true self. Hence, spontaneity is replaced by a defensive rigidity or passive compliance. This compliance may mask as social maturity; but, as Winnicott (1960) puts it, this self "lacks something, and that something is *the essential element of creative originality*" (p. 152) that is the mark of the true self. Hence, stressful events occurring in the family may give rise to the kind of holding environment whereby children have been let down or "dropped" in Winnicott's terms (Winnicott 1971). Central to the concept of the holding environment is the idea of the "good-enough parent" – an approachable, specific, and delicately shaded view of the parenting interactions occurring over the lifespan. These interactions shape identity development and in doing so, help to distinguish between a positive or severely compromised developmental outcome (Winnicott 1956).

The Good-Enough Parent

In elaborating his theory, it is clear that Winnicott (1971) believed that perfect parents could not facilitate development. Only through "failing" in doses that the developing child can tolerate, and then making amends for these failures, can parents provide the essential ingredients of adaptive care (Winnicott 1965). Countless cycles of failure and mending of failure ultimately enable the child to develop stable mental representations of others. The everyday predictability of these cycles engenders in the child an expectation of consistency and reliability.

Being "good-enough" implies that parents not only deeply understand their children but that children have the experience of being understood. The variables representing Mindful Parenting (empathy, regard, unconditionality and mattering) provide the vehicle for understanding the consequences of this process. According to Winnicott, it is the child's experience of being "held" or understood by the good-enough parent that makes all the difference in the development of a true self (Winnicott 1956).

More specifically, understanding the child's reality, regardless of the child's age requires an empathic response by the parent to communicate this understanding. Naturally, this communication also involves conditions that lead to the child's experience of mattering in the family. It is important to state that these kinds of experiences (i.e., maturational processes) may be generated in environments outside of the family as well, such as the school, community, and the sociopolitical environment. Winnicott's theory, however, suggests that it is the good-enough parent in the contextual holding environment that is primarily responsible for generating these experiences.

One way that this occurs is through what Winnicott (1971) referred to as the "mirroring-function," mentioned earlier. This mirroring function is a reciprocal process between parents and children. Parents intuitively register in their facial expressions (and other verbal or non-verbal behaviors) that they understand their child's needs. In turn, the child looks to parents' facial responses to his or her requests in order to construct a repertoire of emotions. Regardless of the child's age, this mirror-role of good-enough parenting is essential for the child's experience of empathy, unconditional acceptance, regard, and mattering in that it validates his/her lived experience and serves as a thread of continuity through repeated cycles of failure and reparation.

The Holding Environment During Stressful Events

Emerging adults who are living with their parents' stress may experience these cycles of failure with parents without the necessary reparation that allows them to stay emotionally connected. In addition, for emerging adults, an intact holding environment with good-enough parenting, past or present cannot be assumed. Many may be coping with family conflict as the fallout from family stress, geographic relocation after job loss, stress from ageing or ill grandparents, economic crises, or have been disappointed by even well-intentioned parents who are distracted by any number of events including divorce. Beset by anxiety and depression, divorcing parents may have difficulty maintaining that which Winnicott called "primary parental preoccupation" with the needs of their children (Winnicott 1989; Epstein 1997).

The natural focus toward the child that begins with the transition to parenthood and is cultivated over time may be foreclosed or replaced by turning the focus toward oneself, establishing new social relationships, taking on additional work hours, spur-of-the-moment court appearances or the seeking of social supports outside of the family. These new activities in the parents' lives may easily result in a mis-attunement to the activities occurring in the emerging adult's life. Hence, the interactions resulting from such mis-attunements are likely to contribute to estrangement rather than ego-relatedness. For the emerging adult, these stressful conditions may disrupt the holding environment to the extent that the emerging adult feels "dropped," lost or left to fend for himself/herself. This disruption is hypothesized to alter the natural tendency for exploration associated with this age-group in ways that affect their self-perception and ultimately, long-term development.

Systemic object relations' theory suggests that from the experiences of our earliest holding environments to the ones in emerging adulthood, we construct all subsequent relationships in adult life. How we construct these adult relationships depends upon our perception of self. It is thought that throughout this developmental journey, our inner selves are mapped into the psychic structures or internal models that shape individual adult relationships (Winnicott 1970). The experience of Mindful Parenting underlies the profoundly subtle, unconscious influences that these phenomena have on the human psyche (Kabat-Zinn and Kabat-Zinn 1997). These are part of what Bollas (1987) calls the "un-thought known" (i.e., knowledge that is largely unknown and preverbal). Hence, this information is more accessible through the examination of lived experience than through the observations and abstract interpretations of researchers and clinicians.

Phenomenology is an area of philosophy and psychology developed by a number of theorists including the German philosopher Edmund Husserl. He argued that the goal of phenomenology is to clarify and thereby to find the ultimate basis of all knowledge (Stein 1970, p. 4). Husserl's idea was followed by a series of investigators, up to and including the humanistic psychologist and phenomenologist, Carl Rogers. While the word phenomenon is typically associated with natural events such as lightning, thunder, tornadoes, etc., the words 'phenomenology' and 'phenomenological' refer to internal experiences (Spinelli 1989). Rogers used the term to refer to the reporting of internal experiences or perceptions about relationships with others.

Rogers' definition of phenomenology is the basis for the measures used to study the four dimensions of Mindful Parenting (Barrett-Lennard 1981; Chadwick 2004). Three of the four variables investigated (empathy, unconditionality, and regard) have been highlighted extensively in the phenomenology and humanistic psychology literature (Rogers 1975) as the core conditions that are necessary to establish healthy relationships. It was assumed that the absence of these variables leave children unprepared for the task of self-development encountered during emerging adulthood.

The hallmark of Rogers' person-centered model is that it outlines the "necessary conditions for healthy therapeutic relationships" and the conditions for being "fully present" to the needs of the client (Rogers 1959). As an adaptation of Rogers' model, the Mindful Parenting model shows that these elements are also significant in the context of SLEs and the emerging adults' sense of self.

Summary

Mindful Parenting emphasizes that being fully present to one's child involves empathy instead of self-absorption, regard for the individual child instead of indifference, the sense that one's child matters or is significant, and unconditionality rather than support based upon certain conditions. Mindful Parenting suggests that under conditions of high stress in the family, these variables may be diminished because parents will have less energy or time to "focus attention on the child's needs." It then logically follows that this alteration in a parent's focus may give rise to disrupted relationships that are expected to affect the sense of self in key areas that influence the identity development and emotional well-being for emerging adults.

If, however, a parent can maintain his/her focus on the child's needs, providing them with the experience of empathy, unconditionality, mattering and regard, it is expected that a *secure* holding environment will exist. This holding environment protects the overburdened family from the potential disruptions that result from life stressors. Thus, the concept of the holding environment describes a family context whereby the emerging adult perceives the mindfulness variables to be present in their relationship with parents. Mindful (child-focused) Parenting conveys that a true holding environment incorporates all four dimensions of experience. Applying these dimensions to the parenting process allows parents to be flexible across developmental stages. The idea of flexibility in meeting the needs of developing children is supported in the work of White et al. (1983). They report that it is the parent's adaptability to the child's needs and the "redefinition" of the parent-offspring bond over time that accounts for optimal development. Meeting the child's needs through Mindful Parenting allows him/her to establish trust and to perceive the world of relationships as safe enough to continue growing into adulthood.

References

Arnett, J. J. (1998). Learning to stand alone: The contemporary American transition to adulthood in cultural and historical context. *Human Development, 41*, 295–315.

Arnett, J. (2000). Emerging adulthood: A theory of development from the late teens through the twenties. *American Psychologist, 55*(5), 469–480.

Baron, R., & Kenny, D. (1986). The Moderator-mediator variable distinction in social psychological research: Conceptual, strategic, and statistical considerations. *Journal of Personality and Social Psychology, 51*, 1173–1182.

Barrett-Lennard, G. (1981). The empathy cycle: Refinement of a nuclear concept. *Journal of Counseling and Psychology, 28*, 91–100.

Berkowitz, L. (1989). Frustration and aggression hypothesis: Examination and reformulation. *Psychological Bulletin, 106*, 59–73.

Bollas, C. (1987). *The shadow of the object: Psychoanalysis of the un-thought known.* London: Free Association Books.

Bowlby, J. (1988). *A secure base: Clinical applications of attachment theory.* London: Routledge.

Brazelton, T., & Greenspan, S. (2000). *The irreducible needs of children: What every child must have to grow, learn, and flourish.* Cambridge, MA: Perseus Publishing.

Bronfenbrenner, U. (1979). *The ecology of human development: Experiments by nature and design.* Cambridge, MA: Harvard University Press.

Burbach, D., & Borduin, C. (1986). Parent-child relations and the etiology of depression: A review of methods and findings. *Clinical Psychology Review, 6*, 133–153.

Chadwick, J. J. (2005). Self-development for emerging adults as influenced by mindful parenting during life transitions. Unpublished doctoral dissertation, University of Connecticut, Storrs.

Chadwick, J. J. (2009). Mindfulness-based family life education. Manuscript submitted for publication.

Cohen, L., Burt, C., & Bjork, J. (1987). Life stress and adjustment: Effects of life events experienced by young adolescents and their parents. *Developmental Psychology, 23*, 583–592.

Coleman, J., Henricson, C., & Roker, D. (2000). Parenting in the youth justice context. *Journal of Adolescence, 23*, 763–783.

Compas, B., Howell, D., Ledoux, N., Phares, V., & Williams, R. (1989). Parent and child stress symptoms: An integrative analysis. *Developmental Psychology, 25,* 550–559.

Conger, R., Lorenz, F., Elder, G., Simons, R., & Whitbeck, L. (1993). Husband and wife differences in response to undesirable life events. *Journal of Health and Social Behavior, 34,* 71–88.

Devereux, E., Bronfenbrenner, U., & Rodgers, R. (1969). Child-rearing in England and the United States: A cross-national comparison. *Journal of Marriage and the Family, 3,* 257–270.

Dohrenwend, B. (1974). *Stressful life events, their nature and effect.* New York: Wiley.

Dohrenwend, B., Krasnoff, L., Askenasy, A., & Dohrenwend, B. (1978). Exemplification of a method for scaling life events: The PERI life events scale. *Journal of Health and Social Behavior, 19,* 205–229.

Downey, G., & Coyne, J. (1990). Children of depressed parents: An integrative review. *Psychological Bulletin, 108,* 50–76.

Elder, G. (1974). *Children of the great depression: Social change and life experience.* Chicago, IL: University of Chicago Press.

Elder, G., Nguyen, T., & Caspi, A. (1985). Linking family hardship to children's lives. *Child Development, 56,* 361–375.

Elkind, D. (1994). *Ties that stress: The new family imbalance.* Cambridge, MA: Harvard University Press.

Elkind, D. (2008). *The hurried child.* The 25th Anniversary Edition. Reading, MA: Addison-Wesley Publishers.

Epstein, M. (1997). *Going to pieces without falling apart: A Buddhist perspective on wholeness.* New York: Broadway Books.

Erikson, E. (1959). Identity and the life cycle. *Psychological Issues, 1,* 1–17.

Field, T. (1995). Psychologically depressed parents. In M. H. Bornstein's (Ed.), *Handbook of parenting* (Vol. 3, pp. 34–45). Mahwah, NJ: Erlbaum Publisher.

Furgusson, D., Horwood, L., Gretton, M., & Shannon, F. (1985). Family life events, maternal depression, and maternal and teacher descriptions of child behavior. *Pediatrics, 75,* 30–35.

Garbarino, J. (1992). *Children and families in the social environment* (2nd ed.). New York: Aldine De Gruyter Publishers.

Gottman, J. (1997). *The Heart of parenting: How to raise an emotionally intelligent child.* New York: Simon and Schuster Publishers.

Grotevant, H., & Cooper, C. (1986). Individuation in family relationships: A perspective on individual differences in the development of identity and role-taking skills in adolescence. *Human Development, 29,* 82–100.

Hammen, C., Gordon, D., Burge, D., Adrain, C., Jaenicke, C., & Hiroto, D. (1987). Maternal affective disorder, illness, and stress: Risk for children's psychopathology. *American Journal of Psychiatry, 144,* 736–741.

Harter, S. (1994). Causes and consequences of low self-esteem in children and adolescents. In R. F. Baumeister (Ed.), *Self-esteem: The puzzle of low self-regard* (pp. 87–117). New York: Plenum Press.

Hauser, S. T., Powers, S., Jacobson, A. M., & Noam, G. G. (1986). *Family interiors of adolescent development.* New York: Free Press.

Hill, J., & Maughan, B. (2000). *Disorders in childhood and adolescence.* New York: Cambridge University Press.

Holahan, C. J., & Moos, R. H. (1987). Risk, resistance, and psychological distress: A longitudinal analysis with adults and children. *Journal of Abnormal Psychology, 96,* 3–13.

James, W. (1890). Principles of psychology. In *The encyclopaedia Britannica* (Vol. 26, pp. 607–611). Chicago, IL: Encyclopaedia Britannica.

Kabat-Zinn, J., & Kabat-Zinn, M. (1997). *Everyday blessings.* New York: Hyperion Press.

Kabat-Zinn, J. (2004). In T. Meili (Ed.), *The power of the human heart: A story of trauma and recovery.* New York: The Bridge Fund of New York Press.

Karen, R. (1994). *Attachment theory.* New York: Guilford Press.

Kohlberg, L. (1998). *Essays on moral development* (2nd ed.). San Francisco, CA: Harper & Row.

Lerner, R. M., & Lerner, J. V. (1987). Children in their contexts: A goodness of fit model. In J. B. Lancaster, J. Altmann, A. S. Rossi & L. R. Sherrod (Eds.), *Parenting across the lifespan: Biosocial dimensions.* Chicago, IL: Aldine de Gruyter Press.

Marshall, S. K., & Fleming, L. (2001). Do I Matter? Construct validation of adolescents' perceived mattering to parents and friends. *Journal of Adolescence, 24*(4), 473–490.

Paikoff, R. L., Brooks-Gunn, J., & Carlton-Ford, S. (1991). Effect of status changes upon family functioning and well-being for mothers and daughters. *Journal of Early Adolescence, 11*, 210–220.

Patterson, G. R. (1983). Stress: A change agent for family process. In N. Garmezy & M. Rutter (Eds.), *Stress, coping, and development in children.* New York: McGraw Hill.

Patterson, G. R., DeBaryshe, B., & Ramsey, E. (1989). A Developmental perspective on anti-social behavior. *American Psychologist, 44*, 329–335.

Rindfuss, R. R. (1991). The young adult years: Diversity, structural change, and fertility. *Demography, 28*, 493–512.

Rogers, C. (1959). A theory of therapy, personality, and interpersonal relationships as developed in the client-centered framework. In S. Koch (Ed.), *Psychology: A study of a science, Vol. III Formulations of the person and the social context* (pp. 184–256). New York, NY: McGraw Hill.

Rogers, C. (1975). Empathic: An unappreciated way of being. *The Counseling Psychologist, 5*, 2–10.

Rosenfeld, A., & Wise, N. (2001). *Hyper-parenting: Are you hurting your child by trying too hard?.* New York: St. Martin's Press.

Rudnytsky, P. L. (1991). *Contending kingdoms: Historical, psychological, and feminist approaches to literature.* Detroit, MI: Wayne State University Press.

Rutter, M. (1990). Commentary: Some focus and process considerations regarding effects of parental depression on children. *Developmental Psychology, 26*, 60–67.

Segal, Z., Williams, J. M., & Teasdale, J. D. (2002). Mindfulness-based cognitive therapy for depression: A new approach to preventing relapse. New York, NY; The Guilford Press.

Spinelli, E. (1989). *The interpreted world: An introduction to phenomenological psychology.* Newbury Park, CA: Sage Publications.

Stein, E. (1970). *On the problem of empathy* (2nd ed.). The Netherlands: Wolters-Noordhoff Publisher.

Steinberg, L., & Silk, J. (2002). Parenting adolescents. In M. H. Bornstein (Ed.), *Handbook of parenting* (2nd ed., Vol. 1, pp. 103–133). Mahwah, NJ: Erlbaum Publisher.

Taylor, J., & Turner, R. J. (2001). A longitudinal study of the role and significance of mattering to others and depressive symptoms. *Journal of Health and Social Behavior, 42*(3), 310–325.

Thomson, B., & Vaux, A. (1986). The importation, transmission, and moderation of stress in the family system. *American Journal of Community Psychology, 14*, 39–57.

Thoreau, H. D. (1854). *Walden.* Boston, MA: Harvard University Press.

Wallerstein, J. (2003). *What about the kids? Raising your children before, during, and after divorce.* New York: Hyperion Press.

Wakefield, J. C. (1996). Does social work need the eco-systems perspective? *Social Science Review, 70*, 1–32.

Weissman, M., & Paykel, E. (1974). *The depressed woman: A study of social relationship.* Chicago, IL: University of Chicago Press.

White, K. M., Speisman, J. C., & Costos, D. (1983). Young adults and their parents: Individuation to mutuality. In H. D. Grotevant & C. R. Cooper (Eds.), *New directions for child development: Adolescent development in the family.* San Francisco, CA: Jossey-Bass.

Winnicott, D. W. (1956). *Transitional objects and phenomena. Collected Papers.* London: Tavistock Press.

Winnicott, D. W. (1960). The parent-infant relationship. In *Maturational processes in the facilitating environment.* New York: International Universities Press.

Winnicott, D. W. (1965). *The family and individual development.* New York: Basic Books.

Winnicott, D. W. (1971). *Playing and reality.* New York: Routledge.

Winnicott, D. W. (1989). Psycho-analytic explorations of D.W. Winnicott; edited by Claire Winnicott, Ray Shepherd, and Madeleine Davis. Cambridge, MA: Harvard University Press.

Chapter 12

Sexual Transitions in the Lives of Adult Women

Emily Koert and Judith C. Daniluk

Sexuality is an important and complex aspect of life. It encompasses "physical, psychological, social, emotional, spiritual, cultural, and ethical dimensions of human experience" (Duplassie and Daniluk 2007, p. 263). Sexual expression involves "the sensual pleasure that comes from the stimulation of the body, often with the anticipation of an enjoyable, erotic feeling" (Westheimer and Lopater 2005, p. 24). Sexuality includes attitudes, beliefs, and expectations about self and others. These are inevitably shaped by external forces such as societal and cultural norms, media portrayals of sexuality, and relationships with others who are important. Women's sexuality at all stages of the course of life is developed through and influenced by interactions with others based on a woman's age, life stage, and significant roles (Daniluk 1998). How women experience their sexuality changes and shifts across the lifespan, especially during key transitions such as infertility, pregnancy, mothering, menopause, and physical illness and disability. Not only do these transitions involve biological processes and changes, but the meanings that women attribute to these events and experiences also have implications for women's sexual self-perceptions, expression, and satisfaction (Daniluk 1998).

These and other key developmental transitions will be explored in more detail throughout this chapter. We have adopted a biopsychosocial approach throughout the chapter – focusing on the physiological, psychological, and social factors that shape and influence the sexuality of adult women during young adulthood, middle adulthood, and later life. Although we identify challenges to women's sexuality across the lifespan, the focus of this chapter is on sexual health, defined by the World Health Organization as the integration of the physical, intellectual, emotional, and social aspects of being sexual, in ways that are positively enriching and that enhances the individual, her relationships, and society (Sexuality Information and Education Council of the United States 1996).

Young Adulthood (Age 20–40)

In general, young adulthood is a time of sexual health and well-being for women. Research shows that young women experience few physical barriers to the enjoyment of their sexuality during this life stage, although what is sexually

From: *Handbook of Stressful Transitions Across the Lifespan,*
Edited by: T.W. Miller, DOI 10.1007/978-1-4419-0748-6_12,
© Springer Science+Business Media, LLC 2010

exciting differs across individuals (Boston Women's Health Book Collective 2005; Westheimer and Lopater 2005). One of the most significant factors that shapes the experience of sexuality for women in young adulthood is her fertility status. Women's reproductive choices, and in particular whether or not they become mothers, shape how they feel about themselves as sexual persons and how they are viewed by society in terms of their femininity and sexuality. In most societies, cultures, and religions throughout the world, the link between women's sexuality and reproduction is strongly supported (Ireland 1993). Biology is deemed to be a woman's destiny with motherhood and procreation being seen as natural and inevitable roles for women. Paradoxically, while motherhood and sexuality do not comfortably co-exist within these paradigms, femininity and sexual identity are closely aligned with the ability to reproduce and the adoption of the motherhood role for women (Daniluk 1998).

With this in mind, we now turn to an examination of the reproductive transitions that typically occur for women during young adulthood – specifically pregnancy; the transition to motherhood; infertility; and voluntary childlessness. We then address the important issue of physical illness and disability which also has implications for how women experience and express their sexuality throughout adult life. Each issue is addressed below from a biopsychosocial perspective.

Pregnancy

During pregnancy women experience significant physical and hormonal changes, many of which can negatively or positively affect body image and sexuality (Daniluk 1998). Hormonal changes include increased levels of progesterone, estrogen and adrenocortical hormones, and lower levels of norepinephrine (Unger and Crawford 1992). These hormonal changes often affect women's overall sense of health and well-being, as well as their sexual desire, responsiveness, and functioning (Duplassie and Daniluk 2007; Kitzinger 1985; Westheimer and Lopater 2005). Paradoxically, some women experience greater sexual desire and satisfaction during pregnancy, while others report decreased desire and sexual responsiveness during this transition. These differences would suggest a more complex interaction between hormonal and physical changes during pregnancy, as well as psychosocial variables.

As a pregnancy progresses, women also experience significant changes in their body shape, size, and weight. Some women report that these bodily changes make them feel more attractive and sensual. Others feel unattractive and experience decreased levels of sexual desire (Daniluk 1998; Kitzinger 1985). Additional factors that influence women's sexuality during pregnancy include the stage of the pregnancy and the experience of any health-related issues. Again, it is difficult to separate the physiological changes from the psychosocial experiences of pregnancy in understanding the impact of this transition on any woman's experience of her sexuality (Daniluk 1998).

From a psychosocial perspective within North American society, pregnancy is championed as a key milestone in women's healthy adult development and is seen a symbol of femininity and mature womanhood (Daniluk 1998; Ireland 1993). Research and theory on adult development (e.g., Erikson 1997) includes women's fulfillment of their reproductive capacities as central to normal female development and adjustment (Ireland 1993). Consequently, many women enter into pregnancy and motherhood without thinking that they have a choice due to pervasive social, religious, and cultural pressure and norms. While there is no research addressing the relationship between reproductive choice and sexuality for women, it makes intuitive sense that a woman's experience of her sexuality during pregnancy will to some degree be shaped by her perceptions of having had some control over this decision, if only the timing of the choice (Daniluk 1998).

Once pregnant, women must adjust to the experience of having a living organism within their bodies and the responsibilities that accompany it, referred to by Bergum (1989) as a sense of "embodied responsibility" (p. 89). Women face societal pressure to treat their pregnant bodies with the utmost care with the goal of creating an ideal environment within which the fetus can grow and thrive. Kitzinger (1985) suggests that fear of damaging the baby is one of the reasons that many women and their partners avoid intercourse during pregnancy. It is not surprising then, that women often blame themselves if their child is born with any defects or abnormalities, leading them and sometimes others to question whether they were vigilant enough in maintaining a healthy diet and lifestyle while pregnant (Daniluk 1998).

The Transition to Motherhood

There are considerable physiological changes in women's bodies after child-birth, including a dramatic drop in hormone levels and changes in the size and shape of the uterus, abdomen, and breasts (Kitzinger 1985). These changes can have an impact on a woman's relationship to her body, and by extension, her sexuality. Given the dramatic hormonal shifts it is common for women to experience a period of sadness and mood instability after giving birth. For the majority of women, these emotional symptoms lift within a week to 10 days (Partridge 1996). For 10–15% of women, these symptoms last up to 6 weeks, and for an even smaller number, postpartum depression lasts for a significant length of time (Gruen 1990; Kleiman and Raskin 1994). Compounding these physiological changes which affect women's emotional and mental states are the additional effects of exhaustion, sleep deprivation, and role changes which accompany the transition to new motherhood (Kaplan 1990; Kitzinger 1985; Partridge 1996). Sexual intimacy and pleasure understandably suffer during the postpartum period and transition to motherhood. It is also important to note that a traumatic birthing experience can leave a woman feeling disconnected and alienated from her body. If the birthing experience did not go as planned, which is often the case for a first birth; a woman may feel that she has failed. Kitzinger explains: "It can be a long, painful journey to get on good terms with your body after such an alienating experience, to begin to like it and allow sexual passion to sweep through every pore" (p. 219).

The experience of breast-feeding and the intimacy involved in caring for a newborn child also have implications for women's sexuality. For some women, breast-feeding is a very sensual experience (Kitzinger 1985; Daniluk 1998). However, in North America, the eroticism inherent in the experience of breast-feeding and mothering a child is not sanctioned. Consequently, feelings of sexual guilt and shame are not uncommon for breast-feeding mothers (Adler 1994; Oberman and Josselson 1996; Ussher 1989).

From a psychosocial perspective, new mothers also face societal pressures and expectations about how quickly their bodies should return to their pre-pregnancy size, shape, and weight. The images displayed in the media include celebrities who drop their pregnancy weight in alarmingly short time spans – further fuelling the expectation that new mothers can and should get control over their bodies within weeks of having given birth. Consequently, many new mothers are disappointed and dismayed when they have difficulty living up to this impossible standard.

Ironically, although women today are inundated with images of slim and attractive new mothers, images that connect motherhood and sexuality are relatively rare, implicitly reinforcing the belief that when they become mothers, women lose their sexual desirability and appeal (Daniluk 1998). Ultimately, the absence of attention to the sexuality of mothers perpetuates the distinction between maternal and sexual feelings and behaviors. This is not because mothers are not interested in or capable of sexual or erotic feelings, but because only a narrow range of behaviors and appearances are seen as acceptable for mothers (Boston Women's Health Book Collective 2005; Kitzinger 1985).

As new mothers, women also take on new roles and responsibilities that were not required of them previously – responsibilities and role changes that can have a significant impact on their sexual self-perceptions, desire, and expression. It is not uncommon for the responsibilities involved in providing care for a child to become a stressor in a couple's relationship (Cowan 1999). Although some couples report a satisfactory and enhanced sex life after the birth of their children, in general, time constraints and exhaustion have a significant impact on couples' level of intimacy as the demands involved in caring for a child leave little time and energy for a sexual relationship (Daniluk 1998; Kaplan 1990; Westheimer and Lopater 2005). The presence of a child changes the distribution of affection in the family as the love that was shared between partners now shifts to include the child (Cowan 1999). Couples often lack the resources and energy to re-ignite the passion and intimacy they shared prior to becoming parents. Women are socialized to believe they must balance the needs of everyone in the family including their partner, child(ren), and themselves, and as such, are expected to constantly remain attentive, affectionate, and available – expectations that are unrealistic and often unattainable given the multiple role demands of work, home, and parenting. Although we know that mothering changes a woman's relationship with her body and with her family, more research is needed to determine how mothering directly impacts women's sexuality (Daniluk 1998; Kitzinger 1985; Unger and Crawford 1992).

Infertility

Infertility is experienced by 8–10% of those who try to produce a child and is defined as the inability to achieve a viable pregnancy after 12 months of regular, unprotected intercourse (Tierney et al. 1999). Problems with the female partner account for approximately 30% of fertility problems, male factors account for 30%, while 20% of infertility cases can be attributed to a combination of male and female factor problems, and 10% remain unexplained. Female factor fertility problems are caused by endocrine imbalances or anatomical impairments such as blocked fallopian tubes, ovulatory difficulties, or endometriosis.

Infertility treatments exist across a continuum with less invasive treatments such as hormone therapy or fertility medications on one end of the spectrum and more invasive procedures such as in vitro fertilization (IVF), egg or sperm donation, and gestational surrogacy on the other.

For the most part, women's bodies are the focus of the majority of fertility tests and treatments. Consequently, the invasiveness of countless medical exams, assessments, and treatments can be emotionally and physically taxing and impact a woman's relationship with her body and overall sexuality (Daniluk 2001a; Leiblum 1997). Fertility medications have been reported to cause physiological and psychological symptoms, such hot flushes, night sweats, weight gain, and headaches (Daniluk and Fluker 1995). Apart from these, infertile women often report experiencing an overall decrease in their sexual desire during fertility treatments. However, it is difficult to separate the effects of the hormonal medications and treatments from the negative effects of timed intercourse, invasive medical interventions, and repeated reproductive failures, all of which profoundly affect intimacy and sexual satisfaction for women and their partners (Daniluk and Tench 2007; Leiblum 1997).

From a psychosocial perspective, since motherhood is socially viewed as a "natural" role transition for women, those who have difficulty in conceiving are left feeling like they have failed to fulfill their maternal role (Ireland 1993; Daniluk 1998). Given the close links between motherhood and femininity, and between femininity and sexuality, many infertile women also feel like sexual and reproductive failures. There is considerable evidence to suggest that psychosocial distress increases during fertility treatments (e.g., Berg and Wilson 1991; Daniluk 2001a). Couples refer to the "emotional roller-coaster" of each treatment cycle as they start out feeling hopeful and optimistic, and after failing to produce a viable pregnancy, are left with feelings of grief, loss, and depression. Women describe feeling a loss of control over their bodies while undergoing fertility treatments. Fertility treatments can cause tremendous strain on a couple's relationship, which has implications for their sexual expression, as intercourse becomes more about timing and conception and less about intimacy, enjoyment, and pleasure (Daniluk 1998; Leiblum 1997). This apart, when couples are unsuccessful in conceiving, sexual intimacy becomes associated with loss and failure (Basson 2000; Daniluk 2001b).

The experience of infertility can be a blow to women's sexual self-esteem. Whether infertility is due to male, female, combined factors, or undetermined causes, women often turn the blame inwards, attributing past experiences such as infidelity or abortion as the cause of their infertility (Daniluk 1998). Therefore, the inability to conceive a child and the medical interventions that accompany fertility treatment have significant implications for women's experience of their sexuality, sexual self-esteem, and sexual identities.

Voluntary Childlessness

Research suggests that the estimated 8–10% of women who voluntarily reject the motherhood role have various experiences and reasons for doing so. Some women know from a young age that they want to remain childless, whereas others remain childless through circumstances or a series of delays and postponements (Ireland 1993; Morell 1994). Despite this growing minority group, there is still stigma attached to women who are voluntarily childless.

In particular, voluntarily childless women are seen as selfish and uncaring – lacking in maternal instinct and by association, femininity (Lampman and Dowling-Guyer 1995). These women are met with negative reactions and distrust as they call into question what it means to be a woman separate from motherhood (Gold and Wilson 2002; Ireland 1993; Letherby 2002). They face disapproval and prejudice by society that views their choice not to parent as unnatural (Ireland 1993). Their sexuality and sexual adequacy is also called into question in their refusal to accept their "biological destinies" or maternal role (Daniluk 1998). However, despite the negative views regarding women who choose to be childless, overall, research supports the psychological health and well-being of voluntarily childless women with few women reporting regrets with regards to their decision to forgo motherhood (Morell 1994).

Ireland (1993) suggests that the experiences of women who are childless are not reflected in current psychological theories or theories of adult development. As a result, for those who choose not to make the transition to motherhood, the challenge becomes defining their female and sexual identities as adult women but not-mothers when there are few socially acceptable examples of healthy and normative female identities for women who are childless (Daniluk 1998; Ireland 1993; Morell 1994). As the number of women choosing childlessness increases, more women are left to construct and negotiate their lives and sexual identities within a society that stigmatizes and until recently has marginalized women who are not mothers.

Physical Illness and Disability

At any age across the lifespan, health problems can influence and affect women's sexual expression, perceptions, and attitudes. These health transitions can include but are not limited to chronic illness, pain, and disability, and serious and life-threatening diseases such as cancer, cardiovascular disease, and severe hypertension (Duplassie and Daniluk 2007; McCormick 1996). The symptoms and treatments of these health problems can have far reaching affects on how women relate to their bodies and by extension, their sexuality. For example, people with neurological disorders such as spinal cord injuries or multiple sclerosis may need to find alternative ways of expressing and enjoying their sexuality due to restrictions in their movement and reduced feeling and sensitivity (Tepper and Owens 2007). Also, medications that treat chronic illnesses such as hypertension have been found to contribute to decreased sex drive and difficulty in reaching orgasm (Daniluk 1998). Selective serotonin reuptake inhibitors (SSRIs) and other medications used to treat depression and anxiety have also been found to decrease sex drive and functioning (Association of Reproductive Health Professionals 2005).

Women with chronic illness and disability are also faced with myths and misconceptions regarding their sexuality as the media and society in general perpetuate the belief that disabled people are non-sexual (Mona and Gardos 2001). These misconceptions are also reinforced by medical professionals who are too often ill-informed and inadequately trained with respect to the sexual expression of those with chronic illness and disability, and consequently, refrain from addressing these issues with their patients. Conversely, patients with chronic illness and disability express reservations about asking their physicians about sexual health concerns (Tepper and Owens 2007). Despite these challenges and misconceptions, however, sexual expression is an important part of life for a significant number of those who have chronic illness or disability (Tepper and Owens 2007). The expansion of the Internet and the consequent access to resources that can be easily accessed at home has provided a wealth of resources and information on how to express and enjoy sexuality despite chronic illness and disability and an arena to connect with others in an anonymous, safe, and low risk manner (Tepper and Owens 2007).

The incidence of breast and reproductive cancers for women in early adulthood seems to be growing. Thousands of women in North America lose their breasts each year because of breast cancer (Love 1990; MacPhee 1994), and a significant number of women undergo a hysterectomy each year for ovarian and uterine cancers (Boston Women's Health Book Collective 2005). Treatments such as mastectomy and hysterectomy can drastically impact a woman's sexual self-perceptions and satisfaction. As Kitzinger (1985) writes, "Losing any part of the body in a mutilating operation, however necessary and however life-saving the surgery, involves grieving. This process is long and painful for some of us. It can profoundly affect our view of ourselves and our sexuality" (p. 297).

The loss of one or both breasts or the uterus as a treatment for cancer has psychosocial implications for women's sexuality and sexual identity. Kitzinger (1985) suggests that "25% of women who have mastectomies eventually need some kind of psychotherapy, and for some women sex comes to a stop" (p. 305). After undergoing such mutilating surgery and invasive treatments, women report feeling less feminine, and often see themselves as "neutered" and "empty" (Bernhard 1992; Kitzinger 1985). Societal norms and expectations with regards to what is deemed "sexy" or "attractive" for women can be especially problematic for those have experienced mastectomy or hysterectomy as some women may internalize the dominant view of sexual attractiveness and experience body dissatisfaction when their own bodies do not reflect these norms (Gross and Ito 1992).

Sexually transmitted infections (STI's) and other sexual health concerns can also be problematic for women's enjoyment and expression of their sexuality at any stage of the life course, although the incidence of these concerns is generally greater during young adulthood when women are more likely to have more and varied sexual partners. These concerns include yeast and bacterial infections, Chlamydia, herpes, and genital warts, gonorrhea, syphilis, human immunodeficiency virus (HIV), and Hepatitis A, B, and C (Boston Women's Health Book Collective 2005). The physical discomforts associated with these infections, the stigma associate with STI's can make women feel dirty, resulting in feelings of embarrassment, shame, and guilt. As such, these concerns often have direct implications for women's sexual self-expression and esteem (Daniluk 1998; Westheimer and Lopater 2005).

Middle Adulthood (Age 40–60)

A North American woman's experience of her sexuality during middle adulthood occurs within the context of a society that worships youth and equates sexual attractiveness and desirability with a young, toned body. The few more recent examples pairing sexuality with middle age (e.g., Madonna) continue to reflect a youthful and unrealistic image of middle-age sexual vitality and desirability. It is not surprising then, that many middle-aged women feel sexually invisible and expect that their sexual frequency and enjoyment will decrease or deteriorate during this stage (Daniluk 1998). These expectations can be problematic, given the link between women's attitudes and expectations about their sexuality and their subsequent sexual experiences (Dennerstein and Hayes 2005).

In discussing what constitutes "normal" or "healthy" sexuality for women during this life stage, from a physiological perspective, it is difficult to distinguish between the effects of menopause and the natural changes that occur with aging (Golub 1992). As they age, women experience changes in their physical appearance including increases in body weight, a gradual softening of the muscles on the body, and reduced elasticity of the skin (Daniluk 1998). Diet, lifestyle, and heredity causes are implicated in how women's bodies change during middle adulthood, but certain changes over a period of time are inevitable. Both men and women gain weight as they age but how the fatty tissues are distributed in the body differs across genders, with women typically becoming more pear-shaped over a period of time as weight becomes centralized in the hips and stomach (Stevens-Long and Commons 1992). Other physical changes experienced by women include thinning and graying hair, decreases in bone density, the addition of age spots on the skin, decreases in visual acuity, and changes in the appearance and size of the various components of the face (Daniluk 1998; Stevens-Long and Commons 1992). How women experience their sexuality in light of these changes is necessarily intertwined with the experience of growing older in a society that worships youth as desirable, beautiful, and sexy.

In terms of sexual desire, capacity for arousal and orgasm, and pleasure, during middle adulthood, women characteristically experience reductions in the levels of estrogen and testosterone in their bodies – hormones which are implicated in sexual functioning responsiveness (Crenshaw 1996; Rako 1996). However, given that a clear correlation between reductions in the levels of these hormones and women's sexual functioning has not been demonstrated, it is likely that these hormonal changes interact with common psychosocial changes in the lives of middle-aged women to influence their sexual responsiveness and pleasure (Association of Reproductive Health Professionals 2005; Daniluk 1998).

Middle adulthood is host to a plethora of unique experiences and transitions such as menopause, changes in long term relationships, the pressures of raising young children or of children leaving the family home, the added responsibility for elderly and ailing parents, and societal and media pressures to maintain a youthful, attractive, and sexy appearance. With the context of the natural aging process in mind, we now turn to an examination of the biopsychosocial factors related specifically to menopause, changes in relationships and life roles, and body image that most commonly shape women's experience and expression of their sexuality during middle adulthood. We also address the implications of physical illness and disability for middle-aged women's sexuality.

Menopause

Between the ages of 45 and 55, women begin to transition to the menopause, which is defined as the complete cessation of menses for a period of 1 year (Daniluk 1998; Boston Women's Health Book Collective 2005). The complete cessation of menses generally occurs around age 51 and is the last stage of the menstrual cycle. The phase leading up to menopause is called the perimeno-pausal transition when gradual changes in women's hormone levels begin to occur and the menstrual flow decreases and typically shortens in length. During menopause, the production of estrogen and progesterone hormones in the ovaries decreases. It is during this stage that estrogen levels in the blood return to the baseline levels experienced before puberty. As estrogen levels stabilize, the ovaries no longer release follicles (eggs), signaling the end of women's fertility. The inability to ovulate usually occurs before the complete cessation of menses.

There is a dearth of unbiased research that examines the biological changes women experience during menopause. Previous research has been seen as problematic due to sampling biases, lack of consistent definitions, and meth-odological problems (Daniluk 1998). However, we do know that menopause is a natural part of the aging process that includes physical and hormonal changes similar to, albeit the reverse of puberty. For a significant number of women, the bodily changes experienced during the perimenopausal and menopausal phases can have an impact on their sexuality and sexual pleasure. Painful intercourse and stress incontinence (the leaking of small amounts of urine) commonly occur as a result of increased vaginal dryness and the thinning of the vagina and urethra due to a reduction in estrogen production (Association of Reproductive Health Professionals 2005; Kitzinger 1985). Decreases in estrogen and progesterone levels are also implicated in the loss of women's sexual desire, loss of clitoral sensation, and less/fewer orgasms (Boston Women's Health Book Collective 2005). However, research sug-gests that most women in middle adulthood are still able to be orgasmic and enjoy sexual intimacy during this stage of the lifespan, although some women require the use of vaginal lubricants to increase their comfort and pleasure (Daniluk 1998).

Other symptoms that are common during the menopause transition include hot flashes/flushes, night sweats, bone or joint pain, dizziness, headaches, and sleep disturbances, along with emotional or mood instability including feelings of depression, irritability, and nervousness (Daniluk 1998; Golub 1992; Westheimer and Lopater 2005). For some women, estrogen replace-ment therapy has been found to be helpful in relieving hot flashes/flushes and other menopausal-related symptoms. It is important to note, however, that how women experience these physiological and emotional symptoms varies considerably across individuals. The available literature suggests that only a minority of women experience symptoms so severe that their daily lives are disrupted. Overall, general health and well-being appears to be linked to the positive experience of menopausal health-related symptoms and correspond-ingly, to enhanced sexual functioning (Association of Reproductive Health Professionals 2005; Golub 1992; Kitzinger 1985).

With the cessation of menses, women reach the end of their reproduc-tive cycle and as such are no longer able to conceive a child. Consequently, the onset of menopause may be experienced as a loss for some women who wanted to become mothers but were unable to do so because of infertility or their life circumstances. However, for a significant number of women, the end of their fertility is experienced as freeing and sexually and personally empow-ering (Daniluk 1998). Even those who did not become mothers by choice or circumstance appear to accept the end of their fertility without significant regret or crisis (Ireland 1993).

The relationship between the psychosocial factors and women's expression and enjoyment of sexuality during menopause is complex. There are no definitive answers, but what is apparent is that individual differences exist. As they age and enter menopause, some women appear to experience a decline in their sexual interest and desire. Others report the post menopause period of their lives as being a time of enhanced sexual energy and satisfaction – perhaps because issues of fertility are no longer salient and women can gain a sense of entitlement over their own bodies and sexuality (Daniluk 1998). Dennerstein and Hayes (2005) and Kingsberg (2004) argue that many menopausal and postmenopausal women have more self-assurance, time, and energy at this stage, which positively impacts their sexual expression and enjoyment (Martin 1987).

For those who experience emotional symptoms during the menopause transition, it is difficult to determine whether the mood instability and fluctuations are due to hormonal changes, or are related to the largely negative social and cultural messages regarding menopause, or to the multiple role and relationship demands experienced by women during the middle years (Daniluk 1998). Since research indicates that estrogen replacement therapy is no more effective than a placebo for easing the emotional symptoms related to menopause, it is likely that other factors have more impact on emotional symptoms than do hormonal changes. The stressors and pressures unique to middle adulthood, such as the responsibility of taking care of children and elderly parents, and coping with the illnesses and loss of aging parents and family members may well exacerbate menopausal symptoms (Golub 1992). In fact, "there seems to be evidence that stressful life events are more likely to influence women's menopausal symptoms than the biological event of cessation of menstruation, or the impact of aging" (Ussher 1989, p. 120).

Changes in Relationships and Life Roles

As women age, their sexuality continues to be linked with relationship issues, and as such, can be impacted and influenced by the changing context of their relationships, life roles, demands, and the presence or absence of children in the home (Daniluk 1998). With children typically leaving home much later than in previous generations, women in middle adulthood are often faced with the double-burden of caring for their own children while also assuming the increased responsibility of taking care of their aging parents. Referred to in the literature as "the sandwich generation," middle adulthood for many women is a period of increasing interpersonal demands (Greer 1991). Other pressures on women during the middle decades include career demands and dealing with their own health problems (Cobb 1988; Daniluk 1998; Stevens-Long and Collins 1992).

Relationship issues also play a role in the mid-life woman's experience and expression of her sexuality. Liu (2003) notes that the longer couples are in a relationship, the more negative the impact on their overall sexuality, including the quality and frequency of sexual intercourse. Couples may not realize that they need to attend to their shared intimacy in order to maintain the passion in their relationship (Barbach 1993). Discrepancies between their own and their partner's levels of sexual desire and interest can also impact women's sexuality.

Research shows that women's sexual responsiveness and desire is different than that of men's, in which for women, sexual arousal occurs before sexual desire, and as such, many women need to be aroused before experiencing desire (Basson 2000). For many women emotional intimacy and relationship satisfaction are necessary for sexual desire and enjoyment. Gradual changes in sexual desire and functioning occur in both men and women as they age. However, "few men or women are aware that these changes are a normal part of the aging process" (Daniluk 1998, p. 320). It is not surprising then, that some men may blame their decreased sexual desire and functioning on their partners and women may internalize the blame, believing that their aging bodies are no longer sexually attractive.

Conversely, the changes in sexual functioning during middle adulthood can have a positive effect on the couple's intimacy. Researchers argue that if couples make the effort to reconnect during their middle years they can experience increased sexual intimacy and enjoyment (Liu 2003; Westheimer and Lopater 2005). With increased experience and knowledge of their sexuality and what gives them erotic pleasure, women may experience enhanced sexuality and find that middle adulthood is a time of sexual reawakening. The literature suggests that for women in middle adulthood, "sex can be richer and more honest ... in taking on less urgency, there is opportunity for greater depth and intensity" (Daniluk 1998, p. 335).

During middle adulthood, some women face the reality of being without a partner due to divorce, death, or a lack of available or suitable partners. However, many women are happy with their lives at this stage and do not view being without a partner as negative (Daniluk 1998). Research reveals that some women find it challenging to include safe and satisfying sexual experiences into their lives during middle adulthood, however, others make satisfying sexual arrangements, find other outlets for their sexual expression and enjoyment, or choose to live a celibate lifestyle (Anderson and Stewart 1994; Cline 1993; Daniluk 1998). Women who do engage in new relationships during the middle decades are often rewarded with enhanced sexual desire and pleasure (Greer 1991; Westheimer and Lopater 2005).

Body Image and the Aging Process

As already outlined, the natural aging process during middle adulthood involves gradual changes in women's bodies such as weight gain, loss of skin elasticity, the appearance of wrinkles, and the thinning and graying of hair. In reviewing the research, Daniluk (1998) reports that, "middle aged women see themselves as less attractive than do any other age group" (p. 259). Women's sense of their body image and sexuality in middle adulthood cannot be understood without considering the considerable influence of the context of our youth-oriented culture. Middle-aged women are inundated with media and advertising campaigns promoting products and services to stop the aging process and create a more youthful appearance. Save for the recent Dove Campaign for "real beauty," there is little celebration in the media and popular culture of women's natural beauty throughout the aging process. Rather, there are few popular examples of healthy and realistic models that reflect the diversity of shapes, sizes, appearances, and beauty that characterizes the bodies and appearance of many middle-aged women (Greer 1991; Dowling 1996).

"Midlife women's experience of their sexuality, the sexual choices they feel entitled to make, and their perceptions of their sexual desirability are powerfully influenced by social and cultural expectations" (Daniluk 1998, p. 316). The few images of women in middle adulthood who are deemed sexually desirable and attractive (e.g., Madonna, Sharon Stone) are air brushed, often surgically altered, and employ a team of health, fitness, and beauty experts, and therefore present an ideal that is virtually unattainable for mainstream women. The virtual invisibility in the media of examples of women whose physical realities reflect the characteristics of the majority of middle-aged women contributes to many women feeling sexually invisible, undesirable, and unattractive at precisely the time in their lives when they are more self-assured and confident in many other aspects of their lives (Daniluk 1998; Dowling 1996; Greer 1991).

Physical Illness and Disability

During middle adulthood, women are more likely to acquire chronic illnesses and life-threatening diseases as changes in the immune system make women more susceptible to illness (Stevens-Long and Collins 1992). As already outlined in the previous section on Young Adulthood, these ailments can impact women's sense of their bodies, and by extension, their sexuality (Tepper and Owens 2007). During middle adulthood, cardiovascular disease "accounts for 40% of all premature deaths in this age group" (Stevens-Long and Collins 1992, p. 269). The incidence of cancer also increases for women in this age group. Treatment for uterine and ovulatory cancers often includes hysterectomy, after which many women report intercourse to be painful (Kitzinger 1985). For a full and current discussion of the sexual implications and consequences of various illnesses and disabilities, readers are referred to Tepper and Owens (2007).

Later Adulthood (Age 60+)

Overall, less is known about the sexuality of older women, as they are relatively absent from the research, academic, and popular literature. What little we do know needs to be interpreted with caution due to differences between previous cohorts of seniors as compared to the current generation of older adults who experience significantly better health and quality of life than those of previous generations (Daniluk 1998). Despite popular cultural assumptions that older women and men have little interest in sex, the limited available research reveals that a significant number of men and women over 60 years of age continue to express and enjoy their sexuality – with sexual intimacy continuing to be viewed as an important part of their lives. Even as early as the 1960s, Masters and Johnson (1966) reported that seven out of the ten couples in their study who were over the age of 60 remained sexually active, although most reported a decline in their rate and intensity of intercourse. More recent studies support these findings and suggest that in spite of physical and health barriers to sexual expression and enjoyment, sexuality is still considered an important component of a vital life even by those in late, late adulthood (Johnson 2007; Westheimer and Lopater 2005).

Specific to women, although most women have the physical capacity to continue to enjoy their sexuality into older adulthood, many are faced with a barrage of lifestyle and relationship changes and losses that can have an impact on their sexual expression and intimacy (Gannon 1994). Furthermore, the ageist attitudes and stereotypes perpetuated by society appear to be the greatest barriers to older women's enjoyment and expression of their sexuality (Daniluk 1998). Older women's attitudes and expectations about aging also play a role in their sexuality as attitudes influence women's self-esteem, self-worth, and ideas about what is sexually possible and acceptable for them. These attitudes are inevitably influenced by society and culture. Within the media and popular culture, the few images of older women that do exist portray older women as asexual, nurturing, loving, and wise (Daniluk 1998). Those who are sexual are generally portrayed as eccentric or comical. Kitzinger (1985) argues that in North American culture, "geriatric sex is considered peculiar, laughable, often disgusting and obscene" (pp. 243–244). Rarely are positive images presented that show women in their 60s, 70s, or 80s engaged in loving, sexual, and passionate relationships. As such, older women are less likely to see this as a possibility for themselves. Paradoxically, after being defined by and valued for their sexuality throughout a significant portion of their lives, older women find themselves socially defined by the absence of their sexuality (Daniluk 1998).

There is a dearth of information with regards to the sexual health needs of older women. Furthermore, the sexist and ageist attitudes and beliefs of many medical professionals make it difficult for such women to approach their doctors with questions and concerns regarding bodily changes such as vaginal dryness that have implications for the enjoyment of their sexuality (Dowling 1996; Greer 1991). By denying older women's sexuality, medical professionals' responses can be detrimental to the older women who summon the courage to ask for medical advice. Additionally, older women may be less inclined to accept that sexual enjoyment and pleasure is normal at this stage of their lives (Daniluk 1998).

We now turn to an examination of the biopsychosocial changes related to the post-menopause period as well as changes in older women's relationships, life roles, and contexts that shape women's experience and expression of their sexuality throughout older adulthood. Lastly, we examine the implications of chronic illness, disease, and disability for older women's sexuality.

Post-menopause Sexuality

Women continue to be able to give and receive sexual pleasure into their later years (Kitzinger 1985), however, certain bodily changes that accompany older adulthood can make it more difficult for women to act on their sexual desires and can impede sexual satisfaction. As women transition, into post-menopause and beyond, they continue to experience physiological changes, such as the loss and thinning of body hair, and urinary incontinence, which may negatively impact their self-esteem and comfort with revealing themselves to a lover (Daniluk 1998). Women in this stage also produce less estrogen, which can result in a decrease in vaginal lubrication, which may decrease sexual comfort and increase painful intercourse (Johnson 2007). However, some women find that problems such as vaginal dryness and urinary incontinence can be partially remedied with creams, jellies, and exercises (Boston Women's Health Book Collective 2005; Kitzinger 1985). Also, during this stage women report changes in their experience of orgasm, with orgasms often feeling less intense (Daniluk 1998).

Changes in Relationships, Life Roles, and Contexts

The changes in older women's interpersonal relationships at this stage of the lifespan have a direct impact on the expression of their sexuality. Older women's long-term intimate relationships change and shift over time. At this stage in life, intimacy may take on new meanings as women and their partners cope with the physical realities of their lives and aging bodies (Daniluk 1998). For some older couples, the expression of sexuality continues through intercourse, whereas for others, intercourse is abandoned and intimacy is expressed in ways such as mutual touching and stroking and the enjoyment of each other's companionship (Johnson 2007; Kitzinger 1985). In a study by Adams and Turner (1985), partnered women between the ages of 60 and 85 reported a gradual increase in the enjoyment of their sexuality in older adulthood. Women in their study reported feeling freer to explore and enjoy their sexual encounters.

Older adulthood is also characterized by losses for many women that ultimately have an influence on how they experience, express, and enjoy their sexuality (Daniluk 1998). In general, women are more likely to outlive their male partners or spouses (Dowling 1996). As such, on a practical level, women who may be in good health and still interested in sexual intimacy may not have partners or spouses with whom to share this experience. Women may also be prevented from sharing intimacy because of illness, decline in health, or lack of sexual desire and interest on the part of their partners or spouses (Johnson 2007; Unger and Crawford 1992).

At this stage, women may no longer be able to care for themselves or enjoy the mobility and freedom experienced in young and middle adulthood. Consequently, women may need to enter long-term care. Women in this age group face practical challenges to expressing and enjoying sexual activity like lack of privacy when living in long-term care (Johnson 2007). Rather than acknowledging older women's sexual needs, many facilities have policies that reflect ageism and sexism along with a lack of respect of the sexual needs of the elderly. Although more nursing homes and intermediate care facilities are beginning to acknowledge older adults' sexual needs, few provide the elderly with adequate opportunities and privacy that are necessary for sexual intimacy (Johnson 2007).

The loss of a partner or spouse's income and the inability to work because of declining health may thrust older women into impoverished conditions. The poverty experienced by many women in older adulthood is problematic given that poor living conditions and inadequate nutrition have implications for overall health, and by extension, women's sexual functioning and satisfaction (Daniluk 1998). As is the case at any stage in life, when older women are struggling to support and feed themselves, sexuality may be a low priority (Gannon 1994).

Women in older adulthood may miss the physical aspects and emotional closeness of sexual intimacy (Daniluk 1998). They may have a close circle of family and friends with whom they feel connected and supported, and choose to live a celibate lifestyle (Daniluk 1993; Unger and Crawford 1992). Or, they may seek out another romantic relationship. While a new relationship may bring with it a renewed sense of sexual exciting and pleasure (Nickerson 1992), older women may have to overcome their insecurities about the perceived attractiveness of their aging bodies (Kitzinger 1985). Women who begin new relationships may also find themselves faced with resistance, most notably from their adult children who may be uncomfortable acknowledging and accepting their parents' sexual needs (Daniluk 1998).

Chronic Illness, Disease, and Disability

Faced with their aging and changing bodies, some women reject the notions of the importance of youth and beauty and come to an acceptance and love of their bodies. However, for many other women, loving their aging bodies is a difficult task when faced with chronic illnesses, pain, and disability – all of which are more likely to be experienced in the later years (Johnson 2007; Stevens-Long and Commons 1992; Westheimer and Lopater 2005). Older women report more chronic non-life threatening impairments than do men of the same age. Also, women spend more years living with chronic diseases. As well as the sometimes physically debilitating symptoms associated with many illnesses, the medications used to treat these conditions can have a negative impact on a woman's sexual desire and enjoyment (Boston Women's Health Book Collective 2005). Heart disease, high blood pressure, and treatments for cancer can affect a woman's sexual desire, pleasure, and activity (Johnson 2007).

Women may also need to adjust to the loss of certain body parts (e.g., breast, leg, or hip) or a diagnosis of a life-threatening illness that may impact their perception of themselves as healthy and sexual persons (Daniluk 1998). Consequently, these experiences may affect women's interest in and enjoyment of their sexuality. "Aging may bring physical disabilities that interfere with the way [women] express [themselves] sexually. Stiff joints, and aching back, difficulty in hearing and seeing, loss of taste and smell, may all mean that [women] need to adapt and experiment in lovemaking" (Kitzinger 1985, p. 247).

Overall, the challenges and barriers faced by women in older adulthood are not insurmountable. There are few complete barriers to a woman's continued experiencing of sexual pleasure throughout later life, although what is deemed as sexual and as satisfying may shift and change during this stage of the lifespan (Johnson 2007; Tiefer 1996).

Conclusion

The focus of this chapter has been on women's experiences and enjoyment of their sexuality during key transitions throughout adult life. It is important to remember that healthy sexuality and sexual expression are highly individual and diverse experiences – what is sexually exciting is different across individuals (Boston Women's Health Book Collective 2005; Westheimer and Lopater 2005) based on their own needs and desires and the biopsychosocial transitions they must negotiate at each stage of the lifespan (Daniluk 1998; Johnson 2007; Tiefer 1996). A woman's sense of herself as a sexual person and her experience of intimacy and pleasure shifts and changes during key transitions such as infertility, pregnancy, mothering, menopause, and physical illness and disability. Biological processes such as physical and hormonal changes have been implicated in women's sexual desire and satisfaction. However, it is important to remember that biology is not destiny. Psychosocial factors such as societal and cultural norms and expectations, along with the popular media's portrayals of sexuality can also influence how a woman understands and experiences her sexuality throughout adult life. The meanings that women attribute to these transitions and experiences inevitably shape their sexual self-perceptions, expression, and satisfaction (Daniluk 1998). These meanings are not fixed as they reflect women's attitudes, beliefs, and values that may change over a period of time as a result of new life roles, experiences, and relationships. This overview underscores the necessity of adopting a holistic approach when considering the issues and concerns related to women's sexuality at key transitions across the lifespan, while also highlighting the importance of understanding women's sexuality as an emergent process rather than a fixed experience (Daniluk 1998).

References

Adams, C. G., & Turner, B. F. (1985). Reported change in sexuality from young adulthood to old age. *Journal of Sex Research, 21*, 126–141.

Adler, B. (1994). Postnatal sexuality. In P. Y. L. Choi & P. Nicolson (Eds.), *Female sexuality: Psychology, biology and social context* (pp. 83–99). New York: Harvester/Wheatsheaf.

Anderson, C. M., & Stewart, S. (1994). *Flying solo: Single women in midlife*. New York: Norton.

Association of Reproductive Health Professionals. (2005). *ARHP clinical proceedings*. Washington, DC. http://www.arhp.org.

Barbach, L. (1993). *The pause: Positive approaches to menopause*. New York: Dutton.

Basson, R. (2000). The female sexual response: A different model. *Journal of Sex & Marital Therapy, 26*, 51–65.

Berg, J. B., & Wilson, J. F. (1991). Psychological functioning across stages of infertility. *Journal of Behavioral Medicine, 14*, 11–26.

Bergum, V. (1989). *Woman to mother: A transformation*. Granby, MA: Bergin & Garvey.

Bernhard, L. A. (1992). Consequences of hysterectomy in the lives of women. *Health Care for Women International, 13*, 281–291.

Boston Women's Health Book Collective. (2005). *Our bodies, ourselves: A new edition for a new era*. New York: Touchstone.

Cline, S. (1993). *Women, passion and celibacy*. New York: Carol Southern.

Cobb, J. O. (1988). *Understanding menopause*. Toronto: Key Porter.

Cowan, C. P. (1999). *When partners become parents: The big life changes for couples*. New York: Lawrence Erlbaum.

Crenshaw, T. (1996). *The alchemy of love and lust*. New York: Penguin.

Daniluk, J. C. (1993). The meaning and experience of female sexuality: A phenomenological analysis. *Psychology of Women Quarterly, 17*, 53–69.

Daniluk, J. C. (1998). *Women's sexuality across the lifespan: Challenging myths, creating meanings*. New York: Guilford Press.

Daniluk, J. C. (2001a). Reconstructing their lives: A longitudinal, qualitative analysis of the transition to biological childlessness for infertile couples. *Journal of Counseling & Development, 79*, 439–449.

Daniluk, J. C. (2001b). *The infertility survival guide: How to cope with the challenges while maintaining your sanity, dignity, and relationships*. Oakland, CA: New Harbinger.

Daniluk, J. C., & Fluker, M. (1995). Fertility drugs and the reproductive imperative: Assisting the infertile woman. *Women and Therapy, 16*, 31–47.

Daniluk, J. C., & Tench, E. (2007). Long-term adjustment of infertile couples following unsuccessful medical intervention. *Journal of Counseling & Development, 85*, 89–100.

Dennerstein, L., & Hayes, R. D. (2005). Confronting the challenges: Epidemiological study of female sexual dysfunction and the menopause. *Journal of Sexual Medicine, 2*(Suppl. 3), 118–132.

Dowling, C. (1996). *Red hot mamas: Coming into our own at fifty.* New York: Bantam Books.

Duplassie, D., & Daniluk, J. C. (2007). Sexuality: Young and middle adulthood. In M. S. Tepper & A. F. Owens (Eds.), *Sexual health: Vol. 1. Psychological foundations* (pp. 263–289). Westport, CT: Praeger.

Erikson, E. H. (1997). *The lifecycle completed: Extended version.* New York: Norton.

Gannon, L. (1994). Sexuality and menopause. In P. Y. L. Choi & P. Nicolson (Eds.), *Female sexuality: Psychology, biology and social context* (pp. 100–124). New York: Harvester/Wheatsheaf.

Gold, J. M., & Wilson, J. S. (2002). Legitimizing the child-free family: The role of the family counselor. *The Family Journal: Counseling and Therapy for Couples and Families, 10,* 70–74.

Golub, S. (1992). *Periods: From menarche to menopause.* Newbury Park, CA: Sage.

Greer, G. (1991). *The change: Women, aging and menopause.* New York: Fawcett Columbine.

Gruen, D. (1990). Postpartum depression: A debilitating yet often unassessed problem. *Health and Social Work, 15,* 261–270.

Gross, A., & Ito, D. (1992). *Women talk about gynaecological surgery: From diagnosis to recovery.* New York: Harper Perennial.

Ireland, M. (1993). *Reconceiving women: Separating motherhood from female identity.* New York: Guilford Press.

Johnson, B. (2007). Sexuality at midlife and beyond. In M. S. Tepper & A. F. Owens (Eds.), *Sexual health: Vol. 1. Psychological foundations* (pp. 291–300). Westport, CT: Praeger.

Kaplan, E. A. (1990). Sex, work and motherhood: The impossible triangle. *Journal of Sex Research, 27,* 409–425.

Kitzinger, S. (1985). *Women's experience of sex.* New York: Penguin.

Kingsberg, S. (2004). Just ask! Talking to patients about sexual function. *Sexuality, Reproduction & Menopause, 2,* 199–203.

Kleiman, K., & Raskin, V. (1994). *This isn't what I expected: Recognizing and recovering from depression and anxiety after childbirth.* Toronto: Bantam Books.

Lampman, C., & Dowling-Guyer, S. (1995). Attitudes toward voluntary and involuntary childlessness. *Basic and Applied Social Psychology, 17,* 213–222.

Leiblum, S. R. (1997). Love, sex and infertility: The impact of infertility on couples. In S. R. Leiblum (Ed.), *Infertility: Psychological issues and coping strategies* (pp. 149–166). New York: Wiley.

Letherby, G. (2002). Childless and bereft? Stereotypes and realities in relation to voluntary and involuntary childlessness and womanhood. *Sociological Inquiry, 72,* 7–20.

Liu, C. (2003). Does quality of marital sex decline with duration? *Archives of Sexual Behavior, 32,* 55–60.

Love, S. (1990). *Dr. Susan Love's breast book.* Reading, MA: Addison-Wesley.

MacPhee, R. (1994). *Picasso's woman.* Vancouver, BC: Douglas & MacIntyre.

Martin, E. (1987). *The woman in the body: A cultural analysis of reproduction.* Boston: Beacon Press.

Masters, W. H., & Johnson, V. E. (1966). *Human sexual response.* Boston, MA: Little, Brown.

McCormick, N. (1996). Bodies besieged: The impact of chronic and serious physical illness on sexuality, passion and desire. *Journal of Sex Research: Special Issue, 33,* 175–230.

Mona, L. R., & Gardos, P. S. (2001). Disabled sexual partners. In L. T. Szuchman & F. Muscarella (Eds.), *Psychological perspectives on human sexuality* (pp. 309–354). New York: Wiley.

Morell, C. (1994). *Unwomanly conduct: The challenges of intentional childlessness.* New York: Routledge.

Nickerson, B. (1992). *Old and smart: Women and the adventure of aging.* Madeira Park, BC: Harbour.

Oberman, Y., & Josselson, R. (1996). Matrix of tensions: A model of mothering. *Psychology of Women Quarterly, 20,* 341–359.

Partridge, K. (1996). Beyond the baby blues: Understanding postpartum depression. *Today's Parent,* September, 84–89.

Rako, S. (1996). *The hormone of desire.* New York: Harmony Books.

Sexuality Information and Education Council of the United States. (1996). *Guidelines for comprehensive sexuality education* (2nd Ed.). Minnesota: 3M Education Press. SIECUS@siecus.org, http:www.siecus.org.

Stevens-Long, J., & Commons, M. L. (1992). *Adult life: Developmental processes* (4th ed.). London: Mayfield.

Tepper, M. S., & Owens, A. F. (2007). Access to pleasure: On-ramp to specific information on disability, illness, and changes throughout the life span. In A. F. Owens & M. S. Tepper (Eds.), *Sexual health: Vol. 4. State-of-the-art treatments and research* (pp. 313-328). Westport, CT: Praegar.

Tiefer, L. (1996). Towards a feminist sex therapy. *Women and Therapy* [Special Issue: Sexualities], *19,* 53–64.

Tierney, L. M., McPhee, S. J., & Papadakis, M. A. (1999). *Current medical diagnosis and treatment.* East Norwalk, CT: Appleton & Lange.

Unger, R., & Crawford, M. (1992). *Women and gender: A feminist psychology.* New York: McGraw-Hill.

Ussher, J. M. (1989). *The psychology of the female body.* New York: Routledge.

Westheimer, R. K., & Lopater, S. (2005). *Human sexuality: A psychosocial perspective* (2nd ed.). Philadelphia: Lippincott Williams & Wilkins.

Chapter 13

Family and Spousal Adaptation to Transitioning a Traumatic Event

Thomas W. Miller, Cindy Dunn, and Ila Patel

Death of a spouse was found to be one of the most stressful life experiences as exemplified in the Life Events Scale (Holmes and Rahe 1967). Randy Pausch entered our lives in September 2007. Randy, his wife and family too were facing a stressful life transition and he provided a model for all of us through his personality and through his masterful skill as a teacher at Carnegie Mellon University. His final lecture was titled by him "How to Live Your Childhood Dreams." Professor Randy Pausch is not like most people. He is a special person to share a message for the living that this previously unknown computer scientist delivered through a remarkable lecture to his students at Carnegie Mellon University in Pittsburgh. Thanks to the wonders of today's technology, the hour-long speech did not fade into the Ethernet, but has been heard by millions of us around the world. He was speaking through that lecture to his wife, his children, his students and a world community about his life's journey and the lessons he had learned on that journey. Most of all he was speaking to the children that he loved and to provide them with the guidance he wanted to share as a dad as they grew up. One recalls that he ended his last lecture with a couple of confessions. The lecture wasn't really about how to achieve one's dreams. It was about how to live one's life. His message to these three children was to "lead your lives the right way and the karma will take care of itself"; the dreams will come to you. This author and editor contacted him and was grateful for his kind response to the inspirational guidance that had been shared. It was September 21 and a world community learned from him on the evening news. He provided lessons for life. These lessons are summarized elsewhere. Randy Pausch, a 47-year-old computer science professor at Carnegie Mellon University, was suffering from terminal pancreatic cancer. He has been on palliative chemotherapy which targets its efforts in slowing the growth of the tumors that had formed in his pancreas and elsewhere. The chemotherapy worked for a while until the side effects began causing congestive heart and renal failure, resulting in his hospitalization. Randy returned home and decided to stop the palliative chemotherapy intended to extend his short lifespan for as long as possible. Pancreatic cancer is the fourth-deadliest type of carcinoma. It takes the lives of 75% of those who have it within a year. Only 4% live as long as 5 years. The impact on family, spouse and children is significant and the transitions that they face are often difficult for them.

From: *Handbook of Stressful Transitions Across the Lifespan*,
Edited by: T.W. Miller, DOI 10.1007/978-1-4419-0748-6_13,
© Springer Science+Business Media, LLC 2010

The purpose and scope of this chapter is to address the transition faced by the spouse and family who face major changes in their wife or husband as a result of a debilitating injury and loss due to a spectrum of causes. Examined are a multiplicity of issues which have been recognized through clinical research and experience as relevant to the spouse who is physically disabled. Specific issues related to life change events, their applicability to personality theory and recent clinical research are explored. Finally, issues in the treatment of the spouse who is physically disabled and family members are explored.

We introduced this chapter with the inspiration of Randy Pausch. There are others who, like Randy provide all of us a model for those facing devastating and debilitating illness, disease and infirmity. After suffering from a brain stem stroke at the age of 34, a professional mental health counselor spent months and years in a silent world of depression and despair. He was a quadriplegic, but had some ability to write messages. He could not speak but through the technology of computer technology, he would begin to speak the many thoughts that he had. It was through encouraging him to write about his thoughts and feelings that he produced, with the encouragement of several people who cared about him, and he wrote "*In Deciding to Die, I Found a Reason to Live.*" This book summarizes his journey elsewhere but the significance of his life was to see his son and daughter graduate and return to live in a nursing home near his wife and family where he could navigate the sidewalks to gain some semblance of life. Watching him, and walking with him, navigating the street crossings and sidewalks of this mid western city reflected his determination and adaptation to his family and his family accommodating his medical condition.

The Combat Veteran "Wounded Warrior" and Re-adaptation to Home and Family

The military of any nation at war have often faced similar challenges as have their spouses and children. Much of the research is related to the surviving or care, given to spouses of combat veterans with posttraumatic stress disorder (PTSD) who have higher rates of psychological and marital distress than do spouses of veterans without PTSD; however, very few studies have examined potential mechanisms of this increased vulnerability. The current study examined spouses of National Guard soldiers recently returned from deployments in Iraq. In addition to documenting elevated levels of psychological symptoms in these spouses, the authors found that spouses experienced greater symptom severity when they perceived high levels of symptoms in soldiers but the soldiers endorsed low levels of symptoms. Furthermore, the spouses' marital satisfaction was negatively linked to the soldiers' self-reported symptom severity only when spouses perceived that soldiers had experienced low levels of combat activity while deployed. When spouses perceived high levels of such activity, soldiers' self-reported symptoms had no relationship with spouses' marital satisfaction. These findings highlight the importance of interpersonal perceptions in intimate relationships and are consistent with the notion that uncontrollable attributions for a relative's mental health problems may provide a buffer against relationship distress.

Numerous transitional experiences and disturbances in life can cause stress. Concerns related to the physical environment, social and interpersonal relations, one's perception of various aspects of daily life, and a non-disabled spouse who suffers a debilitating injury that results in paralysis and dependence have all been known to be stressful life experiences. Examined are a multiplicity of factors which have been recognized through clinical research and experience as relevant to the spouse who is physically disabled. Specific issues related to life, change events, their applicability to personality theory and recent clinical researches are explored. In addition, relevance of current measures of stressful life events and suggested revisions are discussed. Finally, issues in the treatment of the spouse who is physically disabled and family members are examined.

Research in the area of family issues and multiple sclerosis has mainly focused on the impact of multiple sclerosis on the spouse (Moser and Dracup (2004). Examined was the relationship between patients' ratings of their spouses' responses to multiple sclerosis patient disability behaviors and the impact on patient psychological and physical functioning. In this study, multiple sclerosis patients were interviewed over the telephone using standardized questionnaires to assess patient physical and psychological functioning, spouse responses to patient disability and well behavior (i.e., how does the spouse respond when you're having difficulties related to multiple sclerosis?), and family environmental factors. The study was set in a large university-based multiple sclerosis clinical setting. The authors noted that 44 of 64 patients approached with definite multiple sclerosis, participated in the study. Physical functioning was assessed by the Kurtzke-EDSS, SIP, SF-36, and psychological functioning was assessed by the CES-D and SF-36. Scores on the SF-36 were generally lower compared with a normative sample of individuals with major medical problems; however, mean Kurtzke scores of 5.60 reflected moderate to severe impairment. Key to this study was examining spouse responses to disability. Correlation analyses revealed that solicitous spouse responses to patient disability behaviors were significantly associated with greater multiple sclerosis-related physical disability. This relationship was stronger for patients who were more depressed. A significant finding was that spouse's negative responses to patient disability behavior were associated with poorer mental health; whereas spouses' encouragement of the patient's well behavior was associated with lower emotional distress. Impaired psychological functioning was found in patients with families who were reported to have higher conflict and/or who were more controlling in the relationship. Higher levels of independence in families were associated with better psychological and physical functioning in the patients. The authors concluded that patient' perceptions of their families' responses to disability and family environment factors may be important areas for further research. The findings may also provide potential targets for clinical intervention in the future.

The wounded warrior's return home may experience some of the same results. From a clinical perspective, this is a time for both combat veteran and spouse to experience a spectrum of thoughts and feelings that contrast with the pre combat experience. While the Eriksonian theory provides a basic model for the patient and family to understand and embrace a sense of direction in the transitioning, of the related traumatic experiences and resultant disabilities, and their many challenges. There are, unfortunately, many departures from the ideal scenario of the loving spouse who provides the foundation of trust and buffers her partner from the isolation that is inherent in disconnecting from a former life and creating a new life. The following case study illustrates these challenges and represents an amalgam of the many readjustment scenarios.

Case Study

Prior to the veterans return, many families have spent a significant amount of time without the presence of the deployed member. A common scenario involves a spouse who has adjusted to and taken on roles and tasks at home out of necessity. As such, the return home involves resetting roles and tasks to accommodate the veteran. It is not uncommon for the spouse who remained stateside, to harbor resentments to the workload and financial hardship that the veteran's absence may have created. Many veterans also return to children who were born while they were away with bonding a challenge due to lack of immediacy in forming connectedness and to witnessing the effects of war on children overseas. One's own children may be the catalyst for painful reminders and thus, in the midst of trying to bond, distancing may occur. New employment or return to old employment is often fraught with interpersonal difficulties due to easy anger and irritability secondary to stress disorder and/or the effects of traumatic brain injury. For other veterans, return to employment, whether a former position or seeking a new position is not possible due to physical wounds or cognitive impairments. The frequent reality also includes the fact that many returning veterans return to a spouse who has met someone else during the deployment and the marriage is terminated shortly after arrival home. Thus, the challenges detailed above and below, fall to the family of origin. If the veteran remains married and seeks readjustment support from spouse or returns to family of origin for this, the interactional style is likely to be markedly different than prior to when they were deployed. For example, since current wartime experiences involve urban situations, civilians may be a source of perceived danger and suspicion. Furthermore, the returning veteran may seek to limit family interaction with "outsiders." Moreover, returning veterans often exhibit a polarity in interactional style with family members. Either they remain emotionally distant or they become overprotective to the point of controlling family members "movements in the larger world." This is not infrequently exemplified by calling a family member who is outside the home at regular, short term intervals to assess for safety. Substance abuse may create additive challenges to all of the above. Therefore, clinicians are often fielding a very complex situational terrain in the midst of assisting with physical, cognitive and psychological disabilities.

While the clinical ideal is to utilize the Eriksonian theory to assist the family of marriage in the adaptation to the impact of traumatic experiences, often the clinician must make a shift. That shift is one where the clinician must work to assuage the loss of trust, isolation and stagnation that the returning warrior feels in the rehabilitation quest. In the less than desirable scenarios, the situation is compounded by symptomatic and situational stress that adds to the readjustment and reintegration challenges.

The Wounded Warrior

While the case study detailed above offers a broad brush picture that many veterans, spouses and family members face with discharge from the military, the following three considerations are also paramount for clinicians and family members to incorporate in their understanding and interventions. It would be understated to suggest simply that the wounded warrior's return home is complex. Wounds coupled with real, permanent changes are, at best complex. More often than not, the changes are unfathomable by spouse, family of origin and many clinicians. The changes wrought by the sheer force of the war zone experience, may include an entrenched battlefield mindset; filial love and longing as well as shattered assumptions about the world. These changes commonly contribute to the presentation of a very different person than the spouse and the family of the origin they knew prior to war zone deployment. With or without the development of PTSD and/or a TBI, these constitute critical life alterations essentially in cognition, behaviors and for many, personality structure. If we add PTSD or TBI, the veteran's, spouses, and families adjustments are exponentially greater.

The Battlefield Mindset

Since the beginning of the Iraq War, the Department of Defense (DoD) has coined the term "battlefield mindset." It refers to ways of thinking and behaving that soldiers are trained to adopt for effectiveness in war zone situations. While the full description can be found at www.battlemind.army.mil three have been selected to introduce the concept and challenges to adjustment for the returning soldier and family.

The first example is termed "mission opsec vs secretiveness." This refers to the fact that in the combat situation, soldiers learn to talk about their mission only with those who need to know i.e., unit members. As such, upon returning home, the veteran may be perceived as "secretive" about deployment time. While a mental shift in openness may take time, it can be greatly complicated if post traumatic stress disorder exists. An outcome of this condition is avoidance of conversations related to traumatic memories. Even talking about memories that surround the traumatic memory can provoke or increase anxiety, anger and irritability.

Another example of the battlefield mindset that is often quite obvious, are driving behaviors. In the DoD description of the battlefield mindset "non-defensive (combat) vs aggressive driving," they note that combat driving is unpredictable and fast. Straddling the middle lane and keeping other vehicles at a distance is designed to maintain safety for oneself and fellow combatants. While combat driving is necessary to avoid hazards such as IED's and making oneself an easy target, the obvious dangers are apparent when one re-enters civilian driving. Speeding tickets can accumulate as well as family fear of the veteran behind the wheel of a car.

Still another linchpin of the battlefield mindset "discipline and ordering vs conflict" has been identified by the DoD. In combat, survival depends upon discipline and obeying orders. At home, this mindset can lend itself to the veteran being seen as issuing orders to family members and thus, perceived as unreasonably demanding and controlling. This stance can inevitably lead to conflict if we also recognize that the spouse who remained at home may now be accustomed to functioning with a greater degree of autonomy than prior to the veteran's deployment. Children too, may be quite resistant to militaristic "demands."

Within each of these examples there is a challenge to readjustment and a potential barrier to family support if not understood. This was aptly described in Letter from Camp Fallujah, Sammons, M.T. in the *Register Report*, Spring, 2007. These mindsets transferred to the civilian format, can render the veteran as being viewed as impulsive, reactive, and controlling. Other battle mind cognitions and related behaviors can occur initially as well as over the course of a lifetime. One in particular that has been observed is a strong preoccupation with being prepared for danger. This focus can shape the veterans, and thus family's, daily life and social functioning. Participation in gatherings or events is often determined by perception of danger. Predictability rather than spontaneity, seriousness rather than lightheartedness may become a key to daily life.

Finally, while family members may recognize serious transitional problems which are not infrequently accompanied by PTSD and or TBI, the now veteran often retains the battlefield mindset that only "weak" soldiers have mental health and transitional problems. As such, encouragement to "get help" can be perceived as derogatory commentary directed toward the veteran creating yet another barrier to the overall veteran and familial adjustment. Summarily, to assist the veteran, the spouse and the overall family with their returning warrior, utilization of Eriksonian theory, coupled with knowledge of the battlefield mind becomes paramount.

Filial Love

Filial love is a type of love that is particular to combatants who have served together. Shay (1994) described this as a type of affection that is unique to what one experiences for one's spouse. He refers to it as a type of love that is noted as being stronger often, than what one experiences for siblings. Spouses and family members often become aware of and are perplexed by the returning combatant's special connectedness to those with whom they served side by side in battle. Frequently, neither spouse nor family members expect connectedness to fellow soldiers beyond that of working with someone. As such, they are often mystified and perplexed by the strong emotional bond to and longing for fellow combatants. It is as if there is another family to which the veteran is a member. It is this filial love that captures a significant part of the returning soldier's heart and may occupy the mind. While it is sometimes understood, it can also be seen as a shadow force that is a rival for full return to civilian affections and thus, a barrier for full civilian reconnecting. This too then, must be explained and understood by family and clinicians who seek to build familial support and assist with adaptations.

Shattered Assumptions

Janoff-Bullman (1992) described internal framework mental changes that may emanate from traumatic experiences. Whether one develops PTSD or not, exposure to life threatening situations, may well lead to changes in the veterans' "assumptive world." At the more severe end, she described a literal shattering of beliefs about oneself and the surrounding world. She identified three major assumptive changes. Her work offers a most useful conceptual understanding for understanding trauma survivor internal cognitions that may lead to observed personality and behavioral changes.

Specifically, Janoff-Bulman suggested that trauma survivors may view the world around them as hostile and threatening. Clinically, this can translate into the veteran who has survived traumatic experiences as creating a family environment of "us against the dangerous world." What ensues is often, cut off from familial social interactions or a severe limiting of these. As such, not only does the veteran experience isolation but moves into a mindset where this isolation is preferred for self and family safety.

A further change in assumptions that Janoff-Bulman noted in trauma survivors, was a shift from the world being experienced as meaningful to one that lacks meaning. Prior to the experience of trauma, the world being seen as meaningful lends itself to a sense of order, predictability and safety in one's daily existence. But, because traumatic events are often difficult to make sense of and typically occur in a random and chaotic situational context, the survivor mentally often shifts to the assumption now that the world lacks meaning and thus has little predictability, order or safety. This may lend itself to family views that the veteran is paranoid, overprotective and stifling with regard to ordinary daily life functions.

Finally, Janoff-Bulman noted potential movement from seeing oneself as possessing self-worth to a strong questioning of one's real value. This is likely to emanate as identity confusion, self and social isolation and ultimately, depressed mood.

These changes are often superimposed upon the battlefield mindset and familial challenges in understanding Shay's concept of filial love. It is this amalgam that often contributes to or shapes the estrangement and detachment seen in PTSD. And thus, the veteran may exude an emotional distance toward the spouse and overall family. This likely stems from the very sense of self-alienation that the veteran feels due to the incorporation of the battlefield mindset and shattered assumptions. The overall world view has become significantly different than that of civilian counterparts and family. While the returning veteran may physically look similar to when they left, the internal cognitions and personality may be vastly and irrevocably changed.

Summarily, too often families and clinicians focus myopically on adjustments to diagnostic entities such as PTSD and TBI. While it is quite important to understand the changes brought forth by these conditions, such singular focus can preclude a more holistic understanding of the stress impinging upon the veteran and family. Without the holistic focus, adjustment to what has recently been termed as "the new normal" is blocked (Blair 2008). Subjective levels of stress can be significantly addressed if both veteran and family understand the actual scope and magnitude of diagnosis (es) and the impact of overall experiences. Expectations of return to the veteran's former self can be extremely frustrating for both the returning warrior and unrealistic for family members to adopt. The most effective clinicians have a broad understanding and can share this with the veteran and family to set realistic expectations from diagnoses to real structural changes in cognitions and behaviors. While some of these changes can be reshaped with awareness, others endure over the course of a lifetime following the profound experiences that one faces in a war zone. If the clinician and the family move toward restoration of cognitions, personality and behaviors prior to deployment, healthy adjustment to the "new normal" will be precluded.

The Transition for Loss Due to Health Related Injury and Disease

Moser and Dracup (2004) studied emotional responses and perception of control of patients and their spouses to myocardial infarction or coronary revascularization. They further examined the relationship between spouses' emotional distress and patients' emotional distress and psychosocial adjustment to the cardiac event. Results of this investigation suggest that spouses had higher levels of anxiety ($p < .001$) and depression ($p < .001$) than did patients, but there were no differences in level of hostility. Patients also expressed higher levels of perceived control than did spouses ($p < .001$). Spouse anxiety, depression, and perceived control remained correlated with patient psychosocial adjustment to illness, even when patient anxiety and depression were kept constant. Patients' psychosocial adjustment to illness was worse when spouses were more anxious or depressed than patients, and it was best when patients were more anxious or depressed than spouses, whereas psychosocial adjustment to illness was intermediate to these two extremes when patient and spouse anxiety and depression levels were similar ($p = .001$). Based on these findings, the investigators concluded that spouses often experience greater anxiety and depression and less perceived control than patients themselves. Attention to the psychological distress experienced by spouses of patients who have suffered a cardiac event may improve outcomes in patients.

The Impact of Forced Retirement

Szinovacz and Davey (2004) examined the effects of type of retirement (forced, early, abrupt) and spouse's disability on longitudinal change in depressive symptoms. The results suggest that depressive symptoms increase when retirement is abrupt and perceived as too early or forced. Women retirees who stopped employment and were either forced into retirement or perceived their retirement as too early report significantly more depressive symptoms with increasing spouse activities of daily living (ADLs) limitations. There is no similar effect for men. In contrast, for working retirees who retired on time, depressive symptoms decrease with increasing spouse ADLs. These results highlight the importance of retirement context on postretirement well-being. They suggest that both the type of retirement transition and marital contexts such as spouse's disability influence postretirement well-being, and these effects differ by gender.

Critical Issues in Psychosocial Development

In an earlier chapter in this volume, Clark (2009) and Marcia (2009) introduced us to the theory of Erik Erikson. It is Erikson who suggests that within the framework of normal human development, there is a process by which an individual moves from a dependent to an independent lifestyle. Similarly, independent living and re-entry into the "real world" are the goals of rehabilitation process. For the patient facing adaptation from independent and productive functioning, the brain injured person not unlike the wounded warrior or the degenerative disease patient must negotiate a variety of psychological conflicts or crises, which are inherent in recovery, adaptation and accommodation to successfully transitioning a traumatic event or experience.

It was Erik Erikson's model that offers several challenges that must be addressed through the rehabilitation process. Most important of all is the realization that one must re gain a sense of identity. While Erikson's model describes a logical series of developmental processes, Erikson argues that a life crisis can lead to a breakdown in that developmental process. Health care professionals and patient families, not unlike the patient, often have an intuitive sense for the psychological conflicts experienced by a number of patients in the rehabilitation process. During their recovery and adaptation, Erikson's model (Erikson 1950) provides a glimpse of the critical challenges in psycho social development. This model provides a conceptual model that clinicians and families often find helpful in understanding the patients' psychological conflicts as they recover through the rehabilitation process. Erikson argues that psychological development progresses through eight stages based on an individual's ability to negotiate satisfactory adaptation at each of the eight stages. For the patient, each conflict suggested by Erikson seems relevant to the adaptation process that may lead to a successful rehabilitation.

What Are the Challenges for Rehabilitation?

Erikson indicates in his theory that trust is the first and essential epigenetic challenge for the rehabilitation process. Once a trusting experience is realized, autonomy within the rehabilitation process can occur. Only after that can the rehabilitating person show initiative, industry and then ultimately achieve one's identity. The human organism initially is totally dependent upon others. Within the context of the wounded warrior, the person with Parkinson's or the person suffering a stroke, life is a search for who I am and who I can be. . Erikson notes that it is critically important for adults to be reliable in providing caretaking functions so that the patient develops a basic sense of trust in the environment and in significant of others in the environment. The early stages of the rehabilitation process often place the patient in a partially or totally dependent state. In severe cases, the patient's basic bodily functions are assisted by other people, usually nurses and other rehabilitation therapists. The goal of rehabilitation process at this stage is to provide these basic caretaking functions in a timely and reliable manner Failure to achieve a sense of trust is likely to impair the rehabilitation tasks necessary to achieve accommodation and adaptation.

Autonomy becomes the key to successful advancement through the next stage of rehabilitation. Because of the limitations realized by the traumatic event, the patient may well develop a sense of shame and doubt. . Shame involves a sense of being exposed, vulnerable and inferior. Inevitably, this involves feelings of doubt about his/her abilities and identity. Such shame and doubt are often the psychological reasons behind depression and social withdrawal which, not surprisingly, is two of the most commonly reported problems in the rehabilitation process. Erikson, in his conceptual model notes that the person who develops an initial sense of autonomy, finds that the environment offers and provides a strong social network, to support the person in the rehabilitation process. This realization triggers the concepts that Erikson refers to as the need for a sense of initiative and for industry which produces life skills and highlights a generation of competencies and skills.

Eriksonian theory suggests that initiative involves the redevelopment of a sense of self-direction. The patient must again re-enter adult life with competencies and skills in accordance with the limitations realized through the traumatic event. Erikson noted in his writings that every person has an innate need to do something of value, and to take on meaningful work. The person who does not take on this renewed sense of industry will likely be left with a sense of inferiority and failure. Such a condition often leads to a functional type of depression, marked by withdrawal and isolation which significantly impairs the achievement of one's identity.

The achievement of a sense of identity modified by the strengths and limitation of the present condition resulting from the traumatic event or experience is the life blood in achieving those critical hierarchical development milestones embedded in intimacy generativity and integrity as a person. Certainly there are those who struggle to regain their former sense of identity or establish any new sense of identity. Successful resolution of this conflict at this level includes the realization that "I now have an identity as a wounded warrior but the competencies and life skills necessary to gain considerable independence at whatever level to embrace intimacy, generativity and integrity as a person".

Erikson's theory provides a roadmap for the patient and family to understand and embrace a sense of direction in the transitioning of this traumatic experience. Throughout the lifespan it is realized that caring, love and affection are critical factors gained through effective interpersonal relationships, particularly the marital relationship during adulthood. Erikson argued that these stages of psychosocial development offer "intimacy" and "generatively" versus the negative outcome of isolation and stagnation. Intimacy and generativity are achieved through several means and are not limited to sexuality. However, Erikson did note the importance of sexuality as a part of a mature intimate relationship. Often occurring in the process are some changes in personality that may include but are not limited to impulsiveness, irritability, and inappropriate social behavior all of which can lead to interpersonal problems even with the most understanding of significant people in the patient's life, and impair the potential to fully realize a sense of intimacy in a relationship. For Erikson, the development of a sense of ego integrity at the end of life becomes the signal of one's success in adapting to life, to the physical, emotional and psychological conditions created by the traumatic experience and provides the person with a feeling that life has been worth living and having an acceptance of a life lived to its fullest capability.

Lessons Learned in Understanding Trauma and Its Consequences

Stressful Life transitions are challenging to victims and to spouses and their families because they force all concerned to let go of the familiar and face the future with a feeling of vulnerability and uncertainty. Most life transitions begin with a loss due to some traumatic event. Physically it could be a limb or bodily function, mentally and emotionally it could be the loss of identity, role and purpose in life. Any significant loss makes most people feel fearful and anxious. That life transition can be positive or negative, planned or unexpected and some transitions occur without warning, and they may be quite dramatic, as in cases of terminal illness, cancer accident, divorce, job loss, or death. Other stressful life transitions may come from positive experiences such as graduating from school or college, getting married, giving birth to a child, obtaining a new job, pays raise or a promotion. Events like these are just as stressful even though they may be and usually are un- planned and anticipated. They often are just as life-altering as the unexpected events. Whether the event or change experience is positive or negative, life transitions are stress provoking and cause us to leave behind the familiar and force us to adjust to new ways of living our lives.

The family is perceived as a unit that shares not only a sense of history, that experiences emotional bonding, that engages in goal directed behavior, and that for the sake of a marriage contract, enters into a relationship with a belief that it will be for better or for worse, for richer, or for poorer, in sickness or in health (Figley and McCubbin 1983; Van Uitert et al. 1989). Separation of family members as through the deployment during war time, an unexpected life trauma that may be the results of wartime experiences or an automobile accident, the diagnosis of a chronic illness, or a physical disability are rarely thought of when two non-disabled, normal people enter into a marital relationship. Our basic human needs are addressed in the theory of Abraham Maslow (1980) and are summarized in Table 13-1 which provides a summary of each of its hierarchical needs and also the stressors related to each of the needs by both the spouse who is disabled and the family members of the person who is disabled. Not unlike Erikson, Maslow emphasized basic human needs along with safety, social, esteem and self actualization needs. Such needs are transformed into the specific aspects of such needs during the rehabilitation process.

Disabled Spouse, Family Impact

These sacrifices are viewed as minimal compared to the suffering of the spouse who is newly disabled. Consequently, emotional liability, impaired judgment, and coping abilities are often products of these sacrifices. The experienced clinician can reframe immediate responsibilities of concerned family members to enhance longer term adjustments for all members. Efforts should be made to minimize disruptions/interruptions in diet, sleep patterns, and other physical, psychological, social, and vocational needs of able-bodied family members throughout the treatment process.

Most individuals will be quite responsive to directives from authority figures during crisis situations, especially when accompanied by supportive rationales. All family members can be told that frequent visits and other forms of emotional support are critical during the initial phases of recovery. Equally important for all family members (including the spouse who is newly disabled), however, are routine activities which provide the need for satisfaction for able-bodied family members and thus have enhanced stability for the family unit.

Issues and Implications for Family Functioning

The impact of having a spouse who is traumatically injured raises several key issues. One of the most significant is the fact that the individual who is disabled may be reluctant to seek support and assistance from family and friends

Table 13-1. Maslow's theoretical need hierarchy as it relates to stressful life experiences in the family who has a disabled member.

Maslow's theoretical stages	Stressors for the disabled spouse	Stressors for family members
Physical needs	Physical pain experienced	Insufficient sleep/rest
	Course of illness	Inadequate diet
	Physical care received	Absence of personal space
	Privacy	Absence of privacy
	Personal space	
	Quality of food	
Safety needs	Security of personal self	Insecurity regarding own mortality
	Security of possessions	Insecurity regarding absence from household/other
	Appropriateness of medication	Household/other family members
	No harm from treatment	Insecurity regarding new responsibilities
	Competency of nursing care/home care	Insecurity regarding harm from treatment to spouse
	Physician available	Insecurity regarding competency of nursing care/home care
		Acceptance of frequent absences and decreased productivity by employees
		Reassurance other family members are safe/well
Social needs	Acceptance by staff and peers	Acceptance by staff, peers and spouse who is disabled
	Concern by family members	Concern by extended and nuclear family members
	Regular contact from friends and significant others	Regular contact from friends
	Recreational Activity	Redefinition of role in relation to spouse/parent who is disabled
	Redefinition of role in the family	Occasional relief from home/hospital pressures (Recreational activities)
Esteem needs	Maintaining a sense of oneself	Maintaining a sense of oneself
	Treatment with respect by staff, family, friends	Self Respect
	Self respect	Treatment with respect by staff, employers, friends, spouse who is disabled
	Clarification of long and short term vocational goals	Clarification of long and short term vocational goals/family relationships
Self-actualizing	Fulfillment of personal and life goals	Fulfillment of personal and life goals

This table appeared in an earlier article by Miller et al. (1993)

as well as from medical personnel. Often, the person who is disabled fears that the requests that might be offered will negatively reflect on his or her self-image. Networks for individuals with a physical disability who may help one another are sometimes available and can provide the emotional support and reality orientation to individuals with a recent physical disability.

Another important issue pertains to family support. The family's reaction to the shock and stress of a permanently disabling injury or disability typically takes a minimum of 4–6 weeks to process after injury occurs or the diagnosis is realized. Early attempts must be made to provide the family with support, education, and understanding. A theoretical framework for family intervention should be offered in which the person experiencing the disability is a part of the unique personal system dealing with abilities, limitations, aspirations, fears, anxieties, and the concerns of family members, friends, and spouse. It is not uncommon for the person who is disabled and/or close family members to experience some personality change in this process. This may involve impaired capacity for social perceptiveness as well as emotional alterations which lead to impulsive outbursts or anger and frustration. This anger and frustration usually needs to be processed by the family members themselves. A third issue deals with the expectations of both the person and the family after the process of grieving over the traumatic experience has occurred. Addressed usually with the benefit of the professionally trained therapist should be the realistic and unrealistic expectations of both the person and the family. In addition to that, the misinterpretation of the person's behaviors as deficits needs to be addressed. The rehabilitation process often requires considerable attention to a slow, but progressive effort toward assuming maximum independence.

There are several important ingredients which both the person and family members need at the time of realizing the implications of a serious chronic or terminal illness or injury. The initial priority of the patient and the individual with a disability is a clear and sensitive explanation of the person's condition. Tied to this should be realistic expectations of what might be expected with respect to the person's progress. Beyond these two core ingredients, emotional support, financial counseling, and the availability of community resources seem to be critically important in meeting the needs of the family as well as the person who faces a critical illness/injury. Losses suffered by the debilitating effects of head injuries, stroke, or central nervous system dysfunction can be conceptualized as a partial death. This fits into the concept of the "chronic living–dying phase" that Pattison (1987) has addressed. It is a phase characterized by the emergence of many physical needs and limitations. Most fears at this phase involve the fear of loneliness and sorrow, and of loss of self control. Continual or increasing impairment and limitations may often be experienced.

Within the framework of personality development, previous personality styles of the individual may become accentuated during the illness phase. This might be marked by a more demanding attitude and stubbornness which can lead to power struggles between the person who is disabled and the family members and/or staff. Providing some structure so that the individual who is disabled can assume as much control as is physically or emotionally possible can help to reduce the internalized anger and frustration that he/she may well be experiencing. One of the most frustrating aspects is his/her realization of impaired capacity for control and self-regulation.

Efforts toward isolation are not usual as persons who are disabled may be intolerant of probing questions regarding their feelings. Even so, short visits which find the visitor empathic rather than sympathetic may be appreciated. Of considerable concern is the anticipatory anxiety and apprehension about the future and what is not known about this illness, disease entity, or disability. The period of grieving is essential for the person who is disabled and for the family members as well who often feel trapped, isolated, and even abandoned by the extended family. To the spouse who is nondisabled, this is a time also where social experiences are in limbo and there may be an inability to openly mourn the patient's condition. For the person who is disabled, the loss of self-control over physical or mental abilities and the process of becoming more dependent on others are difficult hurdles to accept. To experience an individual regressing toward increasingly greater dependence leads to intense internalized anxiety. One might realize that a person who is disabled can become quite egocentric and their thinking focused on losses that they have already experienced and those that they anticipate in the future.

Continuity of rehabilitation personnel is a critically important issue. From an interdisciplinary perspective, this requires good team management which can be to the benefit of not only the person but also the family members, address key issues which include readjusting their goals and their expectations for the disability. In addition, providing practical advice for patient management and establishing an awareness of needs and responsibilities become critically important. The counseling process should foster the family members' catharting of their anger and frustration as well as their sorrow and natural emotions for the patient's condition. In addition, they must realize that the caretaking person must address their own needs before they can be helpful and facilitative to the person who needs their support. This means that they must rely heavily on their own conscience, judgment, and value structure in dealing with conflicts with the person or with other family members. There are numerous role changes which occur when an adult becomes physically dependent and these role changes can be emotionally distressing for all concerned. When the welfare of dependent children may be at stake, family members need to explore divided loyalties and weight their responsibilities as there are no easy answers and each situation must be addressed on an individual, family basis. Clinical observation suggests that most families and/or spouses or persons who have physical limitations consider the physical care of this individual as a task they must assume. This is particularly true when a young adult experiences traumatic injury. Cases are known where spouses resigned occupational positions, mothers of children who have disabilities have lived on campus commuting home to their spouses only on weekends, etc. The point must be made that physical disability does not necessarily entail severe long-term family disorganization. The sense of guilt and perception of burden a person with a disability assumes in such situations can far outweigh any physical care benefit such an arrangement affords. The hidden resentment and sense of guilt the person providing such physical care endures can be equally devastating to the family unit. Medical and rehabilitation professionals are, therefore, obliged to discuss alternate arrangements for the physical care of persons with disabilities. Such professionals must stress that each member of the family must be afforded time and space for individual life goals and personal satisfaction. The physical care needs of the person with a disability cannot overshadow the psychological, vocational, and physical needs of other family members if a longterm satisfactory solution is to be achieved. Alternate arrangements for the physical care of a person who has a severe disability no longer means institutionalization. For obvious reasons, institutional care may be the least desirable long-term solution. Rehabilitation legislation has mandated funding for the establishment of Independent Living Centers (ILCs) across the United States. These centers provide services to persons with disabilities including physical and attendant care. By 1988, nearly 200 such centers were functioning in this country (Sedgwick 1988). And while some of these centers provide residential programs, many also offer to assist families in locating assistance and support with the physical care needs of a person who has a disability. Several states are creating funding programs for assistance of this type so that the family need not bear the financial burden of such physical support. In cooperation with the Office of State Vocational Rehabilitation Services, efforts to provide vocational retraining where possible have also promoted more support for the fully functioning person with a disability. Considerable activities need to be carried out to develop and enhance the network or persons who are physically disabled and their spouses who seek to help one another with adaptive and adjustment difficulties. The health care delivery system has the obligation and responsibility to greater sensitize itself to the needs and requirements of the population addressed here. Intervention strategies to cope with such trauma can assist both the spouse who is disabled and the spouse who is able-bodied to seek all that their relationship can offer.

Acknowledgments: Appreciation is extended to Robert F. Kraus M.D, Walter Penk PhD., Tag Heister LLB, College of Medicine University of Kentucky, Deborah Kessler, Department of Veterans Affairs and Jill Livingstone LLB, Library Science; Department of Psychiatry, University of Connecticut for their assistance in the preparation of this manuscript.

References

Blair, E. (2008). In Ancient Dramas: Vital Words for Today's Warriors. Retrieved November 25, 2008 from NPR "All Things Considered".

Clark, J. (2009). Life as a Source of Theory: Erik Erikson's Contributions, Boundaries & Marginalities In: Miller, T. W. (Ed) *Handbook of Stressful Life Transitions across the Life Span*. New York: Springer Publishers Incorporated.

Erikson, E. H. (1950) *Childhood and Society*. New York: Norton.

Figley, C. R., & McCubbin, H. I. (1983). *Stress and the family: Coping with narrative transitions*. New York: Brunner/Mayel Publishers.

Goodman, R. (1981). *In deciding to die, I found reason to live*. Image Graphics Publishers: Paducah, Kentucky

Holmes, T. H., & Rahe, R. H. (1967). The social readjustment rating scale. *Journal of Psychosomatic Research, 11*, 213–218.

Janoff-Bullman, R. (1992). *Shattered assumptions: Towards a new psychology of trauma*. New York, NY: The Free Press.

Marcia, J. E. (2009). Life transitions and stress in the context of psychosocial development In: Miller, T. W. (Ed) *Handbook of Stressful Life Transitions across the Life Span*. New York: Springer Publishers Incorporated.

Maslow, A. H. (1980). *Motivation and personality* (2nd ed.). New York: Harper & Row Publishers.

Miller, T. W., Houston, L., & Goodman, R. (1993). Clinical issues in psychosocial rehabilitation for spouses with physical disabilities. *Journal of Developmental & Physical Disabilities, 32*(4), 41–48.

Moser, D. K., & Dracup, K. (2004). The role of spousal anxiety and depression in patients' psychosocial recovery after a cardiac event. *Psychosomatic Medicine, 66*, 527–532.

Pattison, E. M. (1987). *The experience of DyhTg*. Englewood Cliffs, New Jersey: Prentice-Hall Publishers.

Sammons, M. T. (2007). Letter from Camp Fallujah. *The Register Report, 33*, 8–9.

Shay, J. (1994). *Achilles in Vietnam: Combat trauma and the undoing of character.* New York, NY: Touchstone.

Sedgwick, R. (1988). *Family mental health: Theory and practice.* St. Louis: Mosby.

Szinovacz, M., & Davey, A. (2004). Honeymoons and joint lunches: Effects of retirement and spouse's employment on depressive symptoms. *Journal of Gerontology: Psychological Sciences, 59B*, P233–P245.

Van Uitert, R., Eberly, R., & Engdahl, B. (1989). Stress and coping of wives following their husbands' strokes. In T. W. Miller (Ed.), *Stressful life events* (pp. 473–494). New York: International Universities Press.

Walter Reed Army Institute of Research (WRAIR) (2006). PDHRA Battlemind Training: Continuing the Transition Home. Retrieved March 08, 2006, from http://www.battlemind.army.mil.

Part IV

Legal, Ethical, and Financial Transitions

Chapter 14

Ethical and Legal Issues in Transitioning the Lifespan

Steven Nisenbaum, Madelaine Claire Weiss, and Daniel Shapiro

Ethics and law are pivotal inventions for managing stress throughout the life cycle, especially at critical junctures of key life event and stage-of-life transitions. Perhaps this proposition seems improbable, if not patently preposterous, in part, because stress is mostly regarded as a medical event and a psychological challenge rather than an ethicolegal problem. Or perhaps the logic appears ironic, as ethical quandary and the entire edifice of law, litigation, and administration of justice is perceived by many of us as a stressor in life, exacerbating anguish at occurrences that beg for resolution and relief.

Nevertheless, in this chapter, in Part One, we will briefly examine the evolutionary origins of law and ethics as a social institution for stress regulation. In Part Two, we will survey and highlight the scope and content of modern law and ethics for life transition stress, because what these institutions regulate will vary at different developmental stages of societal organization. As we will show in Part Three, twenty-first century modernist notions of rights and entitlements for protection, and for access to the advantages of civilization, make imperative that we regularly revisit and refine this institution upon which our stress regulation, if not survival, continues to depend. Finally, we will examine the issue of formidable iatrogenic stress contributed by moral quandary and navigating legal systems, and conclude with the prospects for a better future approach.

Part One: Evolution of Law and Ethics for Stress Management

What Is Ethical Rule and The Rule of Law?

Ethics is the branch of philosophy concerned with the right conduct and good life, or the worthiness and striving for the life worth living. Although some equate ethics and morality, morality may also be distinguished as pertaining to the more internal conscience, or may refer to the extent to which the actual conduct is considered in comparison with right conduct. Law is a system of rules regulating rights and obligations among the members of a society, including ownership of property and contractual agreements, expectations to

From: *Handbook of Stressful Transitions Across the Lifespan,*
Edited by: T.W. Miller, DOI 10.1007/978-1-4419-0748-6_14,
© Springer Science+Business Media, LLC 2010

be compensated for a breach of duty causing injury, criminal sanctions for harmful violations of peaceful order, inheritance and transmission of wealth across generations, responsibilities in relationships within families and social institutions, and so forth. Legal institutions exist to ensure a well-ordered society conducive to security, productive effort, and prosperity. Generally, the apparatus of law achieves the common good by meting out rewards for worthiness and disincentives for wrongdoing.

The cornerstone of ethics and law is a shared commitment to "just" deserts, being treated justly or as deserved. For all rational and "just" (non-arbitrary, non-chance) legal systems, the basis of ethical reason and legal accountability is the commonly held belief (from ad hoc improvised "meeting of the minds" or a presumptive pre-existing "social contract") about an expectation of fairly imposed obligation. Accordingly, "justice" is:

1. Enforcement of agreed offer and acceptance (i.e., by compensatory contractual damages).
2. Fair response to delict (wrongful act) comprised of:
   (a) Disturbing the public peace and decorum (i.e., warranting sanctions of criminal punishment).
   (b) Violating a duty owed to another (resulting in right to compensation for injury from harm, i.e., warranting lawsuit tort damages).

A "Moral Faculty" for Society, Uniquely Human or not?

In non-religious Post-Enlightenment terms, the capacity for law and ethics is an artifact of evolved moral faculty. Whether morality is uniquely human remains a focus of controversy. Charles Darwin (1874/1981) presumed that the moral facet was the result of an evolutionary process across a constellation of social instinctual proclivities:

Any animal whatever, endowed with well-marked social instincts, the parental and filial affections being here included, would inevitably acquire a moral sense or conscience, as soon as its intellectual powers had become as well developed or nearly as well developed, as in man (pp. 71-72)

Darwin found such social instincts that form the "prime principle" of moral sense in various species, including monkeys, pelicans, dogs, and other animals too. Frans de Waals in *Chimpanzee Politics* (1982) has led a team of contemporary researchers who try to illustrate that non-human primates have the capacity to make judgments about harmful consequences of action, and to share and reciprocate in ways that suggest a repertoire of moralistic behavior and perhaps moral reasoning.

Marc Hauser (2006) suggests that these processes are not conscious moral judgments, but the product of an inborn moral faculty (often largely inaccessible to the mind's conscious awareness), although humans at least have the corollary capacity to provide reasoned explanations by contemplating and manipulating explicit principles for justification. Hauser and others even try to localize this cognitive accomplishment as a cortical function that evolved in certain areas of the human frontal lobes, capable of storing and employing a "deep" universal grammar for morality, especially in the region neurologists label Brodman Area 10. Others, like Sherman and Guillery (2005), focus on a two-way relationship between neocortical areas receiving inputs from the thalamus and also sending outputs to lower motor centers, with pathways carrying messages and modulators which can change the pattern of transmission.

On the other hand, Faith-based Creationists (see, e.g., summary by John Gray, "Are We Moral?" in the *New York Review of Books*, 2007) suggest that the bridles on natural aggressive and self-preservative competitive instincts are God-given uniquely human capabilities, just as depicted in the ancient biblical stories. Indeed, certain exponents of Darwinism sometimes use language that suggests morality as a restraint or repression of natural impulses that is uniquely human: "We, alone on earth, can rebel against the tyranny of the selfish replicators" (Dawkins 1981, p. 201).

Evolving a Moral Faculty

In the Carboniferous period 300 million years ago, the world was spanned by warm, shallow seas. The climate was hot, humid, and constant. A line of mammal-like reptile synapsids flourished in the Permian and early Triassic 280–210 million years ago, and were nearly annihilated by the dinosaurs in the Mesozoic Era, but evolved during the Triassic (225–195 million years ago) into true nocturnal mammals that were 5 cm (2 in.) long. The earliest egg-bearing Prototheria evolved over 200 million years ago into live bearing Theria, and 90 million years later split into marsupials and placentals in the Pliocene Era along with the creation of continental climates and grasslands. Placentals began diversifying in the Late Cretaceous, after the drifting tore asunder Pangea (the term for earth's land mass when it was all unified as one), subdivided and the southern landmasses divided and migrated (Rowe et al. 2007).

The first mammals, comparatively smart, perceptive animals with good memory, evolved around 20 million years ago. Mammals are a morphologically diverse class currently comprising 4,680 animal species with astonishing flexibility of individual behavior. They share certain morphological characteristics; such as having backbones, bodies insulated by hair, placental birth, nursing of infants with milk (such that offspring stay close to their mothers), and unique jaw articulation. Size ranges from tiny, e.g., Kitti's Hog-nosed Bat weighing 1.5 g (0.05 ounces) to massive, e.g., the Blue Whale 100,000,000 times bigger. Life span also varies. The life span of some species may be many decades while the male Brown Antechinus dies even before the birth of the litter he fathers. Birthing batches may vary among species from single offspring births to the Naked Mole Rat's litter of 28. The same rat spends its entire life in a single burrow, while a Wolf's territory may be 1,000 sq km (400 sq miles) (MacDonald 2001, p. xvi).

Primates evolved as a group of mammals with special attributes, including enlarged cerebral cortex, complex high acuity binocular color vision, shortened snout with reduced sense of smell, wide range of arm movement, opposable pre-hensile thumb, longer gestation, and fewer offspring who also are more clingy and dependent. There are 634 species and subspecies of primates (International Union for Conservation of Nature 2008). Primates share, as well, the emotion systems common to all mammalians: viz., accessible by various sensory stimuli; can generate instinctual motor outputs; can modulate sensory inputs; positive feedback components can sustain arousal after precipitating events; are modulated by cognitive inputs; can modify and channel cognitive activities. Therefore, according to Jaak Panksepp (1998), mammalian – including primate – emotions promote and modulate incentive salience. As Charles Darwin (1874/1981) reminded us:

We must acknowledge, as it seems to me, that Man with all his noble qualities, with sympathy which feels for the most debased, with benevolence which extends not only to other men but to the humblest living creature, with his god-like intellect which has penetrated into the movements and constitution of the solar system – with all these exalted powers – Man still bears in his bodily frame the indelible stamp of his lowly origin (p. 528)

Jessica Flack and Frans de Waal (2008) have observed the precursors of a sense of social regularity in pre-human primates. Other hominid primates started to develop mechanisms for conflict resolution foreshadowing human ethics and law, a primitive behavioral repertoire. As Flack and de Waal summarized:

Many non-human primates, for example, seem to have similar methods to humans for resolving, managing, and preventing conflicts of interest within their groups. . . . Such methods, which include reciprocity and food sharing, reconciliation, consolation, conflict intervention, and mediation, are the very building blocks of moral systems (pp. 1-65)

The most celebrated finding of earliest remains of a proto-human (hominid) date to 3.2–4.0 million years ago (Johanson and Edley 1981). The remains suggest that early hominids came down from trees and exhibited bipedalism and free hands to manipulate things in the environment, useful for improvisational problem-solving in "negotiating" the challenges of natural world survival. As hominids evolved, they stood more erect, and the birth canal narrowed so infants had to be born earlier (when less fully matured) to allow relatively big brains to pass through. Infants born earlier in maturation were more dependent. Since women with their dependent infants were more vulnerable to predators, human females needed to entice fathers to be around longer to ward off predators, as well as to provide iron replacements (that would be meat).

But how is it possible to keep males around? According to Leonard Schlain (2003), it was by keeping her ovulation a secret, so that no man could be certain of his paternity unless he hung around with one woman to make sure what is his was his – the origin of human family life.

Perhaps in a small insular tribal society where every other person knows each individual member, delineation and enforcement of formulated prescriptive rules is less urgent. In pre-historic human troops and early human clan tribes, moral reasoning and detailed written codes of law were superfluous or else subordinated to more pressing survival needs. According to Jared Diamond (1998), disputes in bands of less than 100 people could be handled informally by leaders who rose to power on personal or physical strengths. So too for tribes of more than 100 people, with kinship ties still helping to keep conflicts from getting out of hand. Once population size grew to thousands and tens of thousands, "…people had to learn, for the first time in history, how to encounter strangers regularly without attempting to kill them" (Diamond 1998, p. 273).

More complex social organizations required explicit formal rules and more objective ethical norms. Rationally understandable (culturally sanctioned) normative behavior became vital to reliably smooth, regular, and efficient functioning, irrespective of personal trust based on prior acquaintance and direct relationship, or immediate leadership supervision. Systems of law and ethics evolve, therefore, in concert with the stage of socio-economic and political organizational development of the society.

Evolved Human Attributes

The last of the Neanderthals became extinct some 40,000 years ago. Human consciousness and human language evolved among a competitor species with superior improvisational problem-solving capabilities, adaptive specifically for social tasks (i.e., innovative "social negotiation"). Humans today are both capable of, and limited by, the specific array of social-emotional skills suitable for conditions that prevailed at the time of rapid cerebral cortex expansion. Our psychological attributes, from emotions to language and reason, can be understood as specific adaptations to ancestral Pleistocene conditions. Human intelligence, therefore, reflects what Paul MacLean (1990) termed the triune organization of mind:

The Reptilian Brain (Archipallium brain). Includes the structures of the brain stem – medulla, pons, cerebellum, mesencephalon, the oldest basal nuclei – the globus pallidus and the olfactory bulbs. In animals such as reptiles, the brain stem and cerebellum dominate. Hence, it is commonly referred to as the "reptilian brain." It has the same type of archaic behavioral programs as snakes and lizards. It is rigid, obsessive, compulsive, ritualistic, and paranoid. It is "filled with ancestral memories": that is, it keeps repeating the same behaviors over and over again, never learning from the past.

The Limbic System (Paleopallium brain), intermediate (old mammalian) brain. Includes the hypothalamus, hippocampus, and amygdala. The old mammalian brain residing in the limbic system is concerned with emotions and instincts: feeding, fighting, fleeing, and sexual behavior. Everything in this emotional system is either "agreeable or disagreeable." As a whole, it appears to be the primary seat of emotion, attention, and affective (emotion-charged) memories. It helps determine valence (whether you feel positive or negative towards something), salience (what catches your attention), unpredictability, and creative behavior. It has immense interconnection with the neocortex, such that the brain functions are neither purely limbic nor purely cortical but a mixture of both.

The Neocortex (Neopallium brain or Neomammalian brain), superior or rational brain. Includes the cerebrum, cortex, and nearly the whole of the hemispheres (made up of a more recent type of cortex, called neocortex) and some subcortical neuronal groups. It corresponds to the brain of the primate mammals and, consequently, the human species. The higher cognitive functions that distinguish Man from the animals reside in the cortex.

Humans, in particular, are capable of the key social emotional phenomena that comprise the rich, complex tapestry of the dynamic human condition including:

- Hoarding, compulsive ritualized behavior, appetitive addictive goal-seeking behavior
- Fear, paranoia, anger, rage retaliatory, competitive, aggressive profane
- Anxiety, panic, phobic, restless, dysphoria, sadness, depression
- Euphoria, humor, high, social facilitative/attractive/cooperative/cohesive
- Fatigue, listless, anergia, abulia, hypoactive, lassitude to arousal, hyperactive
- Serenity, equanimity, relaxation, soothing
- Initiative, spontaneity
- Authority-submission, respect, rule-subordinate/defiance, oppositionalism, sociopathy
- Self-regard, -esteem, -confidence, enhancing, vulnerability, narcissistic, ego-expansive, aggrandizing
- Imaginary, dream work, mythopoetic, narrative, mythic, meaning-making
- Object-seeking, attraction, needless/yearning, attachment/bond
- Directedness, instrumentalist, goal-oriented, organized
- Love

Societal Development and the Human Social Brain

In the aftermath of this cortical expansion and triune brain development, about 10,000 years ago, human societies transitioned from nomadic hunter and food-foraging groups of under 100 individual members to the proliferation of large sedentary agricultural communities of up to 10,000 people. As biological anthropologist Barbara King (2007) reminds us, at some point between the onset of hominids from the ape lineage, between 3 and 7 million years ago and the beginning of farming and settled communities a mere 10,000 or so years ago, the encephalization necessary for empathy, meaning-making, rule-following, and imagination evolved appropriate to the social challenges of then and there, permitting the survival and flourishing of the human species we know now.

The cortical capacity for human language – articulated reciprocal expectation and obligations – made possible prescriptive morality and intelligent discourse beyond rudimentary gestural communication. At this point in evolution, negotiating the perils and threats to survival from the Natural World faded in comparative priority to negotiating the threats of these newer Social World challenges. Internecine clan clashes did not entirely disappear, of course, so peace-making is a continually unfolding and recurrently enacted dynamic ritual endeavor, endemic to and pervading the sum of human history.

Human nature is distinctively "social." At a certain stage in evolution, as Nick Humphrey notes (2002), the problem that most affected human ancestors' differential chances of reproductive success, beyond survival in relation to Nature, was competition with other people. Some key characteristics of the human social animal are:

- Self and other representational world, including a theory of mind and mutuality
- Sense of presence in the flow of conscious experience, in relation to a past and future, to encourage framing time in relation to motivated behavioral goals
- Emotional development: a repertoire for emotional skills learning, capable of civilizing the primordial tendencies to subordinate these in the interests of a common good
- Emotional and practical communication, and the narrative mythopoetic truth storytelling of mythological order and symbolic reasoning
- Instrumental ingenuity and dexterity

The human social brain refers to the application of that innate endowment in the service of instrumental social goals for meaning-making and meeting incentivized socio-biological needs: including but not limited to family tending and work. Again, interfacing, goal-setting, cooperative problem-solving, division of labor and task delegation, leadership, decision-making, and resolution of antagonisms were essential for orderly social communal living.

Negotiating the stressors of Natural and Social World challenges is the *raison d'etre* of the human condition. We are *Homo Negotiander* – the quintessential primate negotiator of the environs in pursuit of the *cumulative-joint-goal-directed-shared-accomplishment* that is civilization. Towards this end, achieving order by regulating intra-group differences about who gets what – and by providing means by which to resolve the inevitable disputes over who gets what – was made possible though reasoned rulemaking of ethical considerations and legal systems.

We may conceive law and ethics as a natural expression of innate human ethical nature, or as a mechanism to control destructive instincts and maintain social order, or as an instrument of power wielded by the state's rulers or on behalf of elite class exploitation of the less privileged. Nevertheless, the development from "primitive" to "modern" societies represents a shift in the underlying *premise* of "community" from what Ferdinand Tönnies (*Community and Society*, 2002) termed *Gemeinschaft* (community of shared values and reciprocal responsibility) to *Gesellschaft* (aggregated self-interest in rational division of labor and economic pursuit). Indeed, Emile Durkheim (1997, 2008) depicted a corresponding shift in the primary *function* of ethics and law from enforcement of binding tradition (preserving unity of values, traditions, collective conscience, and allegiance) to restitutive order-keeping and facilitating protection for such competitive enterprising activities as are necessary for the growth and development of complex modern societies.

Ethics and Law: Our Species "Exoskeleton" of Stress-Resilience

In 1936, Hans Selye (1956) coined the term "stress" in medicine to describe the non-specific response of the body to any demand for change. Selye, whose first language was not English, borrowed the concept from physics, and his analogy gained credence. He had observed a set of general bodily reactions to stress among animals. Animals subjected to acute but different noxious physical and emotional stimuli, (blaring light, deafening noise, extremes of heat or cold, perceptual frustration), exhibited pathological changes. These included stomach ulcerations, shrinkage of lymphoid tissue, adrenal enlargement, and other physiological responses that cumulatively over time seemed debilitating and, in some cases of chronic persistence, causal in such diseases as heart attack, stroke, kidney disease, and rheumatoid arthritis. Selye's work inspired an entire field of stress management involving improved habits of healthy living and coping skills to foster physical and emotional well-being, sometimes referred to as "resilience," also a term borrowed from physics.

Today, the common dictionary definition of "resilience" is: (1) the ability to recover quickly from illness, change, or misfortune; buoyancy; and (2) the property of a material that enables it to resume its original shape or position after being bent, stretched, or compressed. Elasticity (Morris 1978). Selye recognized the body of the individual human organism as a self-regulating mechanism to restore natural rhythmic functioning and to deploy innate adaptive mechanisms for either avoidance of, or for resilience to, stress. The body routinely senses and monitors external signals (changing seasons, length of daylight hours, weather conditions, perceived environmental dangers, etc.); as well as its own internal biological non-normative data on arousal and alarm (pulse, breathing, sweating, swelling, proprioceptive feedback from facial and bodily musculature emotional expression, headaches and other somatic pain or soreness); and other indicators of organ dysfunction and distress (circadian rhythm sleepiness, appetite, body temperature, etc.).

One can then conceive culture metaphorically as an "exoskeleton" of the collective human micro-consciousness, projected outward to deal with the stress of this ever-expanding, ever-changing macro-system that we, as humans, inhabit. Speaking metaphorically, the exoskeleton of culture is like an erected invisible grid of shared understanding and common ways of relating behavior with a unified

Darwinian purpose: viz, to continuously moderate stress. Ethical reasoning, legal guidelines, and decision-making apparatus are a part of the cultural quilt, fostering sufficient prosocial collaboration; that is to say, a social environ conducive to collaborative societal living.

The Ethicolegal Exoskeleton: Defy the Gods

The exoskeleton of culture is a unique human capacity among the living species on Earth because only *Homo Negotiander* has evolved the cortical and subcortical apparatus and neurotransmitter systems permitting the form of intelligence that encompasses all of the requisite dimensions. These include:

- Awareness of self in relation to other, the basis for a coherent sense of identity over time
- Sense of mortality and understanding of finitude of existence
- Visual mapping, symbolization, and symbolic reasoning
- Metaphorical thinking and transformational cognition
- Emotional intelligence of embodied consciousness
- Attentional focus, ability to recall past states and plan future states of embodied consciousness
- Opposing thumb for grasping objects, instinctual urge for creative playfulness and sustained task sequencing
- Capability for verbal labeling categorization; verbal and analogical memory storage, retention and retrieval; grammatical deep structure and syntactical linguistic operations; speaker vocalization and listener auditory apparatus for oral speech communication, and so forth.

Exoskeletal culture is the means of orienting oneself to a coherent identity, and in relation to our human companions similarly situated present, past, and future, in the vast Universe of other life forms and non-living matter. In effect, it is also an assertion against Fate, the factors beyond human control. All aspects of the cultural exoskeleton embody this defiant cosmology: the ornamentalist embellishments glorifying human identity in jewelry, fashion, art, architecture and aesthetics; the myriad engineering marvels of human task ingenuity; meaning-making cultural narratives, including what we mean by religion, the civic polity, our acquisitive strivings (wealth, health, satisfaction), and ethics and law.

Apprehending an exoskeletal ethics and law is an aspect of the ordering device for understanding and experiencing our choices as informed. It is intrinsic to the nature of human attention and intelligence, which itself creates a perceived order in the chaos of bombarding sensory perceptions for the purpose of action on the world, felt as informed and deliberate – as opposed to dumb animal blind. Law and ethics comprise part of the systematized stress-resilience lubrication for smoother social operations. A common culture indeed provides a sort of global positioning system measuring stick, an apparatus that provides each individual a framework to locate himself vis-à-vis the contextual social environs and threats of deviance. It also provides a collective frame of reference for a particular linguistic community's discourse, the cultural language vocabulary in furtherance of the "familial" or "tribal" project of ongoing regular transmission of shared values and expectations. As the folk saying goes, "it takes a village…" to produce, to preserve and to provide well-being and health.

How Does Our Ethicolegal System Reduce Stress and Promote Health?

What Is Health?

For this question, let us look at Shweder's (2008) enumeration of the prismatic factoring of the modern English speaker's presumptions about health. Among some of the parsed variations:

1. *Health as Energy Potential*: impaired health (illness, sickness, disabling condition) referring to a low state or a loss of energy reserve and potential.
2. *Health as Absence of Conscious Distress*: impaired health is whenever distress in bodily function intrudes into conscious awareness of symptoms such as aches, pain, fever, heart palpitations, effortful functioning, and so forth.
3. *Health as Ability to Perform Daily Activities*: impaired health is a disruption in the ability to carry on with enjoyment the ordinary functions, duties, and activities of everyday life. Shweder suggests this may reflect a value of autonomy, in that the concrete meaning of impaired health denotes use of (i.e., dependence on) drugs, technologies, prosthetic devices (e.g., eyeglasses, insulin injections), special assistants or health aides and caretakers.
4. *Health as Not Meeting an Objective Measure of Fitness or Performance*: impaired or suboptimal health means having high body mass index, large waistline for gender height and age, etc., or inability to run a specified distance or perform callisthenic repetitions within a certain period of time. Shweder suggests health might also be viewed as an Absence of Statistical Risk Factors: impaired health would be indulging behavioral health habits which are statistically highly correlated with future diseases or suffering, e.g., obesity, cigarette smoking, limited physical exercise.
5. *Health as Good Diet or Food Intake*: you are what you eat, so poor health is a reflection of a high fat and high cholesterol diet or vitamin-deficient nutrition.
6. *Health as Genetic Hardiness*: unhealthiness reflects poor genetic stock history in resistance to threats to survive and thrive (perceived vulnerable immunological system to thwart germs, viruses, based on family disease history and longevity).
7. *Health as Freedom from Disease*: unhealthiness is a state of contamination or pollution of psyche, soma, or environs by destructive forces (germs, negative emotions, bad thoughts).
8. *Health as Balance among Countervailing Factors*: impaired health is an imbalance among some array of toxins and beneficial factors, so that sustaining equilibrium is fragile and susceptible to disruption or loss by physical or mental trauma.
9. *Health as Balanced Emotional Control and Self-Regulation*: illness is dysfunction in normal and dignified core manner of interaction and right conduct.

In this chapter, we refer primarily to *Societal Health*. Accordingly, and for the duration of our discussion, we speak in line with the latter two presumptions; that is, with *Health* as well-regulated balance, within and among the countervailing forces of which we are all a part. We believe that our species exoskeleton – our projections outward of our accumulated inner wisdom on how to achieve the *Health* of systems replete with countervailing forces – may be applied at any and every level of our existence, from the physiological to the global, and everything in between and beyond. Against this backdrop, we are ready to survey how the ethicolegal exoskeleton reduces stress and promotes health, by examining two fundamental, species shaping, areas in which we humans spend enormous portions of our lives, as we traverse our life spans – *Family* and *Work*.

Family Matters

The family is the pivotal institution for preparing and supporting most people around many predictable life stresses. No human can reach adulthood without social care and nurturance. For most people the family is the earliest and primary provider of this care and prepares the child for life's hard knocks: imposing conformity; enforcing parental discipline; moderating sibling rivalry; teaching values; imbuing respect and aspirational goals; forging practical skills for assertiveness (e.g., against bullying) and coping (e.g., humor); adjusting to change and loss (e.g., leaving home, grieving death).

Because the family always has been and continues to be such a central institution to human life transitions, family law is in many ways the foundational ethicolegal exoskeleton of societal health. With, and within it, came:

- The formation of mating bonds and obligations (to get married)
- Issues arising before, during, and after the bond relationship:
  - Gender politics of authority, including pragmatic concerns, support, and inter-spousal violence; proprietary sexuality, surrogacy, and adultery
  - Child parentage and illegitimacy; parent–child prerogatives and responsibilities; such as care, support and neglect; child discipline and abuse; filial piety; emancipation; and disownership
  - Extended family obligations; family mergers (e.g., dowry and bride price); family alterations and blending (e.g., adoption, stepfamilial bonds)
  - Family dissolution (e.g., divorce, spousal abandonment, spousal death) and post-familial rights and obligations (e.g., custody and visitation with children; child support; alimony; marital assets division)
  - Wealth transfers, gifts, bequests, and inheritances

The family has special deference. Indeed, the ancient Hebrews began the biblical tales with stories about family life; such as, how male and female mates handle joint decision-making and responsibility (Adam and Eve with the apple) and the meaning of brotherly bonds (Cain and Abel). To wit, "The Ten Commandments" is half devoted to respect for family and those cared about in the Clan Tribe (honor father and mother, do not commit adultery, do not covet nor envy, do not lie nor bear false witness, do not steal, do not inflict murderous harm). In a manner of speaking, especially among the intimate relationships of family, secular law has very much tended to defer to the prior superior territorial claim of ecclesiastical law.

We will address the iatrogenic hazards of what has become our current ethicolegal system later in our discussion. For here and now, by virtue of our being here to discuss any of this at all, it can be said that there had to have been important ways in which our ethicolegal system has reduced stress and promoted societal health.

Work Matters

All of civilization derives from the quintessential human capacity to plan, organize, and perform meaningful productive activity. A few species of domesticated animals have been trained (by humans) as beasts of burden to perform tasks. There are innumerable species of animals, and plants for that matter, which respond to favorable environmental conditions to adapt to the opportunities (e.g., sunlight, water, nutrients, gases of a certain composition in the atmosphere, range of temperatures, etc.). Thus, they forge suitable "habitats" to sustain life, to grow and reproduce, although those are mechanical processes rather than intelligent and consciously planned.

Some higher evolved species of mammals, reptiles, birds, and amphibians, share with humans an inborn instinctual behavioral repertoire or perhaps even something akin to at least a rudimentary human-like intelligence. They can build nests and dams, burrow and tunnel caverns and mazes, exude cocoons, or otherwise construct shelter. They can hunt prey, scavenge carcasses, peel and skin fruits, dig roots, and prepare food. Again, these are largely improvisational skills with limited range of flexible creativity in implementation and only limited future plans, perhaps hiding a cache of nuts for the next season or burying some prize in a known location for a few months or even years, but not a long span of the animal's life. Even the astoundingly impressive technical achievement and physical endurance in migrations of huge flocks, herds, and schools of animals appears to us as simply an imprinted repetitively patterned and programmed instinct.

But for humans, goal-directed instrumental behavior, executed with effort, constitutes our most extensive waking activity. According to the Garden of Eden legend, work was a penalty for disobeying God and failing to be satisfied with paradise without effort, with only the Sabbath day reprieve. As with the challenges of family life, the workplace originated virtually simultaneously with Adam, Eve and their offspring, as Cain planted crops and Abel herded sheep. Interestingly, like the family, so too the workplace was apparently a province of such felt paramount primordial significance that it had been largely left outside the province of legal regulation until the last couple of centuries.

As Camus wryly put it, "Without work, all life goes rotten. But when work is soulless, life stifles and dies." Work may take place within or outside of the home; whether home tending, schooling, or financially compensated activity. The workplace, like the family, is therefore a pivotal institution for preparing and supporting most people around many predictable life stresses, and assuming the worker role is one of the most important indicia of adult responsibility.

All is well and good, except when things are not. As before, when we were few, we could rely on our kinship ties to keep us in line and help us along. But as we grew larger and larger, and not everyone was anymore related to everyone else, these more complex social organizations required explicit and objective formal rules and ethical norms. Not without penalty, however, as we are ready to observe. That is, unfortunately, even if unwittingly, sometimes our ethicolegal exoskeleton of rules and regulations, which we erect and project to reduce stress and promote health, instead promotes iatrogenic stress that impairs health, however well we meant for it to serve us all along. Our solutions can create the very problems we mean for them to solve.

Part Two: Institutionalizing Law and Ethics for Stresses of Modern Life

Global Challenges of Law and Ethics in Modern Societies

The forces of modernization are creating novel challenges in law and ethics for our globalizing world, far removed from the mundane concrete daily tasks in ancient, or even contemporary third world, clan tribes. The habitat and terrain for Modern Man is enormous and the considerations are far too numerous and complex for us to "do justice" in succinctly summarizing here. However, we can glimpse the flavor of pervasive challenges through a brief overview in what arguably are the four fundamental domains for most people's ordinary waking experience, viz., family, work, health, and aging.

Family and Community

In the clan tribe, the family was the crucible for all that we humans acquired to prepare us for roles in the community and world beyond. Today, the family, while still perhaps the single most important transmitter of cultural knowledge and skills, nevertheless now clearly shares this role, and is no longer insulated from broader societal influence and expectations. Four key realms of law and ethics now moderate and regulate the meaning and influence of family in relation to children assuming adult identities and responsibilities. We will survey these developments in the United States, which is representative of the trends across modern Western societies, and now becoming the norm for an emergent truly global "world culture of modernity."

Media and Consumerism: Perhaps the best way to frame the altered functions is to highlight the extraordinary permeability of family boundaries today. No child today lives in a family as an island. Almost everything provided to the child, save mother's milk if nursed for some period, is produced outside the home and acquired according to tastes and preferences instilled by the barrage of consumerist marketing of food, goods, and parenting information. Indeed, children themselves are introduced early to media influences packaged in television, radio, music, games and toys, computers, and print publications in direct advertising and in tacit and portrayed fashion and values.

While largely unbridled except by mores and public morality until the most recent decades, now there is considerable attention to these "outside" influences in the form of legal and ethical strictures. Of course, the very access of the family to water, electricity, telephone, TV and so forth is a reflection of public utilities laws and services subject to Federal and State regulation and even pricing controls. Likewise, the family feels the far-reaching impact of the entire field of taxation (income, estate, gift, and sales taxes), bankruptcy, and consumer protection laws dealing with credit, product safety, and service contracts. Banking, insurance, and credit laws create the opportunities for mortgages, credit cards, college and home improvement loans, automobiles and access to consumer appliances and products (as well as vacation homes and travel industries), along with bill collector regulation, debt consolidation and credit reporting, and consumer borrowing.

Varieties of laws at both the federal or state levels regulate consumer affairs. Among them are the Federal Fair Debt Collection Practices Act and the Fair Credit Reporting Act, Truth in Lending Act, Fair Credit Billing Act, and the Financial Services Modernization Act opening up competition among banks, securities companies, and the insurance industry. The Federal Trade Commission and the U.S. Department of Justice mainly enforce federal consumer protection laws. Many States have a Department of Consumer Affairs devoted to regulating certain industries and protecting consumers who use goods and services from those industries, and to licensing professions whose practitioners provide services. States also encourage consumers to police through consumer legal remedies acts and the Courts which enforce tort litigation, including product and professional liability, as well as whistle-blower statutes for reporting wrongdoing.

Childhood and the household conditions for raising them are subject to quality controls, such as through the Consumer Product Safety Commission, which monitors and regulates standards for every household item, garden and automotive equipment, and child toys, as well as car seats, baby strollers, bicycle helmets, and playground equipment. Manufacturers of wearing apparel, products and equipment have themselves created standards, too, in addition to the monitoring by government agencies and consumer advocacy groups of everything from lead toxicity levels to breakage cutting injury and swallowing potential.

Political and religious groups also attempt to steer the child's environment. Movies, CD audio recordings, and videogames are rated for graphic sexual and violent themes and content. Radio and TV broadcasting is restricted, the internet can be filtered, and laws and distribution standards for pornography are intended to control access to products as well as exploitation of minors. Contraceptives and sex education, even aside from the abortion debate, are fiercely debated in public dialogue. Nutritional value content labeling of foods, requirements and practices for universal vaccination against infectious diseases, maternal prenatal and child health programs, and advocacy group campaigns bombard parents with information and warnings. Laws attempt to restrict access by minors to alcohol, cigarette and firearms purchase and illicit drug distribution. But the fashion industry; manufacturers of clothing, snacks, and cosmetics; purveyors of fast food and entertainment, and their advertising industries; also deliberately subvert some messages in the interest of boosting sales because children are a major consumer market along with parents who may be purchasers on their behalf.

Needless to say, consumerism and the McLuhan Media Age have fundamentally transformed the role of the family and its insularity from societal influence (2005). This moderates certain stress for transitioning to adulthood by establishing formal and informal enforcement of homogenized experience, but also creates powerful reciprocal stress on individuals and intrafamilial relationships by exposing and empowering children to define their own appetites and agendas, and to find access beyond the control of parents.

Education: Compulsory school attendance and provision of education at public expense has also transformed the family's role as a vehicle for value and skills transmission, although in recent years a movement toward charter schools and home schooling has supplemented parochial education systems to give parents more choices about the modalities. Certification of approved curricula, along with teacher's credentials and union-negotiated contracts for rates of pay and working conditions, have standardized much of what is transmitted and theories as to how best to accomplish that. Educational testing is an industry mediating access to funding school programs, degrees for completion and graduation, and access to higher education opportunities. After Horace Mann became the first Secretary of the Board of Education in Massachusetts, public education grew to universal proportions. Today State Departments of Education, local school system districts and school boards are key regulators of formal schooling for children at the elementary and secondary level, while public and private colleges and universities have separate accreditation and affiliation organizations, along with technical and vocational skilled training.

Furthermore, racial segregation by law was dismantled after the 1954 U.S. Supreme Court decision in *Brown v. Board of Education* fundamentally redefined rights and expectations and even the notion of neighborhood schools. The GI Bill after World War II vastly enhanced social equalization of access to higher education. Now the multi-cultural diversification of the population and the ethic of the civil rights movement legacies of equal opportunity and affirmative action present new challenges, but also vastly modify the role and influence of the family in exposure of new generations to ideas and experiences. Federal Title IX and Disabled Persons legislation has transformed access of the handicapped to facilities, and the funding of athletic programs for boys and girls. The need for Head Start and other preschool daycare services, both for preparatory and remediative child learning and socialization, and for childcare in families where parents work outside the home, has reconfigured the exclusivity of primarily parent-provided oversight. Furthermore, children of all ages have many more extracurricular activities and involvements outside the household, which augments the importance of peer and extrafamilial external adult influences.

Domestic Conflict and Its Resolution: The family was once practically a bastion of exclusive parental prerogative in childrearing and discipline. Parental discretion was largely unchallenged and unmonitored. But child welfare legislation and public agency concerns about child abuse and neglect have entirely reapportioned the equation between relative power balance between society and family decision-making in relation to the care protection of children. Especially in the last 30 years, mandatory reporting laws for healthcare professionals, teachers, and police have heightened attention to evidence of child abuse and neglect, with corollary new intervention mechanisms for removing and placing children from the family of origin into other venues. Gender politics and the combined effects of the Women's Movement and the sexual revolution spawned by the Pill and access to abortion have also empowered women to make a wider range of life choices, which inevitably has shifted the paradigms for childcare formats and the protections against spousal emotional and physical abuse.

Family Living Arrangements, Patterns and Access to Life Benefits: The institution of marriage has changed. Cohabitation arrangements are more varied than during the first half of the twentieth century, including arrangements outside the legal obligations and benefits of matrimony. Recently, matrimony and civil union laws have modified the typical institutional parameters further by making legal in some places same sex legal commitments with similar implications. Patterns of adoption, new fertilization technologies, the divorce rate and remarriage, and new role opportunities, have also transformed the landscape of the typically sixteenth to seventeenth century European model bourgeois family structure and gender roles, both in the household and in outside workplaces. Stepfamilies and other blended family arrangements, as well as grandparent and other extended family childrearing arrangements have diversified the childhood experiential framework for more children, which is transmitted among and between child peer cohorts and in television and movie depictions.

Along with this, have come changes in child support obligations and enforcement through computerized databases that permit tracking for taxation, employer reporting, drivers' licenses, and many other information sources. Families have access to investment options in the stock and bonds markets and through pension and retirement savings plans not known before, as well as government-sponsored Social Security and Medicare/ Medicaid. The institutions of alimony and dowry, marital assets division, and other marital dissolution arrangements have been shifting along with these pattern changes. Likewise, an industry of domestic relations courts, lawyers, and helping professionals now pervade custody, visitation, and other parenting plan arrangements in the aftermath of family dissolution. Transportation and communication changes, fostering increased geographic mobility around the world have created new challenges and opportunities in post-divorce parent–child relationships, as well as new dangers addressed by the laws in reference to parental kidnapping or restricting access through restraining orders.

Wealth and investments have also created new forms for wealth protection and transfer through estates and trusts tax planning and inheritance laws.

Work, Meaningful Life Activity and Economy

For ancients, life transition stresses concerning work and livelihood were also tied more closely to the productive activity, environmental conditions and available resources at immediate disposal to eke out subsistence or to prosper by comparison to others similarly situated in the clan tribe. Here again, in this life domain, Modern Man encounters a vast arena of altogether new and more complex legal and ethical ramifications. We can briefly summarize three facets of such categories of concern.

Occupational Opportunities: The Industrial Age brought to fruition a wholesale completely transformed scenario for scale and fundamental relationship between life activities and experience concerning productive activity. Karl Marx grasped the dilemma that Modern Man more than ever before faced profound new-felt connection between expenditure of effort and the derivative rewards in both satisfaction and material well-being. Of course, ever since the ancients advanced beyond primitive hunting and gathering activities for mere survival, new industries have emerged. Herding, farming, craft manufacture, construction, military, and transport for commerce heralded never before conceived of social class distinctions, property and wealth accumulation, and possibilities for socio-economic mobility, depending on the particular society's value structure and avenues for entrepreneurship and enterprise under legal protections and political influence. But the advent of powerful new mechanical and energy technologies and machinery created proliferating economic opportunities in new work roles and employment.

The legal system embraced the needs of encouraging and protecting invention, resource exploitation, entrepreneurial activity, marketplace exchange, and capitalization for expanding industrial economies. The specialization and movement of labor in relation to rapidly diversifying and proliferating occupational and trade roles created new opportunity-associated stressors. Unlike agricultural communities, from feudal reciprocal obligations to private ownership family farming and livestock, and unlike small scale and often cottage industry apprenticed crafts and artisan small retail and trade establishments and bazaars, more often work did not take place in a familial firm environment but rather in a competitive employment context, spawning challenges for nascent labor organizing around wages, hours, and benefits. The relationship between worker and benefactor was formal and impersonal, and the gratifications were more monetarized than sentimentally based.

The workday and workplace was totally divorced from the private lives and activities in the home. Extended family structures were more often distant rather than locally available for immediate support and caretaking, and mass transportation and communication opened geographic dispersion within a lifetime to take greater advantage of emergent opportunities and training.

Working Conditions and Benefits: The changes established modern labor law, employment law, and regulation of workplace conditions. Enter the right to organize and the union movement for collective bargaining in the National Labor Relations Board (NLRB), job actions and leverage of strike, the standard 5 day workweek and 8 h workday, minimum wage law (Fair Labor Standards Act), overtime pay and pay for holidays, sickness and vacations, family sickness benefits in the Family Medical and Leave Act (FMLA), restrictions on child labor, and rights and accommodations for the handicapped in the Americans with Disabilities Act (ADA). The employment contract also became subject to various protections against discrimination in hiring and promotions, unfair labor practices and dismissals, and regulation of protection for employee benefits, such as the Employment Retirement Income Security Act (ERISA), portability of health coverage under the Health Insurance Portability and Accountability Act (HIPAA), the continuation of group health benefits under the Consolidated Omnibus Budget Reconciliation Act (COBRA).

In effect, these are stress-coping mechanisms of the legal system to facilitate economic growth while affording societal protections for individuals.

Economic Forces and Protections: Modern economies create pressures and vulnerabilities due to overall economic activity and prosperity which register on individuals and magnify other life stressors, too. Some of these stresses and the corresponding stress-moderators are individual life transitions, such as choosing to change jobs or being terminated for cause or simply due to industry economic conditions. Workmen's Compensation and State unemployment insurance acts provide benefits in the case of industrial accidents and job loss. The stress of being discriminated against in job seeking has been addressed though Equal Employment Opportunity Commission (EEOC) laws and affirmative action or even race quotas to redress minority and ethnic barriers to entry and unfair treatment on the job or in dismissals. Federal and State laws also address harassment on the job based on race, color, religion, pregnancy, gender, ethnicity, age sexual orientation, marital status, and medical conditions and disability.

Health and Well-Being
Fitness and survival had to be the preoccupation of all in subsistence economies. In contemporary societies, modern medical knowledge and public health movement initiatives combine to raise the expectations for healthful living conditions, the accessibility of healthcare for treatment of illnesses and injuries, and for the promotion of fitness and healthy living. Indeed, in the United States, healthcare expenditures paid to healthcare professionals, hospitals

and healthcare facilities, nursing homes, ambulances, diagnostic laboratories, pharmacies, and medical equipment manufacturers constitute well over 15% of Gross Domestic Product. In recent years, this sector of the economy has consistently outpaced inflation. Employers provide private health insurance as a major job-related benefit to improve the fitness of their labor force, and to protect workers and their family dependents against the devastating stress of incidental routine and unexpected or even catastrophic extraordinary health conditions.

The general protection for citizens against the stresses of health problems is actually an intricate fabricate of laws. The original sanitation and public health concerns became a focus of State and local laws and inspections concerning quarantine of disease, safe water supply, indoor plumbing and sewage disposal, garbage and trash collection, control of epidemic diseases, farm and butchery/fishery handling and transport, food and beverage plant bottling, canning, and manufacturing and processing safeguards, food storage distribution and preparation in groceries and restaurants, household and tenancy filth-free living conditions, and inspected building permitting and construction.

Additionally widespread and extensive were public vaccination and public school health programs. Today the Center for Disease Control and Prevention (CDC) tracks epidemiological trends and promotes health awareness. The Occupational Safety and Health Administration (OSHA) in the U.S. Department of Labor sets and enforces safety and workplace condition standards and measures compliance. Fire, electrical, and building and life safety conditions are regulated by local authorities and agencies. The National Fire Protection Association (NFPA) published codes that have standardized sprinkling and fire extinguishing systems and products. Local career and volunteer fire departments and wildlife firefighters address emergency conditions and rescue operations.

Aging and Spiritual Legacy
The advent of universal coverage for living expenses in retirement was the main objective of Social Security (Old Age Survivors and Disability Insurance) for retired elders and Supplemental Security Income (SSI) programs for aged and disabled. These benefits often need to be supplemented from private savings and investment portfolios. People on fixed incomes are especially vulnerable to economic fluctuations and stock market values. The private life insurance industry began around 1760 in the United States and expanded enormously after the Civil War, so that it is now commonplace, and so are accidental death and dismemberment policies and travel insurance. These provide some sense of security to aging family members against the anxiety and worry stress concerning provisions for their loved ones in case of death.

In addition to employer-provided or individually purchased private pension and retirement plans, under expansions of the Social Security laws, Medicare is a United States hospital and medical care coverage insurance program for people aged 65 and older or who meet other special criteria. Medicaid is the largest source of funding of medical and health-related services for people with limited resources. Complex tax laws govern wealth preservation and transfers across generations, with specialized trust and estate lawyers and financial planners comprising a major industry to address elder's security and legacies. Nursing homes, rest homes, and assisted living programs provide residential care suited to special needs in declining years.

Part Three: Problems from Law and Ethics for Modern Stress

How Does Our Ethicolegal System Fail in Reducing Stress and Promoting Health?: Modern Challenges in Ethicolegal Goals

Civilization emerged because the fertility of land between the Tigris and Euphrates Rivers produced a surplus of food that allowed people to settle in one place. The development of irrigation techniques for the seasonal unpredictability and the relatively less moist regions of Mesopotamia fostered even larger and more complex communities, with corresponding implications for the view of humans in the world:

> Mesopotamian men and women viewed themselves as subservient to the gods and believed humans were at the mercy of the god's arbitrary decisions. To counter their insecurity, the Mesopotamians not only developed the arts of divination in order to understand the wishes of their gods, but also relieved some anxiety by establishing codes that regulated their relationships with one another. These law codes became an integral part of Mesopotamian society…(fl.18th century B.C.) (Kreis 2000, p. 5)

Disparities arose because, for example, wealth accumulation depended on how close to the river, and thereby how fertile, one's farm would be.

> At the same time, the construction of canals, ditches and dikes essential to irrigation demanded cooperation between different social groups. Decision-making, regulation and control of all food production and herding meant cooperation. (Kreis 2000, p. 3)

Humans created law not only to relieve the stress associated with producing for survival and security – the stress associated with being unable to control the uncontrollable provisions of God and Nature – but as well to relieve the stress inherent in our relations with one another. Humans created law to keep things fair. We, as a species, care very much about fairness (Wallace et al. 2007; Chiang 2008). We also seek affirmation, standing in the community that tells the world that we are good (Suzuki and Akiyama 2008; Sommerfeld et al. 2008).

Modern societies present even more complex challenges to basic aspirational needs and in fairness to get along, as evidenced by the brief overview in Part Two of ethicolegal institutionalized devices responsive to these fundamental concerns. But for its apparent complexity, twenty-first century societies still essentially respond simply to the same fundamental concerns as the ancients, utilizing the apparatus of contemporary ethicolegal institutions. Often the responses look deceptively different but are fundamentally equivalent in terms of needs served, and yet the specific ethical and legal techniques and their associated problems of course address the more complex intricacies inherent in modern versions of the stressors. As a result, it frequently seems as if the evolved institutional solutions actually iatrogenically create and exacerbate the very stressors we seek to reduce, thereby failing to promote enhanced net health.

A good example of the modern dilemma, possibly even the most emblematic, is the vexing aftermath of divorce and planning for the rest of life, because it is a life transition stressor situated so pivotally at the intersecting fulcrum of family, the production of assets and their reasonable allocation according to personal needs, the childrearing and available institutions of learning for children, security of health and well-being, and concerns for descendants and legacy for posterity. Divorce is widely perceived as failure. Something bad has happened and people will spend a lot of energy and money to make sure that as many people as possible know that they are good – that it was not their fault. Standing in the community was all along how we made sure that we got fed. Having the judge (and the kids, their teachers, your friends, the butcher, the baker and the postman…) rule in "your favor" on the question of right and fault may feel important for some, no matter how great the financial and emotional cost and stress to ourselves and the people we love.

But how good does anyone really look in the heat of a protracted divorce battle anyway? And how fair is it that people's lives and resources are subsumed to the extent that they are by this process meant to help people along? The obligation to provide properly dates back to the ancients, where even in the Code of Hammurabi it was decreed:

If a man wish to separate from a woman who has borne him children, or from his wife who has borne him children: then he shall give that wife her dowry, and a part of the usufruct of field, garden, and property, so that she can rear her children. When she has brought up her children, a portion of all that is given to the children, equal as that of one son, shall be given to her. She may then marry the man of her heart (Hooker 1996)

Wouldn't we all be better off if we could somehow reduce that $33.3 billion spent annually in the U.S. on divorce and its direct consequences (Schramm, 2006). That way there could be more to spend on groceries or whatever else is needed by a divorcing family – talk about making sure people get fed. As it is, what is meant to solve X (the emotional and financial depletion of divorce) does much to cause X for our very reliance on it – "it" being our brainchild, the ethicolegal exoskeleton of the life span transition that is divorce. Likewise, in the workplace. For an example of iatrogenic stress here, let us look at another kind of life span departure or transition; namely, retirement.

Things Have Changed

A virtually toothless 1.77 million year old early *Homo* skull has been found in the small town of Dmanisi in the former Soviet republic of Georgia. This elderly 40 year old (a very old man for those times) must have been given the choicest of soft foods for him to have survived for some number of years with only one tooth in his head. These foods could have included "brain, marrow and succulent berries" (Lordkipanidze et al. 2005). Researchers are wondering whether the community was just being kind or whether he may have received preferential treatment for some non-physical contribution he was able to make, wisdom perhaps.

Things have changed since the days when people worked on the land until they couldn't anymore, at which point families and communities took over their care until death did them part. For one thing, 78.1 is the new 40 for longevity (National Center for Health Statistics 2006). For another, with the Industrial Revolution people left the land for new kinds of employment, calling for new kinds of security than were ever needed before. The 1874 American Express railroad's pension plan was the first in the U.S., resulting in pension plans to follow across an array of industries throughout our nation. However:

...only a small proportion of the employees ever received benefits under these plans. The pension plans had a number of serious defects. They generally paid inadequate benefits and had limited provisions for disability retirement. Credits could not be transferred freely from employer to employer, and the employers could terminate the plans at will. With few exceptions, the plans were inadequately financed and could not withstand even temporary difficulties. The Great Depression of the early 1930's led to movements for retirement plans on a national basis because few of the nation's elderly were covered under any type of retirement plan (*Railroad Retirement Handbook* 2006)

Enter the Social Security Act of 1935, the first national security program in the United States, including but not limited to help for the aged. In the words of Frank Bane, Executive Director of the original Social Security Board on December 10, 1936:

It is designed to protect childhood, to provide for the handicapped, to safeguard the public health, to break the impact of unemployment, and to establish a systematic defense against dependency in old age.... the initial steps completed during this past week, will go into action January 1, with about 26,000,000 workers qualifying for old age protection as a matter of right... (Social Security Online, 1936/2008)

Did he say *matter of right?* How deftly we humans move from the matter of need to the matter of right and, in so doing, render what was meant to solve X a cause of X all over again. How much stress is reduced and how much societal health created by Warren Buffett exercising his right to his social security check. According to Buffet himself:

I get a check for $1,700 to $1,900 or something every month. I'm 74. And I cash it. But I'll eat without it (Dobbs 2005)

Or something? Buffett cashes the check without even knowing how much, because it does not matter how much. He will eat anyway. Buffett is exercising what has become his right, entirely devoid of the need that gave social security its start... the need of children, the handicapped, the unemployed, and the elderly unable to take care of themselves. Again, the solution creates the problem, because the system is out of balance. And, if things continue as they are, Social Security, an ethicolegal exoskeletal feature designed to meet need, now threatens to fail the very need that it was meant to serve, when the funds run dry. Buffett suggests there are answers: "...I would means test" (2005). Maybe the rich should pay higher social security taxes than they do; still Buffett's check gets cashed along with millions of others – with no demonstrated need.

Form Follows Function

What are we thinking? Whose failure is this? If there is a failure to be had, maybe that failure is our own, our own failure to remember that form follows function, as famed American architect Louis Sullivan has said. Sullivan was inspired by such naturalists as Charles Darwin and Ralph Waldo Emerson. Borrowing from American sculptor Horatio Greenough, also inspired by Emerson, Sullivan spoke of form and function in this way:

It is the pervading law of all things organic and inorganic, of all things physical and metaphysical, of all things human and all things superhuman, of all true manifestations of the head, of the heart, of the soul, that the life is recognizable in its expression, that form ever follows function. This is the law (Sullivan and Twombly 1896/1988, p. 111)

Even better for our purposes, Sullivan went on to say this:

…when we know and feel that Nature is our friend, not our implacable enemy ….something so deep, so true, that all the narrow formalities, hard-and-fast rules, and strangling bonds of the schools cannot stifle it in us-then it may be proclaimed that we are on the high-road to a natural and satisfying art…that will live because it will be of the people, for the people, and by the people (Sullivan and Twombly 1896/1988, p. 113)

Sullivan's art is architecture. So too is the ethicolegal exoskeleton, an architectural art of our own creation to help us to function on the best possible "high-road to a natural and satisfying" culture.

We created rules and formalities, if not strangling bonds, for fear that worse might befall us from above, beyond, and within. But we must always be mindful that we do not turn these defensive structures – which we have built with our own minds – into something potentially as false and frightening as the gods in our heads they were meant to defend us against. What, then, will it take to put the horse back in front of the cart toward a better, more naturalistic, "form follows function" approach?

Prospects for a Better Future Approach

Once upon a time, we took care of ourselves. Chimps rarely ate the sunflower plant, Aspilia. Maybe only when they were sick did chimps make long treks to get the antibiotic leaves, with edges rough enough to rough up parasites, folded neatly, not chewed as food, into their mouths and stomachs. Researchers have been collecting data for decades to support this idea that chimps know what to do to self-medicate, always did, and so did we (Sears 1990, pp. 42–44; Fowler et al. 2007). We on the savannah and we The Iceman too. The 1991 discovery of a 45-year-old body from 5,300 years ago revealed evidence for the Iceman's self-medicating ingestion of a natural antibiotic laxative, birch fungus, Piptoporus (Wilford 1998).

For mental illness, we figured out to drill holes in each other's heads, trepanation (Schizophrenia.com 2004). Believe it or not, we still do that, not only deep brain stimulation for depression, but rumors on the internet of trepanation among friends continuing to this day. Of course, pharmaceutical companies are looking into how to parlay the elements of ancient remedies into our modern day medicines. All along our way, we figured out what to do and did it with whatever was at our disposal. This about us is why we are here.

Now, with modern technological advances, in 2007 the U.S spent in excess of $2.2 trillion on health care (Berenson and Abelson 2008). Possibly, at least one-third of that amount is "waste," producing "no value" or worse (*Rand Corporation* 2006). We have our new $1 million dollar CT scanner, potentially exposing us to large enough doses of radiation to increase our risk of cancer, while never having proven itself to be any better than the "older and cheaper tests" (Berenson and Abelson 2008). And we have the cancer drug, Avastin, "with sales last year of about $3.5 billion, $2.3 billion of that in the United States"; prolonging life by "only a few months, if that"; with its own serious side effects, having not yet been proven to be as effective as the Food and Drug Administration had originally thought it was (Kolata and Pollack 2008).

The problem is not that newer treatments never work. It is that once they become available, they are often used indiscriminately, in the absence of studies to determine which patients they will benefit (Berenson and Abelson 2008)

As before, exoskeleton refers to the collective human micro-consciousness projected outward to deal with the stress of the ever-expanding, ever-changing macro-system that we inhabit. Exoskeleton is like an erected invisible grid of shared understanding and common ways of relating and behavior with a unified Darwinian purpose: viz, to regulate balance within and among countervailing forces and, in so doing, to moderate stress, an evolutionary apparatus somewhat like the psychoanalytic field of "Psychogeography" discussed by Howard Stein. The premise here is that we map or project unconscious psychic material onto the external world and then act as if what we projected belongs to the other more than to ourselves. In this way, we are able to project aggression and other unwanted parts of self onto the other, keeping our sense of goodness, completeness, and safety all to ourselves (Stein 1986).

Ernest Becker, too, detected an underlying universal motive serving a biological need:

The fact is that this is what society is and always has been: a symbolic action system, a structure of statuses and roles, customs and rules for behavior....in which people serve in order to earn a feeling of primary value...by building an edifice that reflects human value (Becker 1973, pp. 4-5)

But we caution: an edifice that reflects and is meant to protect human value, but not always does.

In contemporary society, the central issue is that the seemingly unchanging wisdom from time immemorial clashes with new realities, and continues to change and evolve to a degree or in a manner sufficient to be actually perceptible within a single lifetime, so that inherited schemes on which we rely feel dated and no longer workable. Too often, we persist in relying on them, instead of on ourselves, that is, by taking initiative to creatively fashion better options.

Returning to our earlier life transition example, once divorce looms real, the most important call that many people make is to the lawyer. People believe they are unprepared and incompetent, and that somebody out there owes them for the trouble they are in. The law is invoked, the lawyer retained, both as Stein's (1986) parental figure to take care of everything and make everything okay, and as the agent of the aggression that is projected onto the other for the bad that has occurred, in effect to make oneself good and the other blameworthy (Nisenbaum and Weiss 2007). Form follows function. The lawyer is retained to make things fair and right. But the stress associated with the legal transaction itself can often provide a paradoxical result, defeating our real needs concerning financial and emotional health and well-being, for oneself and one's children, throughout the process and on the other side of this potentially stressful life span transition.

It is suggested that this need not be the case, because there are other options. For example, collaborative divorce is a non-adversarial process, employing mediation techniques to help divorcing couples come to an agreement without litigation, but with the assistance of their respective attorneys and other relevant specialists. Divorce mediation, another alternative to more traditional adversarial divorce, employs an unbiased neutral professional (mediator) to bring the couple together to craft a mutual agreement, again with the assistance of outside legal, financial, and other specialists, as needed.

The evidence suggests that both diminished stress and substantial accrual of benefits is possible, if the case is suitable for these consumer friendly alternative dispute resolution methods. The Boston Law Collaborative analyzed 199 cases it handled and found:

...mediation had a median cost of $6,600, followed by $19,723 for collaborative divorce, $26,830 for a divorce settlement negotiated by counsel, and $77,746 for a litigated divorce (Neil, 2007)

As some have ruefully observed, it's your choice: pay for your kids' college education or pay for the kids of your lawyer to go to college? Of course, that presumes hope to reduce stress is sincere. When the primary interest of one or both parties is war at any cost, to inflict stress on the other (and probably unavoidably for oneself, as well), then the time, energy, and money spent on preliminary stress avoidance is wasted because, if so determined, they eventually wind up in court and incur further frustration and expense.

The ethicolegal exoskeleton is an evolutionary innovation to foster adaptation through stress modulation, so certainly it should be amenable to further ingenuity toward that end. No doubt in recent years, increasingly the pattern has been that first we marry and, if that does not work, then we divorce, and the courts will help us. But the players need not become helpless victims of the stress of rigid systemic exoskeletal constraints. For example, new forms have emerged essentially as remedial renovations of the exoskeleton, so that now there are self-determinative options, such as pre-nups (premarital agreements) and post-nups (agreements for partners already married).

According to John Fiske, Cambridge, Massachusetts attorney and family mediator:

People can use this process very flexibly for all kinds of purposes, to revive a marriage or steer it in a different direction....One husband gave his wife $100,000 (tax-free) to acknowledge her worth....When it came to one business in particular, the wife proposed that her husband receive more than half because he had worked extremely hard to build it up. He was so appreciative that he decided to pay her $50,000 in "marital alimony" every year on her birthday (Berfield 2007)

Practical negotiation tools, based on core human concerns, are available to traverse the life span transitions less burdened by imposed stress (Shapiro and Fisher 2005).

Similarly, with the potentially stressful life span transition that is retirement, forethought and creative ingenuity can moderate stress. The Social Security Act of 1935 was meant to protect those in need. A National Bureau of Economic Research study of 7,700 households nearing retirement found:

...over three-fourths of the respondents said they had saved too little, and virtually none said they had saved too much. Most people were worried by their minimal savings: only a quarter of them thought that 'Social Security or employer pensions would take care of my retirement income' (Varian, 2001)

It goes without saying that as the close to 80 million baby boomers leave the workforce, at some point there will be too few workers left to generate the tax revenues needed to fund the program. The purpose of the ethicolegal exoskeletons is stress-resilience lubrication for smoother social operations. For a particular linguistic community's discourse, the vocabulary in furtherance of the "familial" or "tribal" project of ongoing regular transmission of shared values and expectations is the collective frame of reference. But what if the shared values and expectations have outlived their usefulness in time?

As Ralph Waldo Emerson put it in his essay "Self-Reliance":

A man should learn to detect and watch that gleam of light which flashes across his mind from within, more than the luster of firmament of bards and sages (Ralph Waldo Emerson, 1990, p. 149)

Indeed, the ethicolegal exoskeletal structures we inherit must be revisited continually, with forethought and flexibility, in light of the stress reducing and health promoting purposes we mean them to serve. However, change must be mindful, resisting certain inborn natural tendencies that 'flash across our minds' to desire and acquire beyond our need. Early in evolution, when our brains were forming and our resources were scarce, the "drive to acquire... to seek, take, control, and retain objects and personal experiences human's value," had tremendous survival advantage, suggesting that this drive may well be an inherent part of us now (Lawrence and Nohria 2002, p. 57). We now know that the decisions we make can get made up to 10 seconds before we know that we have made them (Soon et al. 2008).

There is more to learn about which kinds of decisions get made by which parts of the brain. Even so, we already know that the brain gets enormously activated over that which it thinks it desires (Kawabata and Zeki 2008). To the extent that desires were more appropriate and necessary to an evolutionary past than they may be to our present, as we set about to review and refine the laws we live by, it is incumbent upon us to capture the emergence of our desires as they flash across our minds and reflect before we act on what we "decide." We live on what evolutionary psychologists call an "hedonic treadmill," always wanting more than we have, and so we must be watchful.

As Darwin himself opined: "The highest possible stage in moral culture is when we recognize that we ought to control our thoughts" (Charles Darwin 1874/1981, p. 123). So we conclude our discussion with these words from the venerable Justice Oliver Wendell Holmes, Jr.:

The law is the witness and external deposit of our moral life. Its history is the history of the moral development of the race....The development of our law has gone on for nearly a thousand years....most of the things we do, we do for no better reason than that our fathers have done them or that our neighbors do them....Still it is true that a body of law is more rational and more civilized when every rule it contains is referred articulately and definitely to an end which it subserves... (Holmes, Jr., 1897)

Or, in these words from the memoir *Zen and the Art of Motorcycle Maintenance*:

My personal feeling is that this is how any further improvement of the world will be done: by individuals making Quality decisions and that's all....We do need a return to individual integrity, self-reliance and old fashioned gumption. We really do. (Pirsig, 1984, p. 323)

References

Bane, F. (1936/2008). Social Security Online. http://www.ssa.gov/history/banesp.html.
Becker, E. (1973). *The denial of death*. New York: Free Press.
Berenson, A., & Abelson, R. (2008). Weighing the costs of a CT scan's look inside the heart, *The New York Times*, June 29, http://www.nytimes.com/2008/06/29/business/29scan.html?_r=1&oref=slogin.

Berfield, S. (2007). Does your marriage need a postnup? *Business Week, 16,* 2007.

Chiang, Y. (2008). A path toward fairness: Preferential association and the evolution of strategies in the Ultimatum game. *Rationality and Society, 20*(2), 173–201.

Darwin, C. (1874/1981). *The descent of man, and selection in relation to sex.* NJ: Princeton University Press, 71–72.

Dawkins, R. (1981). *The selfish gene* (p. 201). Great Britain: Oxford University Press.

de Waals, F. (1982). *Chimpanzee politics.* Baltimore: Johns Hopkins University Press.

Diamond, J. (1998). *Guns, germs and steel.* New York: Norton & Company.

Dobbs, L. (2005). Buffett: 'There are lots of loose nukes around the world'. *CNN.com,* June 19. http://www.cnn.com/2005/US/05/10/buffett/index.html, June 19.

Durkheim, E. (1997). *The division of labor in society.* New York: Free Press.

Durkheim, E. (2008). *The elementary forms of religious life.* Great Britain: Oxford University Press.

Emerson, R. W. (1990). In R. D. Richardson, Jr. (Ed.), *Ralph Waldo Emerson: Selected essays, lectures and poems.* New York: Bantam Books.

Flack, J. C., & de Waal, F. B. M. (2008). Any animal whatever: Darwinian building blocks of morality in monkeys and apes. *Journal of Consciousness Studies, 7*(1-2), 1–65.

Fowler, A., Koutsioni, Y., & Sommer, V. (2007). Leaf-swallowing in Nigerian chimpanzees: Evidence for assumed self-medication. *Primates, 48*(1), 73–76.

Gray, J. (2007). Are we moral? *New York Review of Books, 54*(8), 26–28.

Hauser, M. (2006). *Moral minds: How nature designed our universal sense of right and wrong.* New York: Harper Collins.

Holmes, O. W., Jr. (1897). The Path of Law. *Constitution Society* at http://www.constitution.org/lrev/owh/path_law.htm.

Hooker, R. (1996). *Mesopotamia: The code of Hammurabi,* http://www.wsu.edu/~dee/MESO/CODE.HTM.

Humphrey, N. (2002). *The mind made flesh: Essays from the frontiers of psychology and evolution.* Great Britain: Oxford University Press.

International Union for Conservation of Nature, *Report at XXII International Primatological Society Congress,* Edinburgh, August 5, 2008.

Johanson, D., & Edley, M. (1981). *Lucy: The beginnings of humankind.* New York: Simon & Shuster.

Kawabata, H., & Zeki, S. (2008). The neural correlates of desire. *Public Library of Science ONE, 3*(8), e3027.

King, B. (2007). *Evolving god.* New York: Doubleday.

Kolata, G., & Pollack, A. (2008). Costly cancer drug offers hope, but also a dilemma, *The New York Times,* July 6, http://www.nytimes.com/2008/07/06/health/06avastin.html?partner=rssnyt&emc=rss.

Kreis, S. (2000). The history guide: Lectures on ancient and medieval European history, *The History Guide,* http://www.historyguide.org/ancient/lecture2b.html.

Lawrence, P., & Nohria, N. (2002). *Driven: How human nature shapes our choices* (p. 57). Jossey-Bass: San Fransisco.

Lordkipanidze, D., Abesalom, V., Ferring, R., Rightmire, G., Agusti, J., Kiladze, G., et al. (2005). Anthropology: The earliest toothless hominin skull. *Nature, 434,* 717–718.

MacDonald, D. (2001). *The encyclopedia of mammals* (p. xvi). London: Brown Reference Group.

MacLean, P. D. (1990). *The triune brain in evolution: Role in paleocerebral functions.* New York: Springer.

McLuhan, M. (2005). *The medium is the message.* California: Gingko.

Morris, W. (ed). (1978). *The American heritage dictionary of the English language.* New York: Houghton Mifflin.

National Center for Health Statistics. (2006). *U.S. mortality drops sharply in 2006: Latest data show.* http://www.cdc.gov/nchs/PRESSROOM/08newsreleases/mortality2006.htm.

Neil, M. (2007). Family law: Kinder, gentler collaborative divorce also costs less. *American Bar Association Journal*, December 20, http://abajournal.com/news/kinder_gentler_collaborative_divorce_also_costs_less/.

Nisenbaum, S., & Weiss, M. (2007). The moral of the story: Who will grant the real divorce? *Family Mediation Quarterly*, 6(3), 1–8.

Panksepp, J. (1998). *Affective neuroscience: The foundation of human and animal emotion*. Great Britain: Oxford Press.

Pirsig, R. (1984). *Zen and the Art of Motorcycle Maintenance: An inquiry into values*. New Jersey: Bantam.

Railroad Retirement Handbook. (2006). Development of the Railroad Retirement System, *United States Railroad Retirement Board*, Chapter 1, http://www.rrb.gov/general/handbook/chapter1.asp.

Rand Corporation. (2006). An overview of RAND health's comprehensive assessment of reform efforts (COMPARE) initiative, *Report*, June 2, http://www.achp.org/library/download.asp?id=6679.

Rowe, C. M., Loope, D. B., Oglesby, R. J., Van der Roo, R., & Broadwater, C. E. (2007). Inconsistencies Between Pangean Reconstructions and Basic Climate Controls. *Science, 318*, 1284–1286.

Schizophrenia.com. (2004). "The History of Schizophrenia" http://www.schizophrenia.com/history.htm.

Schlain, L. (2003). *Sex, time and power*. New York: Penguin.

Schramm, D. G. (2006). Individual and social costs of divorce in Utah. *Journal of Family and Economic Issues*, 27(1), 133–151.

Sears, C. (1990). The chimpanzee's medicine chest. *New Scientist, 127*, 42–44.

Selye, H. (1956). *The stress of life*. New York: McGraw-Hill.

Shapiro, D., & Fisher, R. (2005). *Beyond reason: Using emotions as you negotiate*. New York: Penguin.

Sherman, S. M., & Guillery, R. W. (2005). *Exploring the thalamus and its role in cortical function*. Cambridge, MA: MIT Press.

Shweder, R. A. (2008). The cultural psychology of suffering: The many meanings of health in Orissa, India (and Elsewhere). *Ethos, 36*(1), 60–77, special edition by C. Mattingly and N. Lutkehaus, (Eds.), *Cultural psychology meets anthropology: Jerome Bruner and his inspiration*.

Sommerfeld, R. D., Krambeck, H., & Milinski, M. (2008). Multiple gossip statements and their effect on reputation and trustworthiness. *Proceedings of the Royal Society Biological Sciences, 275*, 2529–2536.

Soon, C., Brass, M., Heinze, H., & Haynes, J. (2008). Determinants of free decisions in the human brain. *Nature Neuroscience, 11*(5), 543–545.

Stein, H. F. (1986). The influence of psychogeography upon the conduct of international relations. *Psychoanalytic Inquiry, 6*, 193–222.

Sullivan, L., & Twombly, R. (Ed.). (1896/1988). *Louis Sullivan: The public papers*. Chicago: University of Chicago Press.

Suzuki, S., & Akiyama, E. (2008). Evolutionary stability of first-order-information indirect reciprocity in sizable groups. *Theoretical population biology, 73*(3), 426–436.

Tönnies, F. (2002). *Community and society*. New York: Dover.

Varian, H. (2001). Economic scene: For too many people, including some of the rich, Social Security is the main retirement plan. *The New York Times*. December 20.

Wallace, B., Cesarini, D., Lichtenstein, P., & Johannesson, M. (2007). Heritability of ultimatum game responder behavior. *Proceedings of the national academy of science, 104*, 15631–15634.

Wilford, J. (1998). Peek into the Iceman's prehistoric medicine cabinet, *New York Times*, December, 7, cited at http://www.newnation.org/NCR/reference/NCR-iceman.html.

Chapter 15

Money in (E)Motion Experienced in Stressful Financial Transitions

John V. Boardman

Examining the Stressors in Our Lives

The American Psychological Association (2008) reports a study that indicates one-third of Americans are living under extreme stress and nearly half of them (48%) believe that their stress has increased over the last five years. Stress is taking a toll on people – contributing to health problems, poor relationships, and lost productivity at work, according to a new national survey released by the American Psychological Association (APA). In September 2007, the American Psychological Association commissioned its annual nationwide survey to examine the state of stress across the country. The research measured attitudes and perceptions of stress among the general public, identifying the leading sources of stress, common behaviors used to manage stress, and the impact of stress on our lives. The survey explored appropriate and excessive stress levels; circumstances, situations, and life events that cause stress; activities, resources, and behaviors people use to deal with stress; and the personal costs of stress. This survey was conducted online within the United States by Harris Interactive between August 30 and September 11, 2007, among 1,848 adults (aged 18 and over). Interviews were conducted in both English and Spanish.

Based on the results obtained, family finances, money, and work continue to be the leading causes of stress for three quarters of Americans, a dramatic increase over the 59% reporting the same sources of stress in 2006. The survey also found that the housing crisis is having an effect on many, with half of the Americans (51%) citing rent or mortgage costs as sources of stress this decade.

A Model for Managing Financial Stressors

As a financial planner, everyday is spent relating to people dealing with the stressors of family finance, money, and work in transition. Newly married, a recent retiree, or taking on a new career are just a few of the many transitions encountered in today's world causing stress in our lives. In an almost scripted way, each client tends to share the attitudes, opinions, and outlooks with

From: *Handbook of Stressful Transitions Across the Lifespan,*
Edited by: T.W. Miller, DOI 10.1007/978-1-4419-0748-6_15,
© Springer Science+Business Media, LLC 2010

those who have gone through the same transitions months or years before. The attitudes and stressors related to financial transition are most often determined by two factors; one's personal history with regard to money and financial issues and the actual transition they are going through. A range of emotions exists in each transition and the list of these emotions is somewhat finite. What is not finite is the experience that a person has lived through. More often than not, the initial interview and questions are more focused on a person's financial history versus their current attitude towards the current transition they are experiencing.

A valuable model of financial planning can reduce the stressors experienced by so many individuals and families. A model for financial planning that may reduce the transitions we face and the stressors we experience involves not only working with a qualified professional, but also following a process that deals with both emotion related to current and past financial experiences as well as the hard facts related to the person's financial situation. Most initial meetings with clients happen when they are experiencing a transition. Divorce, retirement, inheritance, business sale, and remarriage are examples of transitions. If I am working with a client who is not going through a particular transition, it is most often due to the fact that they have moved a few years earlier and have not yet changed to a local advisor, or that they have had trouble with previous advisor and are actively looking for a change. Although these clients are not going through life's transition, there is a great deal of stress associated with finding someone new to entrust with your finances. One might well be hesitant to take on a client who tells of experiences with a number of advisors in the past. These stories tend to involve sub-par performance from an investment standpoint or very poor service issue in the past. As in any service industry, some clients will never be pleased with their experience. Thus, the purpose of this chapter is to address life's stressful financial transitions. While not being a psychologist or a scientist, a financial planner is a specialist and a professional who deals with people in transition each and every day. As a CERTIFIED FINANCIAL PLANNER™ practitioner, one is required to follow a highly disciplined process involving both an in-depth analysis as well as significant disclosure. In fact, the standards for this process are specifically listed as (1) establishing and defining the relationship, (2) gathering client data, (3) analyzing and evaluating the client's financial status, (4) developing and presenting the financial planning recommendations, (5) implementing the financial planning recommendations, and (6) monitoring (Certified Financial Planner Association, 2008). Through these steps, the goals of any professional planner should be to bring both enhancement and coordination to a client's financial life.

Through this chapter, the goal is to address the various financial transitions one can encounter, the varying levels of stress measured through emotion in one's clients and prospects, and the relationship between attributes of transition and the level of stress experienced by those going through that transition.

Conceptualizing a Client's Financial Life

When working with a client to create their financial plan, it is always important to establish the stage of financial life the person is in. The three stages of financial life include: accumulation, preservation, and distribution.

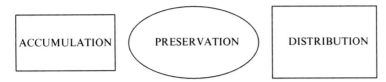

Fig. 15-1 The three stages of financial life

Although these phases occasionally overlap, most clients weigh one goal more heavily than others. The age of a client most often directly reflects the stage they are presently in, i.e., a senior who wants to distribute funds to pay a grandchild's education. However, it is important to not view these stages as mutually exclusive. A young professional is obviously accumulating, but should also recognize that the retirement cash flow implications (distribution) of income, deferral decisions, and investment risk decisions taken (preservation) will have a major impact on his/her financial future (Fig. 15-1).

Accumulation goals encompass persons' working years and investing years, pre-retirement. Accumulation is not only the act of saving for the future, but also the reinvestment of proceeds from previously invested funds. Naturally, younger clients and those still working fall in this category. Transition in a person's financial life tends to be somewhat limited in these years due to the fact that they are deepening their roots in their career. However, transitions in these years tend to be unexpected.

Unexpected financial transitions may well include the death of a family member, an unexpected divorce, an unanticipated windfall, or an inheritance. Job changes, the birth of a child, marriage, or windfall proceeds from a legal settlement fall under the group of transitions deemed to be expected. Expected is used somewhat liberally here to include planned events or those events preceded by some amount of preparatory time. The birth of a child would be the most obvious event included in this group. The difference between planned and unplanned events is very significant and tends to have a direct impact on the emotions expressed and the level of stress experienced in the transition.

The second major factor affecting financial planning is the *preservation* stage. Preservation is mostly thought of as the time when one is not actively working and is a stage when the accumulated assets can be preserved. As one would expect, these clients tend to be older than those looking for accumulation. However, preservation goals tend to be expressed by people in all stages of life. Relative level of wealth is a huge determining factor here. Those with very large sums of money in relation to their lifestyle needs tend to express preservation goals at a much younger age. For example, a 35-year old who inherits $2 million in a situation where interest from the funds supply the proceeds necessary to live, preservation is a typical goal. In contrast, a 60-year old who retires with $100,000 but needs $50,000 a year to live traditionally expresses little to no desire for preservation.

Whether it is a higher tolerance for risk or the understanding that higher returns are necessary for funds to last (more likely scenario), preservation is not an option. Wealth versus needed income tends to be the more important factor than age or career stage for this reason. Preservation goals also come along very frequently in relation to multi-generational planning related to insurance and estate planning. The stresses related to this type of planning are vast.

It is not uncommon that "planning clients" working on estate issues experience very high stress levels because it involves future personal circumstances and the financial environment the client strives to create for his or her spouse, children, or grandchildren. The planning related to preservation often happens as a result of a transition but as stated before, the age range is wide. Detailed later in the chapter are the issues related to passing money to someone else, creating a great deal of stress. The context of the client's personal life tends to most greatly affect the attitudes they maintain related to passing money on.

The third factor that a financial planner works with is in the *distribution* phase. As one would imagine this area of planning most often deals with retirees and older clients. Financial planning most often deals with clients in this phase of their financial life. The stresses are wide ranging and the context of the transition leading to this planning affects the attitude and emotion of the client. In meeting with someone who has been forced to take an early retirement, it is found that their attitudes on distribution differ greatly from someone who sells a successful business voluntarily.

The business owner tends to show higher levels of anxiety due to the fact that their previous income source was under their control. The "early retiree" who has become accustomed to some level of deferral of power over their financial future (to their manager or employing corporation) experiences a stressful life transition. The focus of discussion with planning clients on distribution issues deals with personal circumstances and prior experiences. The anxiety over the amount to withdraw each year from a portfolio is also a major planning focus. Clients are continually pulled between leaving the maximum amount in their account for growth and the counter idea of enjoying what they have earned. In most cases, regardless of circumstances, clients who have hired a financial planner will defer to the hired expert to choose the appropriate withdrawal amount. Without question, the transition from earning income to living off what has been saved is one of the more challenging and stressful times in a person's life.

The distribution phase and preservation phase can overlap in some larger clients but more often than not, a client falls definitively into one of the three categories. Some individuals strive to pass on assets or income to other generations while still living. The emotions expressed in these situations are wide ranging. We have all read of, heard of people squandering inheritance or major windfalls including lottery winnings being exhausted in short order. This notion becomes evident in the level of anxiety people have when planning their finances around their death. How early do we give to our children? Should it be in a trust? Will they stay motivated? Do I owe them anything? All of these are questions clients working on distribution planning can and should ask themselves. Very different from planning for one's own use of the funds, trying to plan to pass funds on is often times much more stressful because it deals with a release of control over the situation either to the spouse, child, or grandchild receiving the funds or to a trustee put in place to manage the funds for the survivor's benefit.

What Are Some of the Stressors Associated with Financial Transitions?

The stressors associated with financial transitions are vast as are the emotions. From my experience with clients, two factors emerge that affect the level of stress and the type of emotion expressed in financial transition.

First, knowledge of a person's prior experiences is vital in understanding a person's attitude towards money. Good or bad experiences shine through in a number of different ways, a case study in itself. For the financial planner and the parties concerned, it is important to not only know the context in which the individual is working in, but also experiences going back to childhood as they relate to money, how their parents thought about and acted with regard to money, as well as both positive and negative experiences in years past. The financial planner will occasionally sit down with someone who has experienced a good number of financial tragedies. This could include job loss, business failure, prolonged unemployment, or parents having struggled for years without? money. These clients show great amounts of stress and anxiety over any level of financial planning. Although this conservatism can work to the detriment of the clients, these prior experiences proliferate through fear in the client's attitudes towards the future resulting in a stressful transition. In working closely with a client who has experienced painful financial situations in the past, they are focusing on the here and now, they have something to clearly plan around. More often than not they are conservative but maintain an uncanny drive for further saving and accumulation.

In *How to be a Billionaire*, Martin Fridson (2005) explores the personal histories of some of the world's wealthiest titans in business history. One commonality that expressed itself was that almost every person she studied experienced some level of financial strain during his lifetime. Most often, it involved his parents, and particularly their father experiencing a business failure. Fridson (2005) suggests, "Rather than pulling themselves up by the bootstraps from poverty, they extended the successes of previous generations. To some extent, perhaps, they were motivated by memories of business reverses that their fathers suffered." He continues by stating, "For some of the great wealth gatherers, periods of financial reversal may have created an intense desire for financial security. This is a thirst that no sum of money can completely extinguish." Fridson (2005) Even if the father succeed in years and ventures to come, the memory and pain of the experience expressed itself in a relentless drive and quasi-hoarding mentality.

Fridson (2005) believes that the concept of failure to these individuals becomes a distant possibility if they spend their lives accumulating, continuing to build fortunes, and not standing still. As for example, although noting its extremity, this illustrates the attitudes around money and their deep-rooted beginnings in an individual. Conversely, the client who has had little if any financial difficulty may also experience a stressful transition.. Parents were successful, money was always available or at least not a continual struggle. Or perhaps, they never paid for furthering their own education as it was funded by scholarships or a parent.

The Zero Knowledge Factor

Regardless, this client almost always sits in front of me with little to no worry or stress over finances because of literally zero knowledge of how things sometimes do not go well. Experience suggests this to be a dangerous attitude because it creates feelings of entitlement and invincibility in a client. Younger clients, particularly early retirees, tend to fall in this category. They may be overly aggressive with their investment style and often times fail to see the value of working with a CERTIFIED FINANCIAL PLANNER™ practitioner.

For those investors and clients under age 50, it seems very few have experienced major financial difficulty during their lifetime. Real estate has consistently gone up in value, markets have quickly regained ground from downward movements, and employment has always been available. Contrast that to a client in her eighties or nineties who experienced the Great Depression as a child, World War II, and major stock market corrections. Clients who were alive and old enough at the time to remember the Great Depression, as one would expect, are the most conservative. Although their age alone justifies a very conservative approach, my conversation with these clients almost always reveals a deep-seeded sense of concern over money, particularly stretching money out to last the rest of one's life. They remember harder times and, having experienced such times, realize it could happen again. Some attribute this difference to the vast difference in what was at the time a "saver's economy" versus today's "consumption economy."

One very interesting consistency observed over time is the emotions and stress realized by clients in similar career paths. Stay at home parents, physicians, lawyers, accountants, engineers, and "blue collar" type workers seem to each maintain attitudes similar to those of their respective colleagues. Engineers, by nature, are the most detail oriented which is often expressed in pessimism over outside opinions. They tend to be the most actively involved in their finances, often times appearing in the financial planner's office with spreadsheets and detailed tracking systems to monitor investment performance.

Although a client that remains involved in their financial planning situation, this level of analysis can act as an obstacle in attempting to stay focused on long-term planning. The detailed nature of an engineer's profession expresses itself in this detailed approach of handling their finances. A physician, on the other hand, although maintaining a career in a hard science, tends to be less involved in their finances but often come to the planner's office with ideas expressed by colleagues. They tend to value using an outside expert due to the time constraints of their job and a mutual respect for professionals. The work of a physician is so involved in staying current that their opinions and ideas tend to be somewhat flawed. They also tend to be more aggressive than other professionals because of their ability to earn. An engineer making $80,000 per year can live off of the income but knows there is little room for error with investments made. As well, a surgeon making $400,000 per year tends to act more aggressively knowing they can earn themselves out of mistakes or investing miscues. This similarity may well be true with investment amounts as well.

The Role and Function of Financial Planning

Financial planners strive to work with wealthier clients. And one would assume that the wealthier clients are harder to persuade to work with you versus other advisors. The experience of this financial planner has been contradictory. Whether it is a lifetime spent using delegation to free up time or a mutual respect for other professionals, business owners and successful professionals are easier to convince of an idea over an average investor with less than $50,000 or so. The relative account size to income need seems to directly affect a client's willingness to do business. A $1 million dollar investor who needs $50,000 per year income is much easier to bring on as a client than an investor with $50,000 who needs $5,000 per year. The need for "over-performance" can paralyze a client into inaction whereas a client requiring modest returns will require less convincing.

The work of a financial planner is most difficult in troubled times. This seems obvious but what is not obvious is that it tends to be the busiest time for new clients and prospects. In 2008, we are experiencing a global financial period of flux and change. Oil is expensive and home prices are falling. The markets struggle and financial pain and stress are widespread. Existing clients want reaffirmation in their approach and prospects are questioning what the "other advisor" is recommending or has previously implemented.

An exceptionally large portion of the financial planner's time is spent with clients managing expectations. It is the expectations of investors that are a major factor in the stress experienced in "rocky" economic conditions. In initial meetings with clients, it is essential that both clients and planners are on the same page in regards to "performance expectations" and overall goals. Many financial advisors will speak of higher returns to attract a client, only to spend future weeks and months convincing them that things will change. A client with unmanageable goals and expectations will experience a much higher level of stress than someone who understands, or more importantly has been taught what to expect. Markets are variable and unpredictable and it is essential to convince clients that we invest the way we do because we cannot predict what will happen.

A competent financial planner prepares for the unexpected. In a world filled with stock pickers on television and in the newspaper or on the radio, people are constantly inundated with financial noise. Or, most recently, the internet has provided a portal for everyone to be an expert. When working with an advisor or financial planner, a client almost always has trouble if he and the advisor have different expectations. Although expectations should be held high, outside influences like the internet can pull client's attitudes off course. A good planner realizes that his job is spent battling client emotions as much as it is spent battling market conditions. In bear markets, defined by most economists as a 20% downward movement in a stock market index, volatility can bring out severe negativity and anxiety in clients. Conversely, a bull market, a 20% up market, brings feelings of confidence, invincibility, and euphoria in clients. Both sides of the spectrum are dangerous. According to a study by DALBAR (2006), the stock market has returned 11.9% over the past 20 years ending December 31, 2005. The average investor returned 3.9% (Fridson 2005). Although some experts will say the fees of professionals have lowered return, almost all of this difference is due to investor reaction and emotion as it relates to volatility. Investors act irrationally when they see their accounts going in the wrong direction and sometimes in the correct direction. Clients may argue "I'm getting out until the market gets going again or once the market hits an all time high." On an interesting note, a study performed by Princeton professor of Psychology Daniel Kahneman and Mark Riepe found that the losses of clients hurt are felt more than gains. They go on further to explain that "investment decisions have both emotional and financial consequences over time. There is potential for worry and for pride, for elation and for regret, and sometimes for guilt" (Kahneman and Riepe 1998).

Marital status may be another stressful factor associated with a financial transition. Single people, to some surprise, act more conservatively, than do married individuals. One could attribute this to the fact that singles do not have a second income to fall back on. Once a married couple has children, they do tend to act more conservatively. In my experience, a number of people's attitudes have changed greatly after the birth of a child. Perspective on money can change to "we don't need all of this" or the opposite which is a provider mentality, stating things like "I need to earn more" for my family.

The Therapeutic Value of Financial Planning

The time and function of the financial planner is spent managing the emotions of clients. There is a therapeutic component to the process of financial planning. The client who desires to "earn more" can be setting himself up for failure by setting goals that are not realistic. On the contrary, as stated before, the birth of a child can exacerbate conservative attitudes towards money. Getting married is a stressful event in itself and much of the emotion can be tied up in giving up some control of one's financial well-being.

One of the most interesting observations are the parallels and attitudes towards money as it relates to social life and status. One often finds a socially diverse group of clients. Some are country club goers, drive the best cars, live in the most exclusive areas of town, and are actively involved in social activities. As one might expect, these are not the "Millionaire Next Door" type and enjoy money earned or saved for the lifestyle it provides. Without question, these clients exhibit the most amounts of stress in all types of financial transition.

In contrast, there are a number of clients who are not socially inclined, and this conservative lifestyle often lends itself to conservative feelings about money and savings. These clients view money as security and are considerably less concerned with the lifestyle it could provide them. Authors Stanley and Danko describes *Millionaire Next Door* stating an affluent person behaves as such. "They become millionaires by budgeting and controlling expenses, and they maintain their affluent status the same way (1996)." This controlled behavior is a significant advantage when facing uncertainty. When facing a financial transition, this group exhibits lower levels of stress and often times does not feel great financial effects from transition due to their conservative, prepared position. Although linked to career choice and personal financial history, the parallels across social lifestyles is quite striking. For critical transitions, it is recommended that both spouses be present for a planning meeting. In married, one earner households, spousal support or pressure can have an overwhelming effect on the stresses experienced in transition. An example of this is in a job loss situation. Supportive spouses are very important for successful transition and this is not always the case. As one would imagine, the level of stress experienced is greatly reduced by a supportive, rather than pressuring spouse. Along the same line, if one spouse is more educated as it relates to financial topics, the stress tends to polarize to one spouse or the other. Interestingly, it could be either spouse. The less-educated spouse, from my experience, has shown signs of deep anxiety or even fear from lack of knowledge while other couples have exhibited stresses focused almost entirely on the "educated" spouse most likely originating from a "caretaker" mentality.

The Do-It-Yourselfer in Financial Planning

The term "do-it-yourselfer" is a commonly used term among the financial planning industry. Undeniably, this is the most difficult group of clients to sell on the value for your services or maintain as a long-term client. Often times based in an intent of frugality, this type of person reads, studies, and/or watches television shows with the intent of learning enough to take care of one's own finances. This type of client based this decision on the idea that they were as qualified as the planners in the marketplace. In recent years, it's a client's attitude towards delegation that often drives this decision. Clients with advanced degrees in far more technical areas than financial planning have the potential to adequately handle the management of their investments. However, they choose to delegate this to someone else, hold them accountable, and spend their time pursuing interests. As well, they tend to appreciate, understand, and value the ancillary benefits of using a professional. In good markets and bad, the emotions of clients become an important ingredient in successfully transitioning difficult times.

The roller coaster of today's financial markets has created a context very stressful to go through the financial transition. The case in point might involve two clients who recently finalized a divorce. For each person in the divorce, their understandable stress level seems to have escalated more when the stock markets in 2008 started going down in the first 8 months. A "do-it-yourselfer" typically does not know or appreciate a sound planner's ability to help manage these stressful times. As stated above, the perception is that money saved in fees is money left to invest but often times ignores the value-added guidance as it relates to decision-making, long-term perspective, and risk management. The stresses of financial transition are exacerbated in individuals who have no one to lean on when economic transition occurs.

There are four definitive groups which emerge. As shown in the chart below, transitions can either be contextual (occurring around someone) or personal. As well, each of these groups has transitions that are anticipated and unanticipated. Based on the above listed characteristics, the levels of stress exhibited are wide ranging. The most stressful events seem to be those that are personal and unanticipated. The death of spouse is the most obvious example of this. In dealing with a number of widows and widowers, the personal tragedy of losing a spouse appears to be the most stressful. The loss of a child is unquestionably as, if not more, tragic but the financial implications are usually lesser than the loss of a spouse. In one instance of working with a widow who lost her husband unexpectedly to a heart attack, her emotions were quite volatile and abrupt. After the first few months passed, her sadness was soon transitioned to feelings of financial inadequacy and anxiety. Her deceased husband was the "bread winner" and although retired at the time of his death, handled all of the finances including working with me as an advisor, paying bills, and assuring their household stood on sound financial ground. As a result of this experience, the lesson learned is that it may not be in the best interests of the client to have both spouses attend our review meetings. Her feelings of anxiety, although impossible to eliminate, could have been mitigated through a basic understanding of their plan prior to his death.

In contrast, where spouses who have lost a spouse to a more expected death, such as a long battle with cancer. Although equally tragic, this survivor usually has made some emotional preparations and most likely some financial preparations should the spouse not make it. As many cancer patients go through a stage of denial in their fight with the illness, so too can a spouse looking to be supportive. Unfortunately, this denial can lend itself to inaction in making sound financial plans in time. I recommend clients update their wills every 5 years if retired and more often if they are in the accumulation phase that is creating complexity. This proactive approach is utilized to combat complacency or unrealistic expectation of a couple battling cancer together. Life insurance is most often the best risk management tool in providing adequate resources to a surviving spouse. It is often very difficult to qualify for insurance when one is retired so early preparations here prove to be quite valuable. A reactive approach to financial planning is very difficult and those who have acted alone in making preparations or worked with an advisor find themselves with many more options when financial transitions occur. In some cases, life insurance can actually complicate the emotions of a survivor.

Ann Kaiser Stearns (1984) describes in her book *Living Through Personal Crisis*, the case she examined included a widow saying, "She never had life so easy financially" and she felt it was "death money." An excessive windfall from insurance can be overwhelming and eventually depressing for a surviving spouse who equates enjoyment of said funds with the loss of his/her spouse. This can lead to issues involving getting remarried as Stearns (1984)elaborates to say her patient said she would "always be married to two men" due to the financial stability her deceased husband had provided (Fig. 15-2).

After the death of a spouse, from my perspective, the second most stressful financial transition is divorce. Where clients have recently completed a divorce, new emotions toward finances do not seem to be created rather existing attitudes are expanded and exacerbated. Those who have traditionally acted conservatively with their money push this conservatism to a new extreme while those who are natural spenders seem to be even more so. If the divorce was pursued because of financial disagreements, this appears to still hold true although a greater sense of responsibility and proactively responding to the transition are established. The stressors of a divorce and the loss of a spouse are quite evident but, much like the expected spousal death versus the unexpected death, a divorce provides, typically, a greater amount of time to cope, prepare, or adjust as it relates to one's finances. In dealing with divorcing clients, the realization that one often creates a good deal of their identity based on their approach to their finances. It becomes a part of your personality just like any other personality trait. In saying this, although the context of the divorce provides adequate circumstances for bitterness or distrust, most divorcing clients feel like their financial discipline or personality has been squashed by their ex-spouse. To combat this, they tend to favor mass, sudden, drastic planning changes matching their own financial personality immediately following. As a responsible planner, there is a duty to assure clients not to be too hasty in making financial decisions. A sense of progress is likely the desired emotion associated with making changes although progress in financial planning is not always associated with immediate action.

After spousal loss or a divorce, according to Holmes and Rahe (1967), marriage itself is a quite stressful event (given a score of 50 out of 100). In fact, it is ranked even higher than retirement (score of 45) as it relates to stress. The birth of a child (score of 39) rates lower than both. Marriage is a major financial

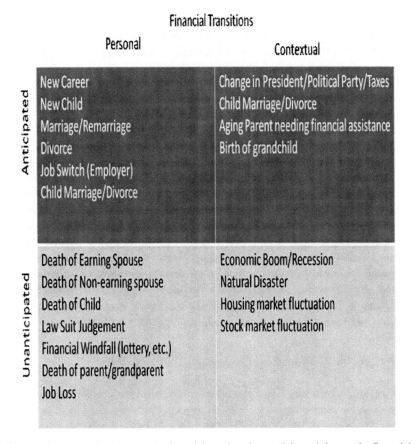

Fig. 15-2 Personal and contextual, anticipated and unanticipated factors in financial transitions

transition because it brings about, not only a substantial increase in the number of issues involved but it also requires a level of compromise and coordination of the two people. As described above, many people have developed a deep identity as it relates to financial matters and any compromise of these traits can be stressful. The added issues, not previously experienced as a single person as it relates to money can include but are not limited to sharing of previously private information, planning around survivor needs and insurance, adequate estate planning. As is often said, money and religion are two areas that lean to marital stress, it is vital to have worked through financial differences prior to getting married to minimize the inevitable stress that marriage provides.

Often times, the transition we experience has nothing do with our own action; we did not make it happen, it happens to us. This type of change could but is not limited to major economic recession or depression, economic boom, change in housing prices/home availability, natural disaster, or the support of a family member moving into a nursing home. In each instance, the change occurred, affected us, but was not necessarily created by us. These transitions and the accompanying stresses maintain a significant range. Due to the anticipated nature of the said events, the stresses experienced are often times greater than those of an anticipated transition. In the economic boom/recession example, there is a direct personal financial change that occurs. In instances like a natural disaster, the change has much to do with the earlier preparations that have been made. In all examples though, the level of stress and anxiety experienced is much lower when adequate preparation has been done. Whether it be insurance coverage, little or no debt, or a large emergency fund, any preparations made for unforeseen events will be beneficial in the long run to combat stresses in the above described transition.

The emotion witnessed in clients going through a stressful transition and their evolution in financial understanding as the transition progresses is undeniable. Like any experience we can learn from, financial transition (unfortunately, in my opinion) is typically the time when people learn most about their finances. Proper preparation would avoid this uncomfortable learning curve. In retrospect, almost all transitions in life have some financial component. It can be a direct effect like a divorce that requires moving forward with lesser assets to support oneself. Or it can be indirect, such as an economic recession. We all handle stress differently but from a financial standpoint, our ability to handle stresses lies more importantly in the preparation we have made to prepare ourselves for change, be it expected or unexpected. The level of emotional stress exhibited by clients is higher in those experiencing unexpected transition (i.e., death of spouse), but the conclusion regarding preparation still holds true.

Take Home Messages for Financial Transitions

In conclusion, there are a few essential factors to consider as take home messages when it comes to successfully transitioning the stressful financial issues facing so many individuals and families. As you analyze your own financial situation and the transition each faces, consider the following key points:

- All transition we experience has some level of financial effect. The stresses related to transition range from very minor to life-altering.
- Secondly, proper preparation for the unexpected is the best way to combat stress in life's transitions. Individuals who have prepared for the unexpected are able to handle the unexpected as if it were an expected event.
- Finally, by utilizing the help of a competent professional who can bring coordination to one's entire financial situation, you will be able to combat the unexpected as well as look to or delegate for help when the unexpected occurs.

References

American Psychological Association (2008) In S. Bethune, & A. Brownwell, (Eds.), Financial Concerns of Holiday Stressors for Women, Families and Children. Washington, DC: American Psychological Association, Office of Survey Research. Retrieved April 12, 2008, from http://www.apa.org/releases/holiday-1208.html

DALBAR Inc. (2006). *Quantitative analysis of investment behavior*. Boston, MA.

CFP® *Practice Standards*, www.cfp.net (2008). Financial Planning Association Understanding Financial Planning. Retrieved April 12, 2008, from http://www.fpa-forfinancialplanning.org/WhatisFinancialPlanning/WhyaCFPProfessional/

Fridson, M. (2000). *How to be a Billionaire: Proven Strategies from the Titans of Wealth*. New York: Wiley and Sons, Inc.

Holmes, T., & Rahe, R. (1967). Holmes-Rahe social readjustment rating scale. *Journal of Psychosomatic Research, 11*, 213–218.

Kahneman, D., & Riepe, M. (1998). Aspects of investor psychology. *Journal of Portfolio Management, 24*(4), 86–106.

Stanley, T. J., & Danko, W. D. (1996). *The Millionaire Next Door*. New York: Pocket Books, a division of Simon and Schuster.

Stearns, A. K. (1984). *Living through personal crisis*. Chicago, IL: Thomas More.

Chapter 16

Dual Cognitive Processes and Alcohol and Drug Misuse in Transitioning Adolesence

Marvin Krank

Adolescence is the time when individuals make the perilous journey from child to adult. Although risk-taking is natural and inevitable, adolescent development is fraught with potentially dangerous situations with choices that can lead to both short- and long-term changes with either positive or negative consequences on healthy development. The developmental imperatives of adolescence include physical, emotional, sexual, social, and cognitive change. The emerging world of adolescents is full of new opportunities, replete with novel and sometimes confusing sensations and experiences. The journey through this wild country comes with potentially dangerous paths that lead to very real risks and rewards. The task of adolescents is to navigate this wondrous landscape and emerge as an adult. Success in adolescence requires that the youth avoid the delays and dead-ends of risky paths. Not the least of the transformative changes that may occur in this developmental phase is the rapid growth of drug and alcohol use. This early substance use occurs in a developmental and social context. Acknowledging the social and developmental context of adolescence, this chapter explores social influences faced by youth through an emerging dual processing cognitive model of choice that helps to explain the vulnerability of youth to alcohol and drug use (Stacy et al. 2009; Wiers and Stacy 2006a; Wiers et al. 2007b).

Adolescent Substance Use

This chapter gives a brief review of adolescent substance use and explores its relationship with social learning and social cognition. The coverage proceeds from a general overview of population statistics on substance use and longitudinal findings taken from the Project on Adolescent Trajectories and Health (PATH).

Many adolescents begin using drugs and alcohol as early as age 12, with the escalation of use through middle and high school years (Cuijpers 2003; Faden and Fay 2004; Johnston et al. 2003; Krank and Goldstein 2006; O'Malley et al. 1998; Wallace et al. 2003; Wallace et al. 2003). Recent Canadian statistics from the National Report on Mental Health indicate that a significant percentage of the population over the age of 15 are current marijuana users and 42.9% of these

From: *Handbook of Stressful Transitions Across the Lifespan,*
Edited by: T.W. Miller, DOI 10.1007/978-1-4419-0748-6_16,
© Springer Science+Business Media, LLC 2010

report failure to control use. The highest level of dependence is among younger users in the 15–24 age range (7%). By the age of 17, most students have used alcohol, many take serious risks (Adlaf et al. 2003), and many are binge drinkers (Krank et al. 2005; Krank and Goldstein 2006; Tucker et al. 2003). Early drug and alcohol use among teens is strongly associated with social problems (e.g. aggression and risky sex) and negative health outcomes (e.g. accidents and STDs). The abuse of substances has been linked to a host of negative outcomes and risky behaviors among youth, including academic problems, dropping out of school, increased mental health problems, risky sexual activity, and unsafe driving practices (Everett et al. 1999; Fergusson et al. 2002; Fergusson 2004; Newcomb et al. 1993; Staton et al. 2001; Stein et al. 1987).

Substance use in youth between the ages of 12 and 17 usually begins with alcohol, followed in some by cigarette or marijuana use, and followed in a few by illicit drug use (Fergusson et al. 2006a; Kandel and Yamaguchi 2002). Whether these typical progressions are causal is controversial (Fergusson et al. 2006a, b; Flisher 2003; Kandel et al. 2006). Nevertheless, the pattern is clear. Alcohol is the initial and most common substance used by youth. Marijuana is the second most commonly used substance. When it occurs at this age, marijuana use normally follows alcohol use, although evidence suggests that other patterns may occur in subpopulations (Flisher 2003). As the trends have developed into the current decade, tobacco use is now somewhat less common than marijuana. Moreover, the order of initiation is less certain as tobacco use may proceed or follow marijuana use. Finally, illicit hallucinogen (LSD, psilocybin, mescaline, and club drugs) and stimulant (amphetamine and cocaine) use is initiated by some in early adolescence. This illicit drug use is much less common, and is almost always preceded by alcohol and marijuana use.

Project on Adolescent Trajectories and Health

The PATH study was a longitudinal study of 1,303 students in early adolescence using a cohort sequential design. Three cohorts were defined by grade at the start of the study: grade seven, grade eight, or grade nine. Each of these cohorts was surveyed for three successive years. Thus, PATH obtained data spanning grades seven to eleven.[1] This developmental period was chosen because it reflects the period of substantial change with new developmental tasks; a vulnerable time when youth are at great risk for risky behavioral trajectories and potential short- and long-term harm. PATH covered several domains of risk and a number of social context and individual risk and protective factors. The present chapter will describe trajectories of substance use in relation to social learning and cognitive measures in PATH.

Prevalence of Substance Use in PATH

Figure 16-1 shows past year use as a function of grade at the time of test for each of the three cohorts. Consistent with many population surveys, alcohol use including self-reported drunkenness, a correlate of binge drinking, is more common than all other drug use (*Overview of findings from the 2003 national*

---

[1]For a detailed description of the methodology used in PATH see http://web.ubc.ca/okanagan/psycomp/faculty/mkrank/research/path.html .

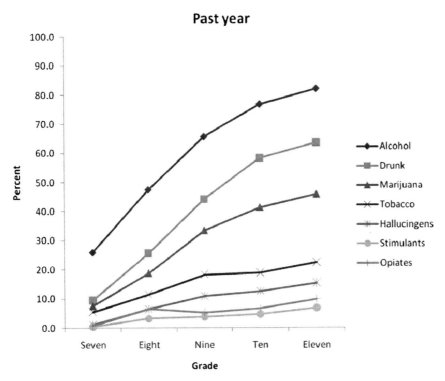

Fig. 16-1. The growth of various substance use in the longitudinal PATH study in British Columbia, Canada. Past year use averages of each of the three cohorts. In the main these usage levels are consistent with population estimates. One exception is the higher level of marijuana use in the sample. This observation is, however, consistent with national Canadian surveys showing higher levels of marijuana use in British Columbia

survey on drug use and health 2004; Scheier et al. 1997; Schulenberg et al. 2005; Tucker et al. 2006; Windle and Wiesner 2004). In addition, the levels of use in the past month are similar to other national surveys in the US (*Overview of findings from the 2003 national survey on drug use and health* 2004; Schulenberg et al. 2005) and Canada (Flight 2007; Adlaf et al. 2006; Ivis et al. 1997), including BC (McCreary Centre Society 2005). The relatively higher use of marijuana in the sample is consistent with both local survey findings (McCreary Centre Society 2005) and provincial comparisons in national surveys (Flight 2007).

Early Substance Use and Prevention

Developmental transitions in substance use reflect a stage of vulnerability that is critical for effective prevention (D'Amico et al. 2005b; O'Leary Tevyaw and Monti 2004). Early substance use is particularly important as it predicts later substance abuse, substance dependence, and progressions to other types of drug use (D'Amico et al. 2005a; Fergusson et al. 2006a; Grant et al. 2006; Kandel and Yamaguchi 2002; Yamaguchi and Kandel 2002). The present research targets this vulnerable developmental stage as a window of risk and a critical period to intervene and prevent the development of and harms from early substance misuse and its associated negative consequences (O'Leary Tevyaw and Monti 2004; Pacula et al. 2001; Spoth et al. 2001; Spoth et al. 2002; Spoth et al. 2004). Prevention efforts in this age group can be effective to

(1) prevent or delay the initiation of substance use, (2) eliminate or reduce extant substance use, and (3) prevent or delay transitions to escalated use and abuse. Thus, effective prevention in the early stages of potential substance use initiation is expected to redirect harmful trajectories in their early stages or before they occur and should be especially cost effective. Much evidence indicates that substance use in adolescents is strongly influenced by social learning and social cognitions. This social learning leads to substance use associations that predict future transitions to substance use (Krank et al. 2005; Krank and Wall 2006; Stacy et al. 2009; Stacy 1995, 1997; Wiers and Stacy 2006a). It stands to reason that effective prevention should include measures that address these cognitions (Krank and Goldstein 2006; Wiers et al. 2004, 2006).

Dual Processing Systems and Decision-Making in Youth

The research reported here focuses on basic cognitive processing, and how it interacts with developmental processes and social learning occurring in adolescence. One very useful dichotomy for understanding cognitive processing is the distinction between reflexive, implicit, or automatic processing and reflective, explicit, or controlled processing (Deutsch and Strack 2006; Graf 1994; Shiffrin and Schneider 1984). In the first instance, responses are elicited by current context and arise from a natural associative process. For example, associative memories just spring to mind in reflexive retrieval without any clear effort to remember. This process is not only reflexive, but may also occur without awareness. Processing at this unconscious level is often referred to as implicit cognition (Gawronski and Bodenhausen 2005; Greenwald et al. 2003). By definition, implicit processing occurs without awareness of the memories that give rise to it. Automatic and reflexive processing are defined somewhat differently, but overlap considerably with implicit processing (Deutsch et al. 2006; Strack et al. 2006). Automatic processing occurs without the intervention of deliberate executive control. Reflexive processing is elicited by stimulus conditions and also assumes the lack of executive control. The lack of awareness is not specifically assumed, but is often inferred for automatic and reflexive processing. At the very least, these three theoretical terms refer to cognition that is rapid, effortless, and spontaneous (Bargh and Ferguson 2000; Bargh et al. 2001).

The second type of processing assumes executive control (Baddeley and Logie 1999; Logan 1985). This explicit, reflective, or controlled processing involves more cognitive effort and occurs more deliberately. Such processing includes working memory (Baddeley and Logie 1999; Hester and Garavan 2005), inhibitory attention (Hester and Garavan 2005; Levy and Anderson 2002), and goal-directed behavior (Royall et al. 2005; Tanji et al. 2007). Considering retrieval as an example, reflective retrieval might recruit intentional mnemonic strategies to aid memory (Shimamura 2002). The goal might be to recollect a specific event or piece of information, such as a specific telephone number. Thus, cognitive processing would be guided by its outcomes and continued mental activity would be engaged until the goal is accomplished or abandoned. Although not necessarily required, awareness is usually assumed. Controlled, reflective, and explicit processing takes longer, requires effort, and is more deliberate. These processes involve different regions of the brain, particularly the frontal cortex (Badre and Wagner 2007; Rolls 2008;

Tanji et al. 2007). Although there are many definitions, for the remainder of this chapter we will refer to implicit cognition as processing that is reflexive, automatic, and normally without awareness.

The importance of the distinction between implicit and explicit cognitive processing is documented by many studies that show cognitive and neurological dissociations (Badre and Wagner 2007; Bechara and Martin 2004; Tanji et al. 2007). Some memories affect performance in different ways, depending on whether they are retrieved implicitly or explicitly (Jacoby and Kelley 1992; Yonelinas and Jacoby 1995). For example, Jacoby and colleagues (Jacoby et al. 1989a, b) showed that exposure to a list of names in a manner designed to reduce explicit memory results in feelings of unattributed familiarity. This familiarity feeling is then misinterpreted, in this case as famous names seen in the past. The familiarity is attributed to past experience with a famous name. In contrast, procedures designed to improve explicit memory produce attributed familiarity. The name is familiar because it was just seen on the list. With explicit memory, there is no need to misattribute familiarity to past learning. This finding is just one example of the dissociations based on memory with or without awareness.

In recent years, the distinction between implicit and explicit cognition or controlled and automatic processing has been applied to the study of addiction (Stacy et al. 2009; Tiffany 1990; Wiers et al. 2007a). The emphasis of this new application has been the unique contributions of implicit cognition or automatic behavior to understanding the basis for addictive behavior. That is, while recognizing that some actions are determined by effortful executive control, this approach acknowledges that actions are often unconscious and based on automatic processing. This observation may be particularly relevant to addiction because it can explain the seemingly irrational basis of self-destructive addictive behaviors (Stacy et al. in press). For example, why do smokers, who often recognize the serious health consequences of tobacco use, continue to smoke in the face of this knowledge? One might argue that they discount negative effects, but this discounting is more naturally a reaction to the conflict between continued smoking and this information. If smoking behavior is largely based on implicit cognitions, such as strong association with reward, then explicit knowledge of negative health consequences has less influence on this behavior.

Figure 16-2 describes a simple schematic of implicit and explicit memory processing. Central to the model is the multitrace long-term memory system (Hintzman 1984; Hintzman 1986; Rolls 2008). This multi-trace network, in accordance with many representational theories (Humphreys et al. 1989), is an exemplar or episodic associative memory network which is connectionist and distributed across a large number of attributes. Such a network is highly contextualized and contains information about seemingly irrelevant details. This rich detail is assumed even when it cannot be directly accessed during the retrieval process. This representation allows the memory system to effectively contain exemplar or episodic information and still produce summary judgments, such as relative frequency (Hintzman 2001), likelihood (Dougherty et al. 1999), or schema abstraction (Hintzman 1986). The general retrieval process is called a global matching process in which activation of individual traces by a memory probe are combined into a single value (Hintzman 2001; Humphreys et al. 1989). Figure 16-2 represents this summary value as the memory image. Many associations may be activated to form an image from memory. Memory retrieval is viewed

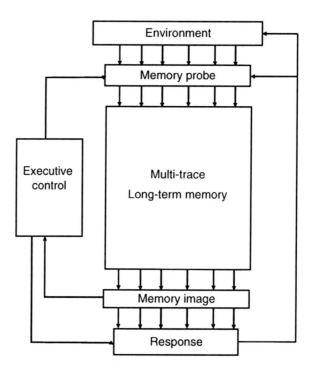

Fig. 16-2. This diagram shows a simple dual processing model of cognition. The model builds from a multi-trace long-term memory containing integrated and associative traces of examplers or episodic events. The model represents dual processing by including executive control with working memory, attention, and goal-directed processing

as a reconstruction of this composite information. The level of detail accessed during retrieval is dependent on both the nature of the long-term memories and the memory probe. Retrieval in these systems is based on a similarity metric. Processing at any given point in time activates associations through a distributed and parallel process. A memory system that contains episodic details of whatever processing occurs at the time of learning and uses a global matching process is useful to explain context effects (Dougal and Rotello 1999; Krank and Wall 2006). Such a system is important to substance use because it can be linked directly to behavioral decision-making (Dougherty et al. 2003; Rolls 2008; Stacy 1997)

It is beyond the scope of this chapter to review the detailed cognitive evidence for this approach. Nevertheless there are some important features of the proposed cognitive structure that capture essential features of memory. First, learning involves storing associations from past experience based on the nature of processing at the time. Secondly, it is naturally contextual; associations contain specific details from encoding that influence the retrieval process. Thirdly, retrieval can be automatic without executive control. This latter feature represents an implicit form of processing that does not require controlled or explicit processing. Explicit processing in Fig. 16-2 assumes an executive control process that monitors cognition and intervenes strategically. The diagram represents executive processing as a distinct way of monitoring and influencing the retrieval of information from associative memory. It is consistent with recent neurocognitive findings of frontal cortex effects on memory and decision-making (Rolls 2008).

The implicit system represents the default or more primitive system where perception of the environment automatically triggers or elicits an image from memory. The classical example of this is Pavlov's dogs salivating in response to a bell that has been associated with food. In more cognitive examples, the implicit memory is an image activated without effort and awareness of remembering. It is the first neural response when experiencing a particular stimulus condition. Explicit memory is more deliberate and assumes an executive function. This function monitors cognition and intervenes with strategies designed to accomplish goals. For example, "what did I have this morning for breakfast" might not produce an immediate result. The executive control system could monitor the images produced and decide whether additional processing is required to resolve the image and confirm a satisfactory level of recall. Another important function of executive control would be to follow logical consequences beyond the immediate reflexive associations. Thus, reflection would consider further options and consequent outcomes not immediately apparent. Such executive control is critical to planning, especially for long-term goals.

Implicit Processing, Incentive, and Substance Use

Many theories of substance use are based on their incentive properties (Glasner 2004; Krank 2003; Krank et al. 2008; Robinson and Berridge 2001, 2004). By incentive, we mean that use is anticipated to have positive or rewarding consequences. Drugs and alcohol that are commonly used by adolescents are usually perceived to have positive effects (Goldman et al. 2006; Krank and Goldstein 2006; Krank and Wall 2006). These rewarding outcomes are learned through both direct and indirect experience. Social learning is a major force. Films, TV shows, music videos, advertising, friends, and family may provide much indirect information about the consequences of drug or alcohol use. Many of these social sources portray drug and alcohol use as a rewarding experience. Youth who have never used alcohol or marijuana often have very positive associations prior to even trying the drug (Krank et al. 2005; Krank and Goldstein 2006; Krank and Wall 2006; Smith and Goldman 1994; Smith et al. 1995). Once the drug is used, direct experience is expected to contribute to further incentive learning. Youth who have positive experiences, especially those that confirm their vicarious learning, strengthen these positive associations with drug use (Stacy 1995, 1997; Stacy et al. 2009).

Incentive and expectancy theories posit that substance use is governed by the strength of anticipated positive consequences (Goldman et al. 1999, 2006; Krank et al. 2008; Robinson and Berridge 2004). It is easy to see how anticipation can work automatically in such a model. Stimulus conditions, such as being invited to a drinking party, activate associations between drinking and its consequences. When these associations are mostly positive (e.g. having fun, forgetting problems,), the invitation generates positive images, increases anticipatory incentive, creates attraction, and elicits attentional bias, and is more likely to be accepted. Here is the point at which the executive control system might be engaged either in support or against the automatic decision. For example, knowing that you have a test the next day and that drinking will interfere with studying may temper your choice. Alternatively, considering other less positive options, such as sitting at home alone may increase the attractiveness of drinking. The executive system allows us to consider the long-term consequences of our choices. Automatic associative memory assumed by implicit processing is impulsive and immediate. Explicit processing under executive control is more deliberate. The question addressed here is how does this dual processing system help explain the major substance use transitions that occur in early adolescence.

Developmental Vulnerabilities to Substance Use in Youth

Youth are particularly susceptible to substance use because of their stage of physiological, neurological, cognitive, and social development and its interaction with their environment (Schulenberg et al. 2001; Stacy et al. in press; Wiers et al. 2007a). First, youth during this time of exploration have a natural tendency to seek new and different experiences. It is part of their developmental task to break away from the protective constraints of childhood and become an adult participant in the greater world around them. At the same time, breaking away from family and venturing into the larger world exposes them to increased information and opportunities to make dangerous choices. In North American culture, positive messages about the benefits of drug and alcohol use permeate the popular media (Grube 1993; Hanewinkel and Sargent 2007; Wallack et al. 1987). In our communities, opportunities to consume drugs are available in many common social contexts (Sussman et al. 1998). In addition, as youth break away from their family, parental influences wane and peer influences increase. This emphasis shifts control from adult influences to adolescent influences that are inherently less reflective and long-term in orientation.

Adolescent Development, Dual Processing, and Substance Use

How do adolescent development and adolescent social environments interact with the dual processing cognitive system outlined here to create increased vulnerability? Adolescents are exposed to a variety of social learning experiences that have positive messages about substance use. Sources include parental and community use, peer use, advertising associations, and use in the popular media (music, TV, movies etc.). Social learning is assumed to lead to long-term memory traces that include detailed information about context, behaviors, and outcomes. Further, these memories include much affective information and are particularly relevant to incentive motivation and behavioral decision-making. Early negative substance use – outcome associations from childhood are often replaced by more positive associations during adolescence because of the changes in social exposure to positive substance use messages during this time. Positive substance use associations enhance incentive motivation to be used as a reflexive, implicit, or automatic response to opportunities. Individual differences in exposure to social stress and dispositions interact with this dual processing system by creating additional reasons to use (i.e. coping or enhancement motivations). Last but not least, adolescents have a relative lack of executive or reflective control to counteract incentive motivation generated by the reflexive associative system. The combined effect of these developmental changes is that youth have more exposure to and more motivation to make risky choices. At the same time they have less cognitive control (executive function) over their behavior.

Individual differences among youth as they enter this critical exploratory phase interact with the general vulnerabilities of adolescent development. Individuals differ in their motivations for substance use according to their personalities and their social environments. For example, sensation seeking youth exaggerate the normal exploratory motivation in adolescence (Conrod 2000; Conrod et al. 2000). Avoiding boredom becomes a dominant goal. Given the many opportunities for substance use and the potential absence of equally stimulating alternatives, sensation seeking youth are particularly susceptible to experimenting with substance use. These youth seek ways of making life more rewarding and exciting (enhancement motivation).

A second important individual difference in risk comes from social environments that increase susceptibility to the effects of drug and alcohol. Families or communities with substance use problems model inappropriate use. Social learning in this context leads to unrealistic norms about how much and when people drink or use drugs. Other social environments expose youth to stressful conditions that create psychological conditions, ripe for self-medication. For example, youth exposed to relatively higher levels of violence or neglect experience more negative emotions and less social connection. Drug and alcohol use can be seen as a quick fix for feelings of hopelessness and anxiety. Substance use can also be seen as a remedy for boredom, a means of reducing anxiety or sadness, and a short cut to social success. Using with others can make them feel part of a group, more relaxed, and more socially connected and successful. These quick solutions are often readily available in the adolescent social environment. Other more adaptive coping strategies are less available because adolescents either have not learned them yet or do not have access to these options in their environment. Thus, negative social conditions can lead to additional motivations for substance use to cope with stress (coping motivations). Although there are many potential risks and protective factors for substance use in teens, the present review will focus on several measures of individual differences studied in our longitudinal work with this population. This chapter will summarize the role of these factors to illustrate the impact of negative social contexts and certain personality tendencies on substance use in adolescents.

Measuring Individual Differences Contributing to Substance Use in Youth

Given the natural level of risk inherent in adolescence, the most pressing question for prevention science is what factors determine whether an individual gets involved with substance use and progresses to abuse. Transitions in substance use are largely determined by individual differences set in the context of biological, dispositional, and social developmental constraints. From this perspective, individual differences are partly genetic and maturational, but also arise from social and cultural experience. Measuring individual differences based on social experience can be done in several ways. We divide these into three classes: those aimed at measuring the experiential history, those measuring dispositional factors such as personality, and those aimed at measuring the social learning impact of experience on memory associations. The first two measures are examples of risk and protective factors (Hawkins et al. 1992). The latter measures are inferential with respect to social learning. That is, measures of memory association are assumed to arise from certain learning experiences (Krank and Goldstein 2006; Krank and Wall 2006; Stacy et al. 2009). This learning assumption is plausible and consistent with animal models of additive behavior (Goldman et al. 1999, 2006; Krank et al. 2008; Robinson and Berridge 2004), but remains to date largely untested in adolescents.

Social Experience

Social experience measures are those designed to assess the level of exposure to certain social conditions. For example, we might ask about the nature of family or friend's use of various substances to gain an indication of the exposure to potential models of these behaviors. Similarly, we could ask about media exposure to modeling of substance use. What types of TV or movies do they watch and how often? More specifically, we might measure the relative exposure to alcohol advertising with its frequent portrayal of positive social situations associated with alcohol use. Many family and demographic measures are directed at experiential history. We assume, for example, that living in a single parent family or one with greater economic means exposes youth to conditions that vary systematically from two primary parent families or lower income families. The goal of these measures is to identify environmental conditions that either directly or indirectly influence the likelihood of substance use transitions.

In his development of risk and protective factors, Hawkins identifies areas of social influence including characteristics of communities; family, school, and peer group experiences (Hawkins et al. 1992). It is beyond the scope of this chapter to review this literature, but there are several excellent reviews of this literature (Choi et al. 2006; Corrigan et al. 2007; Fagan et al. 2007). The present review will focus on a few of these social influences as they were measured in the PATH study. The goal is not a comprehensive review; rather the intention is to set the stage for examining the impact of social experience on memory associations that are relevant to substance use decisions.

Social Exposure to Substance Use Role Models

Social exposure is one of the primary methods of acquiring new learning about substance use contexts and effects, especially prior to actual use (Wall and McKee 2002). Important role models include parents, other significant adults, media personalities, and peers. Among younger children, parental influences dominate. During adolescent development, peer influence increases. The general correlations of parental use reported by adolescents in the PATH study and their current use are shown in Table 16-1. Substance use by mother and father correlates, but weakly. In a standard regression analysis for each substance, the parental use only accounts for five to ten percent of the variance in use. By contrast, peer influence is much stronger in this age group accounting for up to 50% of the variance. In part, the strength of peer use correlations is due to a combined effect of peer influence by modeling and peer selection (Bauman and Ennett 1994). That is, peers influence not only the likelihood of substance use, but also substance use influences the selection of peers. Youth who have

Table 16-1. Correlations between parental and peer use of alcohol, tobacco, and marijuana with use of each respective substance in youth from grades 7–9.

	Mother	Father	Closest friends
Alcohol	.209	.203	.590
Tobacco	.205	.157	.580
Marijuana	.215	.269	.675

friends who are engaged in substance use are more likely to start and increase using, but youth who are engaged in substance use are also more likely to choose friends who use the same substances they use. These dual effects of influence and selection are difficult to disentangle. Nevertheless, careful longitudinal analysis of social networks and substance use documents the effects of both (Bauman and Ennett 1994; Kirke 2004; Pomery et al. 2005).

Additional modeling of social exposure to others engaged in substance use come from media including television, movies, and advertising (Grube 1993; Madden and Grube 1994). Substance use is either portrayed or implied in a variety of media. Although alcohol advertising does not normally show drinking, use and its positive consequences are clearly implied in many "life style ads." These ads commonly show young attractive individuals in a party or bar setting with alcohol in prominent display. Everyone is clearly having fun, often with subtexts of increased sexuality. Although strong causal relationships have not been demonstrated, the level of exposure to alcohol advertising is correlated with youth drinking (Atkin 1990; Collins et al. 2007; Grube 1993; Saffer and Dave 2006; Zogg 2005). Some recent studies have shown longitudinal effects of advertising on drinking, supporting the social influence interpretation of the correlations (Ellickson et al. 2005; Zogg 2005).

Less scientific work has been done to establish the relationship between substance use in movies and television and youth use. Nevertheless, ample opportunities present themselves (Miller et al. 2007; Van den Bulck and Beullens 2005; Wallack et al. 1987). For example, one need only watch one or two episodes of the "That 70's Show" to see the "circle," a clear portrayal of teens smoking marijuana and laughing. Exposure to cigarette smoking in movies is positively correlated with smoking in youth (Dal Cin et al. 2007; Hanewinkel and Sargent 2007). Longitudinal work suggests that this effect includes social influence (Titus-Ernstoff et al. 2008; Wills et al. 2007).

Social exposure effects support a general social learning approach to adolescent substance use. In the context of a cognitive model of substance use, they suggest that social exposure leads to changes in the long-term memory system. In the model proposed here, they are expected to contribute memory traces that contain information about social context and outcomes of substance use. Many of these vicarious experiences fit this view well, containing rich detail about situations in which drugs or alcohol are used with often positive consequences (or perceived positive consequences). As a result, these observational episodes are expected to increase the positive valence of substance use memory associations and incentive motivation to use.

Social Environments

Past studies of substance use in adolescents have indicated many demographic factors that may influence initiation or escalating use (O'Leary Tevyaw and Monti 2004). We focus on three factors here: family status, parental education, and income. Each of these has been shown to influence substance use, but the data has been controversial. In part, differences in interpretation are definitional. Some studies have combined these variables into a single factor. For example, parental education and income when considered together are positively correlated and protective factors (Fergusson et al. 2006a). The evidence from income data alone is less clear; studies show positive, negative, or no effects.

Smart et al. (1994) suggest that this problem may reflect accuracy of adolescent self report on income. They show that adolescents living in areas with higher regional income data are less likely to engage in risky substance use. Alternative interpretations, however, are possible. Area-based incomes may reflect parental education. Variations in individual family income may have an independent influence on substance use. Moreover, adolescents may not be misreporting their income, but basing their report on a different aspect of income, such as the relative income or personal disposable income. The latter may actually provide increased means to obtain alcohol and other drugs and could, at least in the early transitions, contribute to increased risk. These observations suggest that adolescent perceptions of income may be an important independent risk factor for substance use transitions.

Family status has also been shown to influence adolescent substance use. Divorce can have negative effects on psychosocial adjustment in adolescents and is associated with increased substance use in young adolescents (Breivik and Olweus 2006; Doherty and Needle 1991; Locke and Newcomb 2003; Needle et al. 1990). The timing of these effects interacts with sex (Locke and Newcomb 2003) and varies as a function of post-divorce family structure (i.e. single versus two parent family and presence of step parent (Breivik and Olweus 2006).

Child and Youth Maltreatment: Violence and Neglect

Child maltreatment creates vulnerability. Children who have been victims of physical abuse, emotional abuse, physical and emotional neglect, or sexual abuse are at greater risk for many forms of socially deviant behaviors in adolescence, including conduct disorder (McCabe et al. 2005), early and risky sexual behavior (Wilson and Widom 2008), violence (Wall 2003), and substance abuse (Edmond et al. 2002; Hamburger et al. 2008; Hyman et al. 2006; Stein et al. 2002; Wall and Kohl 2007). Most of this literature has focused on the more extreme forms of abuse, physical and sexual abuse, that bring the child or youth to the attention of social services. Less extreme forms of emotional abuse and neglect, however, are more likely and increase the risk of substance abuse (Hyman et al. 2006; Kirisci et al. 2001; Rodgers et al. 2004). We ask here whether lesser levels of violence and neglect influence early substance use in a general population, which includes few youth who have been identified as victims of abuse.

Violence in several forms is common in early adolescence. Violence exposure does not need to reach the criteria for abuse to have a strong influence in youth (Taylor and Kliewer 2006; Wall 2003). Bullying is one main vehicle by which many experience or perpetrate violence at this age (Houbre et al. 2006; Pepler et al. 2002; Smokowski and Kopasz 2005). Bullying may take traditional forms, but new forms, such as internet bullying (Mitchell et al. 2007) and newly recognized forms of relationship violence are also prevalent (Pepler et al. 2002; Wall 2003). As youth begin to enter puberty, dating begins. Accompanying this new interest in sex is dating violence, which while relatively infrequent is nonetheless important. Neglect in its extreme forms is a reportable form of child abuse. Many youth, however, experience neglect to a lesser degree or go unreported, and yet also experience negative outcomes (Hyman et al. 2006; Moran et al. 2004; Rodgers et al. 2004).

The PATH study analyzed substance use in a population of in-school youth. The requirement for parental consent to participate potentially biased the population toward higher functioning families. This sample included a very small number of in-care youth (2%). Nevertheless, we asked whether community and family exposure to violence and perceptions of familial neglect impacted substance use. Our measure of violence exposure was ratings of the level of: violence in my life, fighting normal, violence in neighborhood, violence in school, and people older than me are mean. These items held together well with a Cronbach's alpha of .772. The neglect items were reverse-coded based on ratings of: family always there for me, family looks after me, family cares about me, affectionate family, and treated well by people (Cronbach's alpha=.815).

These measures of violence exposure and neglect were strong independent predictors in a multilevel analysis across a broad range of substances including alcohol, marijuana, tobacco, hallucinogens, and stimulants. The effects of both measures were especially strong for illicit substance use. The sample of PATH youth was divided into three levels of each variable to illustrate the nature of these effects. In each case the upper third was designated High, the middle third as Mid, and the bottom third as Low. Figure 16-3 shows the effect of these levels of violence exposure on the trajectories of the amount of alcohol use teens from grade seven to eleven indicated was normal for them. Although all three curves grow across this time frame, the High violence exposure group reaches an average of about six drinks per occasion by grade ten. This quantity is clearly indicative of a binge drinking pattern in many of these youth. By contrast, the Low exposure group reaches half this level by grade eleven indicating many fewer heavy drinkers in this group. This pattern is consistent

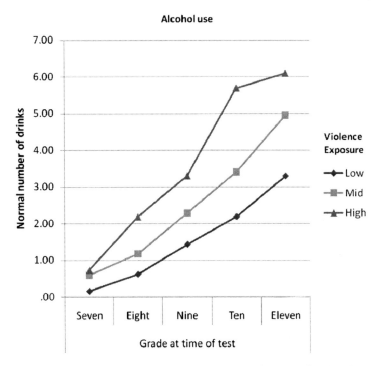

Fig. 16-3. The effect of violence exposure on the growth of the quantity of typical alcohol use in teens from grade seven to eleven. The upper third on the violence exposure measure of the sample was designated High, the middle third as Mid, and the bottom third as Low

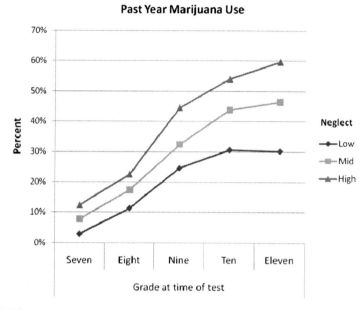

Fig. 16-4. The effect of neglect on the growth of marijuana use in teens from grade seven to eleven. The upper third on the neglect measure of the sample was designated High, the middle third as Mid, and the bottom third as Low

across a variety of alcohol use measures, tobacco use, and various forms of illicit drug use.

Levels of neglect also define an increased risk for substance use. Again the groups were classified by thirds into Low, Mid, and High levels of neglect to illustrate the relative increase in risk. Figure 16-4 shows the growth trajectories of past year marijuana use as a function of perceived neglect. The High neglect group reached 60% use in the past year by grade eleven, whereas fewer than 30% of the Low neglect group had used marijuana. Although neglect and violence exposure are moderately correlated, $r=.401$, the risk effects of each are independent and additive. In youth, these effects are consistent across a number of measures and substances.

The independent and additive effects of violence and neglect are apparent in alcohol, marijuana, tobacco, hallucinogen, and stimulant use, but they are most dramatic for illicit drug use. Shown in Fig. 16-5 is the combined effect of violence exposure and neglect on hallucinogen use. The five groups in the figure were defined by adding the level of risk together. The High group represents those who reported high levels of both violence exposure and neglect. Similarly, the Low group represents those who reported low levels of both risk factors. The Mid-High group reported one measure as high and one as mid and the Low-Mid group reported one measure as mid and the other as low. Finally, the Mid group usually consisted of those who reported middle levels on both risk factors. There were, however, a small number in this group that reported high levels on one factor and low levels on the other. The figure clearly demonstrates the combined risk of violence and neglect. Over 30% of youth who were high on both of these risk factors had used hallucinogens in the past year by grade 10. Lower levels of combined risk showed correspondingly lower effects on the growth

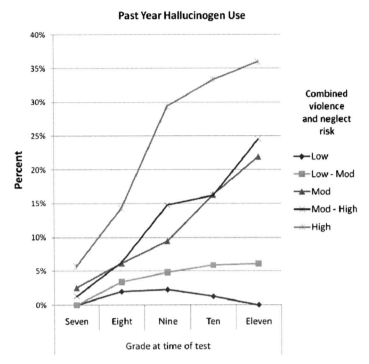

Fig. 16-5.   The combined risk of both violence and neglect on the growth of hallucinogen use in teens from grade seven to eleven. The Low group was low on both measures. The Low – Mod group was Low on one measure and Mid on another. Finally, the Mod group usually consisted of those who reported middle levels, either both Mid or Low – High. The Mod-High group reported one measure as high and one as Mid. The High group represents those who reported high levels of both violence exposure and neglect

of hallucinogen use. The most dramatic finding is in the combined Low group where the growth trajectory both starts in grade seven and ends in grade eleven at zero use. These findings confirm that typically unreported higher levels of neglect and violence experiences are risk factors for youth substance use.

Dispositional Risk Factors

Individuals differ substantially on personality factors. Personality may have a genetic component or be influenced by social experience. Recent advances in genetic science have begun to identify markers for not only biochemical, but also for personality factors that affect substance use. Some personality factors, however, are also influenced by social experience. For example, exposure to violence, neglect, or other features of child maltreatment would be expected to influence dispositions such as hopelessness. Personality measures are important to substance use, whether genetic or social in origin, because they influence the reaction substance use situations and contribute to the reasons for substance use. For example, an individual who has high levels of hopelessness or anxiety sensitivity may be more likely to use drugs to cope with negativity, whereas those with high levels of sensation seeking would be more motivated to enhance positive experiences. These tendencies would be expected to contribute not only to the likelihood of abuse but also to the risk of abuse to specific substances.

Theories of drug abuse vulnerability propose that certain dispositions reflect individual differences in susceptibility to drug reinforcement (Conrod et al. 2000; Cooper et al. 1995; Pihl and Peterson 1995). The PATH study included the Substance Use Risk Profile Scale (SURPS) (Krank et al. submitted; Woicik et al. 2009). The SURPS is a brief scale that was designed to measure four dimensions of personality that are particularly relevant to substance abuse vulnerability. The PATH study confirmed the concurrent and predictive validity of these four dimensions: anxiety sensitivity, hopelessness, impulsivity, and sensation seeking.

Anxiety sensitivity (AS) is the tendency to respond to symptoms of anxiety with greater distress. AS predicts higher levels of a variety of substance-related behaviors in older adolescents, young adults, and high risk populations. The pattern of results suggests that these individuals use drugs for the purpose of managing anxiety (see reviews by Stewart et al. 1999; Stewart and Kushner 2001). Nevertheless, in our sample AS was a protective factor. Higher sensitivities predicted lower levels of use. This difference probably reflects an early avoidance of drug use in particularly sensitive individuals when normative levels of use are fairly low.

Hopelessness (H) and other personality traits related to depression vulnerability, such as low self-esteem and introversion increase the risk for alcohol dependence and opiate use (Conrod et al. 2000). Consistent with these findings, H predicted higher concurrent levels of past year alcohol use, opiate use, drunkenness, and binge drinking. H also predicted future increases in the use of hallucinogens, and two measures of substance misuse, CRAFFT scores, a brief measure of drug and alcohol problems (Knight et al. 2003) and Index of Use scores, a measure of multiple drug use.

Impulsivity (IMP) is associated with polysubstance use, stimulant use, and problem drinking (Conrod et al. 1998; Conrod 2000; Jackson and Sher 2003). Consistent with previous findings, impulsivity was the most consistent and the strongest predictor of substance use and misuse criterion. Higher levels of impulsivity were associated with greater use of alcohol, tobacco, marijuana, hallucinogens, and stimulants. Also consistent with previous work, suggesting impulsivity as a factor associated with polysubstance use and polysubstance problems, impulsivity predicted multiple drug use (Index of use measure) and the number of drug and alcohol problems (CRAFFT).

Sensation seeking (SS) has been related to quantity and frequency of alcohol consumption in adult and older adolescent samples (Conrod 2000; Cooper et al. 1995). In the PATH study with a younger sample of adolescents, sensation seeking independently predicted past year alcohol use and binge drinking. In addition, sensation seeking predicted future increases in drunkenness, binge drinking, past year marijuana, tobacco, and hallucinogen use. Consistent with previous findings, sensation seekers appear at greatest risk for more specific forms of substance use and misuse including heavy drinking.

Social Learning, Disposition, and Substance Use Memories

An indirect, but useful, way to measure social influences is its associative impact through social learning. Social experience leads to the acquisition of learned associations between situations, behaviors, and outcomes. According to social learning theory, substance use associations or expectancies are formed not only through direct experience with substance use, but also through observing others. For example, alcohol outcome expectancies defined as outcomes associated with drinking can be measured in early adolescence, prior to any direct experience in drinking. Implicit substance use associations, memory associations with substance use that are measured implicitly without awareness, are also formed prior to substance use itself. We assume that in early learning about substance use, expectancies and memory associations are particularly useful indices of the net result of social learning opportunities. Effective measurement of the net associative results of social learning provides a proximal set of indices that have proven to be good predictors of substance use transitions.

The preceding sections review some areas of social learning and dispositional factors that contribute to an increased risk of substance use in adolescents during the critical developmental period for substance use initiation and escalation as revealed in the PATH study. Youth, given their social and neurological development, are particularly vulnerable to individual differences in these influences (Bechara and Martin 2004; Luciana et al. 2005). In the next section, the role of memory is considered as a proximal factor in individual substance use transitions in youth. One main assumption in the dual process model proposed here is that social and dispositional influences on substance use decision-making is largely governed by the substance use memories in a multi-trace memory system. These memories may be assessed in several ways that reveal the relative risk of substance use and reflect particular social and dispositional influences. Some of these predictions are tested in the PATH study and will be used to illustrate cognitive influences.

The second assumption, inherent in the dual processing model, is executive control. Executive control has the potential to moderate, both positively and negatively, the impact of social learning and disposition on substance use. This section will conclude by reviewing the evidence that youth have an incompletely developed executive control and the relative level of executive functioning exerts a moderating influence on substance use.

Substance Use Cognitions, Implicit Memory, and Substance Use Transitions

A number of approaches have been developed to assess substance use cognitions. For example, the Modified Drinking Motives Questionnaire asks direct questions about reasons for drinking (Grant et al. 2007). More extensive work has been done on measures of substance use expectancies, especially with alcohol (Goldman et al. 1999). Expectancy and motive approaches target specific areas of cognition that influence behavioral decisions. They should provide a window on the structure and content of the memory system (Goldman et al. 1999). Both approaches have proven valuable, concurrent, and prospective predictors of alcohol use (Goldman et al. 1999; Grant et al. 2007). Expectancy measures have also been shown to be valuable indices of adolescent risk for alcohol use (Dunn and Goldman 1998; Krank and Wall 2006; Smith and Goldman 1994; Smith et al. 1995). One explicit expectancy measure was used in the PATH study.

Despite their utility in predicting alcohol use, these direct methods of interrogating memory have been criticized as having alternative interpretations (Ames et al. 2006; Stacy et al. 2006, 2009; Wiers and Stacy 2006b). Direct measures of substance use expectancies or motives explicitly ask about substance use. Such methods may produce good readouts from long-term memory, but they are also liable to interpretational biases in memory processing. For example, asking about the expectancies of drinking will immediately bring to mind the frequency of drinking. It is possible that demand characteristics may influence the decision to endorse positive statements about drinking. Such possibilities do not eliminate the value of direct measures of expectancies or motives in assessment of risk, but alternative indirect or implicit memory tests provide a different window on the memory system that uniquely predicts substance use transitions (Stacy et al. 1996, 2006; Wiers et al. 2002).

Implicit association tests of substance use memories reduce the potential confounding influences from demand characteristics because they do not ask about substance use. Instead an associative cue is used that will retrieve substance use memories only if the memory system contains the appropriate associative traces (Krank and Wall 2006; Stacy et al. 2006). In the PATH study, two implicit memory assessments were used based on free association measures developed by Stacy (1995, 1997). The *behavior associates* task presents common positive outcomes that may be associated with drinking, such as "having fun" or "relaxing" and asks the subject to write the first word or phrase that comes to mind. In the second task, *homograph associates*, rapid free association responses to ambiguous words, such as "draft" or "pot" are obtained and scored for relevance to their potential associates, in this case alcohol and marijuana respectively. Stacy found that latent constructs based on the accessibility of alcohol-related behavioral and homograph associates strongly predict current and future alcohol use controlling the explicit alcohol outcome expectancies and other risk factors. Other recent work implicated alcohol associations with social situations (Ames et al. 2006), and resulted in the development of new and more sophisticated analytic tools, such as the Implicit Association Test (Greenwald et al. 1998, 2003). The importance of these measures rests on two points; implicit measures predict unique variance not captured by other measures (McCarthy and Thompsen 2006; Stacy 1997; Wiers et al. 2002) and provides a more direct test of long-term memory associations (Stacy et al. 2009).

The potential value of implicit memory associations in the prediction of adolescent risk for substance use transitions is most dramatic when applied to the prediction of future use in young adolescents. In the first year of the PATH study (grades seven to nine), about half of the participants had not ever previously had one or more standard drinks of alcohol. In addition, 76% had never used marijuana. Longitudinal assessment of this population tests risk factors for critical first steps in substance use, the initiation of alcohol and marijuana use. Figure 16-6 shows the frequency of alcohol use as a function of the number of alcohol-related responses to ambiguous words (homographs) in the first year of the study. Clearly seen here are the differential rates of use as a function of these simple implicit associations. Youth with more memory associations with alcohol or marijuana in the PATH study were at significantly greater risk for the initiation and escalation of use of each, respectively. These associations develop during adolescence before youth, and have direct experience with substance use and may provide an implicit measure of the strong prosubstance use social influences faced by many youth.

Reduced Executive Control and the Impact of Implicit Memory

In addition to the messages promoting use that youth experience, they face an additional challenge that reduces their ability to reflectively counter the impulsive influence of substance use associations. Much evidence indicates

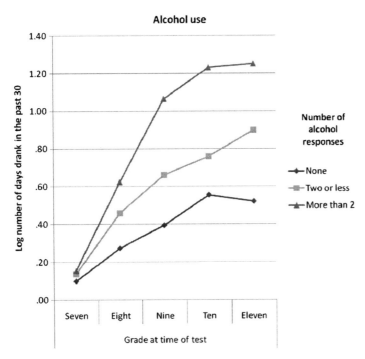

Fig. 16-6.   The prediction of drinking by implicit memory associations. The groups were defined by the number of alcohol related responses to eight ambiguous words that were tested in year one of the study. The log frequency of drinking in the past 30 days (+ 1) is ploted over the five grades covered by the study

that executive control systems in the adolescent brain lag behind the physiological and social changes that accompany adolescent development (Ellis et al. 2004; Luciana et al. 2005; Rubia et al. 2006). Youth have a relative lack of executive control, have a more immediate focus, and are more impulsive than adults. Thus, youth focus socially more outside the family with consequent increased risks before critical reflective control processes develop. Evidence also indicates that adolescents with relatively less executive functioning are more at risk for substance use and abuse (Bechara and Martin 2004; Ellis et al. 2004; Nigg et al. 2006). According to the dual process model outlined here, this differential risk is due to reduced ability to control automatic influences. Thus, executive functioning is important as a moderator of cognitive influences (Stacy et al. 2009). The direct support for this relationship comes from studies that measured indicators of executive control and implicit association in relation to substance use. These studies demonstrate that the prediction of drinking by implicit associations is stronger in adolescents with reduced levels of executive control (Grenard et al. 2008; Thush et al. 2008).

The PATH study did not measure the executive control directly; however, impulsivity is a likely surrogate measure (Whitney et al. 2004). Thus, individuals with higher levels of impulsivity will be more susceptible to social influences leading to substance use. As we reviewed above, the PATH study confirmed the general finding that impulsivity is linked to increased risk of substance use in youth. Finally, we briefly ask the question does the relative level of impulsivity moderate the relationship between implicit memory and substance use. In individuals with higher levels of impulsivity, simple correlations between alcohol homograph scores in year one correlated significantly with all measures of alcohol consumption in year 2. A similar difference occurred in correlations between marijuana homographs and marijuana use. Although these observations may have alternative interpretations and require further study, they are consistent with the findings that executive function may moderate the impact of memory on addition (Grenard et al. 2008; Thush et al. 2008).

Summary and Conclusions

This chapter presented a recently developed approach to adolescent substance use that builds on dual processing models of cognition. Adolescents are assumed to have developmental and individual differences in areas of social experience, dispositional traits, and cognitive functioning that predispose them to the relative risk for transitions to substance use. Social experience factors include exposure to social modeling of positive substance use outcomes and normative substance use, exposure to less supportive family environments, exposure to violence, and experience of neglect. In addition, the present review emphasized three dispositional factors: impulsivity, sensation seeking, and hopelessness that lead to an increased risk of adolescent substance use. Finally, the growing evidence supporting the role of substance use associations as proximal mediators of substance use decisions was presented. Of interest is the evidence that automatic, reflexive, and implicit memories may be particularly relevant to the development of early alcohol and marijuana use. The dual processing model is consistent with this outcome because adolescents seem to have reduced levels of executive control relative to adults. Increased vulnerability occurs because social and developmental influences on automatic memories occur before executive control matures. The dual processing approach is important because it suggests new ways of assessing vulnerability through tests of executive function and memory associations. This approach promises new tools for prevention science (Krank and Goldstein 2006; Stacy et al. 2009; Wiers et al. 2006).

References

Adlaf, E. M., Korf, D. J., Harrison, L., & Erickson, P. (2006). Cross-national differences in drugs and violence among adolescents: Preliminary findings of the DAVI study. *Journal of Drug Issues, 36*(3), 597–618.

Adlaf, E. M., Mann, R. E., & Paglia, A. (2003). Drinking, cannabis use and driving among ontario students. *Canadian Medical Association Journal, 168*(5), 565–566.

Ames, S. L., Franken, I. H. A., & Coronges, K. (2006). Implicit cognition and drugs of abuse. In R. W. Wiers, & A. W. Stacy (Eds.), *Handbook of implicit cognition and addiction* (pp. 363–378). Thousand Oaks, CA, USA: Sage Publications, Inc.

Atkin, C. K. (1990). Effects of televised alcohol messages on teenage drinking patterns. *Journal of Adolescent Health Care, 11*(1), 10–24.

Baddeley, A. D., & Logie, R. H. (1999). Working memory: The multiple-component model. In A. Miyake & P. Shah (Eds.), *Models of working memory: Mechanisms of active maintenance and executive control* (pp. 28–61). New York, NY, USA: Cambridge University Press.

Badre, D., & Wagner, A. D. (2007). Left ventrolateral prefrontal cortex and the cognitive control of memory. *Neuropsychologia, 45*(13), 2883–2901.

Bargh, J. A., & Ferguson, M. J. (2000). Beyond behaviorism: On the automaticity of higher mental processes. *Psychological Bulletin, 126*(6), 925–945.

Bargh, J. A., Gollwitzer, P. M., Lee-Chai, A., Barndollar, K., & Trötschel, R. (2001). The automated will: Nonconscious activation and pursuit of behavioral goals. *Journal of Personality and Social Psychology, 81*(6), 1014–1027.

Bauman, K. E., & Ennett, S. T. (1994). Peer influence on adolescent drug use. *American Psychologist, 49*(9), 820–822.

Bechara, A., & Martin, E. M. (2004). Impaired decision making related to working memory deficits in individuals with substance addictions. *Neuropsychology, 18*(1), 152–162.

Breivik, K., & Olweus, D. (2006). Adolescents' adjustment in four post-divorce family structures: Single mother, stepfather, joint physical custody and single father families. *Journal of Divorce & Remarriage, 44*(3), 99–124.

Choi, Y., Harachi, T. W., & Catalano, R. F. (2006). Neighborhoods, family, and substance use: Comparisons of the relations across racial and ethnic groups. *Social Service Review, 80*(4), 675–704.

Collins, R. L., Ellickson, P. L., McCaffrey, D., & Hambarsoomians, K. (2007). Early adolescent exposure to alcohol advertising and its relationship to underage drinking. *Journal of Adolescent Health, 40*(6), 527–534.

Conrod, P. (2000). Personality, sensitivity to alcohol reinforcement and family history of alcoholism: Different sources of motivation for substance use in high-risk and substance abusing individuals. *Dissertation Abstracts International: Section B: The Sciences & Engineering, 60*(12-B), 6356.

Conrod, P. J., Pihl, R. O., Stewart, S. H., & Dongier, M. (2000). Validation of a system of classifying female substance abusers on the basis of personality and motivational risk factors for substance abuse. *Psychology of Addictive Behaviors, 14*(3), 243–256.

Conrod, P. J., Pihl, R. O., & Vassileva, J. (1998). Differential sensitivity to alcohol reinforcement in groups of men at risk for distinct alcoholism subtypes. *Alcoholism: Clinical & Experimental Research, 22*(3), 585–597.

Cooper, M. L., Frone, M. R., Russell, M., & Mudar, P. (1995). Drinking to regulate positive and negative emotions: A motivational model of alcohol use. *Journal of Personality and Social Psychology, 69*(5), 990–1005.

Corrigan, M. J., Loneck, B., Videka, L., & Brown, M. C. (2007). Moving the risk and protective factor framework toward individualized assessment in adolescent substance abuse prevention. *Journal of Child & Adolescent Substance Abuse, 16*(3), 17–34.

Cuijpers, P. (2003). Three decades of drug prevention research. *Drugs: Education, Prevention & Policy, 10*(1), 7–20.

Dal Cin, S., Gibson, B., Zanna, M. P., Shumate, R., & Fong, G. T. (2007). Smoking in movies, implicit associations of smoking with the self, and intentions to smoke. *Psychological Science, 18*(7), 559–563.

D'Amico, E. J., Ellickson, P. L., Collins, R. L., Martino, S., & Klein, D. J. (2005a). Processes linking adolescent problems to substance-use problems in late young adulthood. *Journal of Studies on Alcohol, 66*(6), 766–775.

D'Amico, E. J., Ellickson, P. L., Wagner, E. F., Turrisi, R., Fromme, K., Ghosh-Dastidar, B., et al. (2005b). Developmental considerations for substance use interventions from middle school through college. *Alcoholism, Clinical and Experimental Research, 29*(3), 474–483.

Deutsch, R., Gawronski, B., & Strack, F. (2006). At the boundaries of automaticity: Negation as reflective operation. *Journal of Personality and Social Psychology, 91*(3), 385–405.

Deutsch, R., & Strack, F. (2006). Reflective and impulsive determinants of addictive behavior. In R. W. Wiers, & A. W. Stacy (Eds.), *Reflective and impulsive determinants of addictive behavior* (pp. 45–57). Thousand Oaks, CA, USA: Sage Publications, Inc.

Doherty, W. J., & Needle, R. H. (1991). Psychological adjustment and substance use among adolescents before and after a parental divorce. *Child Development, 62*(2), 328–337.

Dougal, S., & Rotello, C. M. (1999). Context effects in recognition memory. *American Journal of Psychology, 112*(2), 277–295.

Dougherty, M. R. P., Gettys, C. F., & Ogden, E. E. (1999). MINERVA-DM: A memory processes model for judgments of likelihood. *Psychological Review, 106*(1), 180–209.

Dougherty, M. R. P., Gronlund, S. D., & Gettys, C. F. (2003). Memory as a fundamental heuristic for decision making. In S. L. Schneider, & J. Shanteau (Eds.), *Emerging perspectives on judgment and decision research* (pp. 125–164). New York, NY, USA: Cambridge University Press.

Dunn, M. E., & Goldman, M. S. (1998). Age and drinking-related differences in the memory organization of alcohol expectances in 3rd-, 6th-, 9th-, and 12th-grade children. *Journal of Consulting and Clinical Psychology, 66*(3), 579–585.

Edmond, T., Auslander, W., Elze, D. E., McMillen, C., & Thompson, R. (2002). Differences between sexually abused and non-sexually abused adolescent girls in foster care. *Journal of Child Sexual Abuse, 11*(4), 73–99.

Ellickson, P. L., Collins, R. L., Hambarsoomians, K., & McCaffrey, D. F. (2005). Does alcohol advertising promote adolescent drinking? Results from a longitudinal assessment. *Addiction, 100*(2), 235–246.

Ellis, L. K., Rothbart, M. K., & Posner, M. I. (2004). Individual differences in executive attention predict self-regulation and adolescent psychosocial behaviors. In R. E. Dahl & L. P. Spear (Eds.), *Adolescent brain development: Vulnerabilities and opportunities* (pp. 337–340). New York, NY, USA: New York Academy of Sciences.

Everett, S. A., Lowry, R., Cohen, L. R., & Dellinger, A. M. (1999). Unsafe motor vehicle practices among substance-using college students. *Accident Analysis & Prevention, 31*(6), 667–673.

Faden, V. B., & Fay, M. P. (2004). Trends in drinking among americans age 18 and younger: 1975–2002. *Alcoholism, Clinical and Experimental Research, 28*(9), 1388–1395.

Fagan, A. A., Van Horn, M. L., Hawkins, J. D., & Arthur, M. (2007). Using community and family risk and protective factors for community-based prevention planning. *Journal of Community Psychology, 35*(4), 535–555.

Fergusson, D. M. (2004). Marijuana and madness. *Addiction, 99*(11), 1480–1481.

Fergusson, D. M., Boden, J. M., & Horwood, L. J. (2006a). Cannabis use and other illicit drug use: Testing the cannabis gateway hypothesis. *Addiction, 101*(4), 556–569.

Fergusson, D. M., Boden, J. M., & Horwood, L. J. (2006b). Testing the cannabis gateway hypothesis: Replies to hall, kandel et al. and MacCoun (2006). *Addiction, 101*(4), 474–476.

Fergusson, D. M., Horwood, L. J., & Swain-Campbell, N. (2002). Cannabis use and psychosocial adjustment in adolescence and young adulthood. *Addiction, 97*(9), 1123–1135.

Flight, J. (2007). *Canadian addiction survey: A national survey of canadians' use of alcohol and other drugs: Substance use by youth*. Ottawa: Health Canada.

Flisher, A. J. (2003). Review of stages and pathways of drug involvement. Examining the gateway hypothesis. *South African Journal of Psychology, 33*(4), 269–270.

Gawronski, B., & Bodenhausen, G. V. (2005). Accessibility effects on implicit social cognition: The role of knowledge activation and retrieval experiences. *Journal of Personality and Social Psychology, 89*(5), 672–685.

Glasner, S. V. (2004). Motivation and addiction: The role of incentive motivation in understanding and treating addictive disorders. In W. M. Cox, & E. Klinger (Eds.), *Handbook of motivational counseling: Concepts, approaches, and assessment* (pp. 29–47). New York, NY, USA: John Wiley & Sons, Ltd.

Goldman, M. S., Darkes, J., & Del Boca, F. K. (1999). Expectancy mediation of biopsy-chosocial risk for alcohol use and alcoholism. In I. Kirsch (Ed.), *How expectancies shape experience* (pp. 233–262). Washington, DC, USA: American Psychological Association.

Goldman, M. S., Reich, R. R., & Darkes, J. (2006). Expectancy as a unifying construct in alcohol-related cognition. In R. W. Wiers, & A. W. Stacy (Eds.), *Handbook of implicit cognition and addiction* (pp. 105–119). Thousand Oaks, CA: Sage Publications, Inc.

Graf, P. (1994). Explicit and implicit memory: A decade of research. In C. Umiltà & M. Moscovitch (Eds.), *Attention and performance 15: Conscious and nonconscious information processing* (pp. 682–696). Cambridge, MA, USA: The MIT Press.

Grant, J. D., Scherrer, J. F., Lynskey, M. T., Lyons, M. J., Eisen, S. A., Tsuang, M. T., et al. (2006). Adolescent alcohol use is a risk factor for adult alcohol and drug dependence: Evidence from a twin design. *Psychological Medicine, 36*(1), 109–118.

Grant, V. V., Stewart, S. H., O'Connor, R. M., Blackwell, E., & Conrod, P. J. (2007). Psychometric evaluation of the five-factor modified drinking motives questionnaire – Revised in undergraduates. *Addictive Behaviors, 32*(11), 2611–2632.

Greenwald, A. G., McGhee, D. E., & Schwartz, J. L. K. (1998). Measuring individual differences in implicit cognition: The implicit association test. *Journal of Personality and Social Psychology, 74*(6), 1464–1480.

Greenwald, A. G., Nosek, B. A., & Banaji, M. R. (2003). Understanding and using the implicit association test: I. An improved scoring algorithm. *Journal of Personality and Social Psychology, 85*(2), 197–216.

Grenard, J. L., Ames, S. L., Thush, C., Sussman, S., Wiers, R. W., & Stacy, A. W. (2008). Working memory moderates the effects of drug-related associations on sub-stance use. *Psychology of Addictive Behaviors, 22*(3), 426–432.

Grube, J. W. (1993). Alcohol portrayals and alcohol advertising on television: Content and effects on children and adolescents. *Alcohol Health & Research World, 17*(1), 54–60.

Hamburger, M. E., Leeb, R. T., & Swahn, M. H. (2008). Childhood maltreatment and early alcohol use among high-risk adolescents. *Journal of Studies on Alcohol and Drugs, 69*(2), 291–295.

Hanewinkel, R., & Sargent, J. D. (2007). Exposure to smoking in popular contem-porary movies and youth smoking in Germany. *American Journal of Preventive Medicine, 32*(6), 466–473.

Hawkins, J. D., Catalano, R. F., & Miller, J. Y. (1992). Risk and protective factors for alcohol and other drug problems in adolescence and early adulthood: Implications for substance abuse prevention. *Psychological Bulletin, 112*(1), 64–105.

Hester, R., & Garavan, H. (2005). Working memory and executive function: The influ-ence of content and load on the control of attention. *Memory & Cognition, 33*(2), 221–233.

Hintzman, D. L. (1984). MINERVA 2: A simulation model of human memory. *Behavior Research Methods, Instruments & Computers, 16*(2), 96–101.

Hintzman, D. L. (1986). 'Schema abstraction' in a multiple-trace memory model. *Psychological Review, 93*(4), 411–428.

Hintzman, D. L. (2001). Similarity, global matching, and judgments of frequency. *Memory & Cognition, 29*(4), 547–556.

Houbre, B., Tarquinio, C., Thuillier, I., & Hergott, E. (2006). Bullying among students and its consequences on health. *European Journal of Psychology of Education, 21*(2), 183–208.

Humphreys, M. S., Pike, R., Bain, J. D., & Tehan, G. (1989). Global matching: A comparison of the SAM, minerva II, matrix, and TODAM models. *Journal of Mathematical Psychology, 33*(1), 36–67.

Hyman, S. M., Garcia, M., & Sinha, R. (2006). Gender specific associations between types of childhood maltreatment and the onset, escalation and severity of substance use in cocaine dependent adults. *American Journal of Drug and Alcohol Abuse, 32*(4), 655–664.

Ivis, F. J., Bondy, S. J., & Adlaf, E. M. (1997). The effect of question structure on self-reports of heavy drinking: Closed-ended versus open-ended questions. *Journal of Studies on Alcohol, 58*(6), 622–624.

Jackson, K. M., & Sher, K. J. (2003). Alcohol use disorders and psychological distress: A prospective state-trait analysis. *Journal of Abnormal Psychology, 112*(4), 599–613.

Jacoby, L. L., & Kelley, C. M. (1992). A process-dissociation framework for investigating unconscious influences: Freudian slips, projective tests, subliminal perception, and signal detection theory. *Current Directions in Psychological Science, 1*(6), 174–179.

Jacoby, L. L., Kelley, C., Brown, J., & Jasechko, J. (1989a). Becoming famous overnight: Limits on the ability to avoid unconscious influences of the past. *Journal of Personality and Social Psychology, 56*(3), 326–338.

Jacoby, L. L., Woloshyn, V., & Kelley, C. (1989b). Becoming famous without being recognized: Unconscious influences of memory produced by dividing attention. *Journal of Experimental Psychology: General, 118*(2), 115–125.

Johnston, L. D., O'Malley, P. M., & Bachman, J. G. (2003). Monitoring the future national results on adolescent drug use: Overview of key findings, 2002

Kandel, D. B., & Yamaguchi, K. (2002). Stages of drug involvement in the U.S. population. In D. B. Kandel (Ed.), *Stages and pathways of drug involvement: Examining the gateway hypothesis* (pp. 65–89). New York, NY, USA: Cambridge University Press.

Kandel, D. B., Yamaguchi, K., & Klein, L. C. (2006). Testing the gateway hypothesis. *Addiction, 101*(4), 470–472.

Kirisci, L., Dunn, M. G., Mezzich, A. C., & Tarter, R. E. (2001). Impact of parental substance use disorder and child neglect severity on substance use involvement in male offspring. *Prevention Science, 2*(4), 241–255.

Kirke, D. M. (2004). Chain reactions in adolescents' cigarette, alcohol and drug use: Similarity through peer influence or the patterning of ties in peer networks? *Social Networks, 26*(1), 3–28.

Knight, J. R., Sherritt, L., Harris, S. K., Gates, E. C., & Chang, G. (2003). Validity of brief alcohol screening tests among adolescents: A comparison of the AUDIT, POSIT, CAGE, and CRAFFT. *Alcoholism, Clinical and Experimental Research, 27*(1), 67–73.

Krank, M. D. (2003). Pavlovian conditioning with ethanol: Sign-tracking (autoshaping), conditioned incentive, and ethanol self-administration. *Alcoholism, Clinical and Experimental Research, 27*(10), 1592–1598.

Krank, M. D., & Goldstein, A. L. (2006). Adolescent changes in implicit cognitions and prevention of substance abuse. In R. W. Wiers, & A. W. Stacy (Eds.), *Handbook of implicit cognition and addiction* (pp. 439–453). Thousand Oaks, CA: Sage Publications, Inc.

Krank, M. D., O'Neill, S., Squarey, K., & Jacob, J. (2008). Goal- and signal-directed incentive: Conditioned approach, seeking, and consumption established with unsweetened alcohol in rats. *Psychopharmacology, 196*(3), 397–405.

Krank, M. D., Stewart, S. H., Woicik, P. B., Wall, A., & Conrod, P. J. (submitted). Concurrent and predictive validity of the substance use risk personality scale in adolescents.

Krank, M. D., & Wall, A. (2006). Context and retrieval effects on implicit cognition for substance use. In R. W. Wiers, & A. W. Stacy (Eds.), *Handbook of implicit cognition and addiction* (pp. 281–292). Thousand Oaks, CA: Sage Publications, Inc.

Krank, M. D., Wall, A., Stewart, S. H., Wiers, R. W., & Goldman, M. S. (2005). Context effects on alcohol cognitions. *Alcoholism, Clinical and Experimental Research, 29*(2), 196–206.

Levy, B. J., & Anderson, M. C. (2002). Inhibitory processes and the control of memory retrieval. *Trends in Cognitive Sciences, 6*(7), 299–305.

Locke, T. F., & Newcomb, M. D. (2003). Gender differences and psychosocial factors associated with alcohol involvement and dysphoria in adolescence. *Journal of Child & Adolescent Substance Abuse, 12*(3), 45–70.

Logan, G. D. (1985). Executive control of thought and action. *Acta Psychologica, 60*(2), 193–210.

Luciana, M., Conklin, H. M., Hooper, C. J., & Yarger, R. S. (2005). The development of nonverbal working memory and executive control processes in adolescents. *Child Development, 76*(3), 697–712.

Madden, P. A., & Grube, J. W. (1994). The frequency and nature of alcohol and tobacco advertising in televised sports, 1990 through 1992. *American Journal of Public Health, 84*(2), 297–299.

McCabe, K. M., Lucchini, S. E., Hough, R. L., Yeh, M., & Hazen, A. (2005). The relation between violence exposure and conduct problems among adolescents: A prospective study. *American Journal of Orthopsychiatry, 75*(4), 575–584.

McCarthy, D. M., & Thompsen, D. M. (2006). Implicit and explicit measures of alcohol and smoking cognitions. *Psychology of Addictive Behaviors, 20*(4), 436–444.

McCreary Centre Society. (2005). *Healthy youth development: Highlights from the 2003 adolescent health survey III.* Vancouver, Canada: McCreary Centre Society.

Miller, V., Lykens, K., & Quinn, J. (2007). The effects of media exposure on alcohol consumption patterns in African American males. *Substance Abuse, 28*(2), 41–49.

Mitchell, K. J., Ybarra, M., & Finkelhor, D. (2007). The relative importance of online victimization in understanding depression, delinquency, and substance use. *Child Maltreatment, 12*(4), 314–324.

Moran, P. B., Vuchinich, S., & Hall, N. K. (2004). Associations between types of maltreatment and substance use during adolescence. *Child Abuse & Neglect, 28*(5), 565–574.

Needle, R. H., Su, S. S., & Doherty, W. J. (1990). Divorce, remarriage, and adolescent substance use: A prospective longitudinal study. *Journal of Marriage & the Family, 52*(1), 157–169.

Newcomb, M. D., Scheier, L. M., & Bentler, P. M. (1993). Effects of adolescent drug use on adult mental health: A prospective study of a community sample. *Experimental and Clinical Psychopharmacology, 1*(1–4), 215–241.

Nigg, J. T., Wong, M. M., Martel, M. M., Jester, J. M., Puttler, L. I., Glass, J. M., et al. (2006). Poor response inhibition as a predictor of problem drinking and illicit drug use in adolescents at risk for alcoholism and other substance use disorders. *Journal of the American Academy of Child & Adolescent Psychiatry, 45*(4), 468–475.

O'Leary Tevyaw, T., & Monti, P. M. (2004). Motivational enhancement and other brief interventions for adolescent substance abuse: Foundations, applications and evaluations. *Addiction, 99*, 63–75.

O'Malley, P. M., Johnston, L. D., & Bachman, J. G. (1998). Alcohol use among adolescents. *Alcohol Health & Research World, 22*(2), 85–93.

Overview of findings from the 2003 national survey on drug use and health (2004). Bethesda, Maryland, US: US Department of Health and Human Services, Substance Abuse and Mental Health Services Administration; Office of Applied Studies.

Pacula, R. L., Grossman, M., Chaloupka, F. J., O'Malley, P. M., Johnston, L. D., & Farrelly, M. C. (2001). Marijuana and youth. In J. Gruber (Ed.), *Risky behavior among youths: An economic analysis* (pp. 271–326). Chicago, IL, USA: University of Chicago Press.

Pepler, D. J., Craig, W. M., Connolly, J., & Henderson, K. (2002). Bullying, sexual harassment, dating violence, and substance use among adolescents. In C. Wekerle & A. Wall (Eds.), *The violence and addiction equation: Theoretical and clinical issues in substance abuse and relationship violence* (pp. 153–168). New York, NY, USA: Brunner-Routledge.

Pihl, R. O., & Peterson, J. B. (1995). Alcoholism: The role of different motivational systems. *Journal of Psychiatry & Neuroscience, 20*(5), 372–396.

Pomery, E. A., Gibbons, F. X., Gerrard, M., Cleveland, M. J., Brody, G. H., & Wills, T. A. (2005). Families and risk: Prospective analyses of familial and social influences on adolescent substance use. *Journal of Family Psychology, 19*(4), 560–570.

Robinson, T. E., & Berridge, K. C. (2001). Incentive-sensitization and addiction. *Addiction, 96*(1), 103–114.

Robinson, T. E., & Berridge, K. C. (2004). Incentive-sensitization and drug 'wanting'. *Psychopharmacology, 171*(3), 352–353.

Rodgers, C. S., Lang, A. J., Laffaye, C., Satz, L. E., Dresselhaus, T. R., & Stein, M. B. (2004). The impact of individual forms of childhood maltreatment on health behavior. *Child Abuse & Neglect, 28*(5), 575–586.

Rolls, E. T. (2008). *Memory, attention, and decision-making.* Oxford, England: Oxford University Press.

Royall, D. R., Palmer, R., Chiodo, L. K., & Polk, M. J. (2005). Executive control mediates memory's association with change in instrumental activities of daily living: The freedom house study. *Journal of the American Geriatrics Society, 53*(1), 11–17.

Rubia, K., Smith, A. B., Woolley, J., Nosarti, C., Heyman, I., Taylor, E., et al. (2006). Progressive increase of frontostriatal brain activation from childhood to adulthood during event-related tasks of cognitive control. *Human Brain Mapping, 27*(12), 973–993.

Saffer, H., & Dave, D. (2006). Alcohol advertising and alcohol consumption by adolescents. *Health Economics, 15*(6), 617–637.

Scheier, L. M., Botvin, G. J., & Baker, E. (1997). Risk and protective factors as predictors of adolescent alcohol involvement and transitions in alcohol use: A prospective analysis. *Journal of Studies on Alcohol, 58*(6), 652–667.

Schulenberg, J. E., Merline, A. C., Johnston, L. D., O'Malley, P. M., Bachman, J. G., & Laetz, V. B. (2005). Trajectories of marijuana use during the transition to adulthood: The big picture based on national panel data. *Journal of Drug Issues, 35*(2), 255–280.

Schulenberg, J., Maggs, J. L., Steinman, K. J., & Zucker, R. A. (2001). Developmental matters: Taking the long view on substance abuse etiology and intervention during adolescence. In P. M. Monti, S. M. Colby & T. A. O'Leary (Eds.), *Adolescents, alcohol, and substance abuse: Reaching teens through brief interventions* (pp. 19–57). New York, NY, USA: Guilford Press.

Shiffrin, R. M., & Schneider, W. (1984). Automatic and controlled processing revisited. *Psychological Review, 91*(2), 269–276.

Shimamura, A. P. (2002). Memory retrieval and executive control processes. In D. T. Stuss & R. T. Knight (Eds.), *Principles of frontal lobe function* (pp. 210–220). New York, NY, USA: Oxford University Press.

Smart, R. G., Adlaf, E. M., & Walsh, G. W. (1994). Neighbourhood socio-economic factors in relation to student drug use and programs. *Journal of Child & Adolescent Substance Abuse, 3*(1), 37–46.

Smith, G. T., & Goldman, M. S. (1994). Alcohol expectancy theory and the identification of high-risk adolescents. *Journal of Research on Adolescence, 4*(2), 229–248.

Smith, G. T., Goldman, M. S., Greenbaum, P. E., & Christiansen, B. A. (1995). Expectancy for social facilitation from drinking: The divergent paths of high-expectancy and low-expectancy adolescents. *Journal of Abnormal Psychology, 104*(1), 32–40.

Smokowski, P. R., & Kopasz, K. H. (2005). Bullying in school: An overview of types, effects, family characteristics, and intervention strategies. *Children & Schools, 27*(2), 101–110.

Spoth, R. L., Redmond, C., & Shin, C. (2001). Randomized trial of brief family interventions for general populations: Adolescent substance use outcomes 4 years following baseline. *Journal of Consulting and Clinical Psychology, 69*(4), 627–642.

Spoth, R. L., Redmond, C., Trudeau, L., & Shin, C. (2002). Longitudinal substance initiation outcomes for a universal preventive intervention combining family and school programs. *Psychology of Addictive Behaviors, 16*(2), 129–134.

Spoth, R., Redmond, C., Shin, C., & Azevedo, K. (2004). Brief family intervention effects on adolescent substance initiation: School-level growth curve analyses 6 years following baseline. *Journal of Consulting and Clinical Psychology, 72*(3), 535–542.

Stacy, A. W. (1995). Memory association and ambiguous cues in models of alcohol and marijuana use. *Experimental and Clinical Psychopharmacology, 3*(2), 183–194.

Stacy, A. W. (1997). Memory activation and expectancy as prospective predictors of alcohol and marijuana use. *Journal of Abnormal Psychology, 106*(1), 61–73.

Stacy, A. W., Ames, S. L., & Grenard, J. L. (2006). Word association tests of associative memory and implicit processes: Theoretical and assessment issues. In R. W. Wiers, & A. W. Stacy (Eds.), *Word association tests of associative memory and implicit processes: Theoretical and assessment issues* (pp. 75–90). Thousand Oaks, CA, USA: Sage Publications, Inc.

Stacy, A. W., Ames, S. L., Sussman, S., & Dent, C. W. (1996). Implicit cognition in adolescent drug use. *Psychology of Addictive Behaviors, 10*(3), 190–203.

Stacy, A. W., Ames, S. L., Wiers, R. W., & Krank, M. D. (2009). Associative memory in appetitive behavior: Framework and relevance to epidemiology and prevention. In L. M. Scheier (Ed.), *Handbook of drug use etiology* (pp. 165–182). Washington, DC: APA Books.

Stacy, A. W., Leigh, B. C., & Weingardt, K. R. (1994). Memory accessibility and association of alcohol use and its positive outcomes. *Experimental and Clinical Psychopharmacology, 2*(3), 269–282.

Staton, M., Mateyoke, A., Leukefeld, C., Cole, J., Hopper, H., Logan, T., et al. (2001). Employment issues among drug court participants. *Journal of Offender Rehabilitation, 33*(4), 73–85.

Stein, J. A., Burden Leslie, M., & Nyamathi, A. (2002). Relative contributions of parent substance use and childhood maltreatment to chronic homelessness, depression, and substance abuse problems among homeless women: Mediating roles of self-esteem and abuse in adulthood. *Child Abuse & Neglect, 26*(10), 1011–1027.

Stein, J. A., Newcomb, M. D., & Bentler, P. M. (1987). An 8-year study of multiple influences on drug use and drug use consequences. *Journal of Personality and Social Psychology, 53*(6), 1094–1105.

Stewart, S. H., & Kushner, M. G. (2001). Introduction to the special issues on 'anxiety sensitivity and addictive behaviors'. *Addictive Behaviors, 26*(6), 775–785.

Stewart, S. H., Samoluk, S. B., & MacDonald, A. B. (1999). Anxiety sensitivity and substance use and abuse. In S. Taylor (Ed.), *Anxiety sensitivity and substance use and abuse* (pp. 287–319). Mahwah, NJ, US: Lawrence Erlbaum Associates Publishers.

Strack, F., Werth, L., & Deutsch, R. (2006). Reflective and impulsive determinants of consumer behavior. *Journal of Consumer Psychology, 16*(3), 205–216.

Sussman, S., Stacy, A. W., Ames, S. L., & Freedman, L. B. (1998). Self-reported high-risk locations of adolescent drug use. *Addictive Behaviors, 23*(3), 405–411.

Tanji, J., Shima, K., & Mushiake, H. (2007). Concept-based behavioral planning and the lateral prefrontal cortex. *Trends in Cognitive Sciences, 11*(12), 528–534.

Taylor, K. W., & Kliewer, W. (2006). Violence exposure and early adolescent alcohol use: An exploratory study of family risk and protective factors. *Journal of Child and Family Studies, 15*(2), 207–221.

Thush, C., Wiers, R. W., Ames, S. L., Grenard, J. L., Sussman, S., & Stacy, A. W. (2008). Interactions between implicit and explicit cognition and working memory capacity in the prediction of alcohol use in at-risk adolescents. *Drug and Alcohol Dependence, 94*(1), 116–124.

Tiffany, S. T. (1990). A cognitive model of drug urges and drug-use behavior: Role of automatic and nonautomatic processes. *Psychological Review, 97*(2), 147–168.

Titus-Ernstoff, L., Dalton, M. A., Adachi-Mejia, A. M., Longacre, M. R., & Beach, M. L. (2008). Longitudinal study of viewing smoking in movies and initiation of smoking by children. *Pediatrics, 121*(1), 15–21.

Tucker, J. S., Ellickson, P. L., Orlando, M., & Klein, D. J. (2006). Cigarette smoking from adolescence to young adulthood: Women's developmental trajectories and associated outcomes. *Women's Health Issues, 16*(1), 30–37.

Tucker, J. S., Orlando, M., & Ellickson, P. L. (2003). Patterns and correlates of binge drinking trajectories from early adolescence to young adulthood. *Health Psychology, 22*(1), 79–87.

Van den Bulck, J., & Beullens, K. (2005). Television and music video exposure and adolescent alcohol use while going out. *Alcohol and Alcoholism, 40*(3), 249–253.

Wall, A. (2003). *Violent experiences and adolescent substance abuse among high-risk youth.* Washington, District of Columbia, USA: American Psychological Association.

Wall, A., & McKee, S. (2002). Cognitive social learning models of substance use and intimate violence. In C. Wekerle, & A. Wall (Eds.), *Cognitive social learning models of substance use and intimate violence* (pp. 123–149). New York, NY, USA: Brunner-Routledge.

Wall, A. E., & Kohl, P. L. (2007). Substance use in maltreated youth: Findings from the national survey of child and adolescent well-being. *Child Maltreatment, 12*(1), 20–30.

Wallace, J. M. J., Bachman, J. G., O'Malley, P. M., Schulenberg, J. E., Cooper, S. M., & Johnston, L. D. (2003). Gender and ethnic differences in smoking, drinking and illicit drug use among american 8th, 10th and 12th grade students, 1976–2000. *Addiction, 98*(2), 225–234.

Wallack, L., Breed, W., & Cruz, J. (1987). Alcohol on prime-time television. *Journal of Studies on Alcohol, 48*(1), 33–38.

Whitney, P., Jameson, T., & Hinson, J. M. (2004). Impulsiveness and executive control of working memory. *Personality and Individual Differences, 37*(2), 417–428.

Wiers, R. W., Bartholow, B. D., van den Wildenberg, E., Thush, C., Engels, R. C. M. E., Sher, K. J., et al. (2007a). Automatic and controlled processes and the development of addictive behaviors in adolescents: A review and a model. *Pharmacology, Biochemistry and Behavior, 86*(2), 263–283.

Wiers, R. W., Bartholow, B. D., van den Wildenberg, E., Thush, C., Engels, R. C. M. E., Sher, K. J., et al. (2007b). Automatic and controlled processes and the development of addictive behaviors in adolescents: A review and a model. *Pharmacology, Biochemistry and Behavior, 86*(2), 263–283.

Wiers, R. W., Cox, W. M., Field, M., Fadardi, J. S., Palfai, T. P., Schoenmakers, T., et al. (2006). The search for new ways to change implicit alcohol-related cognitions in heavy drinkers. *Alcoholism, Clinical and Experimental Research, 30*(2), 320–331.

Wiers, R. W., de Jong, P. J., Havermans, R., & Jelicic, M. (2004). How to change implicit drug use-related cognitions in prevention: A transdisciplinary integration of findings from experimental psychopathology, social cognition, memory, and experimental learning psychology. *Substance Use & Misuse, 39*(10), 1625–1684.

Wiers, R. W., & Stacy, A. W. (2006a). Implicit cognition and addiction. *Current Directions in Psychological Science, 15*(6), 292–296.

Wiers, R. W., & Stacy, A. W. (2006b). Implicit cognition and addiction: An introduction. In R. W. Wiers, & A. W. Stacy (Eds.), *Handbook of implicit cognition and addiction* (pp. 1–8). Thousand Oaks, CA, USA: Sage Publications, Inc.

Wiers, R. W., Stacy, A. W., Ames, S. L., Noll, J. A., Sayette, M. A., Zack, M., et al. (2002). Implicit and explicit alcohol-related cognitions. *Alcoholism, Clinical and Experimental Research, 26*(1), 129–137.

Wills, T. A., Sargent, J. D., Stoolmiller, M., Gibbons, F. X., Worth, K. A., & Cin, S. D. (2007). Movie exposure to smoking cues and adolescent smoking onset: A test for mediation through peer affiliations. *Health Psychology, 26*(6), 769–776.

Wilson, H. W., & Widom, C. S. (2008). An examination of risky sexual behavior and HIV in victims of child abuse and neglect: A 30-year follow-up. *Health Psychology, 27*(2), 149–158.

Windle, M., & Wiesner, M. (2004). Trajectories of marijuana use from adolescence to young adulthood: Predictors and outcomes. *Development and Psychopathology, 16*(4), 1007–1027.

Woicik, P. B., Conrod, P. J., Stewart, S. H., & Pihl, R. O. (2009). The substance use risk profile scale: A scale measuring traits linked to reinforcement-specific substance use profiles, *Addictive Behaviors*, DOI 10.1016/j.addbeh.2009.07.001.

Yamaguchi, K., & Kandel, D. B. (2002). Log linear sequence analyses: Gender and racial/ethnic differences in drug use progression. In D. B. Kandel (Ed.), *Stages and pathways of drug involvement: Examining the gateway hypothesis* (pp. 187–222). New York, NY, USA: Cambridge University Press.

Yonelinas, A. P., & Jacoby, L. L. (1995). Dissociating automatic and controlled processes in a memory-search task: Beyond implicit memory. *Psychological Research Psychologische Forschung, 57*(3), 156–165.

Zogg, J. B. (2005). *Adolescent exposure to alcohol advertising: A prospective extension of strickland's model (donald E. strickland)* Univ Microfilms International.

Part V

Life Threatening Transitions in Maturation and Health

Chapter 17

Life Stress and Managing Transitions Unanticipated Change of Course: The Diagnosis of Chronic Progressive Neurological Disease: No Deal!

William D. Weitzel and Judith K. Carney

The first author is a physician and psychiatrist, and the subject of this chapter. It is, thus, related in the first tense. Some two decades ago, he began to develop symptoms. His transitional journey as both a physician and a patient is the focus of this chapter. The second author is an occupational therapist whose career involved working with persons with Parkinson's disease.

The Transition Through an Unanticipated Change of Life Course

James Parkinson described the disease in 1817 in an article "Essay on the Shaking Palsy" or "Paralysis Agitans." It was then published as a monograph by Sherwood, Noely, and Jones. Parkinson's disease is a movement disorder. In the brain there is a small center known as the basal ganglia. Abnormal movement is inhibited by this center. So when the substantia nigra proteins, which alter how the basal ganglia control movement, begin to die the movements are no longer inhibited. There are hundreds of thousands of substantia nigra cells, and these cells begin to die before the first symptoms of Parkinson's disease occur (80%). Hence, the symptoms are the clue to determining the diagnosis. At first, the disease commonly involves one or more of the following symptoms: resting tremor, bradykinesia or slow movement, rigidity, and postural instability. As described by the Mayo Clinic, Parkinson's disease develops gradually, with symptoms varying from person to person and worsening as the disease progresses. There are two scales generally used to understand the progression of the disease -- The Hoehn and Yahr (1967) Staging of Parkinson's and the Unified Parkinson's Disease Rating Scale (UPDRS). Generally, five stages of the disease are considered.
Stage One

1. Signs and symptoms are on one side of the body only
2. Symptoms are mild. Symptoms are inconvenient but not disabling. Usually the symptoms present with tremor of one limb.

From: *Handbook of Stressful Transitions Across the Lifespan,*
Edited by: T.W. Miller, DOI 10.1007/978-1-4419-0748-6_17,
© Springer Science+Business Media, LLC 2010

3. Friends have noticed changes in posture, locomotion, and facial expression

Stage Two

1. Symptoms are bilateral
2. Minimal disability
3. Posture and gait affected

Stage Three

1. Significant slowing of body movement
2. Early impairment of equilibrium while walking or standing
3. Generalized dysfunction that is moderately severe

Stage Four

1. Severe symptoms
2. Can still walk to a limited extent
3. Rigidity and bradykinesia
4. No longer able to live alone
5. Tremor may be less than earlier stages

Stage Five

1. Wheelchair-bound or bedridden unless assisted
2. Cannot stand or walk
3. Requires constant nursing care

Despite extensive studies on the subject, the actual cause is unknown. Some experts think that there may be a combination of genetic and environmental reasons. It is possible that genetics may play a role, but for others it may be a head injury, or an illness, or some environmental factors.

My (WDW) symptoms began in the spring of 1987, when I developed paresthesias in my left lower extremity. At the time, I was involved in a high profile forensic psychiatry case in Eastern Kentucky. My first explanation for my strange new symptom was that I was experiencing a lot of anxiety associated with the trial (Elsie Deskins v Hazel Deskins 1/23/25/1987; Pike Circuit Court).

I tell you that my symptoms began in 1987 but actually they began in the mid 1980s. It was my habit to reward myself with a new suit or sport coat every spring from Hunt Club Clothiers in Cincinnati, which is a men's clothing shop at Fountain Square. I remember being aggravated to learn that my left arm was shorter than my right arm, and this had become an issue every time I would be fitted for a new sport coat or suit. Actually, the left arm was not shorter than the right arm. It just could not be extended straight. It was constantly a little bit flexed at the elbow. So there was a lack of body symmetry between the left side and the right side with respect to my upper extremities. At that point the symptom was known only to me (or so it seemed).

Since I originally blamed my symptom of left extremity paresthesias on anxiety, I expected it would go away after the trial ended, but it lingered. Also, I noticed a tremor beginning in my hands which I attributed to my excessive intake of caffeine with coffee. I tried to pretend that I had no symptoms. But my friends began to pester me to get myself evaluated when my left lower extremity limp became difficult to ignore. In fact, it was there for everyone to notice.

In 1990, I went for a physical exam with my family physician, and he made the initial diagnoses of Idiopathic Parkinson's Disease. Then, I was 47 years old. I remember asking him not to write that conclusion in the chart, and to allow me to see a neurologist for that diagnosis since that would be his specialty. I did so 3 months later in April of 1990 and was told again that I had Idiopathic Parkinson's Disease. I was started on Parkinson's syndrome medications (Sinemet and Amantadine) and my symptoms became less noticeable for the next several years. Then the symptoms returned with more tremors, more rigidity, and more slowness of movement.

My reaction to the diagnosis by the neurologist for Idiopathic Parkinson's Disease was tempered by my own anticipation of the diagnosis. Idiopathic Parkinson's disease means that the etiology is neither understood nor identified. It is a progressive and chronic disorder, which leads to increasing impairment and usually death after the initial diagnosis secondary to aspiration pneumonia or blood clots from the lower extremities after a fall or fracture of the hip. Falls are a frequent and a big part of this disorder as it progresses. The most devastating part of the diagnosis is that there is no cure, and there is no way to arrest the progression of the disease, but there are ways of treating the symptoms as the deterioration continues.

I now find myself in the position of knowing the diagnosis which will probably be the end of me (Parkinson disease and its complications). I am aware of the usual time frame for the course of the disease, and the increasing impairments that develop as one moves closer to the end of the allotted time. An issue will be exiting with dignity. The information that I now have makes each day worth living. I am now quick to rebuke myself for complaining and not taking full advantage of the time that I have.

As a psychiatrist, I have in the course of my practice of 40 years, taken care of many Parkinson's patients for treatment of their depression and insomnia (co-morbidity). I have even cared for some of my friends, as they lived through the final months. I have often heard the bromide "Parkinson's disease is not for sissies." Yet I know that this script and similar scripts are lived out by many other adults in my community, the explanation can be cancer, stroke, multiple sclerosis, COPD, or one of a multitude of other chronic progressive diseases. For me and others, the challenge is to make the most of time left, which with Parkinson's disease can be many years from the time of initial diagnosis.

Primary ego defense mechanisms that I have used to cope with my illness have been denial and bargaining. Looking for guidance from a theoretical model to deal with loss, one is regularly referred to Elizabeth Kubler-Ross M.D. and her work on Death and Dying. You remember that she said that the initial reaction to terminal illness news is shock, then there is denial, then there is bargaining, followed by depression and preparatory grief, and then there is finally acceptance and decathexis.

One of the attractions of the medical profession is that after one achieves an M.D. degree one has the assumption that one has a better control over what happens to one's self. That runs counter to the observation made by a good friend. He found that most of the big decisions made in his life were determined by circumstances outside of his control, and that seems more true than false to me.

Elizabeth Kubler-Ross M.D. (in pages 174–179 of her book), "I think that physicians have it much harder. We are trained to heal, cure, to prolong life and I think that many of us feel like if a patient dies on us it is defeat or failure. Emotionally it is extremely important to appreciate that in terms of the unconscious, we cannot conceive of our own death and in addition we do not differentiate between the wish and the deed. Our society has changed and has become increasingly a death denying society."

We live today with the illusion that since we have mastered so many things we are able to master death also. All patients know when they are terminally ill, whether they have been told or not. Patients usually state that they would like to be told whether it is serious but not without hope. Most, but not all patients pass through the seven stages: Shock, denial, anger, bargaining, depression, and acceptance and decathexis. When these stages occur it's during the interval between the first awareness of serious illness and aware-ness of a foreshortened future. This to me represents the fear of death: "the catastrophic destructive force that comes upon you and you cannot do anything about it."

Bargaining is an especially difficult issue for a physician to deal with. "The most typical part of bargaining is that of promises that are never kept." Patients say that if I could only live long enough for my children to get through high school and then they add college, and then they add I just want to see a grandchild and the list goes on. If in the denial stage they would say no not me. In the anger stage they would say why me. In the bargaining stage they say "yes, me, but" when they drop the "but" it becomes "yes me", then many patients become in touch with their depression and soon the patients accept the inevitable, and experience decathexis from other people and the environment.

1990–1996 were good years for me. My practice was successful and I stayed busy. In 1996, I was asked to be a speaker at a local lawyer's confer-ence involving the use of psychiatric data, including structured tests of psy-chiatric measures. However, by then, my symptoms had become prominent and I developed dyskinesia as my most obvious symptom, which continued to bother me and all the people who had the occasion of working with me. In an attempt to sell myself, one more time, I advocated by presenting the requested material and in the process exposed my symptoms to my special audience.

The years of 1996–2007 were a time of continuing deterioration and a struggle with my own denial. To the point at which there developed a great dichotomy between how I saw myself and how others saw me. I thought that I was fooling a large group of people, but I was only fooling very few. During that time interval, my impairment increased with falls, weakness of the legs, impaired gait, and increasing reliance on a wheelchair and a walker.

In April of 2007, I reached my nadir when I was unable to leave a restaurant under my own power and had to be helped to the car. I then found myself unable to climb up the stairs to my room on the second floor of my house. It became apparent that something needed to be done. I investigated the Deep Brain Stimulation program at the University of Kentucky Medical Center. I then underwent three different brain surgeries including placement of the electrodes – beginning with the left side and followed by the right side, and finally the connection of all the equipment to the pacemaker. I had a good response to this Deep Brain Stimulation technology and my bradykinesia faded, and I became more supple and my mood improved.

I developed a hospital-based staphylococcus infection (M.R.S.A.) after the third surgery. An attempt was made to deal with this situation with IV antibiotics and a PICC line from November 2007 until February 2008. However, it then became apparent that the antibiotics were not going to work, and so the equipment in my brain was taken out in two procedures, first below the neck and then secondly, after a positive culture of a probe in my brain, above the neck. The equipment was removed because of the fear that it would facilitate the spread of the infection. As of April 2008, I had completed a 6-week course of antibiotics and awaited the decision ("after a decent interval") to see if I could remain uninfected, if so, then the procedures were to be started again. There were planned a total of three further surgeries with the placement of the electrode pacemaker, on the left side of my chest rather than the right side where it started. I awaited that implementation with hope, because it worked so well before.

On July 14, 2008 I underwent the first placement of the deep brain electrode and there was a complication. As a result of the procedure, I developed a receptive and expressive aphasia and special treatment was needed at Cardinal Hill Rehabilitation Hospital for treatment of my aphasia. In December of 2008, the surgery (two more brain procedures) was completed. I have spent the subsequent months recovering from my expressive aphasia and learning again how to handle multiple tasks at the same time. My overall physical condition has improved. I can feel a remarkable improvement, and I feel like a "poster boy" for the procedure (deep brain stimulation). My medical course had many serious detours, but at this time, I feel the satisfaction of experiencing an increased quality of life for the immediate future.

A debt of gratitude goes to my sister (Maureen W. Heckman) and my brother (Daniel Weitzel), both for their encouragement and assistance during these times. Murphy's Law seemed to be in the environment and it seemed that if something could go wrong, it would go wrong. Heartfelt gratitude is also expressed toward my Neurosurgeon (Byron Young, M.D.).

After I had been told of my diagnosis, I remember making a fantasy deal with God "bargaining." I agreed that I would do my best to exercise and keep my health up to speed if He would delay the development of symptoms. We never shook on it and so the deal was never consummated.

Another text that I reviewed is called *Managing Transitions: Making The Most of Change* authored by William Bridges 1991, Addison Wesley Publishing Company, Reading Massachusetts. I found the distinction between transition and change as useful ideas, which seemed to have application to me (giving up being a practicing psychiatrist). The starting point for transition is not the outcome but the ending that you will have to make to leave the old situation behind.

Situational change hinges on the new thing, but emotional transitions depend on letting go of the old reality and the old identity that you had before the change took place. Failure to identify and be ready for the ending and losses that changing produces is a large and very singular problem according to the author. Once you understand that transition begins with letting go, you have taken the first step in transition management. The second step is in understanding what really comes after letting go: "the neutral zone." This is the no man's land between the old reality and the new. It is the limbo between the old sense of identity and the new. It is the time when the old way is gone and the new way does not feel comfortable yet. Change happens fast, emotional transition happens much more slowly. The author explained that the neutral zone kind of feels like an emotional wilderness, when it is not clear who you are or what is real. The neutral zone is both a dangerous and a very opportune time. It is the very core of the transition process. It is the time and place when old habits which are no longer adaptive to the situation are extinguished and the new and better patterns of habits begin to take shape. It is the night during which we are disengaged from yesterday's concerns and prepared for tomorrows. It is the chaos in which the old form of things dissolves and from which the new form emerges. It is the seedbed of the new beginning that we seek.

Differentiating "Change and Transition"

Dr. Bridges writes that change is not the same as transition. Change is situational -- the new site, the new boss, the new team, the new rules, and the new policy. Transition is an emotional process that people go through to come to terms with a new situation. Unless transition occurs, the change will not work. Every new beginning has a consequence and every beginning ends something. Change and endings go hand in hand. All changes, even those most longed for, have their melancholy for what we leave behind – a part of ourselves. We must die to one life before we can enter into another. Historic continuity with the past is not a duty, it is a necessity. The first task of change management is to understand the destination and how to get there. The first task of transition management is asking people to leave their homes. One of the most difficult aspects of the neutral zone for most people is that they do not understand it. They expect to be able to move straight from the old to the new. But this trip is not from one side of the street to the other, it is a journey that is not yet understood because it is constantly evolving. A new mindset requires a very significant transition as the old expectations are painfully abandoned and a long difficult journey is made though the neutral zone before a reliable new beginning is in sight.

The greatest challenge is figuring out what is actually changing for you. Remember that changes have both secondary and side effects. Think about your situation and how it could be changed by the indirect fallout from current events. You cannot be sure about such things, for unseen events could change everything further. Decide what is really over for you, what are you going to have to let go of? What are you likely to lose in the transition you face? Not only because the effects of change are complex, but also because one is likely to react with denial when first faced with loss. These thoughts applied to me as necessary when one runs into the "brick wall" of "can't be done" and we are tested to see how much we want to survive and change. Because when one meets the change defining event, one has to transition through the neutral zone to a new identity after giving up the old one, rather than perseverate with old maladaptive habits.

In an interview with Arthur Jones in The National Catholic Reporter in November of 2003 on pages 11–43, Dr. M. Scott Peck (2003) reflected on his experience with Parkinson's disease, which had been diagnosed in 1999, although he reported he certainly had noticeable symptoms by at least 1996. He revealed his feelings and ways of coping in his own solitary fight. He reflected on his own judgment on himself as a parent, he stated "I paid a lot of attention to my writing and my speaking career." "I paid less attention to my children than I should have." During his 25 years of celebrity status he did stick by his vow never to expose his children to the publicity that surrounded him. Peck separated their private and personal lives from his own public writing and his lectures. When asked if he was afraid of death, Peck replied "less than I use to be, but yes, I am still afraid." He has a general message for Parkinson's patients, "if the hand writing on the wall is extremely clear, read it." In other words pick apart your denial, pay attention to the changes that are occurring in your person and body. Peck is concerned about denial because it tends to create difficulties for those who would otherwise willingly love and/or be supportive of the dying person. Dr. Peck discusses his symptoms with scientific distance and curiosity. Dr. Peck's discussion of his Parkinson's disease was introspective, literal and very personal.

This is to be distinguished from the way Dr. Randy Pausch handled his terminal disease, pancreatic cancer. *Wall Street Journal* Saturday/Sunday May 3–4 2008 pages R1 and R3. Dr. Randy Pausch was in his mid-life and a College Professor at Carnegie Mellon University (Pittsburgh), and had received much media attention. The attention was drawn to him by the way he chose to say goodbye to his students and his colleagues. His final lecture to them delivered in September 2007, turned into a phenomenon viewed by millions of people on the internet. Dying of pancreatic cancer, he showed a love of life and an approach to death that many people have found inspiring. For many of his listeners, the lecture has become a reminder of our own future destiny if not as drastically brief. His fate is ours just – sped up. What is remarkable is the zest and positive outlook on life that Dr. Pausch still exhibited when he spoke. He was not involved in self-pity. Dr. Pausch directed his last lecture toward his work family and it seemed difficult for them to imagine a future without him. Since his last lecture, he focused on his actual family, his wife and his three young children aged 6, 3, and 1. He passed away in September 2008.

Dr. Pausch received his actual diagnosis in August of 2007. At the time he had published his book, he had not told his children that he was dying because he still looked pretty good, but he felt an internal urgency that he was trying not to let them pick-up on. Despite childhood dreams and the fortitude needed to overcome set-backs he opined "brick walls are there for a reason and that is to prove how bad that you want something." He celebrated mentors and protégées during his last lecture. He acknowledged how his lecture had inspired others to spend more time with loved ones, to quit indulging in self-pity and to even shake off suicidal urges. Dr. Pausch's advice to his children is "tell the truth" and his addition to that – "all the time" and to "keep having fun every day" and then he recommended the flight attendants advice to us "put on your own oxygen mask before assisting others." Dr. Pausch was an unusual fellow. He certainly presented a creative model for dealing with his terminal illness. His secret seemed to be that he was sublimating his energy by giving back to his family and he was not spending his time pondering his own future and his unfortunate fate. His experience serves as a reminder of our own futures, which will be similar in dénouement if not as drastically brief as his. His fate is ours – just sped up.

Processing this Transition Through Stages of Change

In attempting to understand transition, numerous coping styles emerge. Elizabeth Kubler-Ross M.D., William Bridges, PhD., M. Scott Peck, M.D. (once introduced by Melvin Sabshain, M.D., Medical Director of American

Psychiatric Association as the most famous psychiatrist in the world) and the thoughts and behaviors of Randy Pausch PhD, the Carnegie-Mellon University professor from Pittsburgh. Each has a converging lesson to teach. Dr. Pausch's secret seems to be that he has allowed himself to become focused on his children and his wife. Getting back to them and storing up memories, videos, and interviews to convey his wishes and dreams for them. He has made a list for each child containing some of the fine memories that they have had together. He continued to make memories so that they would continue to remember him a little bit longer as they grow toward adult life and in this way he will continue to have some influence in shaping them even after he is gone (the not unusual wish for immortality).

The model found to be most useful for understanding what is happening to me is Dr. Elizabeth Kubler-Ross's thoughts summarized in her book on *Death and Dying* (Kubler-Ross 1950). However, Dr. Pecks advice "if the hand writing on the wall is extremely clear, read it" is good advice for Parkinson's patients about how to adapt and plan for changes that will take place inevitably, as the disease progresses.

Also, Dr. Randy Pausch's advice to "carpe diem" and "enjoy life as much as you can!" Certainly, the ego defense mechanisms of denial and bargaining as one is coping with this transition and with the loss of certain functions are adaptive in this situation.

The Transitional Journey with Parkinson's Disease

No one wants to hear it, ever. But then one day, there it is, the answer to the puzzling circumstances that have presented themselves to the body. The body is under attack with brain cells dying off daily and creating mean tricks on the body. It is a diagnosis that is supposed to explain why the leg does not move the way you want or why the hands shake when you bring the cup to your mouth. It is a mean trick on the body. So what is the answer to any mean trick on the body, trick it back. It is the kind of trick that does not happen overnight and cannot be cured totally. It can be controlled to a certain extent with medication and therapy but it is still there. It is still able to attack, always. After all, Parkinson's disease is a progressive neurological disease. As the basal ganglia are altered, the substantia nigra cells die, the symptoms intensify. At this point there are medications that allow for more flexibility and mobility, especially in the early stages. But eventually, enough of the cells have disintegrated and the loss is beyond repair. It is becoming more hopeful that a cure will come. Research continues. However, in order to keep the mobility and function, the resistance for now on a daily basis is best served with a form of combined medication timed with mobility and daily functional tasks. There are surgeries as well, deep brain surgeries, to limit some of the symptoms. Before the first symptom is noted, 60–80% of the substantia nigra nerve cells have already died. These keep dying. A combination of medications can help therapy that will allow for a maximum of independence, and participation in activities of daily living can keep a person moving in normal patterns. That is the goal. That is the head fake.

Simple pleasures, daily tasks like getting up from bed or dressing are major tasks of the day. Just trying to raise the arm to the mouth can end in food dropping everywhere, once the tremors begin to take place. Or losing one's sense of gravity and falling backward in space without realizing it feels like a major trick and a huge safety risk. The biggest danger is falling and hitting the head or a head injury. The tricks to the body begin, often starting slowly with a slight tremor of the hand or even the finger that over time runs rampant and furiously as it distances the ability to perform the easiest of tasks. Using adaptive devices, such as a Safety Transfer Pole that can be found now at most medical supply businesses, are simple early solutions to maintaining stability when getting out of bed or on or off the toilet. Most importantly, this simple pole which is spring loaded and extends from the floor to the ceiling combat the difference as the center of gravity is challenged. This simple device provides outside the body stability and allows for continued function. It is also a wonder for the family member or caregiver who is at risk for their own injuries related to assisting their loved one.

My (JKC) first encounters with Parkinson's disease are usually after the disaster, the point at which a second or third fall has happened and the person has still not been told that this disease might have accounted for it. I see it but they do not know it, yet. It is rarely on the first fall, most often a later one. I am the intervening professional, the Occupational Therapist, who specializes in treating people who have suffered falls or have tendencies toward falling, often ending in some orthopedic tragedy, like a broken hip or arm. That is when I am asked to come up with solutions to allow the broken body part to heal and the desire to keep upright and moving. The most important task is maintaining maximum independence and sometimes that is not just walking. But mostly, initially, a person fears most losing that human skill of uprightness and movement. It is the movement sensation that most represents humanness versus other mammal positions. It is, of course, the most difficult to lose along with the ability to feed oneself and verbalize.

So we start with where the person is. Are they walking, bi-pedalness? It is usually reported to me as "I'm not aware of falling backward. I just tripped over something." This is often reported as if the person has no awareness at all of that sensation, until I ask. And, they usually really do not seem to have that sensation. I believe them. The sensation of falling backward is not what they experience. The fall is what they fear, anticipate, and it can be very stressful and anxiety provoking. Sometimes they can recognize that they did fall backward but it does not occur to them, until that moment that I ask, that that was the sensation, in fact. They cannot tell because the center of gravity has moved and the mind perceives it as normal but the body does not. It is the difference between a normal base of support stance where feet are not so far apart and that of a wide base of support and a shuffle gait of the Parkinson's patient. The mind thinks that these small steps are less likely to cause a trip and a fall when in reality it is in fact just what causes the trip over something. I usually start with "initiating and cueing" that it is, in fact, the big steps that will get them there faster and more safely. What I am learning is that it is the cueing that matters almost as much as the size of the steps.

Tackling Everyday

"Cueing" is a verbal trick for the mind. It is like telling the mind to do one task but the end is meant to trigger a different result. It is a trigger to change the mind's idea. To me, it is like a person with a disease like Parkinson's who is focused on movement and continues not to know that their movement skills have been altered. They will often get focused on unsticking their foot from the floor and no matter how hard they try it will not come unglued. Many Parkinson's people describe that their foot feels literally glued to the floor. Often the diagnosis is still unknown to them. I can see it and I can make it conscious to allow that person to continue to keep from allowing the worsening and stiffening to happen. By providing a sensory stimulation, then a gentle pressure to the ankle joint and then pumping the ankle, the foot unglues and a move forward takes place. Using a walker at this stage is critical to prevent falls. There are, of course, the real neurological reasons but what is important here are the practical interpretations of those inner body actual physical changes. That is cuing. This involves the relearning of everything. In separating stiffness and sticking to the floor, there is also the matter that the person's center of gravity has actually gone. Another cue is to focus toward an object further down the hall at the horizon and keep focusing back to that can assist the freezing that is noted especially at doorways.

"Cueing" comes in a variety of forms, and all forms should be used. Cues are not just verbal. Cues can be attention connecting, forcing a person to think about movement. Cues can be auditory. Cues can be visual, like placing a bright piece of red tape on the floor to step over and trick the mind to accomplish a simple goal of stepping over the tape rather than focus on moving a leg. While it might seem slight it is actually quite a large cue to the person. It generates a movement that appears normal, then it works. Cues can make movement less dependent on the automatic pilot. That is the point. Cues force a different route through the brain. That is good. That is the goal.

The resistance of the broken movement patterns to adapt is what is happening everywhere in the body. Walking is, of course, the initial concern. Usually the fall occurs when the person is trying to move forward or turn to get onto the toilet or get into bed. That is when the "freezing" occurs. That is when the body moves and the feet are stuck. It is usually reported as feeling like glue or gum on the bottom of their foot. Whenever suggesting that this is how it feels, the light seems to go off and the patient gives recognition to that symptom. The follow up to this is to offer simple solutions. Keep the ankles flexible. Do ankle pumps before even beginning to stand. Lift the toes and then the heels while sitting. Trick the mind! Rather than making the toe go up first, the trick is to make the body think that the heel will start first. This works every time. Or, step "over the line" tricks the mind to think it is performing a lifting movement not just walk. For freezing, as one passes the doorway I challenge the trick to look far down the horizon to the end of the hallway. Use music, use the beat of music to generate a movement. Request the feet to take "big steps" not little shuffle ones. Get the focus changed. The mind is tricked again. It works. It takes a cue every time but it is possible to find the desired result for the patient.

The Spectrum of Symptoms and Impairments

There are motor and non-motor symptoms. There is depression and executive dysfunction that shows as cognitive impairment. There are sleep disorders where the sleep behavior is fragmented and does not allow full relaxation of the growing rigidity and deprivation of the mind. There is pain and numbness and tingling and low endurance and anxiety. Changes are happening and adaptations cannot always keep up.

First, however, the skill is in assessing, with the diseased person or the caregiver who is taking care of that person. Learning as much as possible about the patient and their symptoms and condition is essential. Being very interested in how all of the sensations are experienced is essential. It matters both to the patient and to the therapist. Knowing where they are in the stage of the disease is so critical to planning for any form of intervention. It is at the earlier stages that one can be most helpful. Stage I and Stage 2 still have unique abilities that one can be trained to adapt, for a while, sometimes a long while. As the disease progresses, it is as much about the caregiver understanding the process as it is about the patient. In the beginning the trick is all about the ability to maintain flexibility, agility of movement, and adaptations to the environment that is critical to allowing for maximum independence. In later stages of the disease the trick is about protecting the joints from their own rigidity that cause fixed contractures. By using simple splints, a shortening of the muscles and tendons can be reduced, probably not totally prevented but reduced.

Interventions with Purpose

Among interventions with a unique purpose for aiding the patient with Parkinson's disease is a new walker, called a U-Step. It was designed and developed by Dr. Jonathan Miller (2007). This patented front caster system provides a unique stabilization for walking. There is a unique U-shape to the walker and a special ability to differentiate tensions for walking in order to adapt to each individual. It is sturdy and allows the person to maintain a more shoulder forward approach for mobility. Because of the stable U-Shape and the sturdiness the person can literally step inside the walker and move with a stronger sense of security. Options to add a laser light as a trigger line to guide against "freezing" actually works. Any kind of physical cueing to eliminate the grips of the disease can be helpful. Other ways to do this same kind of idea include putting red or bright color tape on the floor to "step over" or across the front wheels for the same idea. The cue to "step over" seems to release the glue-like feeling or stuck to the floor sensation that many Parkinson's subject describe.

Eventually, however, the grips of it all take hold and physical mobility is more of a struggle. That is when the use of adaptations and orthotics or splints comes into play. These tools are sometimes ideas and cues but usually involve an actual tool that either assists the prevention of tightening of muscles that eventually can become serious contractures in key joints, such as those affecting fine motor control that allow a person to grasp in order to pull up their pants or lift a spoon or walk. Adapted built up and slightly weighted feeding utensils to combat tremors and flexibility of hand to mouth abilities allow for self-feeding skills as well as preventing spills. Eating can take time but is important for self-esteem and confidence as long as possible. Use of covered cups or nosey cups or divided plates with partitions that allow for scooping food onto a spoon or swing-like spoons sometimes weighted provide another method to combat the tremors with intentional movements. Keeping flexibility and independence in all aspects of the day gives confidence and allows for a quality of life that is slowly being taken away. Of course, this varies depending upon the person and stage of the disease. Tilt-in-space wheelchairs or wedge cushions with gel materials allow for safe positioning and can assist prevention of skin breakdown during the day. Sitting in an upright centered position with arms supported at level height to the table can give just the support needed for self feeding. These kinds of devices serve to keep flexibility and allow for functional lifestyles.

Learning ways to maximize the benefits of therapeutic intervention can be most helpful in transitioning this stressful life experience. The tricks become more aggressive as the Parkinson disease progresses. It is worth the try. It is always worth the try as the medicines and surgeries continue to adapt and offer support. A cure has not been found yet but research continues for this and other chronic progressive neurological diseases. Here are some thoughts on what health care professionals, the patient and family caregivers can do to help provide the best level of care for the patient with chronic degenerative neurological disease.

Take Home Messages for the Patient, Therapist, and Family Members

Learn as much as you can about the disease. New studies and ideas are developing almost as rapidly as the disease itself. Key to maintaining mobility and holding off the inevitable stiffening is physical flexibility and stress reduction. Physical flexibility includes a regimen of moving each joint of the body starting with the neck, shoulders, and moving through the arms and down to the ankles daily. Doing ankle pumps, which means slowly raising the toes and holding for 1–3 s and then placing the foot back on the floor, keeps ankle flexibility which is necessary for balance as well as signaling the mind to move. While the disease itself will try to tighten the muscle tone and control the body movement, a regular exercise routine that counters with flexibility and uses energy conservation techniques to keep active is essential. Some people find that using rhythm such as moving to music assists the mobility attempts, in fact, using a cane when walking or music with a strong beat assists mobility. There are even some programs that use Tai Chi or ballroom dancing, especially in the earlier stages, as a technique for mobility. Try a metronome and move to it whether sitting in a chair or standing. Try the fox trot with someone nearby and use a walker. Energy conservation techniques that lessen the strain on the muscles and allow for continued activities of daily living are another form of maintaining flexibility. Use of tools, such as reachers and sock aids for dressing keep a person engaged on a daily basis. And this, in turn, keeps a person fighting against depression and fear, and allows for use of muscles for other important skills for the day.

Messages for the Patient

Keep moving. Keep every joint flexible. It is a constant struggle but do not give up. Use your strength every day and throughout the day. Get rest and conserve your energy for important moments of the day. Listen to music. Listen because music gives a "beat" which will allow your joints and muscles to move. Enjoy your family and your friends and keep in touch with them. Keep talking. Keep your mind as active as possible. They are your strongest asset. Use them and get your strength from them. Take your medication and time it for a flexible mobility routine every day. Keep trying. No one has one technique that works, but clearly using multiple mobility skills will help maintain what you have.

Messages for the Therapist and Caregiver

Be there. Listen carefully. There is a lot to be learned and gained in paying attention to the daily struggle that families go through with this disease. Consider it as a way to build your own repertoire of skill sets. Learn everything you can about the disease. There are new ideas all the time. Pace any therapy or activity to be timed closely with the medication. There is often a delay from the time of taking the medication to the actual movement result. While medications are important, the emphasis of using these medications in conjunction with regular flexibility and exercise programs in addition to energy conservation techniques cannot be emphasized enough. Pace the day. Do not try to do everything in the morning. Pace it throughout the day. Keep track of all activities and then pace medication and activity and therapy for frequent stress reduction periods. Stress reduction is key to movement relaxation and the ability to move. Keep social. Allow plenty of time before getting to a doctor's appointment or going to the store to prevent rushing which will just interfere in your attempts to assist. Allow the person to do as much as they can and this might mean pushing them to do it also. Start each mobility effort with a simple stress reduction and cueing for moving or even for eating. This serves multiple purposes. While it might be easier to just get the clothes on someone, for example, it defeats the real purpose of providing some confidence and encouragement for growing independent and additionally moving the body in the process. Stress reduction is important for Parkinson's person but it can do wonders for people working with the disease as well. Allow time for yourself for stress reduction. Find a friend to share your stories and successes with. These are invaluable for self strengthening. Keep yourself strong.

Messages for the Family Members

Learn everything you can about Parkinson's Disease. And then, be there. Listen carefully to the person with the disease. They usually are able to communicate quite well about what they are experiencing. There is a lot to be learned and gained in paying attention to the daily struggle. Most importantly, you are also experiencing the disease. It impacts the caregiver and the family member. It is just not in your body. But you feel it also. You take it with you wherever you go. Pace yourself. Take time for yourself. Learn everything you can about the disease. There are new ideas all the time. While medications are important, the emphasis of using these medications in conjunction with regular flexibility and exercise programs in addition to energy conservation techniques cannot be emphasized enough.

References

Bridges, W. (1991). *Managing transitions making the most of change.* Reading, MA: Addison Wesley Publishing Company.
Elsie Deskins v Hazel Deskins. (1987). 1/23/25/1987: Pike Circuit Court.

Hoehn, M., & Yahr, M. (1967). Parkinsonism: onset, progression and mortality. *Neurology, 17*(5), 427–42. PMID 6067254.

Jones, A. *National Catholic Reports* "Interview with M. Scott Peck, M.D.".

Kubler-Ross. E. (1950). *On death and dying*. New York: Macmillan.

Miller, J. (2007). In-Step Mobility Products Corp., Skokie, IL.

Pausch, R. (2008). Randy Pausch ABC Special about the "Last Lecture", April 2008. Google Video. 2008-04-11. http://video.google.com/videoplay?docid=26526342800 2185148. Retrieved 2008-08-11.

Wall Street Journal. Saturday/Sunday May 3–4 2008 14 pages R1 and R3.

Chapter 18

Transitions Throughout the Cancer Experience: Diagnosis, Treatment, Survivorship, and End of Life

Dorothy Ann Brockopp, Krista Moe, Judith A. Schreiber, and Sherry Warden

Introduction

Transitions are associated with life events that require individuals to consider the direction and meaning of their lives while moving from one stage or state to another. For most individuals, a diagnosis of cancer is such an event. Success in transitioning from one cancer related event to the next is dependent on a number of factors, including: prognosis, ability to cope, social support, and the care provided. While statistics on morbidity and mortality related to cancer are less than positive, progress has been made and an increasing number of individuals are living longer, more productive lives in remission from their disease. As a result, it is now more important than ever to understand the kinds of transitions that cancer patients face as they cope with the challenges of their condition.

Estimates provided by the American Cancer Society (2008a) suggest that 1.4 million new cases of cancer will be diagnosed in the United States in 2008 and approximately 1,500 Americans will die each day from the disease. The terms cancer and malignancy refer to more than 100 diseases characterized by the uncontrolled growth and spread of abnormal cells. Specific causation is difficult to determine, in part because both internal (e.g., genetic predisposition) and external factors (e.g., tobacco, radiation) are involved and they may occur alone or in sequence. To add to the complexity of causation, various immune conditions can lead to a diagnosis of cancer. In addition, a number of years can pass between the initiation of the malignant process and diagnosis of the disease.

Symptoms, treatments, side effects of treatments, and even longevity of life for a cancer patient can vary greatly. For example, the 5-year survival rate of pancreatic cancer, the deadliest form of the disease, is estimated at 5% or less (Jemal et al. 2008) while relative survival rates for women diagnosed with breast cancer are 89% at 5 years, 81% at 10 years, and 73% at 15 years (American Cancer Society 2008b). Treatments can include radiation, surgery, chemotherapy, immunotherapy, and/or other targeted approaches in combination or alone. Side effects of treatment are often debilitating and usually include fatigue, nausea, weakness, anxiety, and a decrease in the ability to

From: *Handbook of Stressful Transitions Across the Lifespan*,
Edited by: T.W. Miller, DOI 10.1007/978-1-4419-0748-6_18,
© Springer Science+Business Media, LLC 2010

perform the activities of daily living. Patients may also experience hair loss, pain, depression, and diminished appetite (Hanna et al. 2008; Morrow et al. 2002). For some patients, medications can relieve nausea, anxiety, and pain. There are a number of causes of fatigue as well as interventions that will assist cancer patients with this problem. Unfortunately, it remains a prevalent complaint. Variation in both prognosis and treatment among various malignancies adds to the uncertainty at diagnosis.

The cancer experience, from diagnosis through treatment to survivorship, is fraught with numerous challenges and transitions. Individuals receive an anxiety-producing diagnosis and then face treatment options that are often accompanied by serious and debilitating side effects. The journey is usually long and arduous and the threat of mortality is a constant companion. Using the Experiencing Transitions model (Meleis et al. 2000) as a framework, this chapter describes the events that are likely to trigger transitions and their potential sequelae as identified in the literature and occurring in clinical interactions.

Theoretical Framework

A change in health status from apparent well-being to a life-threatening diagnosis can prompt a number of psychological, social, and spiritual transitions. At this point in time, people tend to re-evaluate their lives, and as a result, often make significant changes. Effective coping during these transitions is mediated by the event that triggers the transition, experiences during the transition, interactions with others, and environmental conditions surrounding each trigger. Essential properties of transitions cited by Meleis et al. (2000) in the Experiencing Transitions Model include: awareness, engagement, change and difference, time span, and critical points and events.

Awareness of the transition from health to diagnosis, diagnosis to treatment, and treatment to survivorship is influenced by individuals' perception of the disease. How individuals perceive the impact of a cancer diagnosis on their lives can affect their transitions throughout the cancer experience. Knowledge of their particular condition and recognition of movement from one state of being to another (Chick and Meleis 1986) may also enable positive adjustment to their situation. Their degree of awareness may influence their ability to effectively complete the transition from one set of events to another.

Transitioning from one phase to another may be facilitated by individuals' engagement in the process. Engagement refers to the level of involvement in the situation at hand. Highly engaged individuals actively seek knowledge regarding their condition; look for role models; actively prepare for future events and initiate changes in usual activities as appropriate. For example, a professor at Carnegie Mellon, Randy Pausch, in his book *The Last Lecture* (2008) describes his experience with pancreatic cancer. In his book, he outlines his in-depth search for information that began the day he was diagnosed. When he discovered that his cancer was incurable, he began preparing to leave his family. This preparation for the end of life involved numerous changes, including moving to another city to be closer to extended family and deciding what kind of legacy he wanted to leave his children.

Change is a universal characteristic of transitions in chronic illness. Whether an individual makes a change or is considering a change, the concept of change permeates the cancer experience. For example, a young woman whose cancer necessitated removing her leg below the knee had numerous changes to consider. She was from a culture that would marginalize her because of her disability. She would not marry and would live a life that, from her perspective, was unacceptable. As a result, she refused surgery and died 2 years later.

Transitions in chronic illness, like cancer, include dealing with changes in psychological states. Potential psychological problems include bouts of depression, anxiety, anger, and a sense of helplessness. For example, patients may become increasingly anxious and somewhat depressed while waiting for treatment following diagnosis. During the treatment process, their distress may diminish or worsen. Distress often increases following the end of the treatment until their 6 month follow-up visit.

Cancer patients frequently face changes in social status and relationships. Following the diagnosis, many individuals feel that they are "different" in relation to family, friends, and colleagues. They complain of isolation and report changes in their social circle because of their condition. In addition, partner communication is often impaired, which increases the individual's sense that they are different and perhaps undesirable (Lauver et al. 2007).

Variability over time and inconsistency of response are characteristic of transitions triggered by specific events. For example, loss of body parts may initially bring about feelings of grief and anger that may not completely disappear. These feelings often vary over time even when some form of acceptance is reached (Lauver et al. 2007). Specific events such as diagnosis and/or end of treatment may initiate the beginning of a transition. Triggers for psychological, social and/or spiritual, transitions are not as clearly identifiable. This potential variation over time suggests that assessment of well-being of cancer patients needs to occur at multiple points following diagnosis.

The Diagnosis of a Potentially Life-Threatening Disease

How individuals perceive cancer as a life-threatening disease, how much knowledge they have regarding their diagnosis, and their recognition of probable lifestyle changes can influence their response to a diagnosis. Based on these factors, a diagnosis of cancer can present a crisis of major proportions or simply a challenge to overcome. For most individuals, fear of death and concerns regarding the effects of toxic and difficult treatments and the possible loss of body parts are common responses to the diagnosis. The word "cancer" is commonly equated with death, pain, and suffering. Prognostic uncertainty is a major concern and can evoke feelings of depression and/or prolonged anxiety. Current research notes that psychological distress and diminished quality of life are associated with the diagnosis of a potentially life-threatening cancer (Golant et al. 2003). Some research, however, suggests that the cancer experience can lead to both positive life changes and personal growth (Cordova et al. 2001).

Individual health-seeking behaviors may also affect acceptance of a cancer diagnosis. Awareness in the form of specific knowledge about the disease can be more or less important to patients at the time of diagnosis. There are different personality characteristics related to information seeking. Monitors are those individuals who actively pursue information, while blunters prefer not to know anything more than is absolutely necessary (Miller et al. 2001). Therefore, the task for health care providers is to provide information according to patients' needs.

Engagement in the cancer diagnosis process may be partially dependent on the social context of individuals as well as their personalities. Variation in response to the diagnosis may be related to the amount and/or type of social support available. The less isolated and "different" patients feel, the more likely they are to engage in productive coping strategies. The meaning individuals ascribe to the threat (Linden et al. 2005) is also important to effective coping. How they perceive their disease and understand its effects influences their response. Reassurance from family, friends, and health care providers that they are willing to remain supportive throughout the cancer experience is important to the well-being of the newly diagnosed cancer patient (Holland and Holahan 2003; Spiegel et al. 2007; Burgess et al. 2005).

Ptacek et al. (2002) found that among men diagnosed and treated for prostate cancer, their degree of adjustment was largely dependent on perceived social support. Strong social support facilitated effective coping. Five domains of coping were measured: problem-focused, support-seeking, blaming self, wishful thinking, and avoidance. Men who perceived less support expended more effort across these five domains, while those who perceived more support relied solely on support-seeking and problem-based coping. The conclusion of this and other studies suggests that social support is an important factor in how well individuals cope with the disease.

In addition to family, friends, and healthcare providers, employers can make an important difference in the lives of individuals diagnosed with cancer. Shortly after diagnosis, concerns about employment and the ability to remain productive throughout the treatment often arise. Employers who understand the demands of treatment, the associated distress, and the length of time the treatment will take can provide support for the employee. Given support, changes resulting from diagnosis and treatment, don't seem as overwhelming. It is important to note that it is the individual's perception of support that is related to the well-being and/or adjustment to disease. One close friend can be as meaningful to one individual as ten family members might be to another (Holland and Holahan 2003).

Based on genetic predisposition, some individuals are not surprised by a diagnosis of cancer. Most however, express disbelief due to the absence of symptoms. Randy Pausch, the professor at Carnegie Mellon, commented that "…the greatest thing of cognitive dissonance you will ever see is that I am in really good shape. In fact, I am in better shape than most of you (2008)." Mullen (1985), a physician diagnosed with cancer at age 32 stated that "I had been healthy, athletic and free of pain, but with the diagnosis I became formally sick." Treatment choices, potential side-effects, and prognosis are in the forefront at this point in the cancer experience. A nurse diagnosed with Hodgkin's, comments, "my physical recovery from treatment took about 6 months but my psychological, emotional and social recovery took years." She also stated that "…the emotional trauma of the cancer diagnosis lingered long after the scars had healed" (Doell 2008).

Spirituality is increasingly viewed as an important factor in maintaining physical and emotional health in the face of a life-threatening illness. Contextually, Americans are a religious people with 90% believing in God and 80% claiming they pray weekly. Most cancer patients turn to their faith or their religion to provide them with support at diagnosis and throughout the cancer experience (Krupski et al. 2006). For a few, religion or faith in God doesn't play a role in their disease. For example, findings from a study of men diagnosed and treated for prostate cancer provide evidence of the potential power of religion. These men found religious activities and faith in God or a higher power to be highly valuable as they navigated diagnosis, treatment, and survivorship of their disease (Bowie et al. 2004).

Spiritual awareness relates to the experience of newly diagnosed cancer patients. As individuals recognize their diagnoses as a life transition event, they frequently review their beliefs. Some will alter their world views and some will experience a deepening of their faith. In many instances, a transformation in formal (religious) or informal (faith) belief systems may occur (Vachon 2008). As individuals contemplate their own mortality and revisit the meaning and purpose of their lives, they may need to adjust their theological view (Gall and Cornblatt 2002). Spiritual change may occur immediately at the time of diagnosis or throughout the cancer experience, particularly at points of transition.

The way individuals use their beliefs to cope with cancer is reflected in the construct "religious coping." Religious coping instruments categorize how individuals use their belief in God to cope with life events. Coping strategies that are seen as helpful (e.g., belief in a benevolent God) in this situation are generally associated with greater well-being and health status while non-helpful strategies (e.g., belief in a punishing God) are related to a decline in health (Pargament 2007). Encouraging cancer patients to use helpful religious coping strategies may enable them to deal more effectively with their disease.

The transition from seemingly good health to the diagnostic or acute stage of the cancer experience is often emotionally difficult for the individuals involved as well as their networks of friends and families. Feelings of isolation, helplessness, and anxiety predominate. Most patients want to initiate treatment as soon as possible and look to the time when they can feel "cured" (Mullen 1985). The diagnosis of cancer is the trigger that propels individuals into this life transition from good health to a potentially devastating chronic illness. Awareness, engagement, change and difference, time span and critical points and events are important factors in how well individuals make transitions.

Response to Treatment

Most cancer patients face treatment that is at the very least uncomfortable, and at its worst, debilitating. They move from a frightening diagnosis to an uncertain prognosis. Fatigue and depression are major concerns associated with chemotherapy (Payne et al. 2006; Spelten et al. 2003). Among women treated for breast cancer; nausea, pain, anxiety, depression, difficulty in concentrating, and peripheral neuropathy may also occur (Byar et al. 2006; Smith et al. 2008). Many of these symptoms are difficult to treat and often occur in clusters. When symptoms are severe, concerns regarding ability to work and overall quality of life arise. If the response to treatment interferes with an individual's ability to work, financial worries develop (Rendle 1997).

Negative responses to treatment and incomplete knowledge regarding symptoms can be detrimental to the patient's well-being. There is some evidence to suggest that differing responses to treatment are, in part, psychological. Expectation and anxiety have both been identified as leading to severe symptoms, particularly nausea, following chemotherapy (Montgomery and Bovbjerg 2003; Booth et al. 2007). Research regarding differences in response among cancer patients to the same treatment is limited. Even when demographic variables such as age and overall health status are considered, response differences remain.

Timing is important when examining the treatment trajectory. While most cancer patients look forward to the end of treatment, there is a downside to leaving the continuous support and care provided. Questions can be quickly addressed and reassurance given when patients are carefully monitored and health care providers are readily accessible. In most cases, when treatment is complete patients are given an appointment 6 months from the date of the last treatment. For that 6 month period the access to information they've had during their treatment phase diminishes precipitously. The continual professional support and caring related to their disease is gone. Many individuals with cancer become overly concerned with mild symptoms that may be unrelated to their disease. They want reassurance that the cancer has not returned. This period of time is particularly difficult because remission is not yet certain and for most cancer patients the fear of recurrence is ever present (Boyle 2006).

Critical points related to treatment include; the beginning and ending of the treatment protocol as well as the follow-up appointment at 6 months. During treatment, continued awareness of patients' health status, changes due to the side-effects of treatment, and their feelings about being different due to hair loss or surgery are in the forefront of their concerns. Follow-up should include a survivorship treatment plan that addresses long term treatment effects as well as psychosocial and spiritual needs.

Surviving Cancer

The conceptualization of survivorship in relation to cancer has changed dramatically over the years. As advances in early detection have occurred along with improvements in treatment, the term "surviving" has gone from meaning a prescribed period of time post-diagnosis without recurrence to a process that encompasses all of the problems, needs and challenges facing individuals living with the disease (Farmer and Smith 2002). This phase of the cancer experience is an increasingly important area of research and is a priority for most cancer organizations and foundations across the country (Boyle 2006). In 2005, the Institute of Medicine produced "*From Cancer Patient to Cancer Survivor: Lost in Transition*" (Hewitt et al. 2006) a report giving recommendations for dealing effectively with survivors.

Cancer survivorship is presently thought to extend from diagnosis throughout life. The National Coalition for Cancer Survivorship's definition, coined in 1986, is "From the moment of diagnosis and for the balance of life, an individual diagnosed with cancer is a survivor." Emphasis on survivorship is based on the fact that cancer patients are living much longer. Forty-five percent of individuals diagnosed with cancer worldwide will be alive in 5 years (Cancer Research UK 2008). Given the often disabling aspects of many treatments, living longer with cancer has implications for cancer patients, their families and all aspects of the health care system. As individuals are living longer following diagnosis, long-term physical problems resulting from treatment are more prevalent (Bird and Swain 2008). Depending on the diagnosis and type of treatment, cardiac difficulties, urinary incontinence, sexual problems, and chronic pain are potential long term sequelae (Viale and Yamamoto 2008; Yu Ko and Sawatzky 2008). These long term physical difficulties can lead to a variety of psychological problems such as chronic stress and depression.

The concept of survivorship as it relates to cancer is not universally accepted. While the literature is filled with reports regarding the importance of survivorship as a journey that starts with a diagnosis of a potentially life-threatening disease, some individuals disagree with this concept. Shelley Lewis (2008), author of *Five Lessons I Didn't Learn from Breast Cancer*, has a different perception of the cancer experience. She doesn't want to be labeled in any way that reflects an association with her disease.

Lewis' perceptions contrast significantly with the prevailing literature. She states that individuals shouldn't be described as "survivors" when the possibility of recurrence is always present. Lewis prefers the label "no evidence of disease *NED*" to survivor. She sees survivors as those people who make it through one time life events; for example individuals who live through a plane crash. She talks not about "battling" breast cancer, but rather about "hosting" a chemical and radiological assault on her body. She wasn't aware of being "attacked" by cancer, as described by other patients, until her doctors told her she had the disease. While some may take issue with the concept of survivorship, an awareness of the challenges associated with a longer lifespan following diagnosis remains an important shift in focus for health care providers. An emphasis on consistent follow-up and investigation of long term effects of treatment are two positive results of the "survivorship" movement. The awareness of the transition from treatment to survivorship that has occurred among health care providers is described by Aziz and Rowland (2003). They cite a paradigm shift that takes the care of cancer patients beyond treatment; away from a medical-deficit model to an approach that involves all disciplines over the lifetime of the individual.

Life change is another transition characteristic that is inherent in the movement from conclusion of treatment to survivorship. Over the years, considerable research has addressed the problematic nature of living with cancer. Numerous investigations have addressed the depression, anxiety, isolation, and helplessness that result from a cancer experience (Aziz and Rowland 2003). For many years research has focused on the problems and challenges associated with the diagnosis and treatment of cancer. More recent investigations have examined the possibility that this crisis, as with other crises, could lead to personal growth. Patients with a variety of cancer diagnoses claim that the experience has led to positive life changes. They evaluated their lives following this particular crisis and chose to move in new directions. There is empirical evidence, although limited, regarding positive changes following a diagnosis of cancer. Though many patients experience positive growth, it is unlikely that all individuals will grow from the experience. Clinicians are cautioned not to convey to patients directly or indirectly that they are "expected to make positive changes" (Cordova et al. 2001). In addition to Lewis' (2008) concerns regarding the notion of survivorship she claims that her experience didn't bring her wisdom or positive change. She felt an expectation from others that she should grow personally. For her, it was enough to just get through the diagnosis and treatment.

Patients' views of life after a cancer diagnosis, is of particular importance to the concept of survivorship. Questions like: when do individuals believe they are survivors? Do people want to be referred to as "survivors"? remain unanswered. While health care providers view diagnosis as the critical point or trigger that initiates survivorship, cancer patients may not agree. Randy Pausch (2008) was told that he had three to 6 months of good health left. Would he have considered himself a survivor during that period of time? The paradigm shift from cancer victim to survivor suggests that individuals may be facing a chronic rather than an acute condition. While it has helped health care providers and patients stay involved in a process of care beyond immediate treatment, cancer patients themselves may not welcome the label.

The components of the Experiencing Transitions Model (Meleis et al. 2000) can be identified in the survivorship period. Awareness of the meaning of survivorship and its implications, events that may or may not trigger the notion of survivorship, long term changes that often occur, and the level of engagement are integral components of the cancer journey from diagnosis, through treatment, and into the post-treatment or survivor stage.

End-of-Life

Prior to the work of Elizabeth Kubler-Ross (1975), many individuals diagnosed with cancer were not told of the seriousness of their disease. She discovered that patients dying from cancer were usually aware of impending death at some level, but were unable to get confirmation from their health care providers. She notes some patients felt relief as their intuition was confirmed even though the news was not positive. This was true for Randy Pausch (2008) who, when diagnosed with one of the most lethal forms of cancer, stated that he had no feelings of gratitude for his diagnosis but was grateful for the advanced notice of his death.

The critical event or trigger that initiates the dying phase of the cancer experience usually occurs when it is clear that treatment will no longer halt the progression of disease. In some instances, cancer patients will ask their physician to withhold further treatment and thus initiate the dying phase themselves. An awareness of quality of life implications often determines an individual's actions. Knowledge regarding physical deterioration, pain control, and support available factors into whether or not patients want to live each day with enthusiasm or end their lives as quickly as possible (Chochinov et al. 2006). Pausch (2008) wanted to live every minute enjoying what was most important to him; his family.

Multiple concerns frequently arise throughout this transition. Patients may see themselves as a potential burden to others. As they deteriorate physically, they may feel that their dignity as a human being is compromised on a regular basis. Maintaining optimal quality of life during this period is a challenge for family members and healthcare providers. Given the complex medical problems most dying patients experience along with the emotional difficulties inherent in dying, the transition to the dying phase of the disease may be the most difficult of the four transitions. Changes in relationships, grief related to loss of further opportunities to complete life tasks, and the experience of a variety of disabilities are only a few of the potential difficulties.

In the past, care for individuals at the end-of-life received considerable criticism (Institute of Medicine 1997). Medical care was described as too aggressive as well as non-responsive to the needs of patients and families. National committees on care at the end of life stated that the values and preferences of patients and families were not respected. As a result of these reports, along with concerns expressed by national organizations and funding agencies, improvements in end-of-life care have occurred.

In 2002 a definition of palliative care, along with guidelines for care, emerged from the work of several organizations around the world including the World Health Organization (Person 2004). Since that time, palliative care has been recognized as both a philosophy and a structure for providing effective care. The goal of palliative care, for both in-patients and out-patients, is to achieve optimal quality of life for dying patients and their families as well as individuals suffering from debilitating chronic illnesses. The patient and family are seen as the unit of care because death and dying have such a profound effect on all individuals involved. As cure is no longer an option, physical interventions are routinely used to improve comfort levels (Kernohan et al. 2006). While symptom management is a major focus, other services are readily available. Support to diminish, emotional, social, and spiritual concerns is provided. Palliative care can assist cancer patients to die in a manner that is in keeping with their preferences. Hopefully death comes with emotional peace and physical comfort.

Summary

The model Experiencing Transitions (Meleis et al. 2000) is useful in understanding the movement from diagnosis to treatment and treatment to survivorship or death in relation to cancer. Major concepts of the model; awareness, engagement, change and difference, time span, critical points, and events are characteristic of each transition. Knowledge and perception may differ across individuals, but are important to the patient's search for optimal quality of life. Engagement in the cancer journey is dependent on one's social context, personality, and diagnosis. Change is universal throughout each transition. Societal expectations and cultural dictates can moderate the individual's perception of being different as a result of the disease. Critical points that precede a transition may be clearly defined, as in diagnosis, or occur gradually as in survivorship.

The complexities of the cancer experience are difficult to describe in full and responses to the experience are equally complex. Physical, social, and spiritual changes frequently occur, and "life-changing" is a common descriptor for the journey. While variation in response to a diagnosis of cancer is typical, the Experiencing Transitions model helps to articulate commonalities within the cancer population.

Cancer patients frequently have questions for health care providers from diagnosis through survivorship. Questions at the time of diagnosis include: How bad is this really? Now what? What are my options? Who is the best doctor? Which is the best clinic? How will this diagnosis affect my life? Now? In the future? Health care providers need to answer questions to the best of their ability, as they arise. As treatment begins more difficult questions must be addressed. Patients want to know how to handle the side-effects of treatment, what lifestyle changes they may need to make and how they will know if the treatment is effective. Given the variation in physical and psychological responses to treatment, health care providers are limited in their ability to provide useful information. They can provide general information or descriptions of how most people respond.

Survivors ask "Now what?" They need to move on and yet having considered the possibility of dying; their lives may never be the same. They fear recurrence of the disease and need the support of the health care community to provide reassurance regarding their condition. For parents, there are concerns about raising their children should cancer return. Others worry about an uncertain future.

When cancer patients learn that remission from disease is no longer possible, their questions turn to concerns for those left behind. They want to know how family members will manage, what plans need to be made and what kind of care will be required as death approaches. Can you control my pain? How long do I have? Can I remain at home? These are the frequently asked questions as patients contemplate the end of their lives.

Health care providers can assist their patients at any point in the cancer experience by answering questions as honestly as possible, providing information regarding needed psychosocial resources, and giving reassurance as to the kind of physical care that is available to control pain and maintain optimal quality of life. In keeping with the philosophy of survivorship, the relationship between health care providers and cancer patients need to be seamless and ongoing for the remainder of patient's lives following diagnosis.

References

American Cancer Society. (2008a). *Cancer facts and figures 2008*. Retrieved March 1, 2008, from http:www.cancer.org/downloads/STT/2008CAFFfinalsecured.pdf.

American Cancer Society. (2008b). *Breast Cancer Facts and Figures 2007-2008*. Retrieved September 28, 2008, from http://www.cancer.org/downloads/STT/BCFF-Final.pdf.

Aziz, N. M., & Rowland, J. H. (2003). Trends and advances in cancer survivorship research: Challenge and opportunity. *Seminars in Radiation Oncology, 13*(3), 248–266.

Bird, B., & Swain, S. (2008). Cardiac toxicity in breast cancer survivors: Review of potential cardiac problems. *Clinical Cancer Research, 14*(1), 14–24.

Booth, C. M., Clemons, M., Dranitsaris, G., Joy, A., Young, S., Callaghan, W., et al. (2007). Chemotherapy-induced nausea and vomiting in breast cancer patients: A prospective observational study. *The Journal of Supportive Oncology, 5*(8), 374–380.

Bowie, J. V., Sydnor, K. D., Granot, M., & Pargament, K. J. (2004). Spirituality and coping among survivors of prostate cancer. *Journal of Psychosocial Oncology, 22*(2), 41–57.

Boyle, D. A. (2006). Survivorship. *Clinical Journal of Oncology Nursing, 10*(3), 407–416.

Burgess, C., Cornelius, V., Love, S., Graham, J., Richards, M., & Ramirez, A. (2005). Depression and anxiety in women with early breast cancer: Five year observational cohort study. *British Medical Journal, 330*(7493), 702–710.

Byar, K. L., Berger, A. M., Bakken, S. L., & Cetak, M. A. (2006). Impact of adjuvant breast cancer chemotherapy on fatigue, other symptoms and quality of life. *Oncology Nursing Forum, 33*(1), E18–E26.

Cancer Research UK. (2008). *Cancer Worldwide*. Retrieved September 2008 from http//www.cancerresearch.uk.org.

Chick, N., & Meleis, A. (1986). Transitions: A nursing concern. In P. H. Chinn (Ed.), *Nursing research methodology: Issues and implantation*. Gaithersburg, MD: Aspen Publishers.

Chochinov, H. M., Hack, T., Hassard, T., Kristjanson, L. J., McClements, S., & Harlos, M. (2006). Dignity therapy: A novel psychotherapeutic intervention for patients near the end of life. *Journal of Clinical Oncology, 23*(24), 5520–5525.

Committee on Cancer Survivorship: Improving Care and Quality of Life, Institute of Medicine and National Research Council. (2005). *From cancer patient to cancer survivor: Lost in transition*. Washington, DC: The National Academies Press.

Cordova, M. J., Cunningham, L. C., Carlson, C. R., & Andrykowski, A. (2001). Posttraumatic growth following breast cancer: A controlled comparison study. *Health Psychology, 20*(3), 176–185.

Doell, H. J. (2008). Three little words no one wants to hear. *Clinical Journal of Oncology Nursing, 12*(4), 551–554.

Farmer, B. J., & Smith, E. D. (2002). Breast cancer survivorship: Are African American women considered? A concept analysis. *Oncology Nursing Forum, 29*(5), 779–787.

Field, M.J., & Cassel, C. K. (1997). Approaching death: Improving care at the end of life. Washington, DC: National Academies Press.

Gall, T. L. & Cornblatt, M.W. (2002). Breast cancer survivors give voice: A qualitative analysis of spiritual factors in long-term adjustment. *Psycho-Oncology, 11*, 524–535.

Golant, M., Altman, T., & Martin, C. (2003). Managing cancer side effects to improve quality of life. *Cancer Nursing, 26*(1), 37–44.

Hanna, L. R., Avila, P. F., Meteer, J. D., Nicholas, D. R., & Kaminsky, L. A. (2008). The effects of a comprehensive exercise program on physical function, fatigue, and mood in patients with various types of cancer. *Oncology Nursing Forum, 35*(3), 461–469.

Hewitt, M. National Research Council, Institute of Medicine, Ganz, P. A. (2006). From cancer patient to cancer survivor - Lost in transition: An American Society of Clinical Oncology and Institute of Medicine symposium. Washington, DC: National Academies Press.

Holland, K. D., & Holahan, C. K. (2003). The relation of social support and coping to positive adaptation to breast cancer. *Psychology and Health, 18*(1), 15–29.

Jemal, A., Siegel, R., Ward, E., Hao, Y., Xu, J., Taylor, M., et al. (2008). Cancer statistics, 2008. *CA: A Cancer Journal for Clinicians, 58*(1), 71–96.

Kernohan, W. G., Hasson, P., Hutchinson, P., & Cochrane, B. (2006). Patient satisfaction with hospice day care. *Support Care Cancer, 14*, 462–468.

Krupski, T. L., Kwan, L., Fink, A., Sonn, G. A., Sonn, G., Maliski, S., et al. (2006). Spirituality influences health related quality of life in men with prostate cancer. *Psycho-Oncology, 15*, 121–131.

Kubler-Ross, E. (1975). *Death: The finals stage of growth*. New York: Simon & Schuster.

Lauver, D., Connelly-Nelson, K., & Vang, P. (2007). Health-related goals in female cancer survivors after Treatment. *Cancer Nursing, 30*(1), 9–15.

Lewis, S. (2008). *Five lessons I didn't learn from breast cancer*. London, England: New American Library.

Linden, W., Dahyun, Y., Barroetavena, M. C., MacKenzie, R., & Doll, R. (2005). Development and validation of a psychosocial screening instrument for cancer. *Health and Quality Outcomes, 3*(54), 1–7.

Meleis, A. I., Sawyer, L. M., Im, E., Messias, D., & Schumacher, K. (2000). Experiencing transitions: An emerging middle-range theory. *Advances in Nursing Science, 23*(ii), 12–28.

Miller, S. M., Fang, C. Y., Diefenbach, M. A., & Bales, C. B. (2001). Tailoring psychosocial interventions to the individual's health information-processing style: The influence of monitoring versus blunting in cancer risk and disease. In A. Baum & B.

Anderson (Eds.), *Psychosocial interventions for cancer* (pp. 343–362). Washington, DC: American Psychological Association.

Montgomery, G. H., & Bovbjerg, D. H. (2003). Expectations of chemotherapy-related nausea: Emotional and experiential predictors. *Annals of Behavioral Medicine, 25*(1), 48–54.

Morrow, G. R., Andrews, P. L., Hickok, J. T., Roscoe, J. A., & Matteson, S. (2002). Fatigue associated with cancer and its treatment. *Supportive Care in Cancer, 10*(5), 389–398.

Mullen, F. (1985). Seasons of survival: Reflections of a physician with cancer. *The New England Journal of Medicine, 313*(4), 270–273.

Pausch, R. (2008). *The last lecture.* New York: Hyperion.

Pargament, K. I. (2007). *Spiritually integrated psychotherapy: Understanding and addressing the sacred.* New York: The Guilford Press.

Payne, J. K., Piper, B. F., Rabinowitz, I., & Zimmerman, M. B. (2006). Biomarkers, fatigue, sleep, and depressive symptoms in women with breast cancer: A pilot study. *Oncology Nursing Forum, 33*(4), 775–783.

Person, J. L. (2004). Palliative care: The development of clinical practice guidelines. *The Kansas Nurse, 79*(9), 4–6.

Ptacek, J. T., Pierce, G. R., & Ptacek, J. J. (2002). The social context of coping with prostate cancer. *Journal of Psychosocial Oncology, 20*(1), 61–81.

Rendle, K. (1997). Survivorship and breast cancer: The psychosocial issues. *Journal of Clinical Nursing 6*: 403–410.

Smith, E. L., Beck, S. L., & Cohen, J. (2008). The total neuropathy score: A tool for measuring chemotherapy-induced peripheral neuropathy. *Oncology Nursing Forum, 35*(1), 96–111.

Spelten, E. R., Verbeek, J. H., Uitterhoeve, A. L., Ansink, A. C., van der Lelie, J., de Reijke, R. M., et al. (2003). Cancer, fatigue and the return of patients to work: A prospective cohort study. *European Journal of Cancer, 39*, 1562–1567.

Spiegel, J. A., Butler, L. D., Giese-Davis, J., Koopman, C., Miller, E., DiMiceli, S., et al. (2007). Effects of supportive-expressive group therapy on survival of patients with metastatic breast cancer: A randomized prospective trial. *Cancer, 110*(5), 1130–1138.

Vachon, M. L. (2008). Meaning, spirituality, and wellness in cancer survivors. *Seminars in Oncology Nursing, 24*(3), 218–225.

Viale, P. H., & Yamamoto, D. S. (2008). Cardiovascular toxicity associated with cancer treatment. *Clinical Journal of Oncology Nursing, 12*(4), 627–638.

Yu Ko, W., & Sawatzky, J. A. (2008). Understanding urinary incontinence after radical prostatectomy: A nursing framework. *Clinical Journal of Oncology Nursing, 12*(4), 647–654.

Chapter 19

Loss of the Safety Signal in Childhood and Adolescent Trauma

Thomas W. Miller and Allan Beane

Introduction

Bullying experiences in the schools is something most children encounter in one form or another during school age, but too many children are persistently mistreated for extended periods of time and find it devastating (Miller and Beane 1997). Children struggle with being called names, being picked upon, and with being rejected or excluded among peers and in the school environment. Even though bullying has been around since time began, little attention has been given to the long-term effects of bullying behavior on both the victim and the perpetrator. Research studies, mostly conducted in European countries, including England, Ireland, and Sweden, are beginning to address the long-range consequences of bullying behavior on children.

Bullying behavior is a form of hurtful behavior toward another child that is disruptive to the physical and emotional well-being of the victim. Olweus (1992) suggests that there are three main features present when bullying occurs: (1) deliberate aggression; (2) an asymmetric power relationship; and (3) the aggression results in pain and distress and loss of a safety signal in the school environment. The safety signal is a critical ingredient in understanding the implications of threatening-type experiences that are realized at every level in our lives.

Olweus (1994) argues that bullying is basically the repeated intimidation of a victim that is intentionally carried out by a more powerful person or group in order to cause physical and/or emotional hurt. Bullying can take many forms, including physical, relational/emotional, and/or verbal abuse. It may involve one child bullying another, a group of children against a single child, or groups against other groups. It is not unlike other forms of victimization and abuse that it involves: (1) An imbalance of power; (2) Differing emotional tones – the victim will be upset, whereas the bully is cool and in control; (3) Blaming the victim for what has happened; and (4) Lack of concern on the part of the bully for the feelings and concerns of the victim.

From: *Handbook of Stressful Transitions Across the Lifespan*,
Edited by: T.W. Miller, DOI 10.1007/978-1-4419-0748-6_19,
© Springer Science+Business Media, LLC 2010

A Safety Signal in Our Lives

Seligman (1975) introduced the concept of a "safety signal" in his examination of learned helplessness as a form of depression in human beings who believe that they are in a no-win situation, in which they have been traumatized, and that future traumatization is still likely. He later added the importance of "learned optimism" in recovering from traumatic events and experiences as a transitional factor that can breed successful adaptation and accommodation (Seligman 1990). Seligman at the time was questioning why victims of the holocaust failed to fight back against their oppressors. What was it that kept them in a constant state of fear? Through several animal experiments, he came to the conclusion that there was no safety signal for the individual. Individuals who were faced with long-term exposure to a lack of safety in their environment had conditioned or learned depression. He realized that people remembered other people and places that created extreme levels of anticipatory anxiety. Thus, the safety signal hypothesis is that people vividly remember places in which they have been anxious and associate such locations or situations with symptoms of anxiety, while seeking out situations associated with lowered anxiety. A person who is traumatized will be fearful all the time except in the presence of a safety signal. Human beings who have been traumatized through some form of bullying will likely find the safety signal a meaningful and relevant concept for understanding why they experience fear that the trauma experience will be re-experienced; they are reminded that the cause of the trauma may still exist. We all search for a safety signal in a number of ways every day in our lives. When that safety signal is absent or we are reminded of something or someone that causes us to revisit our original traumatizing experience, we may be re-traumatized.

Scope of the Problem: Incidence and Prevalence

The research on bullying has produced results that show a wide range in how often it occurs. Much of this variability is due to differences in the way bullying is defined and how the data are collected. Some researchers, (Olweus 1992) in Scandinavia, have used a definition that requires bullying to be repeated, which therefore excludes the single episode, no matter how severe.

Swedish structures on Cuflying (Olweus 1992) notes that researchers at the University of Bergen has have found that 11% of primary school children experienced significant bullying and by secondary school age, the number of victims had been reduced by half. On the other hand, the number of children identified as bullies stayed fairly constant at around 7% at both primary and secondary school age. An overall figure of 15% of Scandinavian children involved in bullying as victims or bullies is lower than that of some comparable findings. For example, Elliot (1986) found that almost 40% of British children had experienced bullying and Stephenson and Smith (1988) found that bullying in some primary schools was as high as 50% of children, but some children – usually in much smaller schools – reported no bullying behavior at all.

In Great Britain, *Kidscape* has attempted to study how widespread incidences of bullying are. In a 6-month period after the Kidscape National

Conferences on Bullying held in 1989 and 1990, Kidscape received over 12,000 letters and 4,000 telephone calls from parents, children, and teachers about the problems of bullying. *Childline* set up a special bully line for 3 months in 1990. According to Hereward Harrison, the Director of Counseling, they answered 5,200 calls and counseled approximately 2,000 distressed children and teenagers. In 1984, a 2-year study was conducted by Kidscape with 4,000 children. Sixty-eight percent had been bullied at least twice or had experienced a particularly bad incident. Eight percent of the students felt that it had affected their lives to the point that they had tried suicide, run away, refused to go to school, or had been chronically ill. Although it is impossible to know the true extent of bullying, it is probably safe to say that it is one of children's major concerns. Most of the incidents occurred when traveling to or from school or in school. The bullying usually took place when no adult was present.

A recent study was organized by the Department for Education-funded Sheffield bullying project (Whitney and Smith 1993) which found that 55% of students in junior/middle schools in Sheffield, England were bullied at least once during term time, and 10% said they were bullied once a week. Figures for secondary schools were lower, although still far from negligible; 10 and 4%, respectively. The 1989 report on discipline in schools (Pearce 1991) found that bullying includes both physical and psychological intimidation. Recent studies of bullying in schools suggest that the problem is widespread and tends to be ignored by teachers and school administrators. When they ignore or fail to respond when it is reported to them, fear, anxiety and a sense of hopeless increases.

According to the National Association of School Psychologists, one in seven children – male and female – is either a bully or victims of bullying (Foltz-Gray 1996). According to the American Medical Association, 3.7 million youths engage in bullying, and more than 3.2 million are victims of "moderate" or "serious" bullying each year (Cohn and Canter 2002). Some studies have shown that between 15% and 25% of US students are frequently bullied while 15–20% report that they bully others frequently (Nansel et al. 2001; Melton et al. 1998; Geffner et al. 2001). Over the course of a year, nearly one-fourth of students across grades reported that they had been harassed or bullied on school property because of the race, ethnicity, gender, religion, sexual orientation, or disability (Austin et al. 2002). Almost 30% of youth in the United States (or over 5.7 million) are estimated to be involved in bullying as either a bully, a target of bullying, or both. In a recent national survey of students in grades 6–10, 13% reported bullying others, 11% reported being the target of bullies, and another 6% said that they bullied others and were bullied themselves (Nansel et al. 2001). Seventy-four percent of 8- to 11-year-old students said teasing and bullying occur at their schools (Kaiser Family Foundation and Nickelodeon 2001).

Teachers' estimates of the incidence of bullying behavior among school children suggest that teachers greatly underestimate the amount of bullying that goes on in their schools (O'Moore and Hillery 1989). For example, teachers identified only 17 (22.1%) of the 77 self-confessed pure bullies and 38 (25.2%) of the 151 bully-victims in a study of victims and perpetrators. Thus, only 24% of the total number of bullies were identified by their teachers. One can only speculate as to why teachers are so unaware of bullying. It might be because of the covert nature of bullying and the subtle manner which bullies use to intimidate their victims. Much information is lost to teachers as a result of pupils' reluctance to inform teachers about bullying incidents that they have witnessed. They are often afraid that adults will only make the situation worse. Unfortunately, many teachers and principals are unsympathetic to pupils telling tales. Rather than seeking solutions within their schools, some principals have even suggested that victimized children be transferred to a different school.

Victimizer Profile

Studies of children who have exhibited bullying type behavior have found that children who bully can be high-spirited, active, energetic children. They may be easily bored or envious and/or insecure. They may be jealous of another's academic or sporting success, or they may be jealous of a sibling/new baby. They may have a learning disability which makes them angry and frustrated (though this may have the opposite effect and make them a target for bullies rather than being a bully). They may be angry or down-trodden from abuse they themselves have suffered (Olweus 1992).

In a 20-year study, Olweus identified the child-rearing practices of the bully's family as very significant (Olweus 1992). Patterns of perpetration may emerge from the following profiles.

The Neglected Child: If the child is neglected, picked on, or punished excessively at home, he may develop a very negative self-image. The child may become frustrated, anxious, and insecure. They may then start to bully others in order to gain respect and to prove that they are worthy of notice.

The Aggressive Family: The family may be aggressive or quick-tempered with lots of loud arguments and shouting. As this is the child's first behavior model, they will tend to reproduce this type of aggressive behavior when they are with other children.

"Anything Goes" Family: The child may be given a great deal of license at home and so have trouble recognizing what is appropriate with other people. They may react badly to discipline. They may be spoiled and used to being the center of attention at home.

More recently, Olweus (1992) identified three main types of bullies:

1. The Aggressive Bully – majority of bullies are in this group (poor impulse control, positive view of violence, desire to dominate, insensitive to feelings of others).
2. The Anxious Bully – about 20% of bullies seem to have anxiety-related problems. This tends to be the most disturbed group (low self-esteem, insecure, friendless, emotionally unstable).
3. The Passive Bully – Child perpetrators become involved in bullying as they become followers of the bully. This occurs to protect themselves and to have the status of belonging to the dominant group (easily dominated, passive and easily led, not particularly aggressive, empathize with others, may feel guilty after bullying).

Victim Profile

In analyzing the victim profile, it is important to realize that bullied children tend to have positive self-esteem. Self-esteem is a critical factor in understanding both the victim and the perpetrator of bullying. The most prominent cause of bullying is the child who needs victims upon which to build their own self-esteem. However, it is so very important to realize that bullying is rarely caused by the victim. Victim profiles often include children who are gentle, physically weaker than bullies, appear to lack confidence, intelligent, lack social skills, disruptive, and who cannot understand why they have been singled out. According to Byrne (1994), the personality type which puts a child at risk of bullying is the shy, sensitive type. Such individuals tend to take everything to heart and personalize all negative comments. They look and act like easy targets. Of course, not all victims fit this profile. This truth may be most evident when someone is cyber bullied. The truth is no one deserves to be bullied, nor are they being weak for being bullied. In fact, anyone who is not willing to be assertive and stand up for him or herself could become a victim. Therefore, even large and strong individuals can be bullied by small and physically weaker individuals. Also, sometimes the motivating factor with girls is simply jealously, so they spread rumors about someone or socially reject them. Bullies usually spend the first week of school looking (shopping) for individuals to bully until they satisfy their need dominance and control. However, the research of Olweus also suggests that physical attributes that are considered different/deviant may contribute more to short-term and indirect bullying (social isolation, spreading rumors, etc.) than long-term and direct bullying (hitting, shoving, etc.). These characteristics attract the attention of the bully when he or she is shopping for targets. The bully then sits out to test the individual as a potential target of mistreatment. Even though these characteristics may not initiate direct bullying, bullies often use them to maximize their mistreatment of others. However, bullying *mainly* occurs because the bully wants to have power and control over the victims, not because the individuals look different. Of course, another main reason bullies mistreat others is that they are able to do it without adequate adult intervention.

From the profiles of those at risk for becoming involved in a bullying incident, Besag (1989) found that victims tend to fall into the category of passive "watchers" who remain on the sidelines of the playground, whereas bullies tend to be the "doers," confident and fully involved in a variety of activities. Finally, Olweus (1989) has identified some common objects of bullying. They include, but are not limited to race, language, culture, sex and religion.

Bullying results in immediate consequences for both the victim and the bully, (Olweus 1989). The consequences to the victim may be:

- Lose of confidence
- Lower self-esteem
- Withdrawal from social experience
- Problems in concentrating
- Falling grades
- Missing school and classes
- Exhibiting School-phobic responses
- Anger, internalized or against others
- Fear and overwhelming anxiety
- Depression or feelings of sadness
- Self-harm and ideation of suicide
- Show suicidal ideation or intent

The bullies may:

- Learn that using aggression/violence is a successful strategy for getting what you want;
- Realize that they can "get away with" violent and cruel behavior and school discipline may be eroded;
- Become divisive as a dominant group coalesces
- Become more disruptive – perhaps eventually testing school administration and teachers to see how far they can push them.

Elliot and Kilpatrick (1994) surveyed young offenders in Britain. Seventy-nine young offenders, in two institutions, surveyed revealed their experiences of school bullying. They ranged in age from 16 to 21. They were asked whether bullying happened often in their school, whether they were involved in bullying, and what they thought schools should do to tackle bullying effectively. The majority of the young offenders (62%) had themselves been bullies at school. Twenty-three percent were involved as bystanders or witnesses who egged the bullies on, and 15% had been the victims of bullying. Of these victims, 7% subsequently became bullies, 5% committed crimes under the influence of bullies, and 3% remained victims.

O'Moore and Hillery (1989), who studied similar Irish populations of young offenders, indicate that (1) feelings of inadequacy, such as were expressed in relation to academic and school status and (2) popularity among peers, could be strong contributing factors in their subsequent behavior as bullies. The authors suggest that it is to be expected that as long as these factors remain, the compensatory behavior will not cease. There is an existing strong body of evidence which indicates that self-esteem is the single most influential factor in determining behavior (Burns 1982). However, it may be wrong to assume that all bullies have poor self-esteem, as mentioned earlier. Bullies who have not been victims or who may have not been victims may have self-esteems. According to Marano (1995), bullies may feel good about themselves because they are clueless as to how little they are liked.

Transitioning Trauma Through Accommodation

The child confronted with intimidations through bullying often passes through a series of stages dealing with this trauma (Veltkamp and Miller 1994) (Fig. 19-1). The initial stage of the victimization, which is recognized as the stressor, usually brings about acute physical and/or psychological trauma. The child's response is usually one of feeling overwhelmed, intimidated, and powerless. It is not uncommon for the child to think recurringly of the stressful experience and to focus on the intimidating act as well as physical pain associated with the act. This acute stage of trauma is followed by a stage involving more cognitive disorganization and confusion.

The second stage involves a denial or avoidance which can take two directions and may vary in its choice at various within-phase considerations. The first is a phase of conscious inhibition during which the child tries actively to inhibit thoughts and feelings related to the bullying. This can involve a recurrence of the cognitive disorganization phase and the earlier memories and flashbacks to the acute physical trauma. The second phase is one of avoidance, involving unconscious denial.

**Loss of the Safety Signal &
Trauma Accommodation Syndrome**

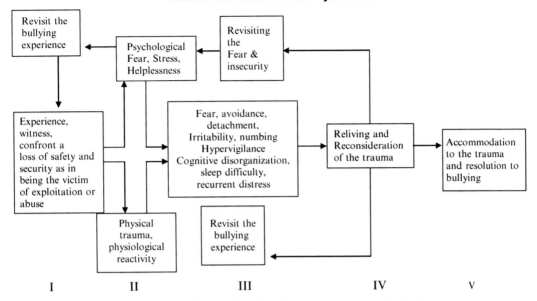

Five Phases of Processing the Trauma experienced in Bullying

Fig. 19-1.   Loss of the Safety Signal & Trauma Accommodation Syndrome

The cognitive disorganization or confused thinking phase is followed by a stage of therapeutic reassessment during which a parent or significant other usually supports the child's reevaluation of the psychological and physical trauma associated with bullying. At this phase, the child victim may begin to disclose the abuse through drawing, fables, or specific content relevant to the experiencing of the abuse. The phase of therapeutic reevaluation and reasoning is significant because it indicates that the child is passing from the avoidant phase to the actual issues, activities, and the trauma of being bullied.

The final stage is one of acceptance and resolution wherein the child has been able, through the support of parents, professionals, or significant others, to deal with the issues. The child will arrive at a better understanding of the abuse and its significance. He or she will develop coping strategies that will allow self-acceptance without shame, doubt, or guilt, and progress to a stage of resolution. At this stage, the child is (1) more open and talks about the incident, (2) able to express thoughts and feelings more readily, and (3) able through assessment and play therapy to discharge some of the aggressive feelings toward the perpetrator, which are a healthy part of the child's response. It is at this phase that the child develops an alliance with significant others and/ or professionals in (1) exploring the original traumatic experience, (2) dealing with both the physical and psychological stressors involved, (3) attending to the repressed material and the process of either conscious inhibition or unconscious denial utilized during the avoidant phase, and (4) focusing on self-understanding.

Clinical issues which must be addressed in treating victims of bullying behavior include:

Fear and helplessness: The child is often afraid of future bullying as a result of reprisals from the perpetrator. These fears often take the form of nightmares or sleep disturbance. It is helpful in the course of treatment to identify the fears, have the child express them and move in the direction of making the child's environment safe.

Depression: Depression is a common reaction in most victims. Clinically, it is necessary to look for signs of depression, to anticipate suicidal thoughts, and to support and believe the victim.

Low self-esteem and poor social skills: These are additional symptoms that are frequently seen in victims. Treatment can help the child identify and ventilate their feelings and offer support to the child. In addition, group therapy is helpful in teaching the child new social skills.

Repressed anger and hostility: Victims are frequently angry at the perpetrator, at significant others who have failed to protect them, and at others in the community who did not respond to their disclosures about the abuse. Treatment aimed at helping victims get in touch with their repressed rage in a healthy and constructive manner and to learn not to be afraid of their own anger.

Inability to trust self or others: If the child has been bullied, problems regarding trust can be expected. Frequently, this is linked to low self-esteem, feeling of helplessness, and problems in forming relationships in the future. Trust can only begin to develop when a child gradually experiences more satisfying relationships with others through guided therapeutic interventions.

Transitioning the Bullying Experience

In summary, there seems to be evidence to suggest that the incidence of behavioral difficulties has a stronger association with the quality of the teacher–pupil relationships in a school than with the pupils' socioeconomic background (Rutter 1967). Schools do make a difference. It is no longer justifiable for schools, when faced with behavioral difficulties such as victimization or bullying, to apportion all the blame on the child's home background. The evidence is clearly in favor of the view that a positive school ethos does contribute significantly to the good behavior of pupils.

Many schools have failed to create a school culture and atmosphere that communicates that bullying will not be tolerated and that there is adequate protection and support for the victims. There is a lack of safety signals in the school such as posted anti-bullying rules, anti-bullying posters, quality and sufficient adult supervision, etc. Some schools have not established anti-bullying rules and behavioral expectations with progressive consequences and pro-social strategies for dealing with bullying behavior. Also, in some schools there is no effort to implement an anti-bullying program and the training provided often focuses only on awareness and not on the nature of bullying and the destructiveness of bullying, or how to prevent it and intervene when it is seen. Also, there is sometimes no adult supervision in the high-risk areas (e.g., inside bathrooms, stairwells, between buildings, etc.), or not enough adult supervision, and/or the quality (passive) of supervision provided is poor. In addition, unstructured times have also been left unstructured, so students are more likely to be bullied. In addition Smith and Brain (2000) and Elliot and Kilpatrick (1994) have discovered a variety of school involvement factors that may contribute to bullying. Some of these factors are: (1) low self morale;

(2) high teacher turnover; (3) unclear standards of behavior; (4) inconsistent methods of discipline; (5) poor organization in classrooms, on playgrounds, etc.; (6) inadequate supervision; (7) children not treated as valid individuals; (8) not enough equipment; (9) lack of support for new students; (10) teachers being lack; (11) intolerance of difference; (12) no anti-bullying policy; and (13) school personnel who use sarcasm. The "bullying experience" heals in the security of a safety signal and that signal is either a person or place that the bullied person feels the comfort of adaptation, understanding and accommodation to the traumatic effects of being bullied.

Acknowledgments: The authors wish to acknowledge the assistance of Jill Livingston M.L.S., Kayla Snow, Tag Heister M.L.S., Deborah Kessler M.L.S., and Katrina Scott, Library Services; and Lane J. Veltkamp M.S.W., Robert F. Kraus M.D., Richard Welsh M.S.W., Department of Psychiatry, University of Kentucky, and Linda Brown, Amy Farmer, Brenda Frommer for their contributions to the completion of this manuscript.

References

Austin, G., Huh-Kim, J., Skage, R., & Furlong, M. (2002, Winter). *2001-2002 California Student Survey.* Jointly sponsored by California Attorney General's Office, California Department of Education, and Department of Alcohol and Drug Programs. San Francisco, CA: California Attorney General's Office, Bill Lockyer, Attorney General State of California

Besag, V. E. (1989). *Bullies and victims in schools.* London: Open University Press.

Burns, R. B. (1982). *Self-concept development and education.* London: Holt, Rinehart, and Winston.

Byrne, B. (1994). *Bullying: A community approach.* Dublin: The Columbia Press.

Cohn, A., & Canter, A. (2002). Bullying: Facts for schools and parents. National Association of School Psychologists. Retrieved February 8, 2009, from at http://www.naspoline.org/resources/factsheets/bullying_fs.aspx

Elliot, M. (1986). *The kidscape kit.* London: Kidscape.

Elliot, M., & Kilpatrick, J. (1994). *How to stop a bullying: a Kidscape training guide.* London: Kidscape.

Foltz-Gray, D. (1996, Fall). The bully trap. *Teaching Tolerance, 5*(2), 19–23

Geffner, J., Genta, M. L., Menesini, E., Fonzi, A. (2001). Bullies and victims in schools in central and southern Italy. *European Journal of Psychology of Education*, 11, 97–110.

Kaiser Family Foundation & Nickelodeon. (2001). *Talking with kids about tough issues: A national survey of parents and kids.* Menlow Park, CA: Kaiser Family Foundation.

Marano, H. E. (1995, September/October). Big bad bully. Psychology Today, pp. 50–57, 62–70, 74–82.

Melton, G. B., Limber, S., Flerx, V., Cunningham, P., Osgood, D.W., Chambers, J., Henggler, S., & Nation, M. (1998). Violence among rural youth. Final report to the Office of Juvenile Justice and Delinquency Prevention.

Miller, T. W., & Beane, A. (1997). A Holistic approach to treating Children who are bullied. Presentation to the Kentucky Psychologal Association. Louisville, Kentucky, November 6–8, 1997.

Nansel, T. R., Overpeck, M., Pilla, R. S., Ruan, W. J., Simons-Morton, B., & Scheidt, P. (2001). Bullying behaviors among US youth: Prevalence and association with psychosocial adjustment. *Journal of the American Medical Association, 285*(16), 2094–2100.

Olweus, D. (1989). Bully/victim problems among school children: basic facts and effects of a school based intervention program. In K. Rubin & D. Pepler (Eds.), *The development and treatment of childhood aggression*. Hillsdale, NJ: Erlbaum.

Olweus, D. (1992). "Bullying Among Schoolchildren: Intervention and Prevention." In R. Peters, R. McMahon and V. Quinsey (eds.), *Aggression and Violence Throughout the Life Span*. Newbury Park, Calif.: Sage Publications.

Olweus, D. (1994). *Bullying at school: What we know and what we can do*. Oxford: Blackwell.

O'Moore, A. M., & Hillery, B. (1989). Bullying in Dublin Schools. *The Irish Journal of Psychology, 10*(3), 426–441.

Pearce, J. (1991). *Bullying: A practical guide to coping for schools*. London: Kidscape.

Rutter, M. (1967). A children's behavior questionnaire for completion by teachers: Preliminary findings. *Journal of Child Psychology and Psychiatry, 8*(1), 1–11.

Rutter, M., Maughan, B., Mortimore, P., Ouston, J., & Smith, A. (1979). *Fifteen thousand hours*. Cambridge, MA: Harvard University.

Seligman, M. E. P. (1975). *Helplessness: On depression, development, and death*. San Francisco: W.H. Freeman. Paperback reprint edition, W.H. Freeman, 1992, ISBN 0-7167-2328-X. ISBN ISBN 0-7167-0752-7.

Seligman, M. E. P. (1990). *Learned optimism*. New York: Knopf. Reissue edition, Free Press, 1998, ISBN 0-671-01911-2.

Smith, P., & Brain, P. (2000). "Bullying in Schools: Lessons From Two Decades of Research." *Aggressive Behavior* 26, 1–9.

Stephenson, P., & Smith, D. (1988). Bullying in the junior school. In D. Tattum & D. Lane (Eds.), *Bullying in schools*. Stoke-on-Trent: Trentham.

Veltkamp, L., & Miller, T. (1994). *Clinical handbook of child abuse and neglect*. Madison, CT: International Universities Press.

Whitney, I., & Smith, P. K. (1993). A survey of the nature and extent of bullying in junior/middle and secondary schools. *Educational Research*, 35, 3–25.

Chapter 20

An Unexpected Traumatic Change in Life: Where to Go from Here?

Richard Welsh, Lane J. Veltkamp, Thomas W. Miller,
Ronald Goodman, and Emily Rosenbaum

Introduction

Trauma exists in two, often interlocking forms: psychological and physical. Psychological trauma can be succinctly defined as "a psychic or behavioral state resulting from mental or emotional stress or physical injury" (Ehde and Williams 2006. The *Diagnostic and Statistical Manual of Mental Disorders*, Fourth Edition (American Psychiatric Association 2000) provides the criteria of a traumatic event to involve "either the experiencing or witnessing" of "an event that involved actual or threatened death or serious injury, or a threat to the physical integrity of self or others" (American Psychiatric Association 1994). It is significant to note that a traumatic event will cause only a proportion of individuals who experience such an event to become traumatized. Estimates suggest that 14% of people living in the United States will develop post-traumatic stress disorder in their lifetime (Yehuda 1999). Although this reveals a high prevalence of the disorder, it actually represents only a small sector of people who experience a traumatic life event, given the fact that most people will experience such an event of some kind during their life. For this chapter, the act of "becoming traumatized" will be clinically referred to as "experiencing symptoms of post-traumatic stress disorder or PTSD."

The prevalence of trauma in the United States is examined closely by Lawrence Robinson in his book entitled *Trauma Rehabilitation*. Trauma is the leading cause of death for 1–34-year olds and the second leading cause of death for 35–44-year olds. Death rates, however, are a misleading factor when determining the breadth of the problem. Traumatic injuries accounted for 29 million nonfatal injuries in 2001 (Robinson and Micklesen 2006). Motor vehicle crashes (MVCs) were the most common cause of traumatic deaths (31%). Traumatic brain injury (TBI), largely caused by MVCs, is the most common neurological disability (300 cases per million), yet many of these individuals survive and require either inpatient or outpatient rehabilitation. Patients with traumatic injuries represent approximately one-fourth of the inpatient rehabilitation patient population in the United States according to Robinson and Micklesen (2006).

From: *Handbook of Stressful Transitions Across the Lifespan*,
Edited by: T.W. Miller, DOI 10.1007/978-1-4419-0748-6_20,
© Springer Science+Business Media, LLC 2010

Major traumatic amputation due to vascular disease or diabetic complications is more common than that due to bodily injury (Robinson and Micklesen 2006). The major difference in these two causes of limb amputation is the age of the patient. For traumatic amputation, the estimated prevalence is 1,300 per million. Individuals who experience a traumatic event typically respond with some combination of the following four outcome trajectories: chronic dysfunction, recovery, resilience, or delayed reactions (Bonanno and Mancini 2008). For those who experience a dysfunctional reaction to a traumatic event, the following phases of their response are common:

1. The impact phase
2. Alternation of intrusion and numbing responses
3. Denial and shock
4. Intrusive memories or flashbacks and/or nightmares
5. Autonomic hyperarousal
6. Irritability and sleep problems (Bonanno and Mancini 2008)

Variables that place an individual at a higher risk of responding adversely to a traumatic event are pretrauma, peritrauma, and posttrauma (Hoge et al. 2007). Pretrauma risk factors exist before the trauma occurs which include demographics of an individual such as their "lower education level, lower intelligence, neurodevelopmental delays…, previous history of mental disorders, and female gender" (Hoge et al. 2007). Examples of peritraumatic risk factors are the "magnitude of the stressor and immediate reactions to the stressor, such as fear of threats to one's safety, or dissociation" (Hoge et al. 2007). Posttraumatic variables include "perceived social support, subsequent life stress, and ongoing threat to safety" (Hoge et al. 2007). If any of the above factors are present in a person's life, one can predict that a traumatic event will more adversely affect that person than someone who does not exhibit these factors.

The *Trauma Accommodation Syndrome* (Miller and Veltkamp 1996) argues that traumatized individuals, both children and adults, who experience, witness or are confronted by a traumatic event, may suffer immediately or after some period of time psychological fear, horror and helplessness. Not unlike Hoge et al. (2007), each person moves through a series of stages or phases. In this model, there are five stages and anniversary reactions are likely to occur for some time. Such anniversary reactions trigger a revisiting so to speak of the traumatic event and a re-evaluation of how the person who was traumatized accommodates to the situation. As a result of this, such individuals show signs and symptoms of traumatization that include avoidance, detachment, irritability, agitated behavior, hypervigilance, cognitive disorganization, sleep difficulty recurrent distress, and re-experiencing of the traumatization through flashbacks. It is in this period that individuals retain the helplessness and do little to escape the traumatization. Rather, they feel entrapped within this cycle and accommodate the pain and psychological trauma there. Through some triggering event, is realized and the person can go through a cognitive re-evaluation of the trauma. In this process, they revisit the physical injury, deaths, mourning, and the psychological fear and helplessness that they have experienced. On the basis of the adaptation, support, and response of those who are involved in treatment, they work towards a resolution to the trauma accommodation. The *Trauma Accommodation Syndrome* appears in Fig. 20-1 and summarizes the five stages in which the person transitions in dealing with the trauma.

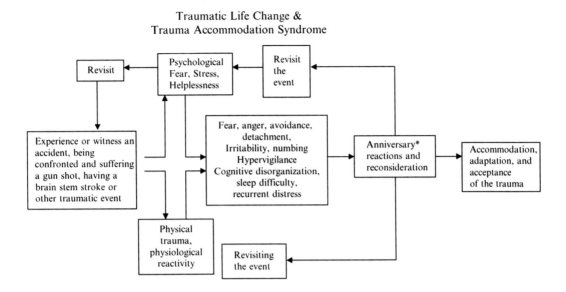

*Anniversary reactions refer to conscious reminders victims of trauma experience

Fig. 20-1. Traumatic life change & trauma accommodation syndrome

The victim may experience an effort to avoid or cope with the trauma through denial that provides relief from both the trauma and confusion experienced in the disease's detection. Denial involves psychological repression as a means of coping with the progression of the victimization, with its periods of apparent denial and avoidance followed by ever more frequent and severe episodes of bullying and victimization. The victim revisits the trauma and any physical pain many times and may move toward acceptance, accommodation or resolution of the traumatic event that initiated this process. *Resolution* would see the victimization and its memories end for the victim, while *accommodation* realizes a revisiting of the trauma periodically whereby the victim never loses the psychological contact with the traumatic event throughout life.

Persons at lower risk for experiencing traumatic stress are said to be resilient. Resilience is a complex phenomenon that is the result of several important factors in a person's life. Factors that promote resilience include person-centered variables, demographic variables and sociocultural factors (Bonanno and Mancini 2008).

Recovery usually results from intensive therapy, including physical therapy, occupational therapy, or speech therapy, to name a few. As for a delayed reaction to trauma, "empirical evidence for delayed grief has never been reported," (Bonanno and Mancini 2008). Reactions to trauma are often conceptualized in terms of pathology versus the absence of pathology, which creates a misleading image that more often than not, people react in an exceedingly adverse way. In reality, research has shown that the majority of people who experience a potentially traumatic event (PTE) in their lives cope with a reasonable amount of functionality and positive mental health.

George A. Bonanno of the University of Michigan's School of Public Health has produced a significant body of research on the phenomenon of resilience, and what he refers to as "potentially traumatic events," or PTEs. Resilience is often associated with individuals who do not experience symptoms of PTSD following a PTE, and is defined by Bonanno as "the ability of adults in otherwise normal circumstances who are exposed to an isolated and potentially highly disruptive event such as the death of a close relation, or a violent or life-threatening situation to maintain relatively stable, healthy levels of psychological and physical functioning…as well as the capacity for generating experiences and positive emotions" (Bonanno et al. 2007). Resilience has been found to result from a combination of several factors in a person's life, including "personality; interpersonal variables, such as supportive relationships; and the type, severity and duration of the stressor" (Mancini and Bonanno 2006). Resilience is also closely related to matters of coping with a traumatic experience. Coping methods can be learned, but they are also largely innate in most people. Ehde and Williams (2006) describe the natural history or psychological responses and their relevant theoretical approaches as follows: "…coping strategies may be learned and reinforced (behavioral approach), psychic distress gradually reduced to a tolerable level (psychodynamic approach), or core beliefs altered and meaning found (cognitive approach)". As a result of coping abilities, many people will "not only show a lack of psychological distress but also show evidence of positive responses such as resilience, positive emotions, and post-traumatic growth during and after the trauma" (Ehde and Williams 2006). Other personality traits that can greatly assist in the coping process are continuity of self and an external locus of control. Support systems in the form of family and friends, and their respective adjustments to the changes in the life of the affected individual also play a large role in achieving resilience.

The resilience phenomenon is one for which there is still a need for further investigation. Bonanno et al. (2007) consider the idea that resilience is "more than the simple absence of PTSD". Some of the variables that researchers were able to see affect resilience were: gender, race and ethnicity, education level, and the absence of depression and substance use (Bonanno et al. 2007). Age of an individual experiencing a PTE was found to be a consistent variable in Bonanno's (2007) research. "Participants over 65 years of age were least likely to have PTSD and more than 3 times as likely to be resilient compared with the youngest (18- to 24-year-old) participants".

Much of the existing literature and research regarding an individual's response and adjustment to an unexpected traumatic life event pertain directly to the first author's accident, response, and recovery.

Scenario I: Transitioning Through a Traumatic Accident and Amputation

In March, 1994, my life suddenly changed and would never be the same. As I had done for several years, my day began with some sort of physical exercise, either jogging or swimming. On this particular spring morning, I was out of town, scheduled to give an all-day professional workshop on attention-deficit hyperactivity disorder at a regional university. As I was enjoying the beautiful scenery, I was suddenly hit head-on by an automobile traveling approximately 57 miles per hour. The collision resulted in 14 fractures and the traumatic severing of my lower left leg. My journey to recovery included 8 weeks of hospitalization, 2 weeks in intensive care, 1 week in an orthopedic university hospital unit, 3 weeks in a rehabilitation center, and 12 weeks of biweekly outpatient physical therapy.

As a result of this accident, I was immediately confronted with significant physical and emotional changes, social discomfort, body-image anxiety, and a change in self-identity. Research discusses the physical and psychological adjustment to lower limb loss, and I have to admit, I initially felt all the difficulties it suggests. These included denial, depression, anxiety, body-image distortion, phantom pain, and reduced independence.

Following the accident, I read an article entitled *Preserving Self: From Victim to Patient to Disabled Person*, by Janice M. Morris. I found this article to be very helpful in understanding my traumatic experience and recovery process. The article accurately described my experience and doubtless that of other individuals who have undergone traumatic injuries. Morris describes four stages an individual goes through in the transformation process from person, to victim, to patient, to disabled person.

Stage 1: Vigilance/Being Engulfed. Often, the injured person realizes his life is in peril but is vigilant and able to assist in his care. Finally, the survivor then relinquishes themselves to competent caregivers.

I have little, if any, memory of being hit by the automobile. I was later told by EMTs that I was initially helpful in describing who I was, where I lived, what I was doing, and where I was going. After spilling my guts, so to speak, I believe I felt safe and someone else could now take over.

Stage 2: Disruption. During this stage, the survivor is now hospitalized and remains in a fog because of heavy sedative medication. The patient experiences periods of amnesia, confusion, and the inability to distinguish reality from vivid dreams. During this stage, the continuous presence of significant others are requested in order to counteract the fear of being alone and to give them a sense of self.

My 2-week stay in the Intensive Care Unit was certainly a "foggy" experience at best. The environment was totally unfamiliar and scary. The pain at times was unbearable. The numerous IVs, monitors and strange noises from all the life support machinery added to the disorientation. The heavy sedation to control the pain made it impossible to distinguish time or reality, but instead produced frightening dreams. When lucid, I found myself feeling insecure and lonely. I searched for attachments. The nursing staff provided reassurance and some explanation regarding what happened and what would take place next.

Stage 3: Enduring the Self: Confronting and Regrouping. During this stage, the individual's condition becomes more stable and the extent of the injuries becomes a "fact" and a part of his new identity. Physical pain has been controlled and the psychological suffering is now a reality. The survivor begins to grapple with the realities of the injury and the losses become more apparent. Physical dependence on caregivers increases and environmental continuity is treasured. He begins keeping track of time by remembering which medical procedure was done and in what order. During this stage, he is finally able to recognize the extent of the injury while developing a strong dependency on others for support and encouragement. The reality finally hits that recovery is slow, painful, and exhausting.

The beginning of my new "identity" began to emerge when I was transferred from Intensive Care to the Orthopedic Unit. Pain medication had been discontinued. This allowed me to begin the difficult task of confronting the realities of my injuries. I struggled to accept a new set of dependencies which were totally foreign to me. I certainly was not accustomed to ask for assistance getting out of bed, getting dressed, standing, sitting in a chair, or taking a shower. I had always been able to do my own thing. I now had to accept a new set of dependencies that were difficult and at times embarrassing.

Stage 4: Stiving to Regain Self: Merging the Old and the New Reality. The grueling task of rehabilitation begins in this phase. The individual is transferred from the hospital to the rehabilitation facility. During this phase of recovery, the individual gets to know and trust the altered body, revise life goals, accepts the consequences of the accident, and come to terms with his changed body. He must now struggle with a new set of dependencies.

Learning to accept my disability was further solidified during my 3 week stay at Cardinal Hill Rehabilitation Hospital. With a tremendously supportive staff, I was helped to see myself as different but not disabled. Their belief that I could walk again, with the use of a prosthesis provided enormous boost to my self-esteem. Without their encouragement and assistance, my hunting trips to Alaska, Canada, and Michigan would have been unfulfilled dreams.

I have often reflected upon my recovery process and subsequent adaptation. What were the factors which inspired me to return to work in a wheel chair just 3 months post-hospitalization? What drove me to hunt Caribou and fish in Alaska that fall? In May of the following year, 14 months after the accident, I resumed full-time teaching and clinical responsibilities. In November, I took my yearly trip to the upper peninsula of Michigan to hunt white-tailed deer. There was thigh deep snow and I hunted with the assistance of a walker. Since the accident, my wife and I have purchased a ranch style home and I recently bought a farm. I devote my spare time to typical farm chores and my passion for hunting, and I continue to work as a therapist.

As I have pondered this adaptation process, the factors that helped me to cope were these: (1) I made a conscious effort to focus on what I *can* do rather than on what I *cannot* do; (2) I developed achievable goals; (3) I continue to believe in God as a loving and healing force; and (4) I have a strong support system consisting of family, friends, professional colleagues and rehabilitation therapists.

Although discouragement was present, I soon came to understand that one's true disability is "above the shoulders." Negative thoughts such as "I will never walk again," "What will people think of me?" or "I am no longer a man" were not only depressing but dysfunctional, adding nothing to my acceptance and rehabilitation.

A major factor influencing my recovery is what I have come to call "goal-directed behavior." My goals were to somehow resume my obsession – or perhaps passion – with outdoor recreation, namely hunting, and return to work in spite of recognized limitations. Without a definable goal and a reformulated future, it would have been easier to avoid the pain involved with rehabilitation and become absorbed in self-pity. Instead, I had to reject the notion of permanent disability. In essence, recovery for me required an optimistic attitude, a strong desire to "get better," acceptance of my limitations and constantly refocusing on what I was able to do as opposed to what I could not.

The most important aspect in my recovery process was my belief in God. I have never blamed God for the accident nor have I ever felt He abandoned me. My recovery is not what I would call a "spiritual miracle." I have always felt God's presence in my recovery process as giving me daily strength to withstand painful procedures and comforted me in times of loneliness. There was never a doubt in my mind that God would help me achieve my goals and with his assistance, nothing would be impossible. Working in a hospital has afforded me the opportunity to observe individuals struggling to recover from devastating physical injuries and illness. I continue to be impressed with the positive impact faith has on an individual's rehabilitative process.

Furthermore, the importance of supportive significant others cannot be minimized or overlooked. Without the daily encouragement of family, acceptance of friends and patience of rehabilitation personnel, recovery would have been virtually impossible. They not only offered love, hope, and support, but helped me accept my new needs and assisted in my new identity which was different but not disabled.

Scenario II: Transitioning Personal Trauma & a Therapist Career

Over the years, much has been written about traumatic experiences and the impact of these experiences on the personal life of individuals. However, little has been discussed regarding the impact of trauma on a psychotherapist professional life. As therapists, we have been comfortable listening to our patients expresses the impact of trauma in their life, but we may discount the degree to which trauma impacts our own professional life and personal life.

For 30 years prior to the attack, I had been on the faculty in the Department of Psychiatry at a major university in the Midwest. My primary responsibilities included teaching, a clinical practice, directing a child and adolescent forensic clinic, and writing throughout the years. My teaching involved residents and medical students in the Department of Psychiatry, graduate courses in the College of Social Work and Family Studies as well as lectures on a variety of subjects. My forensic practice, which involves both children and adults, included the assessment of murder cases, reviews of death penalty cases, assault cases involving children and adults, child litigation or child custody cases, domestic violence, as well as other forensic cases. These forensic cases were the most controversial and involve the strongest emotion on the part of the participants, including the evaluator and/or care giver. For example, much has been written about the high level of emotion in child litigation cases, primarily because it involves a parent's relationship with their children and a fear of being cutoff from part or all of their children's future. In one local case, a circuit court judge was shot and paralyzed: a judge who referred many cases to me over the years. Some thought that his victimization and my shooting where possibly caused by the same perpetrator. Was this an individual angered by the Judge's decision and also by my expert testimony? In the end, the perpetrator was never identified.

In addition to my forensic practice, I also, do individual and family therapy. Being a family therapist and understanding human growth and development allowed me to develop a sense of empathy and compassion toward an offender of assault, including murder. The shooting had a major impact on my ability to experiences empathy and compassion, particularly cases involving assault.

The Attack

The attack occurred approximately 10 years ago following a basketball game at the local university. The arena is located downtown where there were approximately 300 policeman providing traffic control and crowd management after the game. We left the game approximately 2 min early with another couple and began walking toward our car. Approximately 24,000 fans were leaving the arena about the same time. The attack occurred within two blocks of the area. While we were walking down the street towards our car, it became clear that we were being followed by two young males. As I realized this, we began running towards our car. I remotely opened the car from a distance, entered the car and locked the door. Between unlocking the car door and leaving the arena, approximately a 60-s period, the gunmen shot four times into the car, hitting me in the left shoulder. The other bullets went into the head rest and into the back door of the car. I quickly drove out of the parking spot and headed down a main artery towards our home. When I realized that I had been shot, I proceeded to an emergency room where I was evaluated, treated and later released. The police also became involved at this point. The shooting received local and national media attention, primarily because of the national reputation of the basketball team. I received approximately 400 phone calls from around the state and the country. Clearly, the incident triggered off anxiety and fear in others. Questions were raised about why this occurred, many blamed the victim in an effort to make sense of a senseless, unprovoked attack.

Subsequent to the Attack

The attack occurred on a Saturday night and normally I would return to work on Monday. I was not aware of any symptoms or problems of any kind and returned to work early Monday morning. I began seeing patients, continuing with my teaching, submitting court reports, and directing my forensic clinic. Within a day or two, I began noticing a variety of symptoms. Since I frequently talked about trauma and its results and consequences and my practice was filled with traumatized patients, I was well aware of the symptoms associated with PTSD. I began noticing flashbacks in a variety of circumstances. For example, when I taught in the University or in clinic class rooms and walked by windows I noticed heightened anxiety. It took weeks for me to realize the connection between walking by windows and sitting in a car where two bullets had gone through my driver's side window, one hitting me and the other lodging in my headrest. I also had a recurrent nightmare involving getting into a car and locking the other three people out of the car. These nightmares occurred 5–6 times a night, interfering with my sleep. In addition, when driving, when I got into a situation involving a car in front of me and another car directly behind me, it caused heighten anxiety, a feeling I was trapped, a situation similar to my parking spot the night of the shooting. In addition, over time I realized a change in my ability to be optimistic regarding patients' ability to mark changes in their life. For 20 years, I had accepted cases for the defense, people who had murdered, committed assault, or other crimes against innocent people. I learned that I no longer had compassion for those who committed violent crimes. Prior to this incident, I had empathy for criminals. Subsequent to the incident, I had very little.

Accommodation

I was fortunate that I worked in a psychiatry outpatient clinic. I had one colleague who had been shot in a double murder case a few years before and had experienced a variety of symptoms not unlike I had experienced. I talked with him on a regular basis over a 6 month period which was extremely helpful to me. In addition, a week after the shooting, a therapist friend of mine, invited my wife and me to dinner downtown, approximately two blocks from where the shooting occurred. We were terrified to go downtown, but pushed ourselves through it. In retrospect I believe this was one of the experiences that were helpful in facing the trauma and being able to move beyond it.

I also have another friend who worked at a VA hospital and invited my wife and me to do a presentation on this stressful life event and answer questions from the audience. About 200 people came for the presentation which was helpful in the sense that we began re-experiencing the event, began to face it, and began to open up about it. In addition, I was able, primarily because of my work, to talk openly about the experiences to my colleagues. The lectures, seminars, classroom discussions, as well as patients frequently asking about the event, and the traumatic experience and how it impacted me, were all helpful in the process of moving on and reducing the symptoms.

I also used medication for sleeping, which worked very well for me. As I mentioned, I had awakened 6 or 7 times a night and the medication stopped this. It has now been over 10 years since the shooting. A day does not go by that the shooting does not cross my mind, but I have learned not to allow it to trigger symptoms I have learned how to constructively deal with symptoms when they do occur.

Scenario III: Transitioning the Trauma of a Brain Stem Stroke

In Deciding to Die, I Found a Reason to Live became the title of a book authored with the help and support of my family and several friends after I suffered a brain stem stroke and felt as if there was nothing to live for in my life. The book became an inspiration because of a loving wife and two children whom I wanted to see grow up and be successful.

After suffering from a brain stem stroke at the age of 34, I spent months and years in a silent world of depression and despair. This is the story of the fourth author as shared with the third author of this chapter. Both of us would meet weekly on Wednesdays at the nursing home where he was living and where we would share our thoughts about his condition and its impact on his life. He wanted to share the transition he faced through this chapter as well as through other writings. As a result of his brain stem stroke, Ron became a quadriplegic, but had some ability to write messages via computer. He could not speak but through the assistance of computer technology, he would begin to speak the many thoughts that he had had through a most difficult and stressful transition in his life.

This transition found him receiving hospitalization and professional treatment for depression along with support psychotherapy, and several adjunct and rehabilitative therapies. Writing his book along with sharing the thoughts in this chapter became for him a form of therapy in itself. It was through encouraging him over time that he wrote his thoughts and feelings and produced with the encouragement of several people who cared about him, his book entitled "In Deciding to Die, I Found a Reason to Live." The book summarizes his journey elsewhere but the significance of his life was to see his son and daughter graduate and return to live in a nursing home near his wife and family where he could navigate the sidewalks to gain some semblance of life. Watching him, and walking with him, navigating the street crossings and sidewalks of this midwestern city reflected his determination.

At the age of 34, he was gainfully employed as a mental health counselor having completed my master's degree in counseling at a nearby regional university. He and his wife had started their family and they had both a son and daughter. It was in that 34th year that he believed that he had the world in order, a beautiful family and a job that he thoroughly enjoyed and that he suffered a massive brain stem stroke that paralyzed him from the neck down and drastically changed his life. He was in his fifth year of gainful employment in mental health counseling. The stroke found him in a coma for some 2 months. When he awoke from the coma, he was told that he was almost completely paralyzed. The fact that he could not talk or walk became overwhelming. Over the next 2 years, a serious state of depression found him moving toward a vegetative state. Being confined to a bed in a nursing home was very difficult to accept. He often revisited so many aspects of his life including the good times before the stroke.

He felt hopeless and helpless as he lay there in a hospital bed and thinking of all that he had and now all that he had lost. He began to think more of his soul and of his spiritual life. Over and over, he thought of how he could die and wished for death rather than life if all that life had was the current state of immobility. His body as his physical life eventually became less important with the realization that life would not be getting better. It became very important for him to focus on what he could control more than what he could not control in his life. In searching for ways he could die, he came to the realization that there were some reasons to live. This eventually came to a book that he wrote with the assistance of others to tell his story. It further led to expressing his competence and skill through writing and publishing papers through which others who worked and guided him in his clinical and therapeutic needs.

From a life of independence and competence, Ron had moved to a life of dependence and institutionalization. This was devastating at first but as he learned what coping really meant, he embraced his motorized wheelchair as a friend. It began to give him some degree of freedom and he could now sit up and see and do some of the things that he had missed over a period of 6 years in this state. While the massive brain stem stroke deprived me of a normal life, it gave him the strength to look beyond his physical capabilities to his inner self and soul and focused on spiritual growth and goals in his life. Through a period of intense psychotherapy, he began to realize that there were "life goals" which he wanted to accomplish in his life limited by stroke. Among those goals was to increase his independence, revisit my home, enjoy some degree of family life, see his children grow up and become all that they were capable of becoming and to share his story and his newly gained optimism to others who faced the same or similar gut-wrenching experience that he had had as a paralyzed person who loved life and was competent and capable in the world in which he lived.

Ron's transition involved embracing his family, his children, his friends and his spiritual life in a very special way. Ron's journey in this life transitioned to his next life through a very rich and understood spiritual love of God!

Lessons Learned from Stressful Life Events

Three human beings faced an unexpected life change, the transitions in coping with the trauma and survived their stressful life experience. One suffered a traumatic accident, the second was shot in a random shooting and the third person suffered a brain stem stroke when he was in his mid-thirties. Each experience serves as a powerful example of serious bodily injury leading to an amputated limb, the pain and scares of a bullet or the consequences of a brain stem stroke, and extraordinary spiritual healing. The amputation falls within 0.4% of the population undergoing this procedure because of either disease or traumatic injury (Robinson and Micklesen 2006). Being wounded in a random shooting carries with it many physical and emotional scars through life.

In summary, for some individuals, recovery from an unexpected traumatic life-threatening event can represent at least a transient disruption in one's functioning. For others, however, recovery and adjustment can be more chronic, resulting in a lifelong disability. Recovery is dependent upon the individual's perception of the injury, personality traits, age, and access to appropriate medical and rehabilitative services. Other factors include a strong family support system, the capacity to redefine life goals, and for some, like myself, belief in a higher power. Further research in the area of individual resiliency is certainly needed since many individuals who encounter a serious traumatic injury do not always experience chronic emotional and/or physical disability.

References

American Psychiatric Association (2000). Diagnostic and Statistical Manual of Mental Disorders, Fourth Edition, Text Revision. Washington, DC.

Bonanno, G. A., & Mancini, A. D. (2008). The human capacity to thrive in the face of potential trauma. *Journal of the American Academy of Pediatrics, 121,* 369–375.

Bonanno, G. A., Galea, S., Bucciarelli, A., & Vlahov, D. (2007). What predicts psychological resilience after disaster? The role of demographics, resources, and life stress. *Journal of Consulting and Clinical Psychology, 75*(5), 571–682.

Ehde, D. M., & Williams, R. M. (2006). Adjustment to trauma. In L. R. Robinson (Ed.), *Trauma rehabilitation* (pp. 245–271). Philadelphia, PA: Lippincott Williams and Wilkins.

Hoge, E. A., Austin, E. D., & Pollack, M. H. (2007). Resilience: Research evidence and conceptual considerations for posttraumatic stress disorder. *Depression and Anxiety, 24,* 139–152.

Mancini, A. D., & Bonanno, G. A. (2006). Resilience in the face of potential trauma: Clinical practices and illustrations. *Journal of Clinical Psychology: In Session, 62*(8), 971–985.

Miller, T. W., & Veltkamp, L. J. (1996). Trauma accommodation syndrome. In T. W. Miller (Ed.), *Theory and assessment of stressful life events* (pp. 95–98). Madison, CT: International Universities Press, Inc.

Robinson, L. R., & Micklesen, P. J. (2006). Epidemiology of trauma-related disability. In L. R. Robinson (Ed.), *Trauma rehabilitation* (pp. 11–18). Philadelphia, PA: Lippincott Williams and Wilkins.

Yehuda, R. (1999). Biological factors associated with susceptibility of posttraumatic stress disorder. *Canadian Journal of Psychiatry, 44*, 34–39.

Chapter 21

The Role of Self-Awareness and Communication in Issues of Health and Aging

Joseph P. Fox

Introduction

Human life is sustained by a continuous interplay between the mind and the body. Without a mind, an able body has no direction. Without a body, an active mind has no way to act. The mind–body reality of most individuals falls between these two extremes. You use your mind to direct your body so that you can reach desired goals during your lifetime. In fact, your goals in life are heavily influenced by the natural strength and skill of your body systems. Likewise, your sense of personal achievement is influenced directly by changes in the performance capabilities of your body.

The first observer of the state of your mind–body relationship is you. It is the purpose of this chapter to discuss how objective self-awareness and effective communication of your mind–body state to your health care providers can reduce stress and improve your quality of life as you experience the effects of aging.

This is done by first defining the behavioral systems underlying human thought and communication through a model of mind–body relationships. This model is presented in a way that aligns functional behaviors (e.g., hearing, touch, cognition, motor programming, etc.) with the neurosensory and neuromuscular systems that support them.

Using this model, you can begin to understand how specific physical deficits affect behaviors in specific ways and how problems in one system can cause "downstream" problems in other systems. For example, hearing loss may be due to middle ear infection (auditory sensory awareness), but it can impair your ability to be aware of the topic of conversation (cognition), which requires intact hearing. These behavioral, structural, and neurological relationships are real and are always working in simultaneous synchrony to bring you what you interpret as life.

The state of your mind–body relationship will determine what is more or less stressful to you during your life as aging occurs. For example, the same person would likely react quite differently on facing the task of changing a flat tire at age 21 than at age 71. If at 71, you approach the task with the same expectations of a 21-year-old, there is a much greater probability you will

From: *Handbook of Stressful Transitions Across the Lifespan*,
Edited by: T.W. Miller, DOI 10.1007/978-1-4419-0748-6_21,
© Springer Science+Business Media, LLC 2010

overexert some muscular system of your body, for example, your back. The age of your body does make a difference regardless of the confidence you have based on past experiences. Controlling your own body's reactions to stress requires you to accept this fact and learn to be objective about the actual state of your mind–body relationship.

Stress can be defined as your body's organic reaction to a difference between what your mind wants to do and what your body is able to accomplish. It is also true that the dynamics of this relationship change as you age. The overall implication is that when your body changes, so must your mind to keep your life at its best.

It has been reported that one of the barriers to routine physical activity among the elderly is "low self-efficacy" (Orsega-Smith et al. 2008). It is understandable that an elderly person may not appreciate the benefits of regular exercise that is currently less vigorous than what he or she experienced when younger. However, these authors claim that routine physical activity is a virtual "Fountain of Youth" for the elderly and ways to overcome such mental barriers should be investigated.

The benefits of self-awareness and communication involves a narrow portion of a wide field of research findings on stress, but it is a view that helps us understand how to respond to the sudden occurrence of new stressor events that appear because of aging. In most cases, you are the first to sense significant body state changes, so it is most reasonable that you be the first responder, for yourself. How you adapt, physically and mentally to these changes of aging will help determine their impact on the quality and length of your life. When your physical or mental functions change, become aware and be ready to communicate openly with your health care providers. What you say about yourself to doctors and therapists can be just as important to them as the results of any instrumental procedures they perform.

Patterns of survival into old age are unique to each individual. What could be detrimental stress leading to illness for one person might be the type of stress needed to stimulate another person into feeling alert and healthy. An example of this could be the routine vigorous exercise just discussed. Someone simply out of shape will react quite differently than a person with serious heart disease. Stress stimulates adaptive responses that can be positive. However, unrelenting stress to which your body cannot adapt wastefully uses adaptive capacity which can only lead to exhaustion and death. This is a fact that makes a difference so it is important to develop a meaningful partnership with your health care providers.

The Stress Response

When you face anything you perceive as a threat, your hypothalamus alerts your entire body by a release of hormones, mostly adrenaline and cortisol. The hypothalamus is part of your limbic system; a collection of primitive brain structures located beneath the cerebral cortex. The limbic system initiates and drives your survival reactions, such as fight-or-flight when facing eminent danger or other protective reactions when experiencing illness or injury.

The rush of hormones from the hypothalamus have very specific effects on the body. Adrenaline causes your heart rate to rise, thereby elevating your blood pressure. It also boosts your energy supplies.

Cortisol is the primary stress hormone and it causes a release of sugars (glucose) into the bloodstream. It enhances the brain's ability to use glucose and increases the amount of substances needed to repair tissues.

Cortisol also inhibits functions not required to meet the current stressor event. It changes immune system responses and suppresses the digestive system, growth processes, and the reproductive system. In other words, if you are attempting to outrun a bear your body will shut down all desire for food or a mate.

The stress response is a complex alarm that also affects regions of the brain that control mood, motivation, and fear. This same array of reactions occurs regardless of the specific nature of a stressor. In other words, your body reacts in a uniform way no matter how dissimilar different stressing events are. Whether you are avoiding a falling tree, or going on stage to make a speech, your body's stress responses are similar.

The stress response is self-regulating. When fight-or-flight is no longer required, the stress hormone levels decline and your body returns to normal functioning. A necessary and beneficial stress response could be described as finding yourself in danger, responding to the emergency by protecting yourself, then returning to a normal, relaxed state.

Problems occur, however, when stressors persist, giving you little or no opportunity to return to normal functioning or your state of homeostasis. Jumping out of the way of a speeding car requires quick and decisive action, but the situation of stress is resolved as soon as the car passes. In those cases, where the possibility of physical harm is present for protracted lengths of time (e.g., soldiers in combat), symptoms of stress disorders commonly develop.

But activities involving psychological threats or risks (e.g., public speaking, business competition, personal challenges, etc.) can result in identical stress responses that persist from day to day until you change your mind or change your life situation. For example, when the personal benefits and the ease of public speaking become greater than the fear of public speaking, the stress response to that activity is reduced in intensity. When you understand that public speaking gives you an advantage, then that awareness changes who and what you are. What you accept in your mind is as real to your mind as any external activity you experience.

The following is a summary outline of the relationship between human activities and our ability to perform them, and how stress reactions to performing these activities change because of aging:

1. Stress reactions increase when learning new skills or routines, or acquiring new sets of information.
2. Stress reactions decrease as you learn and habituate to the behavior patterns required to accomplish these new activities. A state of homeostasis occurs in which the routine physical and mental operations demanded of you become highly automatic. High levels of skill and the resulting sense of confidence tend to reduce harmful, prolonged stress reactions.
3. However, potentially harmful stress reactions increase again as your body, brain, and nervous system age, because aging gradually reduces your functional performance levels. This can create the most stressful situation which humans face; trying to adapt and readapt to constantly changing levels of mental or physical abilities. Reduced performance levels must be objectively identified and accepted, so lower performance levels can become the new standard for normal. For many, however, this adjustment is as difficult to acknowledge as it is to accomplish.

The Human Mind–Body Connection

On the following page is a model (Fig. 21-1) that correlates fundamental human cortical structures and connections with the major functional motor and sensory behaviors they support. Although this model originally evolved as a communication model, it is easily adapted to illustrating learned human

A MODEL OF HUMAN MIND-BODY RELATIONSHIPS
Edited by Joseph P. Fox, Ph.D.

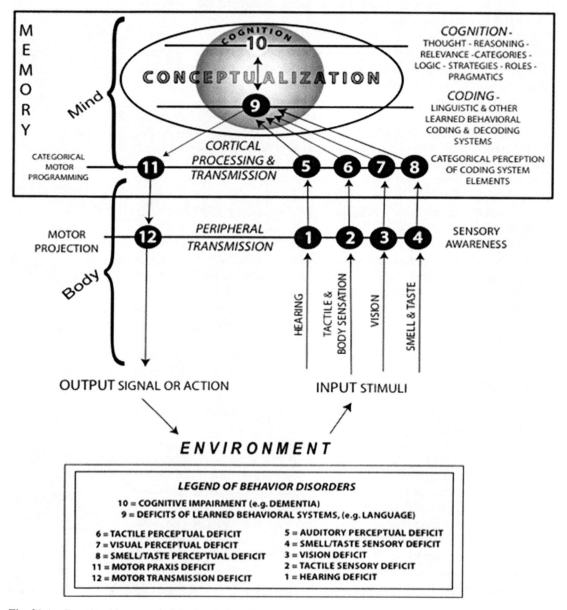

Fig. 21-1   Functional human mind–body relationships

behaviors in general. For example, the motor movements required for good speech, touch typing, and basketball dribbling have much in common. They are all learned, have a functional purpose, are rule-oriented, and are performed reflexively. They are developed and maintained by our desire (mind) to use these behaviors and our ability (body) to perform them. The following are important details of this model that will help make its terminology meaningful in later discussions.

The foundation of the human mind is our brain's ability to form concepts or *conceptualization*. Whenever we organize sensory input into categories and give that category meaning, we have created a concept. For example, something that is spherical and can be bounced and thrown is defined as a "ball." From our first encounter with "ballness", all new sensory experiences with "ballness" are added to that concept to make our own, unique definition of "ball." This includes everything from smell, weight, texture, and sights of balls flying out of baseball stadiums or beach balls bouncing from person to person by the ocean.

In addition to concepts that are the names of objects or actions, you can cluster many concepts together and create new concepts. For example, the concept of ball just described is actually a general concept defined by all the experiences of "ballness" you have ever had. You can combine the concept of ball with bats, bases, fielders, hitters, rules, and ball diamonds, and create a new concept called "baseball." You can keep going. You can link different games together by using the word, "sports." Then you can also create intersecting concepts by talking about such things as "practice," or "exercise," or "motivation," or "equipment." The human mind is almost limitless in its ability to form, revise, and interrelate thousands upon thousands of concepts.

The Unique Human Cortex

This conceptual ability is possible because of the human brain's unique cerebral cortex and its architecture. Only human brains have the sensory interconnections (most specifically among the senses of hearing, vision, and touch) required for nonlimbic, cross-modal associations (Geschwind 1965). This is the foundation for human thought and language.

The brains of all mammals have cortical primary and secondary association areas for these three primary sensory input systems (modalities). The temporal lobe processes auditory signals. The occipital lobe processes visual images and body sensations are received and processed in the parietal lobe.

In each of these lobes of the mammal's brain, there are primary association areas where there is topological localization of modality-specific sensory input. For example, in Heschel's gyrus of the temporal lobe there are specific cortical locations that represent sounds of different frequencies at different levels of loudness.

The occipital pole is an upside down and reversed image of the visual fields that enter the mammal's eye. The anterior margin of the parietal lobe receives sensory input from the body with input from the toes and feet received at the top of the parietal lobe. The body is represented in an upside down fashion as you go down the "sensory strip" to the sensory input from the head and face at the bottom of the anterior parietal lobe.

The purpose of the primary association areas is to make input from the peripheral sensory organs (e.g., the eyes, ears, skin and muscles, etc.) available to the brain. If the temporal lobe system does not work, you have hearing loss or deafness. If the occipital system does not function, you have visual impairment or blindness. If the parietal system is not operating, you have loss of feeling or sensation.

All mammals also have secondary association areas surrounding each primary association area. These secondary association areas begin processing the incoming sensory information and also provide connections to the rest of the brain. If the secondary association area in the temporal lobe does not function properly, then the animal can hear, but cannot tell the difference between different sounds. Perceiving a difference *(auditory categorical perception)* between the mating call of your species and the howl of a predator is obviously an important distinction.

Similar comments can be made about the secondary association areas adjacent to the primary visual and sensory areas. Not being able to detect differences between visual or tactile stimuli *(vision and tactile categorical perception)* could quickly lead to great difficulties or death.

This is the point where human brain structure separates us from all other mammals. Only the human brain has a massive cortical tertiary association area in the inferior, posterior parietal lobe that simultaneously interconnects the secondary association areas of all the sensory modalities. It is an association area of association areas. It is the most recent area of the brain to evolve and the last to mylinate, as humans develop and grow. This is what allows for cross-modal, nonlimbic associations. The cross-modal associations of all other animals require primarily limbic neural integration (Geschwind, 1965).

From an evolutionary perspective, the limbic system is the original primitive brain of all mammals. The limbic structures are situated below the cerebral cortex and function to preserve the individual (fight or flight responses in times of distress) and the species (sexual arousal). Limbic activities monitor everything from the animal's need for food, warmth, shelter, safety, and companionship. For all animals, except humans, cortical sensory stimuli are integrated primarily through the limbic system.

As discussed earlier concerning the stress response, the limbic system is what initiates our reaction to stressors. One might argue that the evolutionary history of our limbic system is better prepared to protect us in the presence of immediate danger than our more fluid and changeable cognition taking place in the cortex.

What does this mean in real life? This means that all animals, other than humans, can hear, see, and feel the same stimuli humans do and can tell they are different, but when it comes to deciding *what these stimuli mean*, it must be related to some primal function of survival. For example, dogs can learn to sit when they hear the word "sit," but only by linking it to a survival behavior (e.g., food, companionship, etc.)

We humans are likewise influenced by our limbic systems, but we have one huge *additional* option. We can and do create nonlimbic concepts (meanings) through direct cortical associations, think about things *(cognition)*, and override our limbic system urges, if we wish. "Current work is verifying the integrative functioning of cortical and subcortical areas (especially, the amygdala) in the organism's response to primitive emotional experiences such as fear (LeDoux, 1994)." This is how a father overcomes his fear of height and accompanies his young son who is begging to be taken on his first roller coaster ride. Behaviorally, it is that one little difference that makes all the difference between humans and other animals.

Cognition is the conscious manipulation of the concepts you have formed to help you think, reason, plan, and act. It creates your sense of awareness and reality, and helps you determine what to do or not do at every moment. It is heavily dependent upon structures and processes carried out in the frontal lobes. You use language and nonverbal symbols *(codes)* to communicate ideas generated by your mind to the minds of others and to *decode* these same kinds of signals from others.

All communications are symbolic. A symbol is one thing that represents something else. For example, the word "chair" represents any object that has a seat, legs, and a back and is sturdy enough to sit on. A wave of the hand could represent a greeting, like saying "Hi" ; or to a football quarterback the wave of the hand could mean "I'm open, pass me the ball." We humans live our lives in an ocean of symbols, which we continually and immediately *code* and *decode*.

An obvious coded system you use is speech and language. Language represents the verbal symbols you use to communicate your thoughts and speech is the perceptual *(phoneme categorical perception)* and motor system *(morpo-phonemic categorical motor programming* and *motor projection)* you use to receive and send your language code within the *environment* that is your life.

All symbolic systems are learned, rule-ordered, and used to the point they operate automatically as conditioned reflexes. You have to learn to perceive and articulate phonemes such as /s/, /k/, /u/, and /l/, so you can understand and use the word "school." The same is true for all other words and verbal and nonverbal symbols.

For example, athletes must learn the detailed movement and observation strategies of their sport until they perform them automatically. Also, going to school provides students a place to practice academic material until it is learned; can be recalled and used without hesitation, especially when applied to new situations.

"Getting through a day" means you successfully and unconsciously (most of the time) string together the proper series of thoughts and conditioned reflexes necessary to perform the activities your schedule requires for that day. You don't have to concentrate on every bodily movement involved in putting on clothes, washing, eating, walking, running, reading, writing, talking, or completing work assignments. You just do them. However, there was a time in your life when each one of these activities was new and impossible for you to accomplish. Practice does, in fact, move us toward perfection because it is the foundation of all of life's activities.

Linguistic and Nonlinguistic Symbols

Speech sounds or phonemes do not convey meaning, but when strung together to form morphemes (e.g., "-ed" meaning past tense) or words (e.g., "chase") they do. Your brain first *perceives* phonemes then *decodes* any meaning units (morphemes, syntax, intonation, etc.) the phoneme strings contain. Your brain does all this almost instantly. If you have not learned the language you are hearing, then it is just noise and your brain will not perceive speech sounds and decodes no words because you have learned neither the vocabulary nor the rules of that language.

The same is true for non-language symbol systems. Think of all the symbols to which we respond throughout a day. There are traffic lights, trademarks on packages, sirens, aprons on cooks, vapor trails across the sky, taps on your shoulder, leashes on animals, and on and on. You interpret (decode) each of these sensory experiences in particular ways depending on what has happened to you in the past and what is happening to you at the moment. If you have not learned these non-language symbols then you may walk right into traffic on a street because you do not understand what it means to be hit by a car or truck. Consider the reaction of mothers when their toddlers run toward a busy street. Toddlers just don't know yet. We were all toddlers at one time.

Mind and Body in Harmony

What is driving your life is a constantly evolving flood of symbolism (mind) and coordinated conditioned responses (body) that you accept as your reality from moment to moment. Whatever you decide is real creates changes in your body and your life which stay that way until you change your mind based on new thoughts or experiences.

As you grow, all of your behavioral input and output systems develop, function with increasing efficiency, and then decline as you age. How you adapt to both the developing and diminishing of these mind/body skills during your life creates the stressful markers (events) with which you will cope. When all your adaptation potential is exhausted, your life ends (Selye 1956). In other words, the more quickly you can identify, understand, and accept significant changes in your body–mind status, the less stressful adapting to these transitions will be and the longer and more satisfying your life.

Learning to cope in ways that reduce the magnitude of stress reactions extends out that final eventuality. This chapter and, indeed, all the chapters of this book contain information that can help you identify and positively cope with the important life events you experience. Clinicians can use this information to assist patients needing to cope with their significant life events.

The Body's Connections to the Mind

Auditory Input System (Hearing)

Hearing is the most important sensory system humans have for developing and maintaining normal human interactions. What makes it so important is that once the fundamentals of language are acquired, oral verbal communication is the quickest and most effective mind-to-mind communication possible between any two humans who speak the same language. The subtlety of vocal inflections, word choice, syntax and the communication situation all meld into an instant message of information, direction, humor, or, perhaps, insult.

So much of the spice of life comes from the verbal shades of meanings we use among ourselves. You instantly understand the intended message and that understanding may provoke you into your own response or retort. Verbal repartee is one of the most intimate and exciting things we do as humans. It seals everything from friendships and business deals to marriages and divorces. It is important everywhere and occurs in virtually all situations when humans are involved.

Presbycusis and Functional Hearing Problems

You are basically unaware of your hearing ability because *what* you understand from hearing speech is much more important to you and your life than *how* you hear the speech. Also, you frequently have no awareness of what you do not hear. However, it is best to understand a few basic concepts about the auditory system and how the brain uses this sensory input modality so that you might identify stressful events related to *presbycusis* (normal hearing loss related to aging).

The middle, and inner ear structures of the ear are essentially adult size at birth. The outer ear continues some growth throughout life. The middle and inner ear structures are actually located in small intricate tunnels and caverns in the left and right temporal bones of the skull. They contain mechanical and neural structures that transduce sound waves into neural impulses. The eighth cranial nerve (auditory nerve) sends these signals to the brain, specifically Heschl's gyrus. There are two Heschl's gyri, one in each temporal lobe of each cerebral hemisphere. As mentioned earlier, these are the sound transmission input centers from the ears to the brain.

Anything that *distorts* the creation or transmission of sound from the outer, middle, and inner ears to the two temporal lobes causes a hearing loss. This includes conditions ranging from too much earwax to middle ear infections to damaged cells in the cochlea.

Anything that *prevents* the creation or transmission of these neural sound signals to the brain results in deafness. This generally means there are devastating lesions in both cochleae or somewhere along both ascending auditory nerves. Cortical deafness rarely occurs since that requires similar and simultaneous destruction of the neurons in both Heschel's gyri, in both cerebral hemispheres.

Normal aging primarily affects the cochlea's ability to transduce the higher frequencies of speech into neural signals. If the cochlea does not transduce those signals, the brain does not know that they exist in the speech to which you are listening.

The practical result is you have difficulty understanding speech. The higher frequencies of speech enable you to hear the consonant sounds and consonants make speech intelligible. The difference between the words "Sue" and "two" is not their final vowel, /oo/, but the initial consonants, /s/ and /t/. By comparison, /oo/ is loud, low-pitched, and longer-lasting whereas /s/ and /t/ are brief bursts of high-pitched sounds that are not nearly as loud.

Therefore, presbycusis makes distinguishing the difference between these two words and all other similar phoneme contrasts more difficult. Your reaction to this natural change in hearing is interesting. Your brain fills in any missing phonemes using a "best guess" strategy. You will have little awareness of the words you incorrectly interpret. It will be your impression that what you understood is exactly what was said even if it was not. These become life-impacting moments for your family and friends also, as they witness you misinterpreting comments that are clearly understood by everyone with normal hearing.

Adaptation to Hearing Loss

There are two steps required in solving this universal problem of aging. First, recognize and accept the loss in high-frequency hearing when it begins interfering with your ability to understand speech. Second, start using hearing aids immediately. The brain needs continual exposure to speech sounds to keep you in touch with your environment and to keep tuned by detecting and decoding speech signals. The longer it goes without receiving some high-frequency speech information, the harder it is to adapt to using hearing aids later. The smaller the steps of adaptation required the easier to accomplish.

This phenomenon accounts for the enormous number of hearing aids some older individuals purchase, but refuse to use, after years of declining hearing sensitivity without hearing aids. Speech is noisy, so if you let your brain adapt to a silent range of high frequencies for many years, then suddenly hearing the full speech sound spectrum again could be intolerable. For many who wait, it is.

Bottom line, each of us is in control of how we adapt as our hearing changes. It is a certainty that we will adapt one way or another because our hearing acuity does decline. On the basis of my clinical experiences, there are two primary adaptation routes individuals take. First, some work with their hearing health professionals and obtain the hearing aids and any aural rehabilitation they need when they need it.

Second, most individuals refuse to admit to hearing problems and insist that the world has simply become noisier and standards of speech articulation lower. This second option is denial. However, this powerful urge to deny is supported by your internal reaction of certainty when your brain makes an interpretation of a word or sentence spoken to you, even when that interpretation is totally incorrect. As far as your brain is concerned, anything it did not perceive was, simply, never said. Also, whatever it decides you heard is what was, in fact, said. We need to view our sensory processing systems as *tools* that we use and they should be verified and countermanded when appropriate.

In terms of stress management, the best tack to take for body–mind balance and positive environmental relationships through your senior years is the first option. This option requires an objective attitude and a willingness to establish new auditory skill sets. In fact, this is the key phrase to working through all the stressful markers of health, which occur during your lifetime. Be open to finding out from the appropriate medical specialists what is really happening within your own mind–body complex, then actively pursue those adaptation skills necessary to maintain the life activities of greatest interest and pleasure to you.

Visual Input System (Sight)

Vision is the most spectacular sense you have. Vision provides huge quantities of stark to subtle graphic details of the environment around you so that you can develop and modify your set of reality concepts. Vision is the sense that most of us would not want to lose, but it is still not as vital to maintaining human relationships as is hearing.

Carrying on a conversation by writing and reading notes is slow and imprecise. Such a conversation is not accompanied with vocal intonation or pauses, which add significant clarity to the intended meanings of spoken words. Have you ever noticed how some of your written comments are misinterpreted in e-mails or text messages? The mood you are feeling does not always get translated correctly when you send your written words out on their own.

Still, vision is highly important in gaining, mastering, and using motor skills. Just ask any seamstress, graphic artist, or basketball point guard. Almost every physical motion we make or master requires visual input and feedback. This viewpoint is supported by current research that describes cortical connections between the occipital pole (primary visual association area) and the parietal lobe (Giorello and Sinigaglia 2007). These sensory pathways are required for grasping objects (a motor function) of various shapes, sizes, and orientations. When these pathways are interrupted, grasping objects is impaired even though they are visually perceived accurately. Visual perception alone is supported by other occipital connections to the inferotemporal cortex.

Vision provides you an almost stable representation of everything around you so that you can learn, practice, and master whatever is yours to do. Infants work on crawling. Toddlers concentrate on walking. Older kids conquer bikes, skateboards, and video games. Adults master skills of their professions and of caring for families. Vision is important in gaining and maintaining most volitional motor skills.

The visual processing system has one major advantage over the auditory processing system. That advantage is time. Auditory signals must be received, perceived, and decoded quickly because they exist briefly. New information follows old information in fractions of a second. However, the visual processing system, in many instances, affords you the luxury of a continuous gaze. You can examine a scene until you can determine what the objects, shapes, and colors are. You can look at poorly scribbled words until they make sense. In contrast, if you misinterpret or completely miss a spoken word it is gone. There is no opportunity to double-check, unless you interrupt the flow of conversation with a well-placed, "Huh?" or "What?"

This difference affects how you adapt to visual decline as opposed to auditory decline. Changes in vision are more noticeable because you are more aware of the time it takes to see something clearly. You may be more willing to wear glasses than hearing aids, though they are directly comparable devices. When you do not hear something, you do not have much time to think about it, so it may br easier to blame the speaker.

Presbyopia and Other Changes of the Eye with Aging

As you age, the lenses of your eyes lose elasticity making it more difficult to focus on fine print or objects that are close-up *(presbyopia)*. This is the change in vision experienced by almost everyone and is usually correctable with glasses or contact lenses.

The lenses of your eyes also yellow as you age. This affects your ability to see colors accurately. As a result, discriminating between shades of blue, green, and violet becomes more difficult.

The pupils of your eyes work less effectively. This reduces the amount of light that enters the eye and makes it more difficult for you to adjust to sudden changes in lighting. You will need more light shining on what you want to see or read than before.

All these subtle, but definite changes, in your eyes combine to create an increased sensitivity to glare. Bright lights tend to blur your vision further, so sunglasses may be needed at times to reduce that effect.

All humans have small particles (floaters) suspended in the fluid within their eyes. Floaters, from time to time, disturb your vision to the point of being annoying, but they are normal and harmless. As you age, there may be more floaters and they may be more noticeable. However, if large floaters suddenly appear and are accompanied with bright flashes of light you should contact your eye care professional (optometrist or ophthalmologist) immediately. Those could be symptoms of an impending or actual retinal detachment.

Some diseases that often impact your vision more seriously as you age are cataracts, glaucoma, and macular degeneration. Cataracts cause your lenses to become cloudy and can progress to the point of near blindness. Cataracts can be removed through surgery.

Glaucoma is the abnormal build up of fluid pressure in the eye that can damage the optic nerve if not treated. It is easily controlled with medication. There are frequently no symptoms until damage occurs, so regular eye examinations help prevent problems from glaucoma.

The macula is the central portion of the visual field in which you see most clearly the details of whatever you are observing or inspecting. Macular degeneration occurs when, for reasons still unknown, the receptors in this area of the retina atrophy and cease to function. It creates central vision blindness while leaving peripheral vision intact. It can be devastating to individuals who, for example, read, sew, drive, or work with tools since the precise vision they need for their activity of interest is impaired or gone. Again, regular visits to your eye care professional are recommended to help detect any signs of macular degeneration.

Peripheral Versus Central Decline

All these changes in vision represent a single functional impairment as shown in Fig. 21.1.. All of these affect only *visual sensory awareness* (A model of mind–body relationships discussed earlier).

This is an example of how peripheral sensory systems are affected functionally more by aging than are cortical systems. Madden et al. (2002a) studied adult age differences in visual word identification *(visual categorical perception)* using PET and found no significant age-related decline between one group of subjects that were 20–29-year-old and another group of 62–70-year-old subjects. They did find differences in how the older brains appeared to process the visual information, but those differences seemed not to matter in terms of functional outcome.

In general, age appears to reduce functioning of all the peripheral sensory and motor systems more than it does the central cortical integrating systems. This may be because the brain has greater functional adaptive options available to it (neural redundancy) than do peripheral motor and sensory systems.

Also, peripheral neuromotor systems involve large masses of muscle, connective, and skin tissues and many hundreds of feet of branching neural connections each of which changes with age (Wickremaratchi and Llewelyn 2006). Because of this peripheral systems also have greater exposure to external trauma. All of these factors may then create greater functional declines in peripheral transmission systems than in central cortical processing systems.

Adaptation to Impaired Vision

As suggested earlier, adaptation to impaired sensory acuity such as vision requires an objective attitude and a willingness to establish new visual skill sets. An example of a new visual skill set would be the use of eyeglasses. The first few days this writer wore glasses for the first time, going up and down stairs and making turns was difficult. I had to retrain my motor systems to new visual input. Knowing and accepting what is happening to your vision is the most important step to reducing your stress reactions to those moments when you realize your vision has changed. When your vision changes your life changes. Being ready ahead of time makes it a less stressful transition.

Routine vision evaluations by your vision health care specialist create a documented history of changes in your vision. This history helps you understand and cope with the functional impact of changing vision. It also provides your vision care specialist the information needed to accurately assess your vision and to determine the probable future course of your eye care needs.

Tactile Input System (Touch)

Your sense of touch *(tactile sensory awareness)* is not as obviously important to you as is your sight and hearing. However, without it you would have serious problems performing the simplest motor tasks. It is a critical feedback system for normal *categorical motor programming* which is required to perform any learned motor task (e.g., writing, speaking, walking, using tools, playing sports, etc.).

Consider the poor control of your speech when Novocain numbs your tongue and lips. Without your sense of touch, precise motor movements become difficult to impossible. Catching a ball would be impossible, if you could not sense where your hands were. Standing and walking would not be simple tasks, if you could not sense when your feet touch the ground. Your sense of touch is so important in almost every movement you make that you are compelled to take it for granted.

A number of changes of sensory thresholds have been reported as being related to aging (Wickremaratchi and Llewelyn 2006). They also describe some major functional behaviors impaired by these changes.

In general, aging results in a rise in sensory thresholds. A rise of a threshold means greater force is required on the peripheral receptor before a neural signal is sent to the brain. Thresholds are higher for light touch, pain, temperature, vibration, and spatial acuity of touch (the closest distance you can sense two points of stimulation). Functionally, these changes are interpreted as feeling more clumsy because you may drop things more often or occasionally have difficulty moving a pencil or pen precisely. As you age, sometimes small cuts and scratches just seem to appear out of nowhere. You do not feel the scrape when it happens.

As you age, you have greater difficulty holding fine motor positions steadily. It is more difficult to manipulate parts so that they fit together. Postural stability is affected. It is not as easy to walk on narrow surfaces. You may trip more and have more difficulty making quick turns or maneuvering between, over, or around barriers.

These are little changes in behavior that can cause concern when you do not know how to explain them. Such behavioral changes may prompt you to speculate that you are just getting older. On the other hand, you may believe you are experiencing the onset of some dreaded disease. The only way to verify the real causes of changes in your body is by a medical evaluation. The least stressful approach to health care as you age is to have regular medical check-ups and to know the truth about how and why your body is changing.

Motor Output System

Learned Motor Movements

So much of what you are is tied to what you teach your body to do. Every profession has a set of motor skills required for both basic competency and expert performance in that profession. Even professions that do not require the overall physical perfection of professional sports still require significant learned motor skills. Attorneys may not have to routinely sprint 50 yards, but the cognition and resulting motor output systems required to support their oral verbal skills are by no means simple.

For all motor skills repetitious motor learning is required. For example, consider using a hammer to drive a nail. When you were young, you did not know how to hold the hammer, how to swing it so that you would hit the head of the nail solidly, and how to repeat the motion until the nail was completely into the wood. You struggled holding the hammer and swinging it until you gained greater control of where it went. You were training your brain to direct the muscles of your body, particularly in your arm and hand, to hit the nail solidly and to drive it down.

The more you practiced, the more quickly you recognized the correct grip, swing, and contact with the hammer that would accomplish your goal. You were establishing automatic motor sequences *(categorical motor programming)* to which your motor system would refer every time in the future when you use a hammer. Anything new you learn about handling a hammer, you adopt by adjusting your motor programming sequence for hammering. Neurologists refer to this function as "praxis" (Yamadori 2002).

The only way you gain expert motor control is by practicing your desired motor movements until they occur automatically. When that occurs, your categorical motor programming system is set with your most current set of directions for that behavior. Every different motor skill you have requires the same development and maintenance of its unique categorical motor programming sequences. This includes batting, ironing, typing, operating video games, talking, dancing, kicking, cooking, operating a cash register…truly, every learned motor skill.

If you are attempting a motor task you have never done before, you have no pre-programmed motor sequences available and you are clumsy despite great attention to every movement. You either give up or start the process of motor learning for that activity until it becomes automatic.

As mentioned earlier, your categorical motor programming system depends heavily on sensory feedback. Therefore, impaired sensory input compromises this motor output system. The body is a balanced sensory-motor system, so everything must work together to get your work and play activities accomplished.

The *motor projection system* represents the peripheral muscles and nerves of the body. When you decide to move, your brain prompts your categorical motor programming system to initiate the proper sequencing of motor movements necessary to perform that action. The proper set of peripheral nerves carry these coordinated signals to the targeted muscles and you perform your planned action as you originally desired. The motor projection system is a transmission system and not a processing system. It connects the brain to the muscles of the body, so what the mind wants to do will happen.

Motor Output Changes with Aging

As discussed earlier, peripheral transmission systems involve many more body structures (muscles, bones, etc. outside the skull) than does the brain (neural tissue and structures inside the skull). Thus, changes due to aging understandably affect the overall performance abilities of peripheral systems more than the functioning of the brain.

Gersten (1991) summarized a number of the changes in the peripheral motor system due to aging. Biopsy of tissues from individuals between 60 and 90 years of age show changes due to aging in all systems and tissues, including both muscle tissue and nerve fibers. Percentage of body fat increases with age while the percentage of muscle mass decreases. As a result, lifting objects weighing as little as 10 lbs. is difficult for 28% of men and 66% of women after age 74.

Adaptation to Motor System Changes

Probably, the most important point about adapting to a changing peripheral motorsystem functioning is that at any age your body's response to increased muscle stress is to build up muscle mass. In other words, increasing muscle mass (strength and endurance) is your body's natural response to the stress of exercise at any age. While it is true that maximum strength attainable may be less than that in previous decades of your life, it is still just as true that improved muscle strength and endurance result from exercise at any age, provided exercise is not contraindicated by other health issues (Gersten 1991).

Wu and Hallet (2005) reported that both younger subjects (average age of 31.5 years) and older subjects (average age of 61.8 years) learned to perform complex, memorized sequential finger movements with essentially equal facility. The older subjects did take longer to practice the sequences until they were automatic, but eventually most of them did as well on the tasks as the younger subjects.

When Wu and Hallet analyzed brain activity of the subjects using MRI, they found significantly different patterns of brain activity between the two groups of subjects. The older subjects had increased neural activity in a number of areas and some reduced activity in other areas. It is as if the older subjects had to create new and expanded neural networks in order to accomplish their desired task performance. This suggests that even though older brains have lost neuron mass, they can still restructure circuits in important areas to accomplish desired tasks. Training takes longer, but automatic proficiency is possible for most.

The body–mind relationship is critical. Your body will adapt to the physical stressors your mind imposes on it through the activities you choose to do. If retirement means taking it easy by sitting around, your body will respond by gaining weight and losing muscle mass. If retirement means keeping active and interested in life activities around you, your body will respond by maintaining muscle mass and slowing or preventing fat accumulation. As the mind guides, the body responds. This means that the first step to changing any condition of your body is changing your mind in some significant way.

The only precaution is to not overdrive your adaptive capacity. Striving to obtain physical goals now beyond your body's capability puts your body under unrelenting stress. Unrelenting stress lavishly consumes overall adaptive capacity and leads to the certain and rapid collapse of organs most affected by the generalized stress response in your body. Finding and maintaining your optimum level of homeostasis is the key to successful aging.

The Mind's Integrating Systems

The Mind and Memory

Looking at the model of human mind–body relationships, there is a box around all the components that constitute "Mind." The box itself is labeled "Memory." This means that every functional aspect of our mind requires some type of memory to function properly. Let us briefly review how memory supports the five major functional systems of the mind.

First and foremost, when the mind develops and understands a new concept *(conceptualization)*, it is remembered. As stated earlier, because of the unique neural architecture of the human brain humans can make nonlimbic, cross-modal associations to create and remember thousands of concepts. Most of these concepts you remember, use, and modify during your life.

The brain's conceptualization ability makes you verbal, self-aware, and human. Part of that humanity is suppressing limbic system impulses through reasoning so that you can live life with a more compassionate and cooperative attitude toward others. The role of the limbic system is survival, not compassion. Your experiences with conscience may well represent the real struggle between your limbic system's role to insure self-preservation and your own cortically driven decisions to reach out and help others. Whatever the final decisions are, you remember them and make them part of your operational view of reality.

The human mind remembers code systems such as languages (including simple, game like codes such as pig-Latin), mathematics, etc. Codes have symbols and rules for their use (syntax). We practice the codes until they are understood and expressed automatically.

The transmitted elements of codes can be sounds (speech), sights (words, hand gestures, etc.) or tactile (Braille). In all the cases, these transmission elements are rule-governed. Phonemes (speech sounds) are specific categories of sounds with unique acoustic characteristics. Braille has a specific pattern of raised dots representing letters of the alphabet.

Your *categorical perceptual* and *categorical motor programming* systems must be trained to *perceive* and produce the appropriate *motor output* equivalents, respectively, for you to use a code system successfully. Thus, both perception and motor programming require specialized memory.

Changes with Aging

The good news is that normal aging does not significantly change the functions of the mind. Serial memory (the number of numbers given in a series that you can recall immediately) may decrease from 7 (±2) to 5 items (±2). Word finding may at times be more difficult. Complicated statements or abstract ideas may be more difficult to grasp, but, despite age, your mind keeps trying to accomplish whatever you direct it to do.

As suggested earlier, the brain appears to have an advantage over the peripheral body systems in compensating for changes due to aging. The older brain appears to operate differently, but still effectively, for performing visual word identification (Madden et al. 2002a), visual search (Madden et al. 2002b), and learning motor movements until they can be performed automatically (Wu and Hallet 2005).

Not to be totally outdone, the body (peripheral motor-neural systems) of over 60-year-old is still capable of improving cardiovascular conditioning through exercise (Gersten 1991) even if not as efficiently as years past.

Also remember, many of the functional problems traditionally associated with aging may have more to do with the need for improving sensory input (glasses and hearing aids) than with any decline in cortical functioning. Denial is strong in a mind that has experienced life and successfully overcome setbacks for three or more generations. However, if the brain does not have quality, intelligible input data, it guesses. When it guesses wrong, the results might mimic dementia to observers and become fodder for anecdotes and jokes about aging.

Adaptation to Cognitive Changes

Reportedly, Aristotle taught, "What we have to learn to do, we learn by doing." This is clear to most adults as we assist our children, but it is equally true for we who are older. Cognitive changes due to aging are minimized by physical activity and conscious mental self-care. Tang et al. (2007) report that even as little as "5 days of meditation practice with the integrative body–mind training method" led to improved scores on the Profile of Mood States scale for their subjects. Their subjects also exhibited "a significant decrease in stress-related cortisol, and an increase in immunoreactivity."

It will require more research to describe the precise physical benefits of meditation and mindfulness training, but signing up for instruction in meditation techniques only requires a personal decision. Each of us is in charge of what we choose to do or not to do. Most adults will not lose their ability to learn, keep in shape, share humor, or appreciate things of value as they age. If anything, the experiences of a lifetime magnify your sense of appreciation. Being objectively informed about your body and keeping proactive in the life that you have created around you is the best plan for keeping the stress in your life balanced.

Aging and Diseases: The Intersect

The Impact of Disease on the Mind–Body Interaction

The discussion to this point has focused on general changes of sensory, motor, and cognitive systems related to aging. I have discussed what these changes are in general and how your awareness of these changes as they occur can help you adapt your life activities to minimize unrelenting stress reactions. These are basically the normal changes most of us can expect. They are different, however, from the impact of diseases or traumatic accidents, which are not normal at any stage of life.

Still, as we successfully negotiate through the expected declines of aging the probability increases that we will experience one or more serious diseases or trauma. This is another way of saying that life has risks, so a longer life means greater exposure to the same risks plus any risks that are uniquely yours (e.g., genetics, family environment, childhood diseases, incidental exposure to pollutants, radiation, toxins, etc.). The need to adapt to local or generalized stressors remains the same when diseases occur, but disease processes may result in sudden, unexpected, and potentially complex adaptation efforts, which may or may not be successful.

The underlying theme of this chapter is about maintaining a positive, proactive attitude. You could reasonably ask, "Fine, but is there any scientific evidence that a positive, proactive attitude really changes anything?" The answer is "Yes." Consider the quick responses to meditation training already described (Tang et al. 2007). Serious research into the "placebo effect" is also gaining momentum. Cavanna et al. (2007) summarize the historical views and current research on the placebo effect, which is a promising area of mind–body control. Thirty percent or more of patients receiving a placebo respond positively. Likewise, those receiving medication believing it to be harmful respond negatively. These results were first noticed in pain management studies, but have since been noted in studies of movement disorders and other neurological conditions. Our mind is potentially our most powerful health ally, but we must keep it properly informed.

Acute Diseases

There are a number of acute diseases commonly related to aging. The list may include stroke, heart attack, diabetes, broken bones, and many others. All of these diseases have one thing in common. They occur suddenly (acute onset), require medical intervention, have a follow-up period of rehabilitation (healing and learning new coping strategies), and require establishing new life survival routines. Every acute disease should result in a decision to make the lifestyle changes necessary to avoid a recurrence. Remember, your body can do only what your mind directs.

None of us can predict with certainty what acute diseases we will ever experience. Living wisely with a balanced diet, regular exercise, and avoiding addictions is the best general prevention plan. However, there are times disease onsets occur anyway. Since you cannot prevent the possible onset of acute diseases, it is best to have general knowledge concerning plans of action for such eventualities.

Being knowledgeable of acute diseases in general and how to respond will help minimize your body's generalized stress reaction if something does occur. It is also important to understand that medical and surgical procedures used to treat acute disorders can seem strange, radical, and inhumane to a patient. This occurs because the goal may have to be stabilizing your bodily functions and overall medical health status and not immediately making you feel safe and comfortable. Ultimately, however, medical and rehabilitation goals focus on finding the proper balance of medications, surgery, physical activity, or behavior change that will re-establish your sense of homeostasis; some sense of comfort and control. If you understand this, then you can help your health care professionals help you. You become one of your own healers and not a victim.

Second, as your body experiences acute changes, you can no longer force it to learn and perform as you did when you were younger. You must be painfully honest about your capabilities and seriously listen to the medical and rehabilitation experts. They are not always correct, but their information is the place to start. You learn from them all that you can, follow their instructions, assess the results, and then, most importantly, report back to them what works and what does *not*. Conversations with your doctors and other health care professionals are crucial. They cannot do their job properly without you as a consultant.

Progressive Diseases

Progressive diseases (e.g., multiple sclerosis, Parkinson's, etc.) create more long-term problems in terms of maintaining lower stress reactions. Progressive diseases tend to have periods where you are sicker followed by periods of feeling better. When bodily functions do not stay stable, then you are put in the position of requiring intermittent rehabilitation in response to new episodes of symptom progression. This is frustrating, but if you are aware of what to expect you can plan your activities accordingly.

It has been this clinician's experience that when working with patients with progressive diseases those who practiced most consistently during periods of disease remission did better working through periods of disease progression. In this case, the learning maxim may not be, "practice makes perfect," but it might be, "practice makes loss, less."

Summary and Conclusions

Life is a continuous string of stressful events. Much of the stress can build us up, keep us healthy, entertain us, help us create lives, careers, communities, and progress. However, viewed from a different mental perspective the same stressors could tear us down, overwhelm our expectations, make us sick and end our lives. The key to mastering which direction you go is becoming aware of your own mind–body systems, learning how to read them, and consciously choosing the least harmful adaptive approaches for yourself from moment to moment.

A mind–body relationship model is presented and the human sensory and motor system connections to the brain are discussed in light of this model. Using this model, you can better understand and more accurately describe the functional changes you experience as you age. The more effective your communications are to your health care providers, the more effective their treatment protocols will be in meeting your needs. However, it is your responsibility to take the lead role in monitoring your own state of health. You are the closest observer.

Also, by understanding how you use your mind–body system to carry out the functional activities of your life you can respond more successfully to each life event and its particular stressors. The particular events that impact your life are unique to you, so your responses to these events will be unique to you. Even though your lifetime adaptive capacity is finite, the more knowledgeable and wiser you become about how to respond to life events as they occur, the greater potential you have for a longer, more productive, and satisfying life.

References

Cavanna, A. E., Strigaroa, G., & Monacoa, F. (2007). Brain mechanisms underlying the placebo effect in neurological disorders. *Functional Neurology, 22*(2), 89–94.

Gersten, J. W. (1991). Effect of exercise on muscle function decline with aging, rehabilitation medicine – Adding life to years [Special Issue]. *The Western Journal of Medicine, 154*, 579–582.

Geschwind, N. (1965). Disconnexion syndromes in animals and man. *Brain, 88*, 237–294 and 585–644.

Giorello, G., & Sinigaglia, C. (2007). Perception in action. *Acta Bio Medica, 78*(Suppl 1), 49–57.

Madden, D. J., Langley, L. K., Denny, L. L., Turkington, T. G., Provenzale, J. M., Hawk, T. C., et al. (2002). Adult age differences in visual word identification: Functional neuroanatomy by positron emission tomography. *Brain and Cognition, 49*(3), 297–321.

Madden, D. J., Turkington, T. G., Provenzale, J. M., Denny, L. L., Langley, L. K., Hawk, T. C., et al. (2002). Aging and attentional guidance during visual search: Functional neuroanatomy by positron emission tomography. *Psychology and Aging, 17*(1), 24–43.

The Stress Response. http://mayoclinic.com

Vision and Aging. http://mayoclinic.com

LeDoux, Joseph E. (1994). "Emotion, Memory and the Brain," Scientific A., 50–57.

Orsega-Smith, E., Getchell, N., Neeld, K., & Mackenzie, S. (2008). Teaming up for senior fitness: A group-based approach; physical activity may be the closest thing to a "Fountain of Youth," but older adults face unique barriers to participation. *The Journal of Physical Education, Recreation and Dance,* 79

Selye, H. (1956). *The stress of life.* New York: McGraw-Hill, Inc.

Tang, Y. Y., Ma, Y., Wang, J., Fan, Y., Feng, S., Lu, Q., et al. (2007). Short-term meditation training improves attention and self-regulation. *Proceedings of the National Academy of Sciences of the United States of America, 104,* 17152–17156.

Wickremaratchi, M. M., & Llewelyn, J. G. (2006). Effects of ageing on touch. *Postgraduate Medical Journal, 82,* 301–304.

Wu, T., & Hallet, M. (2005). The influence of normal human ageing on automatic movements. *Journal of Physiology, 562*(Pt 2), 605–615.

Yamadori, A. (2002). Neurology of praxis disorder. *Rinsho Shinkeigaku, 42*(11), 1082–1084. [Article in Japanese].

Part VI

Cultural, Religious, and Spiritual Influences in Life's Transitions

Chapter 22

Self-Regulation Across Some Life Transitions

Katica Lacković-Grgin and Zvjezdan Penezić

Preparation of this chapter was aided in part by a grant from Ministry of science and technology of the Republic of Croatia, as a part of project 0070002 "Self-evaluation and self-regulation of personal development," by Department of Psychology, University of Zadar, Croatia.

Introduction

Some earlier philosophers and scientists (e.g., in the theory of evolution of Charles Darwin, in the socio-cultural theory of cognitive development of L. Vigotsky, in the symbolic interactionism of G. H. Mead, and in the developmental-cognitive theory of J. Piaget – have brought forth the idea that the development of an individual is the result of the *interaction of a person and the environment.* That idea was best elaborated by K. Lewin (1951) in his *field theory.* From the formula that behavior is the *function* of a person and the environment (B = f(PE)), it follows that the environment influences the person but also that the person influences the environment and changes it. The idea was elaborated later in more detail by U. Bronfenbrenner in formulating the *theory of ecological systems* and R. M. Lerner in his *developmental contextualism.* The biological changes in the organism, as well as the social interactions, exist as a part of the ecological system (Bronfenbrenner 1979), and bi-directional, reciprocal, and dynamic interactions of biological, psychological, and social processes are responsible for development (Lerner and Kauffman 1985). Therefore, development is viewed as a confluence of many mutually linked systems and subsystems, biological, social, cultural, and historical. Under the influence of all this theorizing, in the contemporary *life-span psychology,* changes occurred in the understanding of the principal determinants of development, i.e., the explanation of development in terms of biological changes in the organism that has ceased to dominate. Also, subject of developmental psychology, as the psychology of childhood and adolescence, has been extended after sixties of the twentieth century. Baltes (1983) emphasizes that the German psychology of development in the thirties of the twentieth century the necessity that development should be studied during the whole life-span was

From: *Handbook of Stressful Transitions Across the Lifespan,*
Edited by: T.W. Miller, DOI 10.1007/978-1-4419-0748-6_22,
© Springer Science+Business Media, LLC 2010

emphasized continuously, and takes into consideration the social and cultural factors of development in the process. He points to life events and transitions as important stimuli of development. Historically new phenomena in development, such as prolonged adolescence, the crisis of the forties, the crisis of "the empty nest" as well as the extension of life-span of modern people, they all urge the life-span psychologists to view structures, stages and the dynamics of development with reference to the historical period and with reference to cultural differences.

In viewing the interaction of a person and environment, earlier authors have not emphasized enough the impact of intentional activities of an individual on his personal development. In the eighties and the nineties of the last century, the *plasticity* of a person and his active participation in his own development was emphasized more and more (Lerner 1984, 1996; Brandtstädter 1997; Baltes 1997; Heckhausen 1999, and others). Only little children do not engage intentionally in the promotion of their own development because their development is predominantly under the influence of the action of the grown-ups in the interaction with children. In adolescence and in adulthood, individuals internalize cultural demands and perceive them as their own developmental goals that they strive to attain their own intentional actions. Personal control and developmental self-regulation is then possible because of a relatively stable view of the self and well-articulated future expectations. Therefore, progression in autonomous development occurs in adolescence and adulthood, i.e., greater regulation of ontogenesis.

Developmental regulation involves efforts by the individual to influence the actual development and adapt himself psychologically to the demands of the context in which he lives. These efforts are sometimes called *volition* (Kuhl 1984; Kuhl and Beckmann 1985). According to the *volition theory* of Kuhl and Fuhrmann (1998, p. 15), volition is expressed in two ways. The first kind of volition supporting the maintenance of an active goal is called *self-control* or *action control*, and the second kind, supporting the maintenance of one's actions in line with one's integrated self, is called *self-regulation*.

The concept that these kinds of adaptive processes in adolescence and adulthood consist of emergence, establishment and sustaining of the equilibrium among one's intentions, goals, behavior patterns, and self, will be the analytical framework for the theoretical and empirical studies that will be employed in writing this chapter. It will describe the motivational bases or the regulation of one's own development, constraints on developmental self-regulation across some life-transitions, the organizers of self-regulation, as well as the mechanisms and strategies of self-regulation.

Motivation Bases of the Regulation of Self-Development

The theories of motivation that attempt to answer the question, what is it that urges a person to activity, with reference to the time of their origin, can be divided into theories of the earlier, the middle, and the new generations. While the earlier theories predominantly emphasized the importance of innate and acquired needs (Hull 1943; Maslow 1976), the theories of the middle generation were more directed to the cognitive and affective processes that stimulate, organize and direct human behavior. Some of these theories emphasize that people start and persist in a behavior in a degree that they believe that such behavior will result in the desired end, i.e., to desired outcomes. Among others here are Atkinson's *theory of achievement motivation* (1964), H. Heckhausen's *action theory* (1967), *theories of causal attribution and perceived control* (Rotter 1966; Bandura 1977; and Weiner 1972).

The more recent theories of European origin like volition theory (Kuhl and Fuhrmann 1998), *life-span theory of control* (Heckhausen and Schultz 1995) continue to elaborate certain constructs that dominated in the theories of the middle generation like volition, personal control, and true self-regulation. Also, there are attempt to integrate these concepts from psychology of motivation with the concepts from life-span psychology (Baltes 1987; Heckhausen and Schultz 1995; Carstensen 1995; and Heckhausen 1999). Investigation within the framework of action theory and life-span theory of control is directed toward the selection of developmental goals and the compensation of losses/ errors, and the circumstances and processes that promote the persistence of or withdrawal from developmental goals.

Parallel with the indicated European theorizing, authors in the U.S.A. increasingly emphasize the importance of the goals, or the key constructs that not only induce, lead and organize behavior, but also cognition and affections. These constructs are: *personal strivings* (Emmons 1986, 1992, 1996); *personal projects* (Little 1983, 1989);and *life tasks* (Cantor and Fleeson 1991).

In the context of the discussion of self-regulation and personal development control, the *self-determination theory* (Deci and Ryan 1985) appears to be very relevant, for two reasons. First, the authors of the theory rightly emphasize the difference between the content of the goals or outcomes and the regulatory processes by which these goals are realized. Second, they link the earlier concepts of needs as stimulants of development with the new ideas of the self-regulation of development. They emphasize that the psychological development and the development of well-being could not be realized without innate needs, and they are: (1) *need for competence*, (2) *need for autonomy,* and (3) *need for relatedness*. The social and the cultural contexts and individual differences in these basic needs *stimulate* the processes of growth and development, including the internalization of the regulation of behavior, i.e., the shift from behaviors that are *not* self-determined towards self-determined behavior.

The theory of self-determination emphasizes that internalization of self-regulation is an active process in which a person transforms socially sanctioned habits, norms and demands/tasks into personal values and into self-regulation. Depending on the degree of how much a person has assimilated and reconstructed outer regulation of his behavior to such a degree it can be self-determined. The course of the process of internalization, i.e., the growth of intrinsic regulation moves from non-regulated behavior via external regulation, introjection and identification to integrated intrinsic regulation.

Since human psychological development, according to the self-determination theory, is stimulated by the above-mentioned three basic needs, Ryan (1998) easily recognizes that, in broad terms, these needs are pointed out by certain other theoreticians of self-regulation and personal developmental control. Here, he primarily refers to Kuhl and Fuhrmann (1998) whose term *volition* refers to all intentional and personally caused behaviors, which can be successful when they are autonomous, as the above-mentioned authors have proved exactly. However, in real-life circumstances, person's autonomy is affected by social contexts as well as other needs, which complicate the story of the regulation mechanisms. Further, Ryan (1998) comments on the life-span theory of J. Heckhausen and Schultz (1995), i.e., on the statement about functional primacy of primary control, which is consistent with the innate need for compensation. He warns that in certain situations and/or life periods that control can be optimal strategy while in others it can be counterproductive. Primary control may be in disharmony with the need for relatedness because it does make a person individual but *not* social. Like certain other psychologists (e.g., Brandtstädter and Greeve 1994; Carver and Scheier 1990), Ryan warns of potential maladapted aspects of primary control, particularly in the older life age. Finally, Ryan (1998) considers the work of Higgins and Silberman (1998) where they speak of approach versus avoidance form of action. It seems that the tendency toward these forms of action is formed during childhood depending on the ways of socialization of children in the family. The need of relatedness, i.e., of parental love and rewarding, ensures development of one or the other form of action. In terms of the theory of self-determination, persons whose parents applied excessive control, who insisted on duties and who applied punishment – will tend toward avoidance form of action, i.e., they will use introjected forms of regulation. Introjected regulation marks partial internalization. Regulation is in the individual but it is not yet part of the set of motivation, cognition and affections that construct the self-concept (e.g., the person acts in order to show its abilities or in order to avoid mistakes, to achieve the feeling of correctness). The behavior that follows from introjected regulation is only partly self-determined. It is a relatively unstable form of regulation (Koestner et al. 1996 – according to Ryan and Deci 2000).

Person whose parents emotionally supported and stimulated positive personal attributes will tend to use identification and integrated internal regulation. Integrated regulation means that the person has wholly accepted a certain value and built it into the system of his own values, which thus became part of its identity. Behavior is self-determined, regulation is intrinsic, and the motives of behavior are internal. Numerous studies show greater is the internalization of action, better are the effects of different forms of therapy (e.g., glucose control in the blood of diabetic patients, physical exercise in the elderly and invalids, training of learning and teaching (Chatzisarantis et al. 1997; Gronlick and Ryan 1987 – according to Ryan and Deci 2000).

Self-regulation of development is made possible by the fundamental characteristic of human behavior in relation to other kinds of regulation; this is its great flexibility. Among other things it is reflected in selectivity and in compensation of losses/mistakes (Baltes 1987, 1990).

Selectivity refers to the selection of developmental goals and direction toward the resources that enable the achievements of goals. When relevant goals are selected in adolescence and in adulthood, the shortness of life, as (a) biological constraint does not allow investment in alternative development, which is particularly true of long-term, the so-called life goals. Therefore, for adaptive regulation it is essential to make good choices, make them in-time and insist on them. If the selection of goals is mistaken, it can lead to developmental "stagnation," and if the goals are clear but too narrow the individual may become vulnerable in case of failure, because he does not compensate for the loss of achievements in another field. Development will be optimal in a person who maximizes his achievements selectively in various areas of functioning.

Compensation of losses/mistakes is the effort of a person to make good (for the) negative consequences of wrongly selected goals and strategies of regulation, the consequences of ageing or certain life events, such as the loss of mobility or sensitivity, the loss of the loved ones etc. In advanced age, losses often accumulate in a short time, and this also is the reason that compensation becomes crucial to successful ageing (Heckhausen and Schultz 1995). Compensation may be dysfunctional if it is early. A person may rely on the help of others too early and thus become dependent and helpless. It was shown that inmates of old-age homes show a tendency of weaker psychological functioning from equivalent groups of the elderly people who live alone or without family (Lacković-Grgin and Padelin 1995). Besides losses, compensation is also stimulated by the tendency to errors. While patterns of animal behavior are determined genetically in their form and the time of appearance, human behavior, which is in the function of self-regulation of development, depends on the ability and effort of the individual and his choice when and how to behave. Since in this case, behavior is affected by the situational factors, there is risk of errors on the way to achieving the goal. However, errors can be eliminated by learning better strategies of regulation, which means that the process of learning is crucial in the optimization of development. Some authors stress the value of learning confrontation directed to the problem so as to help the individuals solve their problems during life transitions (Brammer 1992). Confrontation directed to the problem turned out to be a good predictor of adaptation during the first year at the university (Lacković-Grgin and Sorić 1997).

It can be said in conclusion that selection and compensation, in order to be functional, must be regulated by a process of a higher order, which corresponds to the process of *optimization*, which is understood as enrichment of the optimal level of functioning in an area by means of extending internal or external resources.

From the point of view of developmental perspective it should be emphasized that goal-directed actions of an individual, as well as forms of regulation and personal control of development, vary depending on life cycles. These cycles, or life transitions, as well as social and cultural contexts, determine which needs will be salient and more important as initiators of object-directed actions. Actions that promote own development should be distinguished according to whether they are autonomous and self-determined, i.e., whether they are followed with a full sense of volition and a freedom of choice *or* conditioned by outside coercion. This distinction is necessary not only for theoretical reasons but also because it could make possible better operationalization of variables in future attempts of formulating the models of process of developmental regulation in transition periods of life.

The Constraints on Self-Regulation Across Some of Life Transitions

There are several ways of determining life transitions. It is a long tradition in the psychology of development to speak of age-developmental transitions from childhood to adolescence, from adolescence to adulthood, and from adulthood to old age. Some developmental theories offer more precise divisions (e.g., Havighurst 1953; Erikson 1980; and Levinson 1986). In each of these transitions, in predominantly stable societies and cultures, side by side with biological constraints, which are universal, developmental regulation is also affected by socio-structural constraints (Heckhausen 1999). Although these constraints affect development throughout (whole) life, their stimulating force is particularly visible in periods of the aforementioned transitions that are partly influenced by them.

Biological constraints consist of the maturation processes and the ageing processes of the organism. The general biological constraint is the length of human life, which determines the goals of development to a high degree. People live relatively long with a tendency of lengthening recently. Human life is limited to approximately 115 years (Danner and Schröder 1992), so its relatively long duration extends the possibilities of development; in other words, the possibilities of self-regulation of development are extended. However, with men, the processes of decline are relatively long, which limit the self-regulation of development or at least changes the mechanisms and strategies of this regulation. Greater the influence of biological factors on the development of a characteristic or form of behavior, greater is the channeling of development in a certain direction (Plomin 1986), and greater channeling represents restriction of self-regulation of development. The biological resources of bodily and mental functioning mature from the state of helplessness and dependence on the help of others to complete functioning in numerous areas. In adulthood, these resources reach their peak and start declining afterwards (Simonton 1995). Also, the fertility of women, and to a lesser degree in men, shows a specific, biologically determined course: from maximum functioning in youth to minimum in middle age. Developmental psychologists emphasize that biological factors optimize significantly the pre-reproductive stage of life but that, in this sense, affect the adaptive development in post-reproductive life-stage to a lower degree (Finch 1996; Baltes and Graf 1996). It follows that with years adults must include social and cultural benefits accrued till then in order to realize their goals successfully. In older age they make use of the accumulated life experience, which is reflected in wisdom (Erikson 1980), partly because social and cultural benefits for the elderly are nevertheless relatively limited resources. Adults of middle-age, are therefore, compelled to regulate decline and losses more than younger persons. They are obliged to do so also because of social constraints and expectations that also affect self-regulation. In general, in mature adulthood the biological constraints are less significant for self-regulation of development than socio-cultural constraints, while in old age both the biological and social constraints are, roughly, equally significant.

Socio-structural constraints refer to the influence of society and its institutions upon the individual's developmental regulation. Western societies first defined uniform life periods and transitions, and the goals tied to them, with the beginning of the industrial era. In post-industrial societies, there are no tendencies to define age-specific developmental tasks and their sequence are fewer and fewer. This is suggested by biographical reports in which it is increasingly observed that emphasis of individual projects and life goals is more relevant, i.e., the understanding of modern men that they are architects of their lives (Baumeister 1991). Yet, in most societies, institutionalization of life periods with reference to chronological age is still present. That age is important in numerous social systems is affirmed not only by the fact of prescribing the time for performing certain duties but also by the fact that at the same time such societies sanction age-discrimination.

Several aspects of socio-structural constraints upon the regulation of personal development can be identified. One such aspect respects biological facts, and the quantity of developmental goals and their timing are determined in conformity with them (Havighurst 1953). Deadlines, i.e., the right times for certain activities and for developmental regulation are also determined. In this way, also constituted is the second aspect of socio-structural constraints, namely,chronological ordering of life and age-norms.

Age-norms are fairly constant and were not essentially changed in the twentieth century in spite of economic crises, revolutions and wars. Biographical studies of the key life preoccupations of people in Switzerland (Grob et al. 2001) show agreement of three generations of people regarding chronological division of life into the following principal periods: (1) preparation for vocation; (2) working period;and (3) retirement. The fourth part is less unambiguous except for the emphasis on the preparation for death. The sources of limitations of own developmental preoccupations are rather different in different generations. Generations from the first decades of the twentieth century more often stated the social possibilities of continuing education at higher levels, while the younger generations more often stated their personal wishes and possibilities regarding the continuation of their education (e.g., interests, feelings, abilities). This indicates that the younger generations show less respect for social constraints, i.e., that they strive toward greater self-regulation of development, which is congruent with Baumeister's findings mentioned above.

Biological and socio-structural constraints that determine age-developmental transitions are the basis for the derivation and clear prescribing, and also statutory standardization of the so-called *normative life events*, i.e., *normative transitions*. Beside these normative events that mark clearly the transitions in the lives of men, there appear also *non-normative events*, i.e., *non-normative transitions*. These events also cause the dynamics of development, or at least serious changes of behavior. In stimulus-stress models (for stress models cf. Cox 1982) life events are termed stressors. They can be positive and negative. Self-evaluation of transition caused by such events, as positive and negative, will stimulate various actions, mechanisms, and strategies that will influence developmental outcomes. Persons search for strategies to establish new equilibrium, actions, mechanisms, and strategies that will influence the developmental outcomes. Persons search for strategies by means of which they will establish new equilibrium. Transitions such as going to school, transit from one degree of education to another, end of schooling, entry into the world of labor, marriage, having a child – all these are potential increase/gain because they stimulate the establishment of new equilibrium and a higher level of functioning. On the other side are life transitions that are generally regarded as decrease/ loss, e.g., loss of job, retirement, "empty nest," widowhood etc. These losses most often result in constriction, i.e., equilibrium on a lower level of social and psychological functioning. However, what the functional levels will be, i.e., the outcomes of these transitions, greatly depend on the regulation strategies of a person and his social surroundings.

Our research into role stress in family and professional areas of adolescents and adults have shown, among other things, that transition from highschool to university produces considerably higher degree of loneliness in students who are separated more from parents on account of studies than with those who have remained in their family homes. Loneliness decreased at the end of the first year. It was demonstrated that self-esteem, separation from parents, and the style of coping directed to problem are good predictors of adaptation in studies (Lacković-Grgin and Sorić 1995, 1996, 1997). Nurmi et al. (1996) found with Finnish students that pessimistic and avoidant strategies of coping increased their loneliness. It can be said that these strategies remove young persons from successful solution of crisis in stage six, which Erikson terms crisis of intimacy versus isolation. Furthermore, our investigation has shown that unemployment of the young with university degrees (mean age 28) does not affect their life satisfaction if unemployment was shorter than 18 months because they had externalized the causes of unemployment. Because of long-lasting economic crisis and a high level of unemployment in Croatia, to be unemployed after university, means almost a normative life event (Lacković-Grgin 1994). Externalization of the causes of unemployment was also found by Feather (1982), but with Australian workers of lower qualifications. However, in that country where unemployment of persons with university degree was not so high, unemployed graduates are significantly more depressive than the employed (Feather and Bond 1983). It would appear that this indicates that such unemployed people, perhaps, internalize the causes of their unemployment. Contrary to externalization, some cognitive and attributive strategies (e.g., self-handicapping) may increase the harmful consequences of unemployment with the young (Nurmi et al. 1994). It turned out that unemployed women in our sample had greater life satisfaction than men, which we explained with the fact that they had married, that they performed domestic chores, and cared for the members of the family. This points to compensation as the strategy of coping unemployment (Lacković-Grgin et al. 1996). Authors from other countries also find that unemployed women have greater life satisfaction than unemployed men (Warr et al. 1982), which is a probable consequence of different social valuation of the professional work of women and men in the majority of countries. Finally, in our investigation we found that with regard to women of middle-age transition the so-called "empty nest" lessens their life satisfaction compared with the period when children were with them. However, more precise analyses of the data gathered in interviews show that such lessening is more evident with urban than with rural women, and that because their life satisfaction is affected by menopause as well as the loss of youthful appearance. With women from rural areas, however, these "losses" were *not* shown as significant for their life satisfaction (Lacković-Grgin 1993).

Most people go through normative transitions, while non-normative transitions are individually different as to their causes and timing. The strategies of developmental regulation as well as their outcomes are influenced by timing: whether the individual experiences normative transition on-time or off-time. It was established that e.g., too early sex maturing of adolescent girls stimulates intrapersonal and interpersonal dynamics, which may result in weakening of their self-esteem (Steinberg 1988; Lacković-Grgin et al. 1994) or in deviant behavior (Magnuson et al. 1985). Asynchrony of bodily and cognitive maturity does not allow adequate self-regulation. Or, while e.g., parenthood in young adulthood stimulates the growth of the component of personality that Erikson (1980) calls generativity, parenthood in adolescence may make more difficult the development of some dimensions of identity, such as professional identity (Hyde 1994).

Self-regulation of development may also be stimulated by social transitions. These are radical changes of society and its institutions, e.g., such as those that had affected former socialist countries of Europe in early nineties of the last century.

Such social transitions, in which people remain "the same" but the institutions change are potentially stressful as well as transitions of people (migrants, refugees, exiles) who face different institutions, norms and customs in a new environment. It was supposed that social transitions would have more influence on changes in the spheres of schooling/education and work and less in the sphere of family life. After the unification of Germany, Elder and O'Rand (1995) checked out these suppositions with persons from East Germany. They corroborated only partly the quoted presuppositions, not satisfied with the manner in which they operationalized the family variables. In contrast, numerous investigations of stress because of migration show serious changes in life goals and values with migrants, which are different from those of members of different age groups (Berry et al. 1987; Ngyen and Williams 1989; and Liebkind 1996). The pragmatics of life in a new context may require quick adaptation also in aspects of development that do not have central position in the original culture, or were quite marginal (Schmitt-Roderrmund and Sibbereisen 1999).

Organizers of Self-Regulation of Development

Goals, taken as all that an individual considers valuable in his life and to what he strives, may be regarded/viewed as organizers of developmental regulation. An individual's goals may reflect both the age-graded transitions involving normative demands and the developmental tasks typical in their environments (Pulkkinen et al. 2002); also normative transitions and differences in individual's motives related to personality traits.

Developmental goals, in contrast to life-goals, have precisely developmental processes as their aim (e.g., in adolescence: becoming independent of parents, in adulthood: care for the young generation), and because of that are concrete. In the context of time, the goals may be linked with shorter terms rather than life-time goals that are based on abstract foundations, are higher in the hierarchy of goals and linked with longer terms. The concept of developmental goals is sometimes confused with the notion of desires. It is important to distinguish them from the developmental point of view because desires can be determined as aspirations that are not necessarily subject to limitations from the real world. As to regulation of development, desire has no critical force to become volition that stimulates action. Even when it is strong, desire may have yet weaker connection with reality (Chiu and Nevius 1990).

In literature, there are several heuristic procedures in the approach to goals. Some address people with the question to inform about future goals, the chances of their attainment, and the degrees of their attainment at the time of investigation. The answers collected in this way differ in their abstractness and globality. Some developmental goals are age-specific but some of them are age-universal and could be highly *abstract* ideals (e.g., fight for peace, equality, justice) and are reminiscent of Rokeach terminal values (Rokeach 1973). They may be regarded as life-goals. Such goals were investigated in Germany by Pöhlman and Brunstein (1997) by means of a questionnaire, which they compiled themselves. It was composed of items from some earlier questionnaire as well as statements collected from examinees. Theoretically, their work relies on Bakan's idea (1966) of two basic orientations of people: (1) promoting and (2) participating (agency and communion). By means of factorial analysis, the authors identified the following life-goals: power, attainment, changes, altruism, intimacy, and belonging. The first three factors suggest *agency* and the last three *communion* orientation.

Developmental goals are implicitly dealt with in some developmental theories that are better known, such as Havighurst, Erikson, Levinson and Gould's. But, in those theories, however, there are no data for recognizing and distinguishing developmental goals in terms of their content, complexity, and abstractness.

If developmental goals are to be viewed as the organizers of the regulation of own development, then they should be viewed in the manner of modern psychology of personality. As indicated earlier, this is, for example, the concept of "personal strivings" (Emmons 1986) under which the author understands relatively permanent and coherent goal models. Individual goals may be very trivial, and their temporal dimension different from personal strivings. Thus, for instance, an individual's volition to read a story differs from the volition to develop his world-view. Personal strivings unite the functionally equivalent subordinate goals and determine the duration and the direction of action as well as the methods to control personal development. Actually, the striving towards the construction of the world-view may be realized by a systematic consumption of information from different media, evaluating and testing them, and not only by a daily goal of reading a story. Examination of the relation between the daily and the developmental goals shows that subjective well-being is much greater when daily goals are *along* the line of developmental goals than when they serve to avoid unfavorable scenarios in connection with personal development (Brunstein 1993). So, developmental goals are a system of related sub-goals, rather than some separate, isolated units.

Because every period of life has its developmental tasks, it is supposed that with age the importance varies along with the attainment of developmental goals. Some developmental goals are universal and some are age-specific. Universal goals are rooted in permanent motivational dispositions such as personal growth and health, power over others, or are acquired and function as general strivings towards honesty, altruism and so on. Age-specific developmental goals represent the subject's internalization of developmental tasks typical for the age in his surroundings. These are the goals of competences (professional, art, sport), then socio-emotional goals (friendship, love of close persons, emotional stability), and the goals that refer to material achievements (money, valuable property). These enumerated goals are linked with individual facets of self-concept (bodily, material, social, and emotional) as well as with certain key dimensions of self, such as perception of personal competence. We investigated these developmental goals with adolescents and with persons of middle- and older -ages (Penezić and Lacković-Grgin 2001). It turned out that the importance of material and health goals is universal, which points to their deeper foundation in permanent motivational dispositions (in the primary, biological needs). The width and the content of socio-emotional goals, as well as goals of knowledge and competence, vary with age, which indicates their greater foundation in developmental tasks typical of age group. Thus, e.g., with Finnish subjects it was found that persons in mid-thirties generally conceptualize their personal goals in terms of family and profession (Pulkkinen et al. 2002).

Culturally, specific demands and information refer not only to the importance of individual developmental goals but also to the *manner* of their realization. During transition periods, but also before them, personalities learn actions, establish structures that include manners of behavior and their consequences as well as methods of evaluation success in achieving goals. To understand the evolution, transformation, and deactivation of developmental goals, they should be viewed within the framework of recent motivational theories, which take into consideration different phases of action regulation. According to the so-called Rubicon model (Heckhausen 1991), action undertaken by an individual in the direction of realizing a goal is divided into two stages: motivation prior to making decision, and motivation after. In order to become a doctor, prior to decision stage, the individual examines different options (which medical school to attend, whether to leave native place or not, etc). When decision is made, the individual crosses the Rubicon and enters a new phase. He acts toward the goal with dedication, examines opportuneness of his actions, plans their execution, evaluates the outcome of the actions and the way they will reflect on the future. In the process, he takes into consideration many internal and external constraints. Studying the concept of aspiration toward professional identity within the framework of the Rubicon model, Gollwitzer (1987) points out that it requires long-term dedication of an individual. It is the goal that includes efforts over a long period, which contains many sub-goals, and which is always redefined and extended continuously after individual sub-goals are reached. This sort of goal is difficult to abandon because the individual is constantly in the stage of volition. Even when he meets with failure, it is more probable that he will continue in the same direction before seeking alternatives. An individual who is not strongly dedicated to his identity goals, when daunted by obstacles and failures will, likely, reduce his endeavors and perhaps even give up.

The future developmental goals that an individual aims to achieve over medium-term, are usually reflected as aspiration toward gains and avoidance of losses. In the process, the developmental goals are in conformity with the structure of the possibilities and limitations typical of the term. Since age-norms determine the time of action or transition, they provoke the individual's regulation potential to avoid burdening it with developmental choices. Age-norms also point to deadlines when goals are to be attained. In cases when an individual fails age-norm deadline, he will certainly never achieve the goal.

What happens to the behavior of women before and after the deadline for childbirth ("biological clock") was studied within the life-span theory of control (Heckhausen and Schultz 1995). In the study of goals and developmental regulation with women, quasi-experimental design was used. Several age groups of women were selected in one study: age 27–33 without children (the so-called urgent group), age 40–46 without children (past the deadline), and age 19–44 with children. They were asked to name the five most important developmental goals in future 5–10 years. Women with children as well as women without children from pre-deadline phase quoted several goals linked with their parental function than women without children from the post-deadline phase, who quoted more goals linked to self-development, promoting their health and friendship. In another study of five age groups of women, strategies of developmental control were studied in addition to goals by means of OPS scale, which measures the optimization of primary and secondary control. Concerning goals, the results were similar to the first study. As to pre- *versus* post-deadline, strategies of developmental control were different. Pre-deadline group (with children and without) as well as pregnant women, had higher ratings for selective primary control, selective secondary control, and compensatory primary control reflected a greater goal engagement with childbearing. Post-deadline group used compensatory secondary control more often, indicated a disengagement from childbearing goals. The group exhibited the trend to self-protective causal attributions and self-serving social comparison. However, it was found that if women in post-deadline phase use selective primary control, they have more risk of the appearance of depressive symptoms (Heckhausen 2002.) The investigation confirmed the model of adaptive control strategies in different phases of the action. It can also be seen that in transitional period of life, there might be a discrepancy between developmental tasks of personal developmental goals and the actual view of the self or the attainment of those goals. If such discrepancy cannot be decreased with adequate mechanisms and strategies of the regulation of personal development, it can very well lead to alienation and depression. Such a condition is recognized as prolonged stress.

Mechanisms and Strategies of the Self-Regulation of Development

Strategies of the Control of Personal Development

With reference to attempts of explaining intentional actions of an individual to participate in own development, the concept of control is promising, for several reasons. *First*, numerous studies of animals and people show that from the beginning to the end of life the basic motivator of behavior is endeavoring to establish control over environment. *Second*, it is shown that loss of control has negative developmental consequences. *Third*, during lifetime many life events may increase, decrease or even completely damage the existing levels of control. *Fourth*, there are numerous empirical materials about control and similar concepts gathered from persons of all life-ages. Both in experimental and in correlative investigations it consistently occurred that during life-time, individual differences in perceived control are linked with positive outcomes of various areas of human functioning, such as mental and physical health, educational and other achievements, various aspects of social behavior, self-understanding and self-esteem, and life satisfaction. The findings are consistent in spite of the heterogeneity of technical terms used by individual investigators of control. Some of those terms (of related concepts of control) have entered textbooks because of their theoretical foundation and empirical relevance, such as *locus of control* (Rotter 1966), *mastery styles* (Gutman 1964), *hardiness* (Kobasa 1979), *self-efficacy* (Bandura 1977), and recently *personal control of development* (J. Heckhausen and Schultz 1995). On the model of Rothbaum et al. (1982), who preferred the two-process model of control – primary and secondary control, Heckhausen and Schultz also speak of two kinds of control of personal development.

People try to decrease or avoid the discrepancy between the desired and attained in three different ways. *The first* is direct action (cognitive or behavioral), which alters the circumstances leading to discrepancy. Some call it process *assimilation* (Brandtstädter and Greeve 1994) or *active mastery* (Gutmann 1964), and others call it *primary control* (Heckhausen and Schultz 1995; Lacković-Grgin et al. 1999). Primary control is expressed in the process of selection and compensation by means of which the external world is brought to harmony with personal goals and desires. Choices can be made from, for example, enhanced effort, acquiring new skills, time investment of the use of technical devices, asking for expert advice, searching for instrumental social support of a close person, etc. *The second* way is the rescaling of developmental goals and aspirations in terms of their adjustment to the new circumstances. That is the specific "agreement" with the world via *accommodation* (Brandtstädter and Greeve 1994), but at the same time a reassessment of gains and losses or *secondary control* (Heckhausen and Schultz 1995) or *passive mastery* (Gutman 1964). Secondary control is expressed in the selection of goals. It directs action towards possible goals and inhibits action towards unattainable goals; it changes the standards of self-evaluation and social comparisons. In the course of our preliminary interviews, this was described by an elderly female participant as follows: "I can't go shopping to the center of the city any longer ... I do it in the neighborhood instead ... it's good I can do it without anybody's help ... some of my friends can't do it any more ..."

As over life's course, the number of events that cannot be coped with primary control increases (e.g., irreversible losses build up), so assumption is that with age secondary ventral is enhanced. Heckhausen and Schultz (1995) suppose that primary and secondary controls change during life, i.e., that in mature age, and particularly in old age, primary control decreases and secondary control increases. However, aspiration for primary control remains equal throughout life. Some results of transversal investigation indicate that elderly people perceive that their development is less and less under their control (Brandtstädter and Greeve 1994). But, longitudinal studies do not verify these indications but show that perceived personal control does not decrease with age, except in very old age (Brandtstädter et al. 1998). The decrease of the perception of personal control may also appear with middle-aged and even younger people when they experience a radical social or personal transition (e.g., acquired disability). While examining various generations of people from the former East Germany, it was found that a few years after unification the middle-aged had a lower level of self-esteem and pessimistic beliefs of the possibility of control over their lives in the professional and family areas (Heckhausen 1999).

Our research confirmed that accommodation processes increase with age, i.e., that secondary control increases (Lacković-Grgin et al. 1999). The results of the investigation are shown in Fig. 22-1.

It is evident from the figure that although secondary control is enhanced with age, yet it does not outstrip primary control, which speaks in favor of the assertion that people tend to control their surroundings *throughout* life. Our investigation of predictors of primary control (Lacković-Grgin et al. 2001) has also confirmed that secondary control is enhanced with age, although never outstripping primary control. That fact not only confirms primacy of primary control, but also indicates that secondary control is not merely a substitute for the lost primary control. Secondary control is used when the individual is faced with impending future loss. This is confirmed by a highly positive correlation between secondary control and pessimism and a negative correlation between primary control and pessimism.

Whether the elderly will use primary or secondary control depends on several factors. One of them is the surrounding stimulation of the elderly to use primary control (Trimko and Moss 1990). If primary control is lost in old age because of financial losses, it leads to depression and other kinds of

Primary control

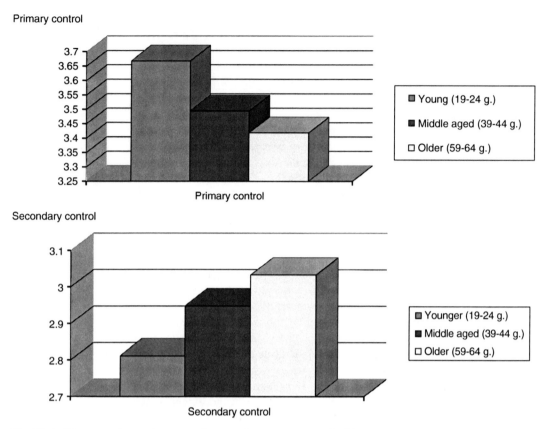

Fig. 22-1 Primary and secondary control among three age groups of subjects

illnesses (Swan et al. 1991). The experience of American investigators that the elderly are generally more stricken by social than by organic problems is interesting. That is because while they cannot control the social environment/surroundings, they can control themselves more successfully. Schulz and Decker (1985) established the impressive possibilities of the elderly with backbone injury to adapt emotionally to the situation, i.e., to prevent the onset of depression. In addition to secondary control, they also use rationalization. The function of secondary control is to maintain stable self-esteem, life satisfaction, and mental health. Some authors note that relentless striving for over-ambitious and unrealistic goals is associated with depression in old age (Carver and Scheier 1990).

Although primary and secondary controls are of equal importance to development and adaptability of the organism, Heckhausen and Schultz (1995) attribute high-status to primary control. The primacy of primary control is corroborated by the evolutionary facts that all living beings exert an active influence on their environment and the fact that primary control ontogenetically precedes secondary control. This standpoint caused critical objections from the circle of developmental and particularly cross-cultural psychologists. The question arose about primacy of primary control in terms of whether in all cultures it is preferred to secondary control and whether it has greater adaptability value. Gould (1999) thinks that the assertion of cultural invariance of the primacy of primary control is not valid because it was not tested in cross-cultural investigation. He asserts that there are indications that in communities where the individual is subordinated to the group and requirements of the collectivity (as is the case in certain Asian cultures), primary control need not be preferred as more adaptive than secondary control. Gould rightly emphasizes that what is perceived in individualistic Western cultures need not be valid for other cultures.

Modern treatises on functional distinction between primary and secondary control point to two basic standpoints. First, *relativistic*, maintains that the two typos of control are equal in their functional values (Baltes 1995). Whether an individual uses one or the other control depends on the availability of primary control, on the values of a society, and also on subjective preference of the person, i.e., stable personality traits. The basic idea of the relativistic standpoint is that the ultimate goal of all human behaviors is to maximize the subjective well-being, either by means of primary or by means of secondary control. According to the other, *universalistic* standpoint, the aim of human behavior is to maximize primary control through life, independent of age, culture, and other contextual factors (Heckhausen and Schultz 1995). According to this standpoint, the higher status of primary control is reflected in that secondary control appears when wishing to reduce harmful effects of the lack or loss of primary control, and because secondary control, in the last consequence, facilitates the return to primary control. If, during a long period of using secondary control it is not possible to realize the desired level of functioning, secondary control ceases to be effective in the sense of returning to primary control. Then, both mechanisms of control collapse. It can be observed that there are limitations to the control of personal development conceived in this way. However, Heckhausen (1999) points out that the theory of the development of personal control did not originate in order to explain developmental regulation under conditions when biological and socio-cultural restraints are so extreme that they produce pathology, i.e., when the mechanisms of control collapse.

That might be one of the reasons why the theory of control of personal development (Heckhausen and Schultz 1995) does not treat the strategy that a person makes use of when neither primary nor secondary control can stabilize the self and life satisfaction. In this case, an individual may make use of a third kind of self-regulation; Gutman (1964) calls it *magic mastery*, Brandtstädter and Greeve (1994) *immunization*, and we suggest the term *tertiary control*. It is the reinterpretation of relevant information, the use of rationalization, fantasizing, and avoidance. In contrast to neurotic defenses, these are mature defense mechanisms, which prove adaptive. The existence of this kind of control of individual development was confirmed by our investigation mentioned above. It is interesting to note that tertiary control does not vary significantly with age, as Fig. 22-2 shows.

Tertiary control is age-universal, which indicates that it is conditioned constitutionally. The maturity of tertiary control is seen in the creation of new possibilities for using secondary or primary control because that kind of control minimizes emotional distress (Baumeister et al. 1998). In this respect, the function of tertiary control is similar to that of emotion-oriented coping (Endler and Parker 1990). There are indications that this style of coping is also conditioned constitutionally.

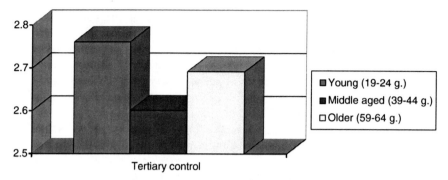

Fig. 22-2 Tertiary control among three age groups of subjects

Our second tentative answer to the question why the possibility of this kind of developmental regulation has been ignored in Heckhausen and Schultz's theory is the state in contemporary academic community. For some members of the academic community of psychologists, defense mechanisms still represent a taboo, because they are affirmed in the area of psychopathology. As is the case with other concepts of Freud's theory, they are denied the possibility of being examined. Nowadays, however, it has been fully proved that some defense mechanisms are part of normal psychological functioning and are not instinctively founded reactions. This is also confirmed by the results of experimental research in contemporary social psychology (see Baumeister et al. 1998). The theory of personal control has been developed to explain development in adulthood, and neglect of empirical facts that immature defense mechanisms decrease with age, and mature mechanisms increase is even more surprising (Cramer 1997). It is precisely the mature defenses that constitute the tertiary control.

Defenses are also treated in the literature on extreme stressors. In searching for the methods of effective adaptation to extremely difficult life events or inexorableness of the end of life, TMT theory points out that people may use distal and proximal defense (Pyszyrinski et al. 2000). In terms of the theory of control, some proximal defenses against lethal illness are primary control (e.g., taking medication, change of diet), immature defense mechanisms (e.g., denial) as well as mature defenses (e.g., rationalization). Proximal defenses are not present when thoughts about death and its close certainty are not in focus, but appear sporadically, as is the case in youth. Distal defenses are used in such cases. They are manifested in an individual's attempt somehow to contribute to the meaning of life, to defend his world-view. The function of these defenses is to *drive away* the fear of transience and death. Since thoughts of death occur with healthy elderly people more frequently than with the young, elderly people search for the universal meaning of life more frequently than the young, which increases spirituality with age. In general, spirituality is a more effective means to control challenges that are brought by the difficult and unchanging facts of life (Emmons 1999). That form of distal defenses appears also in old age when there is no immediate threat of death, but rather *thoughts* of death are in focus.

Besides establishing life-span theory of control, Heckhausen and Schulz (1993) also elaborated the model of OPS, which we mentioned in the preceding section.

With regard to the optimization and the major role of selectivity and failure of compensation, the authors integrated these concepts with the life-span theory of primary and secondary controls. On the basis of two dimensions of control (primary and secondary) on the one hand, and selection and compensation on the other, they could compose four types of control strategies: (1) *selective primary control* (investment of internal resources: effort, time, abilities); (2) *compensatory primary control* (use of external resources: technical aids, other people's assistance); (3) *selective secondary control* (metavolition: enhancement of goal commitment, remaining focused in order to avoid distractions); and (4) *compensatory control* (buffering negative effects of failure: goal change, strategic comparison).

Employment of each of these strategies depends on the possibilities and restrictions in a given developmental context. None of these four strategies is functional by themselves. If any of these strategies is used in a non-optimized manner, it may have maladaptive consequences. Selective primary control, for instance, may become maladaptive when invested in a wrong goal. In the same way, it may become maladaptive when the individual seeks assistance prematurely (compensatory primary control).

Initial investigations within the framework of the OPS model have demonstrated meaningful relationships between these four strategies and developmental outcomes in different age groups (cf. Heckhausen and Schultz 1998). For the purposes of these investigations, the authors have constructed the OPS scales.

Social and Temporal Comparisons as Strategies of Self-Regulation

In addition to the methods self-developmental control described so far, social and temporal comparisons are also regarded as prototype strategies of self-regulation. Their primary aim is protection or growth of self-esteem as well as life-satisfaction in situations that create imbalance. In the beginning of his work on the study of social comparison, Festinger (1954) thought that evaluation of own abilities, knowledge, emotional and other states the principal motive of social comparison. According to recent points of view, which were also confirmed empirically, the motives of social comparison may be of three kinds: (1) *self-evaluation*, (2) *self-enhancement*, and (3) *self-improvement* (Wayment and Taylor 1995). In investigating the reasons why people compare themselves with others, Helgeson and Mickleson (1995) in two independent studies, asked students to investigate these reasons in various hypothetical and real situations. The studies have affirmed the validity of Festinger's assertion, because the need or desire to achieve valid evaluation of own position along a dimension of comparison was the reason quoted most frequently. However, the analysis of the results showed also the presence of two other motives or functions of social comparison – self-enhancement and self-improvement.

The desire or need for self-enhancement as a motive has prompted much interest over the last 15 years. Some of the new researches have suggested that the need for self-enhancement might affect the amount and direction for comparison (i.e., upward *versus* downward comparison) as well as its impact (Wills 1981). Women with breast cancer, sometimes seemed to compare themselves with others as hypothetically having that disease rather than with people who really suffer from that (Wood et al. 1985). Some recent results show that such women compare themselves spontaneously with those whose health is worse than theirs. It allows them to interpret their own health condition as more favorable. In general, it may be said that, depending on the social context and the dimension along which he compares himself with others, a person seeks or interprets information about him in a favorable way. The reason is that this motive of comparison is not intended to assess how we are by ourselves but, how we can draw comfort and feel better, enhance our self-esteem, hope etc. Empirical data made it possible for Wills (1997) to formulate the theory of *downward comparison* in which he emphasizes that that these comparisons are adaptive as strategies of coping unfavorable and/or life-threatening events or unfavorable developmental outcomes. Thus, for instance, Erikson et al. (1986) state that persons in stage 8 of development (integrity *versus* despair) re-interpret their former life to build it into the present life and successfully solve the crisis that is typical of that developmental stage. In the process, they make use of downward social comparison, but also temporal comparison. However, if re-interpretation of earlier life, or of an important life event, is a kind of its mythologization, it may result in pseudo-integration, and the development of integrity will be delayed. Liberman and Tobin 1988 quote that some elderly people use unrealistic evaluation of life as strategy of defense of their self-esteem. Downward comparisons, because they protect self-esteem and hope, represent important resources of secondary control.

The reasons people compare themselves with others is to learn more about their own abilities and skills, and in so doing, improve them(Taylor and Lobel 1989). The motive of self-improvement serves an individual to learn what and how he can change in order to enhance his developmental achievement. Usually, upward social comparison is used for the purpose, that enables obtaining information that may be useful for the realization of a developmental goal. There are indications that in youth, because of numerous requirements for various achievements, upward social comparison is used more frequently. It serves to organize actions by means of which one can achieve that which has a model, i.e., superior person with whom he compares himself. However, with reference to age-norms, it is known in general what are relatively superior and inferior levels in individual transitional life periods. Therefore, in fact, in all developmental periods, people strive to attain superior developmental level, and this suggests that people of all age-periods are in favor of upward social comparisons. Our preliminary results of investigation show that tendency to social comparisons (as a relative stable feature) correlates positively with the frequency of upward social comparisons in areas of achievements, social effectiveness, and physical appearance and fitness in general (Ćubela 2001).

Some stress situations may stimulate the tendency toward upward comparison. Such comparison opens the possibilities of improving own position because we "associate upwards" with people that cope better with threatening situations (Buunk et al. 1997). But, some findings warn that high comparison level can lower self-evaluation or self-esteem. Taylor et al. (1996) state that exposure to upward target of comparison can lower self-evaluations, even when this comparison leads to a better performance. A person, then, can do better but feel worse. In our most recent investigations in the samples of adolescents, the young, the middle-aged, and the elderly it was established that the *frequency* of upward social comparison(s) within the area of achievement is not correlated to general life satisfaction. But, the emotional consequences of these comparisons are significantly correlated with general life-satisfaction, so, more positive the consequences of these comparisons, greater is life-satisfaction. These correlations are the highest with the groups of adolescents and persons of middle age (Penezić 2003).

Besides upward and downward social comparisons, there is also the third type of comparison. These are comparisons with equals, the so-called *horizontal comparisons*. Festinger (1954) thought that people while evaluating their abilities and achievements compare with those who are similar to them or somewhat better. In more recent literature, the term "comparison with similar people" is used not only for lateral comparisons (comparisons with equals) but also for comparing with those that are comparable to us. Brown (2000) emphasizes that investigations show consistently that the majority of people compare themselves with those that are similar to them along analogous attributes. Ćubela (2001) reports that in the areas mentioned above people use upward and lateral comparisons more frequently than downward comparisons.

Individual differences in the frequency of use of individual types social comparisons are also linked with some personality features (e.g., big-five dimensions, depressiveness, self-esteem etc. (Gibbons and Buunk 1999; Olson and Evans 1999).

It is possible to evaluate the adaptive values of individual types of social comparisons on the basis of whether they stimulate or do not stimulate the use of primary developmental control in an area. If controllability of events in a life area is relatively low, individuals objectively have lower possibility of using primary control, and they must establish secondary control. In such cases, downward comparisons are chosen, like in cases when primary control is possible, but it is "too expensive." In cases of serious losses, downward comparisons improve affective states, similar to tertiary developmental controls.

Generally, it can be concluded that if people make use of social comparisons to regulate self-development in a flexible way, these comparisons may produce adequate ways of development. If an individual repeats inflexible use of social comparisons, i.e., if he persists on comparisons that produce negative affects and unfavorable self-evaluation, then as also in the case of overstepping age-normative deadlines, he will have to use tertiary control. Tertiary control may calm negative consequences of inappropriate social comparisons and allow a person to change the ineffective type of social comparison and thus perhaps rehabilitate primary or secondary control in the regulation of own development.

It was emphasized earlier that age-norm requirements represent standards of checking self-development. On the basis of internalized age-norms, the person builds expectations concerning *future* development, but also evaluates *past* development. This is, in fact, the process of *temporal comparisons*, where present self-concept is a point of reference for comparison. Temporal comparison theory (TCT) was originally proposed by Albert (1977). This concept has gained attention within gerontological research. This fact is probably responsible for the assertion of some authors (e.g., Suls and Mullen 1982) that temporal comparison information is particularly salient with the elderly. Later research shows that such comparisons appear equally frequently both with the younger and with the elderly people, but that in different periods of life they may have different functions.

Comparisons with former self are called *downward comparisons*, and with future self they are called *upward comparisons*. When do people use downward and when upward comparisons and what are the consequences of these comparisons? From the developmental standpoint, differences may be expected in preferring the type of temporal comparisons with reference to life period, i.e., with reference to different temporal perspectives, because the young have shorter past and longer future, while it is the reverse with the older. We tested this presupposition in the framework of our research of the integrity of development in adolescence, early adulthood, middle and older adulthood (Lacković-Grgin et al. 2002). The first analysis shows that there is no difference in frequency of downward temporal comparisons between the adolescents and the elderly, but the two groups differ in the frequency of upward temporal comparisons in the sense that the young compare downward among themselves more frequently than the elderly. The young and the old compare themselves with past self equally frequently because the development of integrity presupposes evaluation of past life (Erikson 1982), i.e., because of the sense of self-continuation. Furthermore, the young can compare with past self because the contrast "I now" – "I past" may be rewarding. In the majority of cases it is thought that the progress has been made, which is mainly correct, so the consequences of such comparison are emotionally positive. However, Wilson and Ross (2000) find that if one exaggerates in the evaluation of progress, then one becomes too critical to past self. This might make the development of integrity more difficult. Our results show that integrity is linked relatively with the frequency of downward temporal comparisons in the area of social effectiveness, which could mean that too frequent downward comparisons in the area make the development of integrity more difficult. Integrity is not connected with such comparison in the area of achievement.

More frequent upward temporal comparisons in the young as compared with the elder may mean that for the young such comparisons have the function of self-improvement because they cause and inspire changes of self. Markus and Nurius (1986) think that perception of future selves serves for self-improvement, but only if one has "realistic dreams" about self in the future. Old people, who expect decrease in the future, may be discouraged by such comparisons. That comparisons in old age are more hazardous than downward temporal comparisons is confirmed by our preliminary results, according to which emotional consequences of upward temporal comparison are the most negative in the group of elder subjects in contrast to all other groups. This consistently appears in all examined areas of comparison, and it is especially visible in the area of health. It is interesting that Wilson and Ross (2000), in their experimental research find that with the elderly temporal comparison in general result in unfavorable health estimate, i.e., that those elderly people who avoid temporal comparisons evaluate their health more favorably.

Besides self-evaluation of development in an area, temporal comparisons are also used in the situation of rapid changes (the so-called stress transitions) that are caused by serious illness or loss of the loved ones. Investigations show that temporal comparisons serve as coping strategies with cancer (Klauer et al. 1998). However, also "victims" of life crises (e.g., the forties' crisis) have a stronger tendency toward temporal comparisons, particularly in the area of body image. Temporal comparisons are also used in the case of "attack" on social integrity, such as compulsory retirement. If these comparisons are not combined with the use of adequate strategy control, their consequences may be maladaptive.

Just because of that it was interesting to examine what kind of connection existed between the frequencies of upward and downward temporal comparisons and their consequences with the primary, secondary and tertiary controls. In the research mentioned above, with subjects from four age groups the models of these correlations are different according to age and according to the areas of comparison (academic/professional achievements, social efficiency and health). Since all analyses are not yet complete, we shall report the detailed results of this research in the near future.

The questions being asked for years are: which comparisons people use more frequently, social or temporal, and whether it varies with age. The answers are not unambiguous, which can be explained by means of several factors. First, the investigations mainly use transversal approach. Age spans as well as the determination of age groups are rather different. Some investigated the elderly only, while others students only. Second, discrepancies in findings lie in the fact that social and temporal comparisons were studied in widely different domains and also in different research fields (e.g., some research was done in the field of level of aspiration, some was done in the field of coping with stress experience, some of it in the developmental psychology of childhood). Third, various operationalizations of social and also temporal comparisons were used in research as well as different methods and techniques of investigation, depending on the aims of research.

Because of the reasons just enumerated, some find that social comparisons are in general more frequent than the temporal (Suls 1986). This author supposed that temporal comparisons could be more frequent in the periods of rapid growth and development, such as in childhood and adolescence. Other researchers quote results showing that temporal comparisons are more frequent than social comparisons, particularly in academic and social fields (Wayment and Taylor 1995). Spontaneous descriptions of coping with medical problems indicate that people quote more temporal than social comparisons. Our research of several samples of people of various ages and various levels of education, shows that temporal comparisons are more frequent than social in the fields of academic/professional achievements, social effectiveness, and health.

It is evident that answers to the question of prevalence and adaptive value of social and temporal comparisons, and of their relation to primary, secondary and tertiary control may be offered only by future longitudinal research that will, in a unique way, investigate the factors causing disagreement as indicated in the findings .

Conclusions and Perspectives

The questions of developmental self-regulation in different transition life periods in adulthood are a relative novelty in developmental psychology of life age. Valid theoretical hypotheses have been created for answers to these questions, integrating many former insights in developmental and social psychology, psychology of personality and motivation as well as stress psychology. For the purposes of our research, we have proposed a heuristic model as shown in Fig. 22-3.

In future research of developmental regulation, we should respect the fact that the relation of the variables in the proposed model (social and temporal

PERSONALITY VARIABLES	DEVELOPMENTAL GOALS	SOURCES OF INFORMATION FOR SELF-EVALUATION	ACTION	OUTCOMES
-Traits (Big-five personality dimensions)	IMPORTANCE (want)	OBJECTIVE INFORMATION	PERSONAL CONTROL OF DEVELOPMENT - primary - secondary	LIFE SATISFACTION SELF-ESTEEM
-Self-Esteem	REALIZATION (have)	TEMPORAL COMPARISONS IN RELEVANCE TO PERSONAL STANDARDS (me know, me before, perceived me in future)	- tertiary	COMPONENTS OF PERSONALITY (according to Erikson) - basic trust - autonomy - initiative - industry - ego identity - intimacy - generativity - ego integrity
-Internalized norms and values	DISCREPANCY (difference between importance and realization)	SOCIAL COMPARISONS (downward, lateral, upward – frequency and affective consequences)		

Fig. 22-3 Self-regulation of development across transitional periods of life in adolescence and adulthood (heuristic model)

comparisons, developmental goals, control of self-development as well as the relation of developmental outcomes (self-esteem, Erikson's personality components, life-satisfaction, mental health etc.)) is dynamic, and process-related to feedbacks. Thus, effective primary control may influence the change (preference) of the kinds of comparisons on the restructuring of developmental goals, in equal measure just as restructured goals change the kind of comparison and the kind of control. On the other hand, developmental achievements (e.g., high self-esteem) may also influence the revision of developmental goals, the kind of comparison, and control of self-development. This means that besides character features, which are stable and which act as development moderators in adulthood, all other variables in the suggested model may be mediators of development or outcomes of development. It is quite evident that valid results of the possibilities and the limits of self-regulation can be given by *longitudinal studies* only and new ways of statistical analysis. The methodological literature warns that many process models are tested by means of graded regressive or hierarchical analyses, although the analysis can only evaluate the effects of one variable on another in one period. When there are sufficient valid hypotheses concerning relations among variables, as in the case of this model, it is more advisable to use path-analysis or SEM modeling.

In the end, it is evident that much effort should still be invested in the development of methods of examination and techniques of measuring of some variables included in the outlined model that will be used in examining people belonging to different cultures in order to gain comparable parameters of development regulation in transitional life periods.

References

Albert, S. (1977). Temporal comparison theory. *Psychological Review, 84*, 485–503.

Atkinson, J. (1964). *An introduction to motivation*. Princeton, NJ: Van Nostrand.

Bakan, D. (1966). *The duality of human existence: An essay on psychology and religion*. Chicago: Rand McNally.

Baltes, M. M. (1995). Dependencies in old age: Gains and losses. *Current Directions in Psychological Science, 4*, 14–19.

Baltes, P. B. (1983). Life-span developmental psychology: Observations on history and theory revisited. In R. M. Lerner (Ed.), *Developmental psychology: Historical and philosophical perspectives* (pp. 79–111). Hillsdale, NJ: Erlbaum.

Baltes, P. B. (1987). Theoretical propositions of life-span developmental psychology: On the dynamics between growth and decline. *Developmental Psychology, 23*, 611–626.

Baltes, P. B. (1990). Psychological perspectives on successful aging: The model of selective optimisation with compensation. In P. B. Baltes & M. M. Baltes (Eds.), *Successful aging: Perspective from the behavioral science* (pp. 1–34). Cambridge: Cambridge University Press.

Baltes, P. B. (1997). On the incomplete architecture of human ontogeny: Selection, optimization and compensation as foundation of the development theory. *American Psychologist, 52*, 366–380.

Baltes, P. B., & Graf, P. (1996). Psychological aspects of aging: Facts and frontiers. In D. Magnuson (Ed.), *The life-span development of individuals: Behavioural, neurological, and psychosocial perspectives* (pp. 427–459). Cambridge: Cambridge University Press.

Bandura, A. (1977). Self-efficacy: Toward a unifying theory of behavioral change. *Psychological Review, 84*, 191–215.

Baumeister, R. F. (1991). *Meanings of life*. New York: Guilford Press.

Baumeister, R. F., Dale, K., & Sommer, K. L. (1998). Freudian defensive mechanism and empirical findings in modern social psychology: Reaction formation, projection, displacement, undoing, isolation, sublimation, and denial. *Journal of Personality, 66,* 1081–1124.

Berry, J. W., Kim, U., Minde, T., & Mok, D. (1987). Comparative studies of acculturative stress. *International Migration Review, 21,* 491–511.

Brammer, L. M. (1992). Coping with life transitions. *International Journal for the Assessment of Counseling, 15,* 123–153.

Brandtstädter, J. (1997). Action, culture and development: Points of convergence. *Culture and Psychology, 3,* 335–352.

Brandtstädter, J., Rothermund, K., & Schmitz, U. (1998). Maintaining self-integrity and efficacy through adulthood and later life: The adaptive functions of assimilative persistence and accommodative flexibility. In J. Heckhausen & C. S. Dweck (Eds.), *Motivation and self-regulation across life-span* (pp. 365–389). New York: Cambridge University Press.

Brandtstädter, J., & Greeve, W. (1994). The aging self: Stabilizing and protective processes. *Developmental Review, 14,* 52–80.

Bronfenbrenner, U. (1979). *The ecology of human development.* Cambridge, MA: Harvard University Press.

Brown, R. (2000). Social Identity Theory: past achievements, current problems and future challenges. *European Journal of Social Psychology, 30,* 745–778.

Brunstein, J. C. (1993). Personal goals and subjective well-being: A longitudinal study. *Journal of Personality and Social Psychology, 65,* 1061–1070.

Buunk, B. P., Gibbons, F. X., & Reis-Bergan, M. (1997). Social comparison in health and illness: A historical overview. In B. P. Buunk & F. X. Gibbons (Eds.), *Health, coping and well-being: Perspectives from social comparison theory* (pp. 1–23). London: Lawrence Erlbaum Associates.

Cantor, N., & Fleeson, W. (1991). Life tasks and self-regulatory processes. *Advances in Motivation and Achievement, 7,* 327–369.

Carstensen, L. L. (1995). Evidence for a life-span theory of socioemotional selectivity. *Current Directions in Psychological Science, 4,* 151–156.

Carver, C. S., & Scheier, M. F. (1990). Origins and functions of positive and negative affect: A control process view. *Psychological Review, 97,* 19–25.

Chatzisarantis, N., Biddle, S., & Meek, G. (1997). A self-determination theory approach to the study of intentions and the intention-behaviour relationship in children's physical activity. *British Journal of Health Psychology, 2,* 343–360.

Chiu, P., & Nevius, J. (1990). Three wishes of gifted and non gifted adolescents. *Journal of Genetic Psychology, 151,* 133–138.

Cox, T. (1982). *Stress.* London, Basingstoke: Macmillan.

Cramer, P. (1997). Identity, personality and defense mechanisms: An observer-based study. *Journal of Research in Personality, 31,* 58–7.

Ćubela, V. (2001). Istraživanje procesa socijalnog uspoređivanja (*Research of process of social comparisons*). *RADOVI-Razdio FPSP, 40*(17), 117–142.

Danner, D. E., & Schröder, H. C. (1992). Biologie des Alterns: Ontogenese und Evolution (*Biology of the elderly: Ontogenesis and evolution*). In P. B. Baltes & J. Mittelstrass (Eds.), *Zukunft des Alterns und gesellschaftliche Entwicklung* (pp. 95–123). Berlin: de Gruyter.

Deci, E. L., & Ryan, R. M. (1985). *Intrinsic motivation and self-determination in human behavior.* New York: Plenum Press.

Elder, G. H., & O'rand, A. M. (1995). Adults lives in a changing society. In K. S. Cook, G. A. Fine & J. S. House (Eds.), *Sociological perspectives on social psychology* (pp. 452–475). Needham Heights, MA: Allyn and Bacon.

Emmons, R. A. (1986). Personal strivings: An approach to personality and subjective well-being. *Journal of Personality and Social Psychology, 51,* 1058–1068.

Emmons, R. A. (1992). Abstract versus concrete goals: Personal striving level, physical illness, and psychological well-being. *Journal of Personality and Social Psychology, 62*, 292–300.

Emmons, R. A. (1996). Striving and feeling: Personal goals and subjective well-being. In P. M. Gollwitzer & J. A. Bargh (Eds.), *The psychology of action: Linking cognition and motivation behavior* (pp. 313–337). New York: Guilford Press.

Emmons, R. A. (1999). *The psychology of ultimate concerns.* New York: The Guilford Press.

Endler, N. S., & Parker, J. D. A. (1990). Multidimensional assessment of coping: A critical evaluation. *Journal of Personality and Social Psychology, 58*, 844–854.

Erikson, E. (1980). *Identity and the life cycle.* New York: Norton.

Erikson, E. H. (1982). *The life cycle completed.* New York: W. W. Norton.

Erikson, E., Erikson, J. M., & Kivnick, H. Q. (1986). *Vital involvement in old age.* New York: Norton.

Feather, N. T. (1982). Unemployment and its psychological correlates: A study of depressive symptoms, self-esteem, protestant ethic values, attributional style, and apathy. *Australian Journal of Psychology, 34*, 309–323.

Feather, N. T., & Bond, M. J. (1983). Time structure and purposeful activity among employed and unemployed university graduates. *Journal of Occupational Psychology, 56*, 241–254.

Festinger, L. (1954). A theory of social comparison processes. *Human Relations, 7*, 117–140.

Finch, C. E. (1996). Biological bases for plasticity during aging of individual life histories. In D. Magnusson (Ed.), *The life-span development of individuals: Behavioural, neurobiological and psychosocial perspectives* (pp. 488–511). Cambridge: Cambridge University Press.

Gibbons, F. X., & Buunk, B. P. (1999). Individual differences in social comparison: Development of a scale of social comparison orientation. *Journal of Personality and Social Psychology, 76*, 129–142.

Gollwitzer, P. M. (1987). Suchen, Finden und Festigen der eigenen Identität: Unstillbare Zielintentionen (*Searching, finding and consolidating of one's own identity: Unsaturatable goal intentions*). In H. Heckhausen, P. M. Gollwitzer & F. E. Weinert (Eds.), *Jenseits des Rubikon:Der Wille in den Humanwissenschaften* (pp. 176–189). Berlin: Springer.

Gould, S. J. (1999). A critique of Heckhausen and Schultz's theory of control from a cross-cultural perspective. *Psychological Review, 106*, 597–604.

Grob, A., Krings, F., & Bangerter, A. (2001). Life markers in biographical narratives of people from three cohorts: A life-span perspective in its historical context. *Human Development, 44*, 171–190.

Grolnick, W. S., & Ryan, R. M. (1987). Autonomy in children's learning: An experimental and individual difference investigation. *Journal of Personality and Social Psychology, 52*, 890–898.

Gutman, D. L. (1964). An exploration of ego configuration in middle and later life. In B. L. Neugarten (Ed.), *Personality in middle and late life* (pp. 114–148). New York: Atherton.

Havighurst, R. J. (1953). *Human development and education.* New York: Longman.

Heckhausen, H. (1967). *The anatomy of achievement motivation.* Princeton, NJ: Van Nostrand.

Heckhausen, J. (1991). *Motivation and action.* Berlin: Springer.

Heckhausen, J. (1999). *Developmental regulation in adulthood.* Cambridge: Cambridge University Press.

Heckhausen, J. (2002). Developmental regulation of life-course transitions: A control theory approach. In L. Pulkkinen & A. Caspi (Eds.), *Pathways of successful development – Personality in the life course* (pp. 257–281). Cambridge: Cambridge Press.

Heckhausen, J., & Schulz, R. (1993). Optimization by selection and compensation: Balancing primary and secondary control in life-span development. *International Journal of Behavioral Development, 16*, 287–303.

Heckhausen, J., & Schulz, R. (1995). A life – span theory of control. *Psychological Review, 102*, 284–304.

Heckhausen, J., & Schulz, R. (1998). Developmental regulation in adulthood: Selection and compensation via primary and secondary control. In J. Heckhausen & C. S. Dweck (Eds.), *Motivation and self-regulation across the life-span* (pp. 50–78). Cambridge: Cambridge University Press.

Helgeson, V. S., & Mickelson, K. D. (1995). Motives for Social Comparison. *Personality and Social Psychology Bulletin, 21*, 1200–1209.

Higgins, E. T., & Silberman, I. (1998). Development of regulatory focus: Promotion and prevention as ways of living. In J. Heckhausen & C. S. Dweck (Eds.), *Motivation and self-regulation across life-span* (pp. 78–113). New York: Cambridge University Press.

Hull, C. L. (1943). *Principles of behavior*. New York: Appleton-Century-Crofts.

Hyde, J. S. (1994). *Understanding human sexuality*. New York: McGraw-Hill, Inc.

Klauer, T., Ferring, D., & Filipp, S. H. (1998). "Still stable after all this…?": Temporal comparison in coping with severe and chronic disease. *International Journal of Behavioral Development, 22*, 339–355.

Kobasa, S. C. (1979). Stressful life events, personality and health: An inquiry into hardiness. *Journal of Personality and Social Psychology, 37*, 1–11.

Koestner, R., Losier, G. F., Vallerand, R. J., & Carducci, D. (1996). Identified and introjected forms of political internalization: Extending self-determination theory. *Journal of Personality and Social Psychology, 70*, 1025–1036.

Kuhl, J. (1984). Motivational aspects of achievement motivation and learned helplessness: Toward a comprehensive theory of action control. In B. A. Maher & W. B. MAHER (Eds.), *Progress in experimental psychology research* (Vol. 13, pp. 99–171). New York: Academic Press.

Kuhl, J., & Beckmann, J. (eds). (1985). *Action control from cognition to behavior*. New York: Springer.

Kuhl, J., & Fuhrmann, A. (1998). Decomposing self-regulation and self-control: The volitional components inventory. In J. Heckhausen & C. S. Dweck (Eds.), *Motivation and self-regulation across life-span* (pp. 15–49). New York: Cambridge University Press.

Lacković-Grgin, K. (1993). Socijalno-psihološke odrednice zadovoljstva životom žena srednje dobi (*Socio-psychological determinants of life satisfaction among middle aged women*), Radovi,Razdio FPSP, *31*(8), 95–100.

Lacković-Grgin, K. (1994). Psihološki značaj nezaposlenosti kod mladih visoke naobrazbe (*Some Psychological Conseuences Of Unemployment Of Young Graduates*). *RADOVI-Razdio FPSP, 32*(9), 73–85.

Lacković-Grgin, K., & Padelin, P. (1995). Psihološko funkcioniranje starijih osoba smještenih u različitim uvjetima (*The psychological functioning of elders living in different residential conditions*). *Radovi-Razdio FPSP, 33*(10), 69–79.

Lacković-Grgin, K., & Sorić, I. (1995). Self-esteem and loneliness of freshmen. *VIIth European Conference on Developmental Psychology*, Krakow: Book of abstracts.

Lacković-Grgin, K., & Sorić, I. (1996). Prijelaz i prilagodba na studij: Jednogodišnje praćenje (*Transition and Adjustment of Students to the University Environment: A one year follow-up study*). *RADOVI-Razdio FPSP, 34*, 53–67.

Lacković-Grgin, K., & Sorić, I. (1997). Korelati prilagodbe studiju tijekom prve godine (*Correlates of adjustment to the university amongst first year students*). *Društvena istraživanja, 4–5*(30–31), 461–475.

Lacković-Grgin, K., Deković, M., Milosavljević, B., Cvek-Sorić, I., & Opačić, G. (1996). Social support and self-esteem in unemployed university graduates. *Adolescence, 31*, 701–707.

Lacković-Grgin, K., Deković, M., & Opačić, G. (1994). Pubertal status, interaction with significant others, and self-esteem of adolescent girls. *Adolescence, 29*, 691–700.

Lacković-Grgin, K., Grgin, T., Sorić, I., & Penezić, Z. (1999). Personal control of development: Some correlates, sex, and age differences. *VII European Congress of Psychology, Roma, Abstracts* , pp. 246–247.

Lacković-Grgin, K., Grgin, T., Penezić, Z., & Sorić, I. (2001). Some predictors of primary control of development in three transitional periods of life. *Journal of Adult Psychology, 3*, 149–160.

Lacković-Grgin, K., Nekić, M., & Ćubela, V. (2002). Dobne specifičnosti integriteta s gledišta Eriksonove teorije psihosocijalnog razvoja (*Age specificities of integrity from the point of view of Eriskon's theory of psychosocial development*). *RADOVI-Razdio FPSP, 41*(18), 45–68.

Lerner, R. M. (1984). *On the nature of human plasticity*. New York: Cambridge University Press.

Lerner, R. M. (1996). Relative plasticity, integration, temporality, and diversity in human development: A developmental contextual perspective about theory, process, and method. *Developmental Psychology, 32*, 781–786.

Lerner, R. M., & Kauffman, M. B. (1985). The concept of development in contextualism. *Developmental Review, 5*, 309–333.

Levinson, D. J. (1986). *The Seasons of a Man's Life*. New York: Ballantine Books.

Lewin, K. (1951). *Field theory in social science*. New York: Harper and Row.

Liebkind, K. (1996). Acculturation and stress. *Journal of Cross-Cultural Psychology, 27*, 161–180.

Lieberman, M. A., & Tobin, S. S. (1983). *The Experience of Old Age*. New York: Basic Books.

Little, B. R. (1983). Personal projects: A rationale and methods for investigation. *Environment and Behavior, 15*, 273–309.

Little, B. R. (1989). Personal projects analysis: Trivial pursuits, magnificent obsessions, and the search for coherence. In D. M. Buss & N. Cantor (Eds.), *Personality psychology: Recent trends and direction* (pp. 15–31). New York: Springer.

Magnuson, D., Stattin, H., & Allen, V. L. (1985). Biological maturation and social development: A longitudinal study of some adjustment processes from mid-adolescence to adulthood. *Journal of Youth and Adolescence, 14*, 267–283.

Markus, H., & Nurius, P. (1986). Possible selves. *American Psychologist, 41*, 954–969.

Maslow, A. H. (1976). *Motivation and Personality*. New York: Harper and Row.

Ngyen, A. N., & Williams, H. L. (1989). Transition from East to West: Vietnamese adolescents and their parents. *Journal of the American Academy of Child and Adolescent Psychiatry, 28*, 505–515.

Nurmi, J. E., Salmela-Aro, K., & Routsalainen, H. (1994). Cognitive and attributional strategies among unemployed young adults: A case of failure – trap strategy. *European Journal of Personality, 8*, 135–148.

Nurmi, J. E., Toivonen, S., Salmela-Aro, K., & Eronen, S. (1996). Optimistic approached-oriented, and avoidance strategies in social situations: Three studies on loneliness and peer relationships. *European Journal of Personality, 10*, 201–219.

Olson, B. D., & Evans, D. L. (1999). The role of the big five personality dimensions in the direction and affective consequences of everyday social comparisons. *Personality and Social Psychology Bulletin, 25*, 1498–1508.

Penezić, Z. (2004). Zadovoljstvo životom u adolescentnoj i odrasloj dobi: provjera teorije višestrukih diskrepancija (*Life satisfaction in adolescence and adulthood: The role of multiple discrepancies*). *Doctoral thesis*. University of Zagreb, Croatia.

Penezić, Z., & Lacković-Grgin, K. (2001). Važnost razvojnih ciljeva u adolescentnoj, srednjoj i starijoj životnoj dobi (*Importance of different developmental goals in adolescence, middle aged and older adults*). *RADOVI-Razdio FPSP, 40*(17), 65–81.

Piaget, J. (1952). *The origins of intelligence in children*. New York: International University Press.

Plomin, R. (1986). *Development, genetics, and psychology*. New York: International University Press.

Pöhlman, K., & Brunstein, J. C. (1997). GOALS: Ein Fragebogen zur Messung von Lebenszielen. *Diagnostica, 1*, 63–79.

Pulkkinen, L., Nurmi, J. E., & Kokko, K. (2002). Individual differences in personal goals in mid-thirties. In L. Pulkkinen & A. Caspi (Eds.), *Paths to successful development-personality in the life course* (pp. 331–353). Cambridge: Cambridge University Press.

Pyszyrinski, T., Greenberg, J., & Solomon, S. (2000). Proximal and distal defense: A new perspective on unconscious motivation. *Current Directions in Psychology Science, 5*, 156–160.

Rokeach, M. (1973). *The nature of human values*. New York: Free Press.

Rothbaum, F., Weisz, J. R., & Snyder, S. S. (1982). Changing the world and changing the self: A two-process model of perceived control. *Journal of Personality and Social Psychology, 42*, 5–37.

Rotter, J. B. (1966). Generalized expectancies for internal versus external locus of control of reinforcement. *Psychological Monographs, 80*, 609.

Ryan, R. M. (1998). Commentary: Human psychological needs and the issues of volition, control, and outcome focus. In J. Heckhausen & C. S. Dweck (Eds.), *Motivation and self-regulation across life-span* (pp. 114–137). New York: Cambridge University Press.

Ryan, M., & Deci, E. L. (2000). Self-determination theory and the facilitation of intrinsic motivation, social development, and well-being. *American Psychologist, 55*, 68–78.

Schmitt-Roderrmund, E., & Sibbereisen, R. K. (1999). Determinants of differential acculturation of development timetables among adolescent immigrants in Germany. *International Journal of Psychology, 34*, 219–233.

Schulz, R., & Decker, S. (1985). Long-term adjustment to physical disability: The role of social support, perceived control, and self-blame. *Journal of Personality and Social Psychology, 48*, 1162–1172.

Simonton, D. K. (1995). *Greatness*. New York: Guilford Press.

Steinberg, L. (1988). Reciprocal relative between parent-child distance and pubertal maturation. *Developmental Psychology, 24*, 122–128.

Suls, J., & Mullen, B. (1982). From the cradle to the grave: Comparison and self-evaluation across the life-span. In J. Suls (Ed.), *Psychological perspectives on the self* (Vol. 1, pp. 97–125). Hillsdale, NJ: Lawrence Erlbaum Association, Inc.

Swan, G. E., Dame, A., & Carmelli, D. (1991). Involuntary retirement, Type A behavior, and current functioning in elderly men: 24-year follow-up of the western collaborative group study. *Psychology and Aging, 6*, 384–391.

Taylor, S. E., & Lobel, M. (1989). Social comparisons activity under threat: Downward evaluation and upward contacts. *Psychological Review, 96*, 569–575.

Taylor, S. E., Wayment, H. A., & Carrilo, M. (1996). Social comparison, self-regulation and motivation. In R. M. Sorentino & E. T. Higgins (Eds.), *Handbook of motivation and cognition* (pp. 3–27). New York: Guilford Press.

Trimko, C., & Moss, R. H. (1990). Determinants of interpersonal support and self-direction in group residential facilities. *Journal of Gerontology, 45*, 184–192.

Warr, P. B., Jackson, P. R., & Banks, M. H. (1982). Duration of unemployment and psychological well-being in young men and women. *Current Psychological Research, 2*, 207–214.

Wayment, H. A., & Taylor, C. E. (1995). Self-evaluation processes: Motives, information use and self-esteem. *Journal of Personality, 63*, 729–757.

Weiner, B. (1972). *Theories of motivation: From mechanism to cognition*. Chicago, IL: Markham.

Wills, T. A. (1981). Similarity and self-esteem in downward comparison. In J. Suls & T. A. Wills (Eds.), *Social comparison: Contemporary theory and research* (pp. 243–268). New York: Plenum.

Wills, T. A. (1997). Modes and families of coping: An analysis of social comparison in the structure of other cognitive behavioral mechanisms. In B. P. Buunk & F. X. Gibbons (Eds.), *Health, coping and well-being: Perspectives from social comparison theory* (pp. 167–193). London: Lawrence Erlbaum Associates.

Wilson, A. E., & Ross, M. (2000). The frequency of temporal and social comparison in people's personal appraisals. *Journal of Personality and Social Psychology, 78,* 928–942.

Wood, J. V., Taylor, S. E., & Lichtman, R. R. (1985). Social comparison in adjustment to breast cancer. *Journal of Personality and Social Psychology, 49,* 1169–1183.

Chapter 23

Time, Culture, and Life-Cycle Changes of Social Goals

Helene H. Fung and Tasia M. Y. Siu

Sophie loved meeting different kinds of people and joining various social activities when she was young. Yet, as she grew older, she gradually reduced her social contacts. At Sophie's 65th birthday, her family members suggested inviting the entire neighborhood to her birthday party. But she declined. Rather than having a noisy party packed with people, she preferred having a private dinner with a handful of close relatives.

Paul, at his early thirties, was eager to strive for career success and spent almost all his time on work. However, when he found out that he had lung cancer, he shifted his focus away from his career. He now spent more time with his wife and his close friends.

Though the shifts in social goals in the above two cases are seemingly different, we argue that they both reflect the same underlying motivational process. Gentle and not-so-gentle life events, such as aging or being diagnosed with a terminal illness, remind us of the finitude of life, which in turn affects our priorities and goals. In this chapter, we will first review theories and research on how social goals change across adulthood, and how time perspective may account for the change. Then we will describe how time perspective differs across socio-cultural contexts and review empirical evidences for the effects of these differences on social goals. Finally, we will discuss the theoretical and practical implications of understanding the role of perceived time in social motivation.

Changes of Social Goals Across Adulthood

Goals are ends toward which efforts are directed. They serve as guidelines for intentional self-development (Brandtstädter, 1999). They also serve to direct attention, mobilize effort, increase persistence, and formulate strategies (Locke & Latham, 1994). Studies on adult development find that people at different stages of life focus on different types of goals.

From: *Handbook of Stressful Transitions Across the Lifespan*,
Edited by: T.W. Miller, DOI 10.1007/978-1-4419-0748-6_23,
© Springer Science+Business Media, LLC 2010

441

Jung (1931, 1953, 1960), for example, identifies two major types of goals, which he calls "orientations of the ego." One orientation – "extroversion" – is directed towards the external world while the other orientation – "introversion" – is directed towards the inner, subjective experiences. Based on clinical observations and folklore, he suggests that younger people are more extroverted than are older people.

Later studies confirmed his observation. Neugarten and colleagues (1964, as cited in Neugarten, 1977) conducted a series of studies on people aged 40--80 years over a 10-year period. Using multiple methods including projective tests, questionnaires, and structured and unstructured interviews, they consistently found a change from outer- to inner-world orientation with age. This finding was observed among both middle class and working class adults (Neugarten, 1968). Other researchers found similar results. Gutman (1966) measured extroversion[1] in a large group of people aged 17–94 years. He found that extroversion was negatively related to age. Heron and Chown (1967) also found in a sample aged 20–80 years that older people had a higher level of introversion than younger people. Further evidence was provided by Sealy and Cattell who administered the Sixteen Personality Factor test to people aged 16–70 years and factor-analyzed their scores (as cited in Crown, 1968). They found an age difference in introversion, such that older people were more introverted than were younger people. Likewise, Slater and Scarr (1964) factor-analyzed the Minnesota Multi-phasic Personality Inventory (MMPI) and found that older people scored higher on the dimension of high ego-strength plus introversion than did younger people.

Examining changes in goals from another perspective, Erikson's psychosocial theory of development (1950, 1968; 1982) proposes that tasks change across stages of development. Developmental tasks in adulthood move from establishing intimacy and affiliation with others (intimacy) in young adulthood to developing a sense of concern for the well-being of the world and its future generations (generativity) in middle adulthood, and finally to establishing a sense of meaning in one's own life (integrity) in old age. The developmental transition from generativity to integrity has received empirical support. Ryff and Heincke (1983) asked young, middle-aged, and older adults to rate how well items concerning generativity and integrity described them in young, middle-age, and older adulthood. Young adults made their ratings according to how well generativity and integrity described them in the present, and how well they would describe them in middle and old ages. Middle-aged adults made the ratings according to how well generativity and integrity described them now, had described them in their young adulthood, and would describe them in their old age. Older adults made the ratings according to how well the two developmental tasks had described them in young and middle adulthood, and how well they described them in the present. All three age groups reported

---

[1]Studies in the 1960s defined extroversion--introversion more as a goal orientation (i.e., whether one wants to change the outer world or the inner self) than a measure of sociability; whereas the reverse was true for studies in the 1980s and 1990s, for example, Costa and McCrae (1988). Probably because of this, studies in the 1960s usually found an age difference in extroversion--introversion such that older people were more introverted than younger people. But such a difference was not found in later studies.

the actual and expected generativity in their middle adulthood, and integrity in their old age.

Studies that directly ask adults about their life goals also find age-related changes. Bühler, Brind, and Horner (1968) first asked individuals aged 17-60 years to rate the relevance of 86 life goals. They then factor-analyzed the scores and obtained 12 factors, equally divided into four categories: need satisfaction (necessities of life/pleasure, love and family, and sexual satisfaction), self-limiting adaptation (accepting limitations/caution, submissiveness, and avoidance of hardships), creative expansion (self-development, being a leader/achieving fame and power, and role in public life), and upholding the internal order (moral values, social values, and having success). The relevance scores an individual gave the 12 factors established his/her goal profile. Bühler, Brind and Horner then recruited small groups of younger and older people not included in the original sample and compared their goal profiles. They found that compared with younger people, older people scored higher on the three factors indicating self-limiting adaptation, and lower on "self development," "role in public life" and "having success." In addition, a subgroup of older people scored higher than their younger counterparts on "love and family."

More recent studies on goals further confirm this shift. When asked to complete sentences starting with, "In the coming years...," younger adults focused more on improvements in domains like education, career, family building, and finances while older adults expressed greater concern about having emotionally satisfying social relationships and maintaining achieved levels of functioning and satisfaction (Dittmann-Kohli & Westerhof, 1997). Similarly, when instructed to write down the types of goals, hopes, plans, and dreams they had when they thought about the future, young adults were more likely to mention goals related to their future education and family/marriage than were older adults. Young and middle-aged adults were also more likely to mention property-related goals than were older adults. Older adults, in turn, were more likely to mention goals related to their own satisfaction in health, retirement, and leisure activities (Nurmi, 1992). This age trend is found even among the very old. Staudinger et al. (1999) examined investment, i.e. thoughts and actions, in 10 domains – health, well-being of close relatives, mental performance, relationships with friends and acquaintances, thinking about life, hobbies and other interests, independence, death and dying, occupational or comparable activities, sexuality – among older adults aged 70-103 years. They found that while the relative investment in "hobbies and other interests" was negatively related to age, the relative investment in death and dying was positively associated with age.

In addition, indirect evidence for goal changes throughout adulthood can be found in lay formulations of psychological well-being. Ryff (1989a) interviewed middle-aged and older adults about their conceptions of psychological well-being. She found that while middle-aged adults stressed being confident and assertive, older adults emphasized self-acceptance. Moreover, in responding to an open-ended question about what they would like to change in their life "given the chance," the most frequent response from older adults was "nothing" while that from middle-aged adult was "active self-improvement" (Ryff, 1989b). Indeed, older adults rated themselves lower on personal growth – "see[ing] oneself as growing and expanding" (Ryff, 1989b, 1991), and goal seeking – the desire to achieve new goals, to search for new and different experiences, and to be on the move (Reker et al., 1987), than middle-aged and young adults. Given that what people regard as important to psychological well-being is often what they strive for, the above findings indirectly suggest that older people no longer place great importance on goals that improve their lot. Instead, they seem to pay more attention to maximizing self-acceptance in the present.

In summary, findings from studies that compared people of different ages on self-reported life orientation, developmental tasks, goals, and definitions of psychological well-being suggest that goals change throughout adulthood.

Theoretical Explanations for Age-related Changes of Goals

Theories on adult development have traditionally explained changes in goals throughout adulthood, in terms of changes in experience and life situations that are inherent to the aging process. Erikson's psycho-social theory of development (1950, 1968, 1982) emphasizes the roles of both accumulation of experience with age and situational demands of different life stages. According to Erikson, each developmental stage has a crisis that is defined as a conflict between personal needs and the demands of society. Development entails solving conflicts associated with particular stages and moving on to the next. The progression of developmental tasks represents both the individuals' increased capability of "interacting within a wider social radius" (Hooyman & Kiyak, 1993, p. 190) and age-related changes in societal demands.

Jung (1953) stresses the role of situational demands. To him, younger people attach greater importance to outward orientation because they have a "natural" aim – the begetting of children and protecting "the blood", and the associated acquisition of money and social position. This aim directs their attention to their relationships with the outside world. With increasing age, however, the pressure to attend to the external world lessens. For example, the death of parents frees one from the need of being a dutiful child. The "natural" aim is thus replaced by a "cultural" aim that makes older people focus on appreciation of the internal self.

Also emphasizing situational demands, Neugarten (1968, 1977) explains goal changes as a result of people's recognition and adjustment to their age status. To her, adults alter their goals as they grow older because they perceive changes in their life situations (1977):

> Forty-year-olds, for example, seem to see the environment as one that rewards boldness and risk-taking and to see themselves as possessing energy congruent with the opportunities perceived in the outer world. Sixty-year-olds, however perceive the world as complex and dangerous, no longer to be reformed in line with one's wishes, and the individual as conforming and accommodating to outer-world demands (p. 628).

Hence, forty-year-olds are more likely to focus on goals that are directed towards modifying the outside world while sixty-year-olds place greater emphasis on goals related to changing the inner self.

Although these early theories did not afford greater or lesser value to age differences in goals, later theories came to attribute changes in goals throughout adulthood to losses associated with aging. One such theory is the disengagement theory. The term "disengagement" refers to withdrawal from previous roles and activities. According to the disengagement theory (Cumming & Henry, 1961), it is a function for both older individuals and social world to prepare for the individual's death. On the part of older individuals, pre-conscious awareness of the imminence of death instigates a normal adaptive process characterized by increased self-awareness and social withdrawal. Meanwhile, recognition on the part of the social world that older individuals will soon die leads to a concurrent societal detachment from the individuals, further encouraging their increased self-preoccupation. As a result, people shift their goals with age as a "practicing" of the ultimate loss – death – "through a sense of already being disengaged from immediate relationships" (Henry & Cumming, 1959, p.385).

Activity theory is another theory that explains goal changes in terms of age-related losses (Havighurst & Albrecht, 1953; Maddox, 1963). Theorists argue that barriers to social contact, rooted in an insidious ageism in western societies, are at the root of older people's shift in goals. Such barriers, coupled with deaths of loved ones and poor health, impoverish the social structures of older people and reduce their opportunities for expanding their horizons or even maintaining the level of activity they used to enjoy. Older people are, thus, unable to fulfill some of their goals and eventually drop them.

Social exchange theory (Bengtson & Dowd, 1980–81; Dowd, 1980), a third loss-based theory, explicitly describes how social barriers contribute to age-related changes in social goals, relationships is an equitable power balance. Limited resources in old age force older social network members to contribute less to interpersonal relationships than do their younger counterparts, undermining the equitable power balance and weakening social ties. Older adults, thus, are "squeezed out" of all but the most familiar social relationships and are required to change their social goals accordingly.

Even theories on successful aging attribute goal changes to age-related declines. Recognizing that older adults do not show a reduction in psychological well-being despite the genuine objective losses that accompany aging (George et al., 1988; Herzog & Rogers, 1981; Revenson, 1986), these theories postulate that this is the case precisely because older people downgrade the importance of goals that are unattainable.

For example, Brandtstädter and Greve (1994) propose that people employ three functionally interdependent processes to preserve and maintain a positive view of self and personal development. Two of these processes are: assimilative processes – problem-directed actions which aim at transforming situational circumstances or ways of living in accordance with the values, aspirations, and developmental goals of the individual; and accommodative processes – adjustments of personal goals, values, and aspirations so that they fit more closely with given situations and constraints. Citing evidence that even older people themselves recognize an increasingly negative balance of developmental gains and losses with age (Brandtstädter et al., 1993), Brandtstädter postulates that these declines lead older people to favor accommodative processes over assimilative ones (Brandtstädter & Baltes-Gotz, 1990; Brandtstädter & Renner, 1990), leading to changes in goals with age.

Similarly, Heckhausen and Schulz (1995) account for goal changes in adulthood in terms of older people's adjustment to age-related losses. They distinguish between two types of control, primary and secondary control. Consistent with Rothbaum (Rosenbaum, 1983), Heckhausen and Schulz define primary control as displaying behaviors directed at the external environment. These behaviors aim at changing the world to fit the needs and desires of the individual.

Secondary control, in contrast, refers to internal actions, usually cognitions, that modify the individual's desires to fit with the world. Heckhausen and Schulz postulate that people of all ages exert primary control whenever possible. However, with the increasing negative balance of developmental gains and losses (Heckhausen et al., 1989), secondary control is exercised more often by older people, as compared to their younger counterparts, to buffer emotional well-being and self-esteem from failures to achieve primary control. Empirical findings suggest that older people do use one secondary control strategy, "flexible goal adjustment," more often than do younger people (Heckhausen & Schulz, 1994), contributing to changes of goals in adulthood.

Consistent postulates have been offered by other theorists. Lazarus and Folkman (1984) identify two forms of coping. The first form is known as problem-focused coping which involves managing stress by "trying to change the situation for the better" (Lazarus, 1996, p. 291). While the other form is called emotion-focused coping that entails managing the emotional reaction to stress by changing the meaning of the transaction or by regulating its expression. Lazarus predicts that in situations with uncontrollable stress, like those commonly found in old age, people adjust by shifting from problem-focused coping to emotion-focused coping. Empirical evidences, in general, support this prediction. While older adults engage in both problem-focused and emotion-focused coping, and are more flexible in their problem-solving strategies than younger adults, they are more likely to employ emotion-focused strategies to cope with problems that are more emotionally charged (Blanchard-Fields et al., 1995; Blanchard-Fields et al., 1997).

Other theories on successful aging also imply that people change their goals with age to adapt to age-related losses. Baltes and Baltes (1990) propose a model of aging known as selection, optimization with compensation. According to this model, as people age, they increasingly concentrate their resources and efforts on a handful of selected domains that are most important to them, maintain high levels of functioning in these domains, and compensate for impairments by employing alternative means to achieve the same goal. These adaptation strategies are likely to be associated with changes in goals. Bäckman and Dixon (1992) use the term "compensation" to refer to a similar process. To them, older people respond to a discrepancy between perceived skills and environmental demands by using a range of strategies including changing goals and aspirations.

In summary, theories on adult development postulate that goals shift throughout adulthood in response to changes in experience and life situations that are inherent in the aging process. Early theories do not specify whether these shifts reflect developmental gains or losses. Later theories, however, explain them as direct consequences of, or psychological adjustments to, age-related losses.

Role of Time Perspective in Age-related Changes of Goals

Socio-emotional selectivity theory (Carstensen, 1993, 1995, 1998; Carstensen et al., 1999; Carstensen et al., 2003), in contrast, attributes age-related differences in goals to a motivated process instigated by shifts in time perspective. It argues that rather than experience or life situations specific to the aging process, perceived time left in the future instigates changes in goal hierarchies.

According to the theory, the same essential set of goals operates throughout life, but the relative importance of specific types of goals changes as a function of perceived time left in life. The theory focuses on two broad classes of social motives: knowledge-related goals and emotionally meaningful goals. Knowledge-related goals are those that increase future preparedness by banking information about oneself and the social world. Subsumed under this goal trajectory are information-seeking, social comparison, identity striving, and achievement motivation in educational and occupational endeavors. In contrast, emotionally meaningful goals are present-oriented and are aimed at maximizing emotional satisfaction in the here and now. They include motives to feel good, derive emotional meaning from life, deepen intimacy, and maintain the self. Knowledge-related goals are most salient when time is perceived as open-ended and people allocate considerable resources to prepare for the long and undetermined future. Emotionally meaningful goals, in contrast, assume primacy when perceived time is limited.

Perceived time is inextricably and negatively related to chronological age. Young adulthood is associated with the perception that time is open-ended. The theory predicts that given this time perspective, younger adults are more likely to favor knowledge-related goals over emotionally meaningful goals in situations where the two types of goals are in competition. However, as people grow older, life events, such as the death of an age peer and the birth of a grandchild, prime thoughts of mortality. The long-term payoffs of knowledge-related goals become less relevant than present-oriented emotionally meaningful goals. Older adults are thus more likely to show biases favoring emotionally meaningful goals.

Because social goals direct social behaviors, socio-emotional selectivity theory makes predictions about preferences and behaviors in the interpersonal domain. When knowledge-related goals are accentuated, novel and peripheral social partners are most appealing, because their unfamiliarity increases the likelihood that an individual will learn something new from them[2]. When emotionally meaningful goals assume primacy, however, emotionally close social partners are preferred because they are more likely to provide predictable emotional experiences that facilitate feelings of social connectedness (Carstensen et al., 1997). Hence, the theory predicts that older adults who place greater importance on emotionally meaningful goals prefer to interact with emotionally close social partners whereas younger adults who attach greater importance to knowledge-related goals invest in novel social partners.

Empirical Findings Provide Support for the Theory

Age-Related Prioritization of Emotional Social Goals

Age Differences in Social Cognition
Studies on age differences in social cognition find that old people do pay greater attention to the emotional aspects of their social world than do their younger counterparts, suggesting that they attach greater importance

---

[2]This idea is consistent with Granovetter's theory about the strength of weak ties (Granovetter, 1973). According to Granovetter, people obtain a wide variety of benefits, including new information, from peripheral social partners.

to emotionally meaningful goals. Fredrickson and Carstensen (1990) asked people ranging from adolescents to octogenarians to sort a set of cards, describing various types of prospective social partners according to their perceived similarity. They then employed multi-dimensional scaling techniques to explore the cognitive dimensions that people used to make such judgments and the relative weights placed on each dimension by different age groups. They identified three dimensions that accounted for most of the variance in the mathematical solution: (1) the potential for offering emotional rewards, (2) the potential for providing information, and (3) the possibilities for future contact. Fredrickson and Carstensen found that while younger age groups weighted the three dimensions fairly evenly, successively older age groups placed greater emphasis on the affective potential of social partners. This effect was true for men and women, blue- and white-collar workers, and African-Americans and Caucasian-Americans (Carstensen & Fredrickson, 1998).

The age-related emphasis on emotions also manifests itself in the cognitive processing of social information. Carstensen and Turk-Charles (1994) asked people aged 20–83 years to read a selection drawn from a popular novel. They then tested the participants' memory for the selection using an incidental memory paradigm. They found that older people recollected proportionately more emotional information than did younger cohorts. In another study, Hashtroudi et al. (1990) exposed younger and older adults to a number of everyday situations simulated or imagined in the laboratory. This was followed by a recall test on both types of situations. Hashtroudi and colleagues found that for both types of situations, older adults recollected more associated feelings whereas young adults recollected more non-emotional informations, such as colors, objects, sensory information, spatial information, and actions.

Similar findings were revealed in a series of studies conducted by Labouvie-Vief and her colleagues with diverse age groups ranging from adolescents to the very old. In these studies, they consistently find that older people process information with a greater focus on subjective states and symbolic themes (Labouvie-Vief, 1997), and are more likely to emphasize psychological themes in recalling and interpreting text than are their younger counterparts (Adams, 1991; Adams et al., 1990; Adams et al., 1997; Labouvie-Vief et al., 1989).

Furthermore, our own study found that when presented with different types of advertisements, older adults, compared with their younger counterparts, were more likely to prefer advertisements with emotional slogans like "Capture those special moments" to advertisements with information-related slogans like "Capture the unexplored world." They also remembered a higher percentage of information from the emotional advertisements than from the information-related advertisements (Fung & Carstensen, 2003).

Age Differences in Social Patterns
Probably as a result of the increased focus on emotionally meaningful goals, older people display social patterns that focus more on emotionally close social partners than do younger people. Age-related reductions in social contact have been widely documented in many studies, both longitudinal (Carstensen, 1992; Lee & Markides, 1990; Palmore, 1981) and cross-sectional (Gordon & Gaitz, 1976; Harvey & Singleton, 1989; Lang & Carstensen, 1994; Lawton et al., 1986–87; Montero, 1980). A close examination of

composition of social networks reveals that these reductions are accounted for primarily by a decrease in the number of peripheral social partners. The number of emotionally close social partners is stable throughout adulthood. Colleagues and I (Fung et al., 2001a) examined the social networks of adults aged 18–87 years. We found that compared to their younger counterparts, older people had fewer peripheral social partners but a comparable number of emotionally close social partners. As a result, older people's social networks comprised a greater percentage of emotionally close social partners. This age-related trend has been found among both Caucasian-Americans and African-Americans – two American ethnic groups with well-documented differences in social structures – and a sample of older Germans aged 70–103 years (Lang & Carstensen, 1994; Lang et al., 1998). The age-related trend is not accounted for by personality (Lang et al., 1998) or selective mortality (Fung et al., 2001a, Fung et al., 2001b; Lang & Carstensen, 1994).

Longitudinal studies find a consistent pattern. Cumming and Henry (1961) interviewed a sample aged 48--68 years over a period of 3 years, and found that frequency of social interactions declined with age, except in the case of close family members. Carstensen (1992) analyzed data from adults inter-viewed at ages 18, 30, 40, and 50 years. She found that interaction frequency and relationship satisfaction with relatives increased or remained stable over time but interaction and satisfaction with acquaintances declined during this period. Field and Minkler (1988) also found such changes in late adulthood, suggesting that these changes in social interaction may continue throughout adulthood.

In fact, social interactions in old age seem to be sought almost entirely according to their potential for emotional satisfaction, often at the expense of the potential for new information. Compared to their younger counterparts, older people spend more time in their "most-liked discretionary" activities, including interacting with friends and family members (Lawton et al., 1986–87). The more each of these activities is liked, the more time older people engage in them. Most friends in old age are "old friends" and time spent with them typically involves shared leisure activities or conversations that transcend mundane daily concerns (Larson et al., 1986). This trend is found even among frail elderly. Nursing home residents rate the best days as those that include positive family events and relatively more self-initiated positive behaviors (Lawton et al., 1995).

Studies suggest that this age-associated reduction in peripheral social partners is beneficial to affective well-being. Based on longitudinal interview data, Lang (2000) found that peripheral social partners were dropped from the social networks of older adults mostly out of the latter's own volition. Indeed, average emotional closeness of social networks is positively related to social embeddedness, operationalized as a composite index of social satisfaction, tenderness, and the absence of loneliness (Lang & Carstensen, 1994; Lang et al., 1998).

Age Differences in Social Preferences
The findings described above provide evidences that older people encode social information and categorize social partners along affective dimensions, and their social networks and activities center around emotionally close social partners. In another series of studies, Carstensen and colleagues have shown

that older people typically *choose* social partners who fulfill emotionally meaningful goals. Fredrickson and Carstensen (1990) asked participants ranging in age from 11 to 94 years to imagine that they had half an hour free, had no pressing commitment and would like to spend time with a social partner. The participants were provided with three social partner choices, representing the three dimensions along which people mentally represented prospective social partners (viz., emotional, informational, and future-relevant as described in the section on social cognition). Preferences for particular social partners presumably reflect the desire for the type of experiences typically associated with the prototype. The three social partner choices are: (1) a member of your immediate family (high on emotional dimension, a familiar social partner); (2) the author of a book you have read (high on informational dimension, a novel social partner); and (3) an acquaintance with whom you seem to have much in common (high on future dimension, a novel social partner). Fredrickson and Carstensen found that older Americans were more likely to select the familiar social partner than younger Americans.

Critics may argue that these age differences in social preferences might be, in part, accounted for by the individualistic nature of the American culture. Cultures that are more collectivistic in nature may display a preference for familiar social partners across the entire life span. Refuting this argument, colleagues and I found patterns of age differences in social preferences similar to those shown in the United States among three collectivistic Asian cultures, Hong Kong (Fung et al., 1999, Studies 2 and 4), Taiwan, and Mainland China (Fung et al., 2001b).

Role of Perceived Time in Age-related Prioritization of Emotional Social Goals

Importantly, socio-emotional selectivity theory contends that rather than chronological age per se, perceived time accounts for changes in social goals. Time perspective is defined as a subjective estimation of time left in future (Kennedy et al., 2001). As early as in the 19th century, William James has noted that the subjective experience of time changes with age, such that "the same space of time seems shorter as we grow older" (James, 1980/1950, p. 625). Indeed, older adults report that time seems to pass more quickly with advancing age and consequently, become increasingly precious (Guy et al., 1994). This sense of foreshortening future is captured by the following poem:

> For when I was a baby and wept and slept, time crept;
> When I was a boy and laughed and talked, time walked;
> Then when the years saw me as a man, time ran;
> But as I older drew, time flew.
> (verse by Greg Pentreath, as quoted in Whitrow, 1972).

Indeed, empirical studies that examined age differences in time perspective, as measured by a scale that includes items like "I have a sense that time is running out," found that older people perceived a more limited future than did younger people (Fung et al., 2001b; Lang & Carstensen, 2002).

Socio-emotional selectivity theory argues that it is the recognition that our time is limited that makes us focus on emotional goals as we age. Because of this, the theory predicts that younger people who are placed in situations where perceived time is limited are as likely to favor emotionally meaningful goals and thus emotionally close social partners as are older people. This hypothesis was confirmed. Experimental manipulations of perceived time have successfully changed age differences in social preferences. Recall that younger Americans in Fredrickson and Carstensen (1990)'s study were less likely to choose to spend time with a familiar social partner than were older participants. However, when the same younger participants were placed in a time-limited condition through imagining an impending move across the country, they increased their preferences for the familiar partner to the extent that they were likely to choose the familiar social partner than were their older counterparts. We replicated this finding among three collectivistic, Asian cultures – Hong Kong, Taiwan, and Mainland China – with a different experimentally imposed time constraint, in this case, an imagined impending emigration (Fung, et al., 1999; Fung et al., 2001b).

Conversely, older people's preferences for emotionally close social partners are eliminated when their perceived time is expanded. We (Fung et al., 1999) examined age-related social preferences among people aged 8–93 years in two time contexts. When perceived time was not manipulated, we replicated Fredrickson and Carstensen (1990)'s finding that older people were more likely to pick the familiar social partner than were their younger counterparts. However, when we expanded the perceived time by asking participants to imagine that they had just learned from their medical doctor about a new medical advance that would extend their lives for 20 more years than they had expected, older participants decreased their preferences for the familiar social partner. As a result, the percentage of older participants who picked familiar social partner in this condition was as low as that of younger participants. This study provides strong support for socio-emotional selectivity theory. If older people's preferences for emotionally close social partners and the underlying emotionally meaningful goals were caused by properties inherent in aging, it is unlikely that these preferences would be eliminated by a manipulation of perceived time. The fact that it did underlines the role of perceived time in determining the relative importance of different types of social goals.

Correlation studies also show that age differences in social preferences can be eliminated by statistically controlling for time perspective. We (Fung et al., 1999) measured perceived time left in the future among Taiwanese and Mainland Chinese. We then assessed age-related social preferences by asking participants to choose from among three (one familiar and two novel) prospective social partners, using the paradigm described above. We found that among both Mainland Chinese and Taiwanese, older people (aged 65 years or over) were more likely to choose to interact with familiar social partners than were younger people (aged 18–29 years). However, once time perspective was statistically controlled, these age differences disappeared.

Moreover, there is evidence that the effect of perceived time limitation on social goals is not accounted for by perceived goal obstruction. Recall that many theories on human development propose that some goals are blocked by age-related declines and older people adjust to these losses by downgrading the importance of these goals (Bäckman & Dixon, 1992; Baltes & Baltes, 1990; Brandtstädter & Greve, 1994; Heckhausen & Schulz, 1995; Lazarus & Folkman, 1984). Given that knowledge-related goals are more likely than emotionally meaningful goals to be obstructed by age-related losses, the age differences in social preferences described above may simply reflect the older people's efforts to lower their knowledge-related aspirations. From this perspective, it is even possible to construe time limitation as a form of knowledge-related goal blocking that forces individuals to focus on the more tangible emotionally meaningful goals. To test socio-emotional selectivity theory against this alternative hypothesis, we (Fung & Carstensen, 2004) manipulated constraints on time and knowledge-related goals among young and older adults, and investigated under which conditions people were more likely to prefer familiar social partners. They found that while both time and goal constraints were associated with an increased preference for familiar social partners – which, we argue, reflects an increased emphasis on emotionally meaningful goals, constraints on time showed an independent effect. Moreover, while both types of constraints motivated people to seek comfort, only constraints on time heightened the desire for emotional meaning in relationships.

In summary, socio-emotional selectivity theory has received considerable empirical support in the interpersonal domain. There is much evidence that emotionally meaningful social goals are more important to older people than to their younger counterparts. Compared with younger people, older people attach greater importance to the potential for emotional rewards in categorizing prospective social partners and are more likely to remember emotional information in social interactions. Given the choice, they are also more likely to select emotionally close social partners over novel ones, and consequently, have a higher percentage of emotionally close partners in their social networks.

Moreover, it has been shown that these age differences are not static. When placed in situations that impose constraints on perceived time, younger people mentally represent and choose prospective social partners in the same way as do older people. Conversely, when their perceived time is expanded, older people no longer prefer emotionally close social partners. This pattern of findings strongly suggests that the observed age differences in social goals are at least in part accounted for by differentiated time perspective.

Differences in Time Perspective across Socio-cultural Contexts and Their Effects on Social Goals

The literature reviewed above suggests that cognitive appraisal of time assists people in choosing among goals to adapt effectively to their particular circumstances. With a limited time perspective, people are motivated to focus on emotionally meaningful goals. Since what prompts the goal prioritization is perceived time, not age per se, younger individuals who are suffering from terminal illnesses or are otherwise facing endings in their life situations are likely to place as much emphasis on emotionally meaningful goals as are older individuals.

Facing Personal Time Limitations

In an effort to disentangle the effect of chronological age from that of perceived time on social goals, Carstensen and Fredrickson (1998) examined mental representations of social partners in two samples. One sample comprised

Caucasian- and African-American adults aged 18–88 years. And the other sample comprised three groups of young gay men who differed in their HIV-status (HIV-negative, HIV-positive/asymptomatic or HIV-positive/symptomatic) but were comparable in age. Thus, while the ages of these groups were held constant, their perceived time left in life, varied. Participants from both samples completed a card sort task in which they sorted descriptions of prospective social partners according to their perceived similarity. Multidimensional scaling techniques were again employed to reveal the dimensions along which these categorizations were made and the relative weight subsamples placed on specific dimensions. Once again, the same three dimensions as those found in Fredrickson and Carstensen (1990) accounted for most of the variance: emotional qualities, informational potential, and future prospects. Importantly, the pattern of dimension weights for young, middle-aged, and older adults closely resembled that for HIV-negative, HIV-positive/asymptomatic, and HIV-positive/symptomatic men respectively. Both older and younger people who were HIV-positive and experiencing AIDS symptoms, placed greater weight on emotional qualities of social partners than on informational or future possibilities. These findings support the contention that perceived time left in life influences the way people think about social partners. Moreover, they suggest that perceived constraints on time shift attention from information seeking and future prospects – i.e. knowledge-related goals – to emotionally meaningful goals.

In addition, the literature on stress and coping suggests that younger people with terminal illnesses are more likely to adopt emotion-focused coping strategies than are their healthy peers (Kausar & Akram, 1999). Patients with cancer are more likely to discuss their fear of cancer with others while their mates are more likely to cope with the fear through direct actions (Gotay, 1984). Moreover, our own study found that young adults who had a history of cancer reported a greater number of emotionally close social partners in their networks and a greater need to attain emotional goals than did their age peers without a history of cancer (Kin & Fung, 2004). Further evidences suggest that it is adaptive for terminally ill patients to focus on deriving emotional meaning from their situations. For example, patients with life threatening illnesses who actively find personal meaning in their illnesses can slow down disease progression (Taylor et al., 2000). Prioritization of emotionally meaningful goals seems to be adaptive when people perceive a foreshortened personal future.

Non-life-threatening situations that pose limitations on time perspective also prompt a desire to focus on emotions and to treasure emotionally close relationships. Liu and Fung (2005) found that adolescents who were involved in gangs reported a more limited time perspective and a higher percentage of emotionally close social partners in their networks, compared with age peers who were not gang members. Even mundane endings, such as college graduation, can lead to a prioritization of emotionally meaningful goals. Fredrickson (1995) examined social interaction patterns of students living in university dormitories. She found that compared with students who were not graduating and thus were not facing a social departure, graduating seniors reported greater emotional involvement with close friends relative to acquaintances.

Interestingly, other than personally experiencing an anticipated ending, witnessing the time limitations of other people can also make us realize the finitude of our time. The literature on subjective life expectancy suggests that we induce our perceived life expectancies from the actual life expectancies of those who are similar and are around us. Age of family members at death is highly positively related to perceived personal life expectancy (Denes-Raj & Ehrichman, 1991; Robbins, 1988). In addition, having frequent exposure to deaths of others also leads to a shorter perceived life expectancy. Mortuary science students reported a younger perceived death age than did university students and nursing home administrators (Sabatini & Kastenbaum, 1973).

To assess whether experiencing losses associated with deaths of relatives or friends might affect the time perspective and thus social goals, colleagues and I (Fung et al., 2002) examined the coping strategies of a large sample of college students who had experienced death-related losses to different extent. We found that compared with students who perceived time as less limited, those who perceived time as more limited were more likely to engage in coping that focus on emotions, such as disclosure of emotions to other people, seeing things in a positive light, and trying to leave a mark on this world. Moreover, while emotion-focused coping was not related to meaning and purpose in life among students who perceived time as less limited, it was positively related to meaning and purpose in life among those who perceived time as more limited. These findings suggest that among people who have experienced death-related losses, not all of them perceive their own time as limited. But among those who do, they are more likely to prioritize emotional goals and to benefit psychologically from doing so.

If it is indeed the case that exposure to deaths of others leads at least some individuals to perceive their own time as limited, then groups that have shorter life expectancy may collectively perceive time as more limited than groups with longer life expectancy. When this occurs, systematic group differences in time perspective may emerge, leading to group differences in social goals.

There is qualitative evidence that belonging to an ethnic group with a shorter average life expectancy may give rise to perceived limitation on how long one can live. Life expectancy for African-Americans is shorter than that of European-Americans at all ages (National Center for Health Statistics, 1994). Differences in mortality rate, life-long health conditions and practices, health care accessibility, and financial resources have all contributed to the differences in life expectancy (Manuel, 1988). Many African-Americans are aware of their actuarial shorter life expectancy. Ninety-one percent of the African-American women interviewed by Burton (1990) perceived their life expectancies to be 60 years, shorter even than the actuarial predictions. One 21-year-old woman in the study commented, "I've been seeing people die when they are around 58 all my life. I'm surprised that my grandmother [age 62] is still around" (p.132).

As perceived time limitation is related to prioritization of emotionally meaningful goals, ethnic groups that have shorter life expectancy are likely to show greater emphasis on those goals. In fact, African-Americans do seem to have more emotionally close social networks than European-Americans. African-Americans are more likely to have extended kin networks than are European-Americans (Hogan et al., 1993). Interactions and exchanges among family members are more common among African-Americans than among European-Americans (Mutran, 1985; Stewart & Vaux, 1986; Taylor, 1988). Moreover, the principle of substitution – a phenomenon in which nieces and nephews serve as children when an older person is childless

(Perry and Johnson, 1994) – is more prevalent among African-Americans than among European-Americans (Troll, 1994). In contrast, interactions with acquaintances are less frequent among African-Americans than among European-Americans. African-American college students receive more emotional support from family but have fewer friends and receive less emotional support from friends than do their European-American counterparts (Stewart and Vaux, 1986). Indeed, when we (Fung et al., 2001a) directly compared the social network composition between African-Americans and European-Americans, we found that while the two ethnic groups had comparable number of emotionally close social partners in their networks, European-Americans as a group had more peripheral social partners in their networks than did African-Americans. This pattern of findings suggests that compared with their European counterparts, African-Americans show greater social selection, focusing on the handful of social partners who are truly emotionally significant to them.

Similar group differences in social goals are also found between Taiwanese and Mainland Chinese, two groups who are ethnically identical and share many customs and beliefs, but have different actuarial life expectancy. The life expectancy of Mainland Chinese is 7 years shorter than that of Taiwanese (U.S. Bureau of the Census, 1999). In fact, when we directly measured perceived time among Taiwanese and Mainland Chinese, we found that older Mainland Chinese perceived time as more limited than did older Taiwanese (Fung et al., 2001b). We further found that this group difference in time perspective was reflected in social preferences. Mainland Chinese were more likely to prefer familiar social partners, relative to novel social partners, than were Taiwanese, suggesting that they place greater emphasis on emotionally meaningful social goals.

Facing Macro-Level Time Limitations

The empirical evidences reviewed above suggest that personal life expectancy, individual social endings, and group actuarial life expectancy can all shift time perspective, leading to a reprioritization of social goals. Further studies were conducted to test whether culture-wise, macro-level time limitations also shift age-related social goals and thus social preferences. Fung et al. (1999, Studies 2, 3, and 4) examined age differences in social preferences a year before, two months before, and a year after the handover of Hong Kong from the United Kingdom to the People's Republic of China. We construed the handover as a macro-level socio-political ending and predicted that the perceived limitations on time associated with the ending would make even younger people prioritize emotionally meaningful goals and thus prefer familiar social partners. Our prediction was confirmed. A year before the handover, the typical age differences in social preferences were found: only older Hong Kong people preferred familiar social partners to novel ones; younger Hong Kong people did not. However, two months before the handover when the socio-political transition was more salient, even younger people preferred familiar social partners. There was no longer any age difference in social preferences. A year after the handover when the time constraint no longer existed, once again only older people preferred familiar social partners. Younger people no longer showed such a preference.

Similar shifts in age-related social goals were found around the 9–11 attacks on the United States and the Severe Acute Respiratory Syndrome (SARS) epidemic in Hong Kong (Fung & Carstensen, 2006). On September 11, 2001, two planes hijacked by terrorists crashed into the World Trade Center in New York City, causing thousands of deaths. Even though Hong Kong was half the globe away from the site of the tragedy, Hong Kong people, like the rest of the world, were greatly shaken by the attacks. During the first few days after the attacks, images about human-life and property losses were shown on television 24 hours a day. These images reminded many Hong Kong people of the finitude of life. Moreover, some Hong Kong people worried that America might take revenge and start the third world war (Broom, 2001). Others worried about the inevitable economic downturn that followed the attacks (The Sun, 2001). In short, to many Hong Kong people, the 9–11 incident was as a time marker beyond which life might never be the same. As described above, we examined the age-related social preferences in Hong Kong in 1998, a year after the handover. We also examined age-related social preferences in Hong Kong on September 23–25, 2001 (i.e., right after 9–11), and on January 14–22, 2002 (i.e., 4 months after 9–11). Older participants were more likely to prefer emotionally close social partners to novel social partners than were younger participants in 1998. However, right after 9–11, when the finitude of life was made salient, younger participants increased their preference for emotionally close social partners to the levels of their older counterparts. Four months after the attacks when the war on Afghanistan had ended and the sense of ending associated with the attacks had faded, age differences in social preferences reemerged.

The same age-related shift in social goals was repeated in 2003 during the SARS epidemic. A year and a half after the 9–11 attacks, between March and June 2003, a new form of pneumonia known as SARS spread rapidly to various parts of the world. Hong Kong was severely affected by the disease. One thousand seven hundred and fifty-five cases of infection were reported, resulting in 296 deaths. To reduce the risk of infection, schools and preschools were shut down; industries such as tourism, retail and entertainment collapsed, and international trade was severely affected. There was every reason to believe that under these circumstances, people came to view their futures as precarious. We examined age differences in social preferences at this point (peak of SARS: March 2003) and found that younger people responded like their older counterparts, preferring emotionally close social partners to novel ones. We followed up the same sample several months later when the SARS outbreak had subsided (June 2003; when the World Health Organization had lifted the travel advisory on Hong Kong). At this point when perceived time was no longer limited, the typical age differences in social preferences reemerged.

Taken together, the shifts in age-related social preferences before and after historical time markers described above suggest that macro-level time perspective can influence social motivation in the same way as personal time perspective does. Constraints on time, no matter whether they occur at the individual or group level, prompt an increased focus on the aspects of life that are emotionally meaningful.

Understanding the Role of Perceived Time in Social Motivation: Theoretical and Practical Implications

Theoretical Implications

In this chapter, we have reviewed how goals change across the life cycle and the role of time perspective in the change. Empirical evidences suggest that individuals are likely to perceive time as limited (1) when they age, (2) when they have limited subjective life expectancy due to terminal illnesses or exposure to death of others, (3) when they are facing micro- or macro-level events, such as graduation or a political transition, that symbolize an end to the life as they know it. As the finitude of future time becomes salient, they reprioritize their goals, focusing on the goals that are most important to them. The result of this reprioritization usually leads to a focus on goals that are emotionally meaningful.

Jeppsson-Grassman (1993) found in a study of visually impaired adults that a perceived limited life span was important for understanding "the changing priorities, adaptive strategies, and general life planning of the participants" (p. 371). We argue that a foreshortened future does not influence the priorities of the visually impaired alone. It affects the social motives of everyone. Time perspective, at least in part, accounts for age differences in social goals. It explains why as people grow older, they decrease their social contacts but deepen the ties with the handful of close social partners who are most important to them. It also provides a possible explanation for why older adults are particularly attuned to emotional information in their social environment than are younger adults. These research directions have shed and will continue to shed important light on adult development.

In addition, time perspective, as an individual difference, can account for differences in social cognition, social relationships, and social preferences. Further studies of the influence of time perspective on social phenomena may contribute to the fields of personality and social psychology. Moreover, studies on time perspective can potentially shed light on why terminally ill patients often find personal meaning in their illnesses (Taylor, et al., 2000), thus contributing to health and clinical psychology. Last but not least, further studies on the relationship between historical events, macro-level time perspective, and social motivation may reveal the mechanisms underlying well-documented cultural differences in self construal and values, such as collectivism in Chinese cultures and individualism in North American cultures (Oyserman et al., 2002), furthering the literatures in cultural and cross-cultural psychology. In short, subjective estimation of future time is a promising independent variable for future studies.

Furthermore, the literature we have reviewed clearly illustrates that there are gains and losses at every stage in the life cycle (Baltes, 1997). Being old, having terminal illnesses, and experiencing other time limitations are generally believed to be negative life events. Yet, through them people are motivated to screen their goals and focus on those goals that are truly emotionally significant. As a result, total number of social partners decreases but social networks become tighter and more emotionally close. Memory may be more selective but the encoded information is relatively more positive and emotionally meaningful. Coping may become less problem-focused, but the resulting emotion-focused coping is associated with greater meaning and purpose in life. In fact, when time is perceived as limited, people seem to avoid "spreading themselves too thin." Rather, they selectively construct a social and cognitive world that maximizes emotional payoffs. It should be noted that we, by no means, seek to downplay the physical, cognitive, and sociological losses associated with aging, terminal illnesses, and other time limitations. Some events that lead to constraints on time no doubt exert negative influences on individuals. However, we argue that individuals are not merely passive victims of their environment. They exercise agency (Bandura, 1982) and shape their environments in ways that fulfill the goals that they value most highly, maximizing life satisfaction and maintaining a high level of emotional well-being.

It should also be noted that the reviewed literature implores us to critically examine the definition of achievement. Some argue that Western societies share a cultural legacy that values distal goal attainment as the forefront of achievement, the focus on proximal goals, in contrast, is often conceived as an inability to delay gratification (Nuttin, 1985). The reviewed findings suggest that to individuals and groups who are in life situations that limit their perceived time, proximal goals are more important than distal ones. At least in some situations, enjoying the richness of today and engaging in social interactions that are emotionally meaningful may be as much an achievement as striving for long-term knowledge-related successes.

Practical Implications

In addition, the literature we reviewed above also casts doubt on some common social interventions. Many social services are provided based on the common beliefs that social contacts and information seeking are important for everyone. Based on these beliefs, senior centers or visitation programs are set up to encourage older people to expand their social networks like younger people do. Terminally ill patients are encouraged to go to school and to work in order to lead "normal" life as healthy people do. However, these services, while meaningful, may fail to recognize the needs of individuals with limited time perspective. Older people and terminally ill patients may not want to achieve knowledge-related goals. Like the cases we encountered at the beginning of this chapter, Sophie prefers a family dinner to a meal with neighbors while Paul wants to spend his precious time with his wife rather than striving for further achievement. Meeting novel people and expanding horizons are important to young people and those with expansive time perspective, but they may no longer be centrally important for people with limited time perspective. Instead, emotionally meaningful goals may assume primacy when time is perceived as limited and social services that facilitate the deepening of close social ties may be particularly helpful to people in such a life situation.

We argue that social intervention for those who may perceive time as limited should begin with a detailed analysis of the kind of relationships that these individuals want to strengthen. Crawford (1987) proposed such a strategy for older adults. The strategy requires the individuals to fill out a network diagram to measure the number of very close social partners and the number of peripheral social partners in social networks. Nurses then discuss with the clients the kind of support they want and the potential sources of the support. Together, they plan and work to involve social partners toward desired goals.

Similar inventions can be modified to include educational and career goals, and adopted for terminally ill patients. In essence, it is probably a mistake to assume that the priorities of individuals in time-limited situations are the same as those of the general public. Social service providers should understand the desires and needs of those individuals before conducting any invention on them.

Conclusion

Though we may not be aware of it, time perspective is influencing our choices over many areas. Many life events such as growing old, having a terminal illness, witnessing the death of others, and graduation prime us on the finitude of time, urging us to focus on the goals that are most significant to us. As an older gentleman elegantly describes, "I think when you see the so-called hour glass, and see the sands running out, a kind of panic sets in, or at least an urgency that makes you focus and crystallize on things that are important" (George, 1997, as cited in Caldwell, 1997, p. 6). It is precisely because life is finite that we learn to appreciate its richness and emotional significance.

Acknowledgment: Work by the first author was supported by two direct grants for research from Chinese University of Hong Kong and an Endowment Fund Research Grant from United College, Chinese University of Hong Kong.

References

Adams, C. (1991). Qualitative age differences in memory for text: A life-span developmental perspective. *Psychology and Aging, 6*, 323–336.

Adams, C., Labouvie-Vief, G., Hobart, C. J., & Dorosz, M. (1990). Adult age group differences in story recall style. *Journal of Gerontology, 45*, P17–P27.

Adams, C., Smith, M. C., Nyquist, L., & Perlmutter, M. (1997). Adult age-group differences in recall for the literal and interpretive meanings of narrative text. *Journal of Gerontology, 52*, P187–P193.

Bäckman, L., & Dixon, R. A. (1992). Psychological compensation: A theoretical framework. *Psychological Bulletin, 112*, 259–283.

Baltes, P. B. (1997). On the incomplete architecture of human ontogeny: Selection, optimization, and compensation as foundation of developmental theory. *American Psychologist, 52*, 366–380.

Baltes, P. B., & Baltes, M. M. (1990). Psychological perspectives on successful aging: The model of selective optimization with compensation. In P. B. Baltes & M. M. Baltes (Eds.), *Successful aging: Perspectives from the behavioral sciences* (pp. 1–34). Cambridge, England: Cambridge University Press.

Bandura, A. (1982). Self-efficacy mechanisms in human agency. *American Psychologist, 37*, 122–147.

Bengtson, V. L., & Dowd, J. J. (1980–81). Sociological functionalism, exchange theory and life-cycle analysis: A call for more explicit theoretical bridges. International Journal of Aging and Human Development, 12, 55–73

Blanchard-Fields, F., Chen, Y., & Norris, L. (1997). Everyday problem solving across the adult life span: Influence of domain specificity and cognitive appraisal. *Psychology and Aging, 12*, 684–693.

Blanchard-Fields, F., Jahnke, H. C., & Camp, C. (1995). Age differences in problem-solving style: The role of emotional salience. *Psychology and Aging, 10*, 173–180.

Brandtstädter, J., & Greve, W. (1994). The aging self: Stabilizing and protective processes. *Developmental Review, 14*, 52–80.

Brandtstädter, J. (1999). The self in action and development: Cultural, biosocial, and ontogenetic bases of intentional self-development. In J. Brandtstädter & R. M. Lerner (Eds.), *Action and self-development: Theory and research through the lifespan* (pp. 37–66). Thousand Oaks, CA: Sage Publications.

Brandtstädter, J., & Baltes-Gotz, B. (1990). Personal control over development and quality of life perspectives in adulthood. In P. B. Baltes & M. M. Baltes (Eds.), *Successful aging: Perspectives from the behavioral sciences* (pp. 197–224). New York: Cambridge University Press.

Brandtstädter, J., & Renner, G. (1990). Tenacious goal pursuit and flexible goal adjustment: Explication and age-related analysis of assimilative and accommodation strategies of coping. *Psychological and Aging, 5*, 58–67.

Brandtstädter, J., Wentura, D., & Greve, W. (1993). Adaptive resources of the aging self: Outlines of an emergent perspective. *International Journal of Behavioral Development, 16*, 232–349.

Bühler, C., Brind, A., & Horner, A. (1968). Old age as a phase of human life: Questionnaire study. *Human Development, 11*, 53–63.

Burton, L. M. (1990). Teenage childbearing as an alternative life-course strategy in multigeneration Black families. *Human Nature, 1*(2), 123–143.

Broom, J. (2001, September 13). This is my Pearl Harbor. *The Seattle Times* (LEXIS–NEXIS® Academic).

Caldwell, L. (1997). Time and Aging: An Exploration into the Temporal World of Older Adults. Unpublished manuscript, Stanford University.

Carstensen, L. L. (1992). Social and emotional patterns in adulthood: Support for socioemotional selectivity theory. *Psychology and Aging, 7*, 331–338.

Carstensen, L. L. (1993). Motivation for social contact across the life span: A theory of socioemotional selectivity. In J. Jacobs (Ed.), *Nebraska symposium on motivation* (pp. 209–254). Lincoln, NE: University of Nebraska Press.

Carstensen, L. L. (1995). Evidence for a life-span theory of socioemotional selectivity. *Current Directions in Psychological Science, 4*, 151–156.

Carstensen, L. L. (1998). A life-span approach to social motivation. In J. Heckhausen & C. Dweck (Eds.), *Motivation and self-regulation across the life span* (pp. 341–364). New York: Cambridge University Press.

Carstensen, L. L., & Fredrickson, B. F. (1998). Socioemotional selectivity in healthy older people and younger people living with the Human Immunodeficiency Virus (HIV): The centrality of emotion when the future is constrained. *Health Psychology, 17*, 494–503.

Carstensen, L. L., & Turk-Charles, S. (1994). The salience of emotion across the adult life span. *Psychology and Aging, 9*, 259–264.

Carstensen, L. L., Fung, H. H., & Charles, S. T. (2003). Socioemotional selectivity theory and emotion regulation in the second half of life. *Motivation and Emotion, 27*, 103–123.

Carstensen, L. L., Gross, J., & Fung, H. (1997). The social context of emotion. In K. W. Schaie & M. P. Lawton (Eds.), *Annual review of gerontology and geriatrics* (Vol. 17, pp. 325–352). New York: Springer Publishing Company.

Carstensen, L. L., Isaacowitz, D., & Charles, S. T. (1999). Taking time seriously: A theory of socioemotional selectivity. *American Psychologist, 54*, 165–181.

Costa, P. T., Jr., & McCrae, R. R. (1988). Personality in adulthood: A six-year longitudinal study of self-reports and spouse ratings on the NEO Personality Inventory. *Journal of Personality and Social Psychology, 54*, 853–863.

Crawford, G. (1987). Support networks and health-related change in the elderly: Theory-based nursing strategies. *Family Community Health, 10*, 39–48.

Crown, S. M. (1968). Personality and aging. In K. W. Schaie (Ed.), *Theory and methods of research on aging* (pp. 134–157). Morgantown, VA: West Virginia University.

Cumming, E., & Henry, W. H. (1961). *Growing old: The process of disengagement.* New York: Basic Books.

Denes-Raj, V., & Ehrichman, H. (1991). Effects of premature parental death on subjective life expectancy, death anxiety, and health behavior. *Omaga, 23*(4), 309–321.

Dittmann-Kohli, F., & Westerhof, G. J. (1997). The SELE-Sentence Completion Questionnaire: A new instrument for the assessment of personal meanings in aging research. *Anuario de Psicologia, 73*, 7–18.

Dowd, J. J. (1980). Aging as exchange: A preface to theory. *Journal of Gerontology, 30*, 584–594.

Erikson, E. H. (1950). *Childhood and society.* New York: Norton.

Erikson, E. H. (1968). *Indentity, youth and crisis.* New York: Norton.

Erikson, E. H. (1982). *The life cycle completed: A review.* New York: Norton.

Field, D., & Minkler, M. (1988). Continuity and change in social support between young-old, old-old, and very-old adults. *Journal of Gerontology, 43*, P100–P106.

Fredrickson, B. L. (1995). Socioemotional behavior at the end of college life. *Journal of Social and Personal Relationships, 12*, 261–276.

Fredrickson, B. L., & Carstensen, L. L. (1990). Choosing social partners: How age and anticipated endings make people more selective. *Psychology and Aging, 5*, 335–347.

Fung, H. H., & Carstensen, L. L. (2006). Goals change when life's fragility is primed: Lessons learned from Older Adults, the September 11th Attacks and SARS. *Social Cognition, 24*, 248–278.

Fung, H. H., & Carstensen, L. L. (2004). Motivational changes in response to blocked goals and foreshortened Time: Testing alternatives for socioemotional selectivity theory. *Psychology and Aging, 19*, 68–78.

Fung, H. H., & Carstensen, L. L. (2003). Sending memorable messages to the old: Age differences in preferences and memory for emotionally meaningful advertisements. *Journal of Personality and Social Psychology, 85*, 163–178.

Fung, H. H., Carstensen, L. L., & Lang, F. R. (2001a). Age-related patterns of social relationships among African-Americans and Caucasian-Americans: Implications for socioemotional selectivity across the life span. *International Journal of Aging and Human Development, 52*, 185–206.

Fung, H. H., Carstensen, L. L., & Lutz, M. A. (1999). Influence of time on social preferences: Implications for life-span development. *Psychology and Aging, 14*, 595–604.

Fung, H. H., Kuiken, D., Mcewan, A, & Wild, C. (2002). Time perspective, emotion-focused coping, and spirituality. Manuscript in preparation.

Fung, H. H., Lai, P., & Ng, R. (2001b). Age differences in social preferences among Taiwanese and Mainland Chinese: The role of perceived Time. *Psychology and Aging, 16*, 351–356.

George, L. K., Blazer, D. F., Winfield-Laird, I., Leaf, P. J., & Fischback, F. R. (1988). Psychiatric disorders and mental health service use in later life: Evidence from the Epidemiologic Catchment Area Program. In J. Brody & G. Maddox (Eds.), *Epidemiology and aging* (pp. 189–219). New York: Van Nostrand Rand.

Gordon, C., & Gaitz, C. (1976). Leisure and lives. In R. Binstock & E. Shanas (Eds.), *Handbook of aging and the social sciences* (Vol. 1, pp. 310–341). New York: Van Nostrand Reinhold.

Gotay, C. C. (1984). The experience of cancer during early and advanced stages: The views of patients and their mates. *Social Science and Medicine, 18*(7), 605–613.

Granovetter, M. S. (1973). The strength of weak ties. *American Journal of Sociology, 78*, 1360–1380.

Gutman, G. M. (1966). A note on the MPI: Age and sex differences in extroversion and neuroticism in a Canadian sample. *British Journal of Social and Clinical Psychology, 5,* 128–129.

Guy, B. S., Rittenburg, T. L., & Hawes, D. K. (1994). Dimensions and characteristics of time perceptions and perspectives among older consumers. *Psychology & Marketing, 11,* 35–56.

Harvey, A. S., & Singleton, J. F. (1989). Canadian activity patterns across the life span: A time budget perspective. *Canadian Journal on Aging, 8,* 268–285.

Hashtroudi, S., Johnson, M. K., & Chrosniak, L. D. (1990). Aging and qualitative characteristics of memories for perceived and imagined complex events. *Psychology and Aging, 5,* 119–126.

Havighurst, R. J., & Albrecht, R. (1953). *Older people.* New York: Longmans.

Heckhausen, J. & Schulz, R. (1994). Primacy of primary control as an universal feature of human behavior. Paper presented at the 13th Biennial Meetings of the International Society of the Study of Behavioral Development, Amsterdam, The Netherlands.

Heckhausen, J., & Schulz, R. (1995). A life-span theory of control. *Psychological Review, 102,* 284–304.

Heckhausen, J., Dixon, R. A., & Baltes, P. B. (1989). Gains and losses in development throughout adulthood as perceived by different age groups. *Developmental Psychology, 25,* 109–121.

Henry, W. E., & Cumming, E. (1959). Personality development in adulthood and old age. *Journal of Projective Techniques, 23,* 383–390.

Heron, A., & Chown, S. M. (1967). *Age and function.* London: Churchill.

Herzog, A. R., & Rogers, W. L. (1981). Age and satisfaction: Data from several large surveys. *Research on Aging, 3,* 142–165.

Hogan, D. P., Eggebeen, D. J., & Clogg, C. C. (1993). The structure of intergenerational exchanges in American families. *American Journal of Sociology, 6,* 1428–1458.

Hooyman, N. R., & Kiyak, H. A. (1993). *Social gerontology* (3rd ed.). Boston: Allyn and Bacon.

James, W. (1980/1950). The principles of psychology. New York: Dover Publications.

Jeppsson-Grassman, E. (1993). The short life: The life-span construct of visually impaired adults with diabetes. *Journal of Visual Impairment and Blindness, 87,* 371–375.

Jung, C. G. (1931). Die Debenswende (Life's turning point). In C. G. Jung (Ed.), *Seelenprobleme der Gegenwart (Psychological problems of today)* (pp. 248–274). Zurich: Rascher.

Jung, C. G. (1953). The structure and dynamics of the psych. In: H. Read, M. Fordham, & G. Adler (Eds.), The collected works of C. G. Jung (Vol. 8, pp. 119–410). New York: Pantheon Books.

Jung, C. G. (1960). The stages of life. Collected works (Vol. 8). Princeton, NJ: Princeton University Press.

Kausar, R., & Akram, M. (1999). Cognitive appraisal and coping of patients with terminal versus nonterminal diseases. *Journal of Behavioral Science, 9,* 13–28.

Kennedy, Q., Fung, H. H., & Carstensen, L. L. (2001). Aging, time estimation and emotion. In S. H. McFadden & R. C. Atchley (Eds). *Aging and the meaning of time.* (pp. 51–74). New York: Springer.

Kin, A. M. Y., & Fung, H. H. (2004). Goals and social network composition among young adults with and without a history of cancer. *Journal of Psychology in Chinese Societies, 5,* 97–111.

Labouvie-Vief, G. (1997). Cognitive-emotional integration in adulthood. In K. W. Schaie & M. P. Lawton (Eds.), *Annual review of gerontology and geriatrics* (Vol. 17, pp. 206–237). New York: Springer Publishing Company.

Labouvie-Vief, G., Hakim-Larson, J., DeVoe, M., & Schoeberlein, S. (1989). Emotions and self-regulation: A life span view. *Human Development, 32,* 279–299.

Lang, F. R., & Carstensen, L. L. (1994). Close emotional relationships in late life: Further support for proactive aging in the social domain. *Psychology and Aging, 9*, 315–324.

Lang, F. R. (2000). Endings and Continuity of Social Relationships: Maximizing Intrinsic Benefits Within Personal Networks When Feeling Near to Death? *Journal of Social and Personal Relationships, 17*, 157–184.

Lang, F. R., & Carstensen, L. L. (2002). Time counts: Future time perspective, goals, and social relationships. *Psychology and Aging, 17*, 125–139.

Lang, F. R., Staudinger, U. M., & Carstensen, L. L. (1998). Perspectives on socioemotional selectivity in late life: How personality and social context do (and do not) make a difference. *Journals of Gerontology, 53*, 21–30.

Larson, R., Mannell, R., & Zuzanek, J. (1986). Daily well-being of older adults with friends and family. *Psychology and Aging, 1*, 117–126.

Lawton, M. P., DeVoe, M. R., & Parmelee, P. (1995). Relationship of events and affect in the daily life of an elderly population. *Psychology and Aging, 10*, 469–477.

Lawton, M. P., Moss, M., & Fulcomer, M. (1986–87). Objective and subjective uses of time by older people. International Journal of Aging and Human Development, 24, 171–188

Lazarus, R. S. (1996). The role of coping in the emotions and how coping changes over the life course. In C. Magai & S. H. McFadden (Eds.), *Handbook of emotion, adult development, and aging* (pp. 289–306). San Diego: Academic Press.

Lazarus, R. S., & Folkman, S. (1984). *Stress, appraisal and coping*. New York: Springer.

Lee, D. J., & Markides, K. S. (1990). Activity and mortality among aged persons over an eight-year period. *The Journals of Gerontology: Social Sciences, 45*, 39–42.

Liu, C. K. M., & Fung, H. H. (2005). Gang members' social network composition and psychological well-being: Extending socioemotional selectivity theory to the study of gang involvement. *Journal of Psychology in Chinese Societies, 6*, 89–108.

Locke, E. A., & Latham, G. P. (1994). Goal setting theory. In H. F. O'Neil Jr. & M. Drillings (Eds.), *Motivation: Theory and research* (pp. 13–29). Hillsdale: Lawrence Erlbaum Associates.

Maddox, G. L. (1963). Activity and morale: A longitudinal study of selected elderly subjects. *Social Forces, 42*, 195–204.

Manuel, R. C. (1988). The demography of older adults. In J. S. Jackson, P. Newton, A. Ostfield, D. Savage & E. L. Schneider (Eds.), *The black American elderly: Research on physical and psychological health* (pp. 25–49). New York: Springer.

Montero, D. (1980). The elderly Japanese American: Aging among the first generation immigrants. *Genetic Psychology Monographs, 101*, 99–118.

Mutran, E. (1985). Intergenerational family support among Blacks and Whites: Response to culture or to socioeconomic differences. *Journal of Gerontology, 40*(3), 382–389.

National Center for Health Statistics. (1994). Vital Statistics of the U.S., 1990 (Vol. 2: Mortality, pt. A). Maryland: Public Health Service

Neugarten, B. L. (1977). Personality and aging. In J. E. Birren & K. W. Schaie (Eds.), *Handbook of the psychology and aging* (pp. 626–649). New York: Van Nostrand Reinhold.

Neugarten, B. L. (ed). (1968). *Middle age and aging*. Chicago: University of Chicago Press.

Nurmi, J.-E. (1992). Age differences in adult life goals, concerns and their temporal extension: A life course approach to future-oriented motivation. *International Journal of Behavioral Development, 15*, 487–508.

Nuttin, M. (1985). *Future time perspective and motivation: Theory and research method*. Leuven Belgium: Leuven University Press/Lawrence Erlbaum.

Oyserman, D., Coon, H.-M., & Kemmelmeier, M. (2002). Rethinking individualism and collectivism: Evaluation of theoretical assumptions and meta-analyses. *Psychological Bulletin, 128*, 3–72.

Palmore, E. (1981). *Social patterns in normal aging: Findings from the Duke Longitudinal Study*. Durham, NC: Duke University Press.

Perry, C. M., & Johnson, C. L. (1994). Families and support networks among African American oldest-old. *International Journal of Aging and Human Development, 38*(1), 41–50.

Reker, G. T., Peacook, E. J., & Wong, P. T. P. (1987). Meaning and purpose in life and well-being: A life-span perspective. *Journal of Gerontology, 42*, 44–49.

Revenson, T. A. (1986). Debunking the myth of loneliness in late life. In E. Seidman & J. Rappaport (Eds.), *Redefining social problems* (pp. 115–135). New York: Plenum Press.

Robbins, R. A. (1988). Objective and subjective factors in estimating life expectancy. *Psychological Reports, 63*, 47–53.

Rosenbaum, M. (1983). Learned resourcefulness as a behavioral repertoire for the self-regulation of internal events: Issues and speculation. In M. Rosenbaum, C. M. Franks & Y. Jaffe (Eds.), *Perspectives on behavioral therapy in the eighties* (pp. 54–73). New York: Springer.

Ryff, C. D. (1989a). In the eye of the beholder: Views of psychological well-being among middle-aged and older adults. *Psychology and Aging, 4*, 195–210.

Ryff, C. D. (1989b). Happiness is everything, or is it? Explorations on the meaning of psychological well-being. *Journal of Personality and Social Psychology, 57*, 1069–1081.

Ryff, C. D. (1991). Possible selves in adulthood and old age: A tale of shifting horizons. *Psychology and Aging, 6*, 286–295.

Ryff, C. D., & Heincke, S. G. (1983). Subjective organization of personality in adulthood and aging. *Journal of Personality & Social Psychology, 44*, 807–816.

Sabatini, P., & Kastenbaum, R. (1973). The do-it-yourself death certificate as a research technique. *Life-threatening Behavior, 3*(1), 20–32.

Slater, P. E., & Scarr, H. A. (1964). Personality in old age. *Genetic Psychology Monographs, 70*, 229–269.

Staudinger, U. M., Freund, A. M., Linden, M., & Maas, I. (1999). Self, personality, and life regulation: Facets of psychological resilience in old age. In P. B. Baltes & K. U. Mayer (Eds.), *The Berlin Aging Study: Aging from 70 to 100* (pp. 302–328). New York: Cambridge University Press.

Stewart, D., & Vaux, A. (1986). Social support resources, behaviors, and perceptions among Black and White college students. *Journal of Multicultural Counseling & Development, 14*(2), 65–72.

Taylor, R. J. (1988). Aging and supportive relationships among black Americans. In J. S. Jackson, P. Newton, A. Ostfield, D. Savage & E. L. Schneider (Eds.), *The black American elderly: Research on physical and psychological health* (pp. 259–281). New York: Springer.

Taylor, S. E., Kemeny, M. E., Reed, G. M., Bower, J., & Gruenewald, T. L. (2000). Psychological resources, positive illusions, and health. *American Psychologist, 55*, 99–109.

The Sun (2001, September 16). *Behaviors of War*. Retrieved December 21, 2001, from http://libwisesearch.wisers.net.

Troll, L. E. (1994). Family-embedded vs. family-deprived oldest-old: A study of contrasts. *International Journal of Aging and Human Development, 38*(1), 51–63.

U.S. Bureau of the Census (1999). International Data Base [On-line]. Available at: www.census.gov/cgi-bin/ipc/idbsum.

Whitrow, G. J. (1972). *The nature of time*. New York: Holt, Rinehart, and Winston.

Chapter 24

Refugees' Life Transitions from Displacement to Durable Resettlement

Marie-Antoinette Sossou

Refugees experience various life transitions as a result of armed conflicts and civil wars that lead to emergency displacement in their normal everyday lives. These transitions begin at the onset of a complex emergency and last until a durable solution is found for their safety.

Wars and armed conflicts are one of the main causes of forced migration leading to the creation of refugees and internally displaced persons. According to the Stockholm International Peace Research Institute (SIPRI), there were 59 major armed conflicts in 48 different locations since the post-cold war period.

In 2003, there were 19 major armed conflicts in 18 locations throughout the world, and only two were classified as inter-state conflicts – the war in Iraq and the long-standing conflict between India and Pakistan. Thus, the main type of armed conflict continues to be the intra-state conflict (SIPRI 2004). The causes of forced migration are a complex mixture of political factors, such as gross violations of human rights, economic and environmental disadvantages, and the humanitarian crisis of involuntary displacement of people, mostly civilians and vulnerable people such as women, children, and the elderly.

The UN Convention (1951) on the status of refugees and the New York Protocol (1967) on refugees see a refugee as someone fleeing persecution, torture or war, and is in need of asylum or protection. According to the UN Convention and the UN Protocol, a refugee is defined as someone "who owing to a well founded fear of being persecuted for reasons of race, religion, nationality, membership of a particular social group or political opinion is outside the country of his nationality and is unable or, owing to such fear, is unwilling to avail himself of the protection of that country; or who, not having a nationality and being outside the country of his former habitual residence as a result of such events, is unable or, owing to such fear, is unwilling to return to it."

In addition to the United Nations' definition of a refugee, there are regional instruments such as the 1969 Organization of African Unity

From: *Handbook of Stressful Transitions Across the Lifespan,*
Edited by: T.W. Miller, DOI 10.1007/978-1-4419-0748-6_24,
© Springer Science+Business Media, LLC 2010

Refugee Convention and the 1984 Cartagena Declaration in Latin America that also defined refugees to include people who have fled because of war or civil conflict (UNHCR 2006a). For example, The African Union (1969) preferred definition included "those who have been forced to leave their home country as a result of external aggression or domination, occupation, foreign domination or events seriously disturbing public order." This definition gives consideration to people who are forced to leave their homes and country of origin by aggressors from neighboring countries rather than fearing persecution from their own government.

A total of 146 countries have signed the 1951 UN Refugee Convention and recognized people as refugees based on the definitions contained in these and other regional instruments. UNHCR (2006a) stated the global refugee population to be 8.4 million and this estimated to be the lowest total since 1980. In addition to refugees, it is estimated that there are about 23.7 million internally displaced people worldwide. Internally displaced people (IDPs) are defined as people who are caught in situations similar to refugees, but who continued to stay in their own countries rather than cross an international frontier (UNHCR 2006a). Against the background of massive disruptions to a way of life, such as those brought on by widespread violence, terror, and genocide, this chapter aims to review the life transitions of refugees from their once stable and ordinary lives to that of uprooted citizens seeking refuge and asylum in neighboring countries and resettlement in Western industrialized countries.

The Demographics of Refugees

Globally, it is estimated that there were about 9.9 million refugees by the end of 2006 and 12.8 million who were internally displaced within their individual countries and approximately 5.8 million who were stateless (UNHCR 2006a). Currently, there are 1.2 million people who are internally displaced in Iraq, 400,000 in Somalia, and 841,900 in Darfur, Sudan. The breakdown of the global distribution of refugees is given in Table 24-1.

A number of countries (as shown below) have been identified as the leading creators of refugees and as at the end of 2006 Afghanistan continued to be the leading country of origin of refugees. The three other countries responsible for creating refugees were Somalia, the Democratic Republic of the Congo, and Burundi (UNHCR 2006a) (Table 24-2).

Table 24-1. Global refugee population: continents/regions.

Africa	2,421,300
Central, South, West Asia	3,811,800
Asia and Pacific	875,100
Americas	1,035,900
Europe	1,733,700
Total	9,877,800

Source: 2006 Global Refugee Trends (UNHCR 2006a)

Table 24-2. Origin of major refugee populations.

Afghanistan	2.1 million
Burundi	438,700
Democratic Republic of Congo	400,000
Iraq	2.2 million
Somalia	460,000
Sudan	686,000

Source: UNHCR (2006a)

Refugees and Gender

It is estimated that women and girls make up about 50% of the world's refugee population. Even though demographic information on the populations of concern is not available for all countries, available information on refugees indicates that in mass influx situations the proportion of female refugees tends to be around 50%. It is also estimated that 20 million young people around the world are refugees and displaced victims of other people's wars and conflicts and they have seen atrocities and survived trauma that most of their peers will never experience, and were caught between adult burdens and childhood innocence (UNHCR 2003a, b). About 45% of refugee children are under the age of 18 years, with 11% being under the age of 5 years. In all, half of the refugee population is between the ages of 18 and 59 years, with only 5% being 60 years old or more (UNHCR 2006a).

Life Transitions of Refugees

Life span transitions offer an insight into the development of human beings across the life span, with particular attention to the biological, cognitive, and psycho-social processes that people experience as they adapt to life circumstances. Baltes et al. (1980) argue that developmental processes may begin at any point in life and are not necessarily linear. They recognize three influences on human development which together account for substantial individual variation. First, there are normative age-graded influences, which refer to age and physical maturation, commencement of education, and parents' death. Secondly, there are normative, history-graded influences, which refer to historical events that influence the entire age cohorts leading to economic depressions, epidemics, wars, and social movements and finally, they recognize a host of non-normative influences and events that have great impact on individual lives but that most people escape, such as contracting a rare disease, having a child with a genetic abnormality, or winning a lottery (Baltes et al. 1980).

For the purpose of this chapter, Baltes and his colleagues' normative history-graded influence on life transitions fits the life situations of most refugees. Refugees' normal life development as members of their respective cultures is tragically disrupted by socio-environmental factors, such as ethnic wars, political persecutions, ethnic cleansing, and civil unrest that drive them out of their countries of origin into exile against their will. The effects of this disruption on the lives of individuals may differ depending on a person's age at the time of the event, but most people of a given age and a whole cohort will have similar experiences (Baltes et al. 1980).

Refugee situations are not created in a void but are results of human rights violations, political persecution, torture, harassment, sexual violence, detention, and threats to life, personal freedom and well-founded fear of persecution. These conditions, when out of hand, will drive people to leave their homelands, families, and cultures to seek safety elsewhere. According to UNHCR (1999), persecution occurs during war or armed conflict and also during a time of peace, as a deliberate policy of a state against individuals, a group, or groups. Three main stages, namely, *pre-flight, in-flight,* and *post-flight* or *resettlement* have been identified as the phases that most refugees go through to survive as they face danger and threat to their lives as individuals, a group, or a nation (UNHCR 1999).

Pre-flight Life Situations of Refugees

It is important to remember that before the events of refugees' crisis, the refugees had lived their normal lives in their respective countries of origin as ordinary citizens going about their normal daily activities as any normal human being. Delgado et al. (2005) outlined a number of characteristics of refugees before they flee their respective countries for safety. They assert that refugees either live in urban or rural communities; they have socio-economic backgrounds in terms of standard of living, class, status. In addition, they have different levels of education and some have achieved the highest level of education in their countries of origin; they have employment and some are highly trained professionals, technocrats, and political leaders of their countries. They also have their family structures; enjoy stability and high level of social and economic functioning and at times refugees could be members of majority or minority ethnic groups in their countries, and have some degree of exposure to both western and traditional culture.

They also assert that refugees may have some experience, if any with repression and discrimination and that they have expectations and hopes for the future with regards to their children, family members, and their countries (Delgado et al. 2005). This assertion is supported by a study conducted by this author and her colleagues on Bosnian refugee women resettled in the United States. The participants in this study recounted their pre-flight experiences as very normal, peaceful, enjoyable, and ordinary as that of any normal citizens in any part of the world until the 1994 Bosnian war disrupted their peaceful lives (Sossou et al. 2008).

A number of studies have documented the pre-flight phase of refugees as that characterized at the societal and community levels, with social upheaval and increasing chaos, disruption of education and social development at the family and individual levels, in addition to threats to their safety and that of their family members (Gonsalves 1992; Papadopoulos 2001; Rumbaut 1991). According to Jastram and Newland (2003), refugees run multiple risks in the process of fleeing from persecution, one of which is the real risk of separation from their families. For individuals who, as refugees, are without the protection of their own countries, the loss of contact with family members may disrupt their major remaining source of protection and care or, equally distressing, put out of reach those for whose protection a refugee feels most deeply responsible.

Situations of Refugees In-Flight

One common response to threat to life and safety is for people to simply flee their homes. Such flights frequently lead to a large number of refugees crossing international boundaries often, with nothing more than the clothes on their back. For most refugees, the decision to leave their home countries is not about the dream of finding a better life elsewhere, as implied in the label of economic migrant. Rather, the motivation for flight is for survival and safety. The flight phase is particularly stressful because of its instability and unpredictability as refugees leave their homes either forcibly or involuntarily and most of the time, they are forced to leave their possessions behind. Fleeing refugees seek refuge in the homes of relatives or at refugee camps run by the United Nations High Commissioner for Refugees (UNHCR) or other non-governmental organizations. In flight, most refugees become economically dependent on relief agencies for food aid, shelter, and safety as they are also removed from their everyday cultural and familiar environments and have no way of knowing what their situation will be (UNHCR 1999).

It has been documented that during flight, refugees are forced to travel long distances, through difficult terrain or across open seas, using inadequate means of transportation. Their plight is also combined with harsh climatic conditions that threaten their health and especially the health of children, pregnant women, the sick, and the elderly. During flight, refugees become separated from their families, which increase their vulnerability and exposure to trauma and gender-based violence, attacks by bandits and pirates and sometimes, attacks from unscrupulous elements among those in flight (UNHCR 1999; The State of the World's Refugees 1998).

In flight, refugees also suffer various forms of atrocities and gender-based violence as they are caught in between violence and ethnic cleansing. For example, Human Rights Watch (2002) reports that as many as 3,000 women were raped in the Democratic Republic of the Congo (UNIFEM (2005). Refugees International (2004) estimates that up to 40% of women were raped during Liberia's 14 years civil war and teenagers were the most targeted group. In addition, displaced women face sexual exploitation by aid workers as reports indicated from West Africa (Secretary General's Bulletin 2003).

According to Avega (1999), majority of Tutsi women were also exposed to some form of gender-based violence during the 1994 genocide in Rwanda and it was estimated that between 250,000 and 500,000 women survived rape. It has also been documented that whilst in flight, refugee women are often subject to sexual abuse and harassment by border security guards, customs and immigration officials, and bandits. This violence persistently and increasingly subject refugee women and girls to physical, sexual, and psychological trauma, which is a gross violation of women's human rights (UNIFEM 2005). Studies have indicated that exposure of children to traumatic events during flight could lead to display of aggressive behavior, reduced social competencies, depression, fear, anxiety, sleep disturbances, and learning problems (Harrell-Bond 2000; Groves et al. 1993).

Conditions in Refugee Camps

World refugee survey (2007) indicates that globally, there are 8,809,700 million refugees living in refugee camps and 8,779,700 million have lived in these camps for 10 years or more. The provision of protection and humanitarian assistance to vulnerable refugees amid large-scale migratory movement has become a huge challenge to host governments and international organizations. The creation of refugee camps or temporary settlements has become the norm upon arrival of mass groups of refugees in any international territory or country. As early as 1955, Murphy (1955) notes that although the physical conditions of camps may vary widely, from hell to hotels, the effects tend to be uniform. He describes the most important characteristics of the refugee camps as being segregated from the host population, the need to share facilities, a lack of privacy, plus overcrowding and a limited, restricted area within which the whole compass of daily life is to be conducted. According to him, this situation gives the refugees a sense of dependency, and the clear signal that they have a special and limited status, and are being controlled (Murphy 1955).

Murphy (1955) further explained that it is during the refugees' stay in the camps that refugees really experienced the enormity of what has happened to them as human beings. They assert that apart from the suffering, trauma, and persecution already endured, and the loss of loved ones, the refugees also faced the loss of homeland, identity, and their former lives and the beginning of a new life in a strange land. They, therefore, suffer from anxiety, fear, frustration, and emotional disturbances, and often they regress to a more infantile state, loss of will power, and become apathetic, helpless, or manic and aggressive and they lose their structure, the ability to coordinate, predict and expect, and their basic feelings of competence (Murphy 1955).

According to da Costa (2006), refugee camps and settlements are meant to provide refugees with a safe and secure environment and to serve as a refuge from war, civil strife, personal attacks and other human rights violations and abuse, as well as from a climate of fear and persecution. In addition, refugee camps are expected to provide personal physical security, respect for fundamental human rights, and access to the basics of life such as food, water, shelter, and other essential needs (da Costa 2006). UNHCR (1999) asserts that in the immediate aftermath of flight, refugee camps and settlements do generally provide relief from imminent attacks and persecution. However, from the refugees' perspective, living in refugee camps is fraught with unforeseen problems, such as loss of privacy and sense of control over their lives, lack of routines and responsibilities of daily, independent life, and the difficulty to maintain self-respect, self-reliance, and the belief in their own futures.

Harrell-Bond (2000) analyzes the situation in refugee camps and is of the view that refugee camps have the essential feature of being authoritarian in the character of their administration and that most camps are like "total institutions" as in prisons or mental hospitals, and everything is highly organized, and the inhabitants are depersonalized and become numbers without names. In addition, she states that another characteristic of camps is the persistent shortage of food due to lack of access to land by the refugees. A study conducted by the Center for Disease Control, in nine refugee camps in Sudan found the prevalence of acute malnutrition among children under the age of 5 years to vary between 20 and 70%, as compared to 3 and 5% in various African countries (Harrell-Bond 2000).

Harrell-Bond (2000) also discusses the adverse social, psychological, and economic consequences of involuntary resettlement of refugees in camps. She asserts that resettled people suffered higher rates of mortality and morbidity and that they got poorer and traumatized by being resettled against their will, and the experiences were especially difficult for the elderly and children. In addition, she discusses the breaking up of many refugee families due to displacement leading to children being cared for by only one parent, or without either parent, and sometimes refugee children have to act as head of family, trying to care for their younger siblings. She alleged that refugee parents are deprived of their authority and their roles as care-givers and breadwinners are undermined by their dependence on a system over which they have no control, and parents become degraded in the eyes of their children as they suffer further humiliation of standing in queues to get food, and being forced to manipulate the system to get extra ration cards in order to have enough food to feed their children (Harrell-Bond 2000).

da Costa (2006) conducted a global study of 52 refugee camps in 13 countries of Bangladesh, Cote d'Ivoire, Ethiopia, Guinea, Kenya, Mexico, Nepal, Pakistan, Sierra Leone, Tanzania, Thailand, Yemen, and Zambia, with a total population of nearly a million refugees. In all, she found that refugee populations are often in dire and urgent need of basic necessities such as food, shelter, and non-food items due to restrictive camp regulations or lack of employment opportunities. She asserts that refugees also suffer from an uncertain legal status in the host country, as well as from restrictions on their basic human rights such as freedom of movement and the right to work or earn a livelihood and in addition, they are trapped in situations of dependence and poverty, and there is a general lack of capacity and resources in the camps. The study also discusses the remoteness of many refugee camps and the lack of resources and infrastructure that has led to the isolation of refugee populations rendering them more dependant and vulnerable. In addition, she states that the lack of easy access to services such as medical services, communications, markets, and legal institutions and restricted mobility have left the refugees with fewer options for the resolution of their problems and in the day-to-day management of their lives (da Costa 2006).

Finally, refugee women in some camps are subject to sexual violence when they venture out to collect firewood or go to the water and sanitation facilities located at the edge of the site. Women are also exposed to sexual harassment in the camps by security guards, police, other male refugees, and local residents. In addition, domestic violence is also a common incident in refugee camps as both men and women may be suffering anxiety and depression as a consequence of the hopeless situation in which they live. Substance and alcohol abuse is also common among men and women as they abuse alcohol as a means of forgetting their problems (Harrell-Bond 2000).

One of the main controversies being advanced against refugee camps is the warehousing of refugees in isolated and remote camps across the globe. It has been argued that more and more refugees worldwide are spending longer periods of time in refugee camps to the point that there are currently more than seven million refugees who have been warehoused for 10 years or more in camp situations (World Refugee Survey 2004). Warehousing is defined as the practice of keeping refugees in protracted situations of restricted mobility, enforced idleness, and dependency, with their lives on indefinite hold.

According to Chen (2004), more than half a million refugees from Myanmar have lived without the right to work or travel for up to 20 years in Thailand, Bangladesh, Malaysia, and India, and more than half a million Sudanese are stuck in camps or segregated settlements that have been operating for two decades. In addition, he stated that more than two million Afghan refugees have been in exile in Pakistan and Iran for over 25 years and Palestinian refugees have been warehoused in refugee camps throughout the Middle East since 1948 (Chen 2004). Currently, the genocide in Darfur has resulted in some 250,000 refugees from Sudan living in 12 refugee camps in eastern Chad (Herz 2007). This is an indication that refugee camps, as warehouses will not be discarded in the near future.

Education of Refugees

Women's Commission for Refugee Women and Children (2004) in a global survey on education in emergencies asserts that more than 27 million children and youth affected by armed conflict, including refugees and internally displaced persons, do not have access to formal education. The survey states that only 6% of all refugee students are enrolled in secondary education, and adolescents and youth have the least access to formal education as many have not completed even primary education and so require a range of formal and non-formal educational options. It is also evident that in most emergency situations, the majority of teachers are men and as a result there is low enrollment of girls, and families often do not allow their girls to attend school post-puberty as they fear for their daughters' safety.

In addition, there is evidence of lack of adequate water and sanitation facilities, which poses a health risk, especially, for the adolescent girls' attendance, retention, and completion (Women's Commission 2004). Mehraby (2000) confirms this situation in a Pakistani camp for Survey Afghan refugees. According to him, there was only one school for 15,000 refugee children and the school was only at the primary grade level and girls were not allowed to attend and there were no chairs or tables and students had to sit on the ground.

Physical and Mental Health of Refugees

According to World Health Organization (2008), population movements generally render migrants and refugees more vulnerable to health risks and expose them to potential hazards and greater stress arising from displacement, insertion into new environments, and reinsertion into former environments. They often have to deal with poverty, marginality, and limited access to social benefits and health services. In addition, refugees travel with their epidemiologic profiles, level of exposure to infectious agents, genetic and lifestyle-related risk factors, culture-based health beliefs, and their susceptibility to certain conditions. There is also evidence that certain non-communicable diseases, such as hypertension, cardiovascular diseases, diabetes, and cancer, are an increasing burden on refugee populations and impose considerable demands on health systems of destination countries (WHO 2007).

Connolly et al. (2007) assert that refugees and displaced populations are at particularly high risk of developing tuberculosis, partly as a result of the crowded living conditions of these populations in refugee camps. In addition, they stated that co-existent illness, particularly HIV and poor nutritional status, can also weaken their immune system and make them more vulnerable to developing active tuberculosis. Tuberculosis is an increasingly important cause of morbidity and mortality among refugee and displaced populations. For example, in 1985, 26% of deaths among adult refugees in Somalia and between 38 and 50% of all deaths among refugees in camps in eastern Sudan were attributed to tuberculosis. They also found in 1994 that the incidence of new infectious tuberculosis patients in refugee camps in north-east Kenya was four times the rate in the local population and in 2000, the tuberculosis notification rate for displaced Chechens in Ingushetia was almost twice as high as the resident population (Connolly et al. 2007).

Hunger and malnutrition are also prevalent among refugees and displaced populations, and the mostly affected people are infants, children, adolescents, adults, and the elderly (WHO 2008). According to Moss et al. (2006), the highest mortality rates in refugee populations are children younger than 5 years. They assert that the major causes of childhood morbidity and mortality in complex emergencies have not changed significantly in the past decade. For example, 80% of deaths among Congolese children younger than 5 years in Lugufu camp in the United Republic of Tanzania were due to malaria, diarrhea, and pneumonia (Moss et al. 2006).

Refugees are equally at high risk for mental and other psychological problems. Gureje and Alem (2000) are of the view that wars and strife disrupt social and community life, and these disruptions lead to psychological disorders among large number of people and it is often not sufficiently realized that psychological morbidity accompanies and outlasts the physical morbidity of war and in most cases, the most disadvantaged and economically vulnerable victims are women and children (Gureje and Alem 2000). Mollica and Jeon (2001) assert that historically, the psycho-social problems of refugees were not considered as medical consequences of mass violence in the same way as landmine or battle injuries, and they believe mental health problems are "invisible" wounds that cannot be readily examined.

Refugees in all categories experience psychological problems in the form of torture, trauma, post-traumatic stress disorder (PTSD), depression, sexual and physical abuses, loss of family members, friends, and jobs and their homelands and mental illness. For example, Fazel et al. (2005), in a recent analysis of mental illnesses within refugees residing in developed countries, found that the prevalence of post-traumatic stress disorder (PTSD) was roughly 1 in 10, and major depressive disorder was roughly 1 in 20. Studies by Farwell (2001), Foster (2001), and Dybdahl (2001) have indicated that exposure of children to traumatic events could lead to a display of aggressive behavior, reduced social competencies, depression, fears, anxiety, sleep disturbances, and learning problems and untreated mental disorders and illnesses could lead to unsuccessful integration of refugees back into their societies. Recent studies on the mental health of Bosnian, Sarajevo, and Croatian refugee children seeking asylum in developed countries, concluded that children exposed to armed conflict or the harsh living conditions of refugee camps have high rates of serious psychiatric problems (Allwood et al. 2002).

An epidemiological survey conducted between 1997 and 1999 among survivors of mass violence from Gaza, Algeria, Ethiopia, and Cambodia reported PTSD rates as high as 37.4% (de Jong et al. 2001). There are debates about the consequence of trauma in children. Cunningham (1991) argues that trauma in children has long-term pathogenic effects, while others believe that the developing personality allows trauma to occur with less serious consequences than in adults. However, it is generally agreed that children are more vulnerable than adults, and their future relationships may be threatened if there is not appropriate intervention and treatment (Cunningham 1991).

Durable Solutions to Refugees' Plight

In finding durable solutions to the global refugee problems, the 1951 Convention on the Status of Refugees outlines the rights of refugees to include non-discrimination, freedom of religion, free access to the courts of law on the territory of all States that are parties to the Convention, the right to work, the right to housing, the right to education, the right to public relief and assistance, freedom of movement within the territory, and the right not to be expelled from a country, unless the refugee poses a threat to national security or the public order, and the right to be protected against forcible return, or refoulement, to the territory from which the refugee had fled. The 1951 Convention and the 1967 Protocol make non-refoulement or protection from forced return, a fundamental right of refugees fleeing the threat of persecution (United Nations 1951).

UNHCR (2003a, b) outlines three durable solutions for permanent resolution of refugee exodus. Voluntary repatriation, local integration in the country of first asylum, and resettlement in a third country are the three durable solutions. All three solutions are regarded as durable because they promise an end to refugees' suffering and their need for international protection and permanent dependence on humanitarian assistance.

Voluntary Repatriation

There are two methods of voluntary repatriation – *organized repatriation*, which refers to return by means of UNHCR's assistance of transportation and other assistance package of food and cash and *spontaneous repatriation*, which is return by the refugees' own means, but with some assistance from the refugee agency. In most cases, the two categories of repatriation may occur at the same time (UNHCR 2003a, b).

The principle of voluntary repatriation is the cornerstone of international protection with respect to the return of all refugees to their countries of origin by choice and not by force and repatriation is often regarded as the most desirable durable solution, provided that return is genuinely voluntary and sustainable. According to the State of World's Refugee (2006), the 1990s became the decade of repatriation and more than nine million refugees were repatriated between 1991 and 1996. In 2004, almost 15 million refugees have been repatriated to their countries of origin across the globe. The main countries of origin to which refugees returned were Afghanistan, Iraq, Burundi, Angola, Liberia, and Sierra Leone and the other countries were Somalia, Rwanda, the Democratic Republic of the Congo, and Sri Lanka (State of the World's Refugees 2006; UNHCR 2005).

Ideally, refugees are supposed to be the main actors in their voluntary repatriation as they are expected to make the decision and participate in determining the modalities of their movements based on the safety conditions of their countries. However, refugees have been forced to return under pressure from host governments. For example, in 1996, Rwandan refugees hosted by the Democratic Republic of Congo and Tanzania were forced to return home, and this situation has raised fresh questions about the degree of voluntariness and the role of compulsion in "imposed return" (Loescher 2001).

Repatriation does not end once refugees have crossed the border into their homeland. Most often, refugees return to countries, which have been devastated by conflict and divided communities, physical insecurity, material insecurity, such as lack of access to basic necessities, land and property, and education and legal insecurity such as lack of documentation. UNHCR (1999) has outlined guidelines for the successful reintegration of returned refugees. The guidelines include monitoring and training sessions on human rights for the returnees, local authorities, and the local population. In addition to the registration of returnees and linking them to resources, such as having access to land, their properties, fair trials, education and social services, social and economic projects are launched to assist them with their reintegration. The guidelines emphasized the importance of reconciliation and confidence-building programs and the involvement of returnees and members of the local population in all stages of planning and maintenance of their reintegration (UNHCR 1999).

Local Integration

According to UNHCR (1999), voluntary repatriation is the preferred option for most refugees; however, local integration becomes the second durable solution to some refugees who feel unsafe to return home due to political insecurity and fear. In addition, vulnerable refugees, such as elderly or severely handicapped individuals who have lost all contact with their families and countries of origin and have lived in exile for so many years, are also qualified for local integration on humanitarian grounds. Local integration can only be achieved with the consent and active participation of the national government of the country of asylum. That is, the host governments must fully agree to actively support efforts to integrate refugee populations in their countries. For local integration to be successful, it must be economically viable, in terms of availability of agricultural lands to rural refugee communities, as well as access to markets, employment, and income-generating opportunities.

The refugees should also have sufficient external financial support to assist in their local transitions. Local integration must be voluntary; and refugees must be fully incorporated into their new societies, and have the opportunity to acquire national citizenship to exercise all the rights that citizenship confers (UNHCR 1999). It is noted that developing countries do not usually welcome large numbers of refugees for local integration due to economic, environmental, and demographic problems and some industrialized countries, due to the high cost of welfare services may also shy away from local integration of refugees (UNHCR 1999). However, by the end of 2005, it was reported that 69% of an estimated 6.1 million refugees hosted by developing countries had access to assistance provided by UNHCR for local integration (UNHCR 2006b).

Resettlement of Refugees

Resettlement involves the transfer of refugees from the country in which they sought asylum to another country that has agreed to admit them as refugees for permanent settlement. According to UNHCR (2004), resettlement serves three important purposes. It is a tool to provide international protection and to meet the special needs of individual refugees whose life, liberty, safety, health, or other fundamental rights are at risk in the country where they have sought refuge. Secondly, resettlement is a durable solution for larger numbers or groups of refugees, alongside the other durable solutions of voluntary repatriation and local integration and lastly, resettlement can be a tangible expression of international solidarity and a responsibility sharing mechanism that allows individual countries to help share the global burdens, and reduce problems impacting the country of first asylum (UNHCR 2004).

Resettlement is also used for other refugees at risk, such as survivors of torture and violence, the disabled and other injured or severely traumatized refugees who are in need of specialized treatment unavailable in their country of refuge. In addition, resettlement is often the only way to reunite refugee families who have been separated through no fault of their own. UNHCR (2004) asserts that resettlement of refugees in a third country is a humanitarian gesture and no country is legally obliged to resettle refugees. Hence, only a small number of countries do so on a regular basis, by allocating budgets, devising programs, and providing annual resettlement quotas for refugees. Some countries regularly accept refugees for resettlement, sometimes in relatively large numbers, but with no annual targets. Recently, countries that have not previously accepted refugees for resettlement have established resettlement programs or expressed an interest in doing so (UNHCR 2004).

Historically, the office of United Nations High Commissioner for Refugees has successfully used resettlement, voluntary repatriation, and local integration to protect refugees from political persecutions. For example, in 1956, 200,000 Hungarian refugees who fled to Yugoslavia and Austria during the Second World War were resettled in many countries, and in 1972, some 40,000 Uganda Asians expelled from Uganda by Idi Amin were resettled in a total of 25 countries with assistance of the International Organization for Migration (IOM), the International Committee of the Red Cross (ICRC), and the United Nations Development Program (UNHCR 2004). In 1979, the largest and most dramatic example of resettlement in modern times occurred in South East Asia and 700,000 Vietnamese refugees were resettled in other countries as they were refused first asylum in some South East Asian countries.

In the late 1980s and early 1990s, the major focus of resettlement activity shifted to the Middle East due to the overthrow of the Shah of Iran and the first Gulf war. Ten thousand Iranian Bahais refugees who sought asylum in Turkey and Pakistan were later resettled in the United States of America and 30,000 Iraqi refugees from Saudi Arabia and 450,000 Kurdish refugees have been accepted for resettlement in several third countries after voluntary repatriation and local integration failed in the Middle East. Another major refugee resettlement occurred in 1992 as a result of the ethnic cleansing that took place in Bosnia and Herzegovina and by 1997, some 47,000 refugees were resettled in several third countries (UNHCR 2004).

In 2004, with the assistance of UNHCR, 30,000 refugees were resettled in several third countries from their previous countries of asylum. There were 5,610 refugees from Liberia, 5,050 from Sudan, 4,870 from Somalia, and 2,710 from Afghanistan. There were also 2,190 refugees from the Islamic Republic of Iran, 1,900 from Myanmar, 1,490 from Ethiopia, and 1,290 from the Democratic Republic of the Congo. In all 15 countries, including USA,

Australia, Canada, Sweden, Norway, Finland, and Denmark, the refugees were received and resettled (UNHCR 2005). In 2006, UNHCR's resettlement interventions were directed mainly at 5,700 refugees from Myanmar, 5,200 from Somalia, 2,900 from Sudan, and 2,000 from the Democratic Republic of the Congo, and 1,900 from Afghanistan (UNHCR 2007).

Resettlement of Refugees in the United States

Almost 2.4 million refugees and asylum seekers from at least 115 countries entered the United States between 1980 and 2006, and despite decline in refugee admissions, the United States continues to resettle more refugees than any other country (USCRI 2003). In 2002 fiscal year, 27,100 refugees have been resettled in the United States and this has been the lowest number since the program began in 1980. The largest number of resettled refugees was from the former Soviet Union and this consists of 9,800 refugees, followed by 4,900 Bosnians, 2,900 Vietnamese, 1,900 Cubans, and 1,600 Afghans (World Refugee Survey 2003). The Refugee Act of 1980 gives the United States the legal back for resettlement of refugees. The Refugee Act was significant for establishing a federal policy for continuous admission of refugees, and it also defined the term "refugee" to incorporate with the international United Nations Convention definition and in addition, established the principle of resettlement assistance for refugees (The Refugee Act 1980).

In 2003, President Bush authorized the increase in admission of refugees from the traditional 50,000 per fiscal year to 70,000 from five regions of the world, namely Africa, East and Central Asia, Europe, Latin America and the Caribbean, and the South Asia (USCRI 2003).

During the 2005 fiscal year, the U.S. Refugee Program resettled about 53,800 refugees, which was a significant increase over the 52,900 refugees resettled during the 2004 fiscal year and that of 28,400 refugees in 2003 (O'Hara 2006).

The processing of refugees for admission for resettlement is carried out through a system of priorities outlined by the United States Department of State identifies three categories of priorities. The first priority is carried out by UNHCR or the United States Embassy. This involves persons facing compelling security concerns in countries of first asylum, persons in need of legal protection because of the danger of forced repatriation, and those refugees in danger due to threats of armed attack in an area where they were located. The first priority also applies to refugees who have experienced recent persecution because of their political, religious, or human rights activities, at-risk women, victims of torture or violence; physically or mentally disabled persons and persons in need of urgent medical treatment (Delgado et al. 2005).

The second category of priority involves groups of special concern, within certain nationalities as identified by the Department of State in consultation with Non-Governmental Organizations, UNHCR, and Department of Homeland Security, and other area experts. Examples of this category are former political prisoners from Cuba, Jews, Evangelical Christians, and Ukrainian Catholic and Orthodox religious activists due to fear of religious persecution and the war victims from Vietnam (UNHCR 2004). The third category of priority includes spouses, unmarried sons and daughters, parents of persons lawfully admitted into the country as permanent resident aliens, refugees, and asylees. Refugees accepted for resettlement into the United States must receive medical and security clearances, in addition to cultural orientation (Delgado et al. 2005).

In 2000, under the first priority category, a total of 3,500 Sudanese "Lost Boys" who have experienced years of deprivation, loss of their families, war violence, and life in refugee camps in Kenya were resettled in the U.S., under the Unaccompanied Minors Program. The Unaccompanied Minors program was originally developed in the 1980s to address the needs of thousands of children in Southeast Asia without a parent or guardian to care for them. Since 1980, almost 12,000 minors have been assisted through this program. Currently, the Office of Refugee Resettlement has about 600 children in care and most children are placed in licensed foster homes, licensed care settings, such as therapeutic foster care, group homes, residential treatment centers, and independent living programs (Office of Refugee Resettlement 2007).

UNHCR (2002) defines women at-risk as those women who have protection problems and are single heads of families, or are accompanied by an adult male who is unable to support and assume the role of the head of the family. They may suffer from a wide range of problems including expulsion, refoulement and other security threats, sexual harassment, violence, abuse, torture, and different forms of exploitation. Hence, the United States place women at-risk under the highest priority category for resettlement. Upon approval for resettlement, refugees without sources of income for their travel are eligible for loans from the International Organization for Migration for their air fares to the United States and they are expected to begin repaying within a few months of arrival (Delgado et al. 2005).

Legally, refugees could be denied resettlement in this country due to several factors and among them are health-related reasons, such as communicable diseases, physical or mental disorders, and current drug abuse or addiction; however, health-related denials may be overcome when the problem has been successfully treated, or upon waiver at the discretion of the U.S. Attorney General. A second ground for denial concerns criminal activities, such as crimes of moral turpitude, drug trafficking, multiple criminal convictions, prostitution, murder or acts involving persecution or torture. The third grounds of resettlement denial is based on national security, such as espionage, terrorist activity, membership in Communist or other totalitarian parties, Nazi persecution or genocide, or individuals who would present a serious security threat (UNHCR 2004).

Resettlement of refugees within the United States is officially carried out by several voluntary agencies that are under contract with the Department of State to provide reception and placement services for the refugees (Delgado et al. 2005). These voluntary agencies are responsible for assisting refugees with housing, employment, English classes, medical care, school enrollment for children, and general orientation to public transportation systems, currency, and other daily living activities (Delgado et al. 2005). According to these authors, these voluntary agencies are required to work with refugees for the first 90 days after their arrival. As part of successful resettlement of refugees, most refugees are eligible for accessing some federal social welfare programs as compared to other legal immigrants who migrated into this country after August 1996. According to the refugees are eligible for supplemental security income, food stamps, Temporary Assistance for Needy Families (TANF), Emergency Medicaid, Full-Scope Medicaid, State Children's Health Insurance Program (SCHIP), and Medicare.

Post-resettlement Stressors and Acculturation

Resettlement implies that refugees cannot return to their home countries for years and this means permanent separation from family members and friends in the country of origin. It also means the beginning of a new life with new opportunities, which involves learning a new language, getting a new education and becoming adapted to new cultures and a totally different social environment. Often, there is an assumption that refugees, who are able to adapt to the new environment without any major problems, are more likely to have a successful resettlement experience and become valuable members of their communities.

The challenges faced by refugees during their resettlement in any new country have implications for their eventual successful integration into their new country of asylum.

Several studies have documented the post-migration experiences that affect the general well-being of various groups of refugees. Such studies revealed that refugees frequently encounter pre- and post-migration trauma experiences that might directly undermine their physical and psychological health, and these traumas may also have indirect effects by diminishing the capacity to cope with acculturation stressors, rendering refugees more vulnerable to stress-related disorders (Bhui et al. 2003; Steel et al. 2003). According to these authors, post-resettlement can be a highly stressful experience as loved ones and familiar environments are left behind, to be replaced by diminished social support, loss of status, difficulties with a new language, and immigrants of minority statuses might also become targets of discrimination (Steel et al. 2003).

Berry (2003) defines acculturation as an adaptation process that occurs when a person comes into contact with a culture distinct from his or her own. This process is often experienced by new immigrants, which includes refugees and is associated with changes in cultural attitudes, values, and behaviors. As a process, individuals, families, or groups experience acculturation differently. Some have higher levels of acculturation than others, by the degree to which they have adapted to the majority culture in terms of language use, cultural identity, and integration into the new system. The effects of acculturation on refugees have been found in many different mental health and behavioral outcomes. For example, the lack of English language knowledge slows down the orientation of most refugees from non-English speaking countries in the new environment, and to survive they need to learn the everyday ways of life, the prevalent communication styles, appropriate behavior in the work environment, and many other things that citizens take for granted.

Several studies conducted among Bosnian, Cambodian, and Soviet refugees resettled in this country have indicated the effects of cross-cultural transition and a series of stress-provoking events that could affect refugees' coping resources and lead to complete withdrawal from social life, mental health complications, and incidence of psychopathology (Ward et al. 2001; Birman et al. 2002).

Refugee children and adolescents also face a multiplicity of settlement problems such as language difficulties, loss of identity, adaptation to the new culture and new educational system, and the processing of their traumatic memories. Practically, many refugee children are placed in school within a week after arrival in this country without any period of adjustment to the new country. Their problems are often underestimated in comparison to those of their parents, who are often preoccupied with their own traumatic experiences and post-settlement problems, therefore, children' needs could be overlooked and neglected. Aroche (1998) asserts that refugee children are affected not only by their own traumatic experiences, but also by those of their parents, and this may cause them to exhibit post-traumatic symptoms which create problems at school and elsewhere. Birman (1998) suggests that immigrant children who are more acculturated to the American culture may be able to be more helpful to their parents in the role of culture broker. In this way, American acculturation may contribute positively to parental support rather than negatively (Birman et al. 2002).

Professional Intervention

It is evident that thousands of refugees are accepted into this country for resettlement every fiscal year and most of these refugee groups of children, women, men, and elderly populations are highly traumatized. Their reactions to trauma and torture, and issues relating to their losses of migration and resettlement challenges, may intersect with their own families and personality issues. There is a call now for a holistic understanding of a comprehensive approach to the overall general well-being of refugees by primary care physicians and other professionals who work with refugees. For example, Henderson (2001) asserts that good intentions and sound medical knowledge are not sufficient to provide the health care required by this community of patients, with respect to their history of displacement, persecution, fragmentation of cultural and familial structures, and violation of human rights. He advised health care providers to become more aware of the more complicated bio-psychosocial profile of this population to become better at confronting their acute and long-term health problems.

Mollica (2001) also advised physicians to pay particular attention to the psycho-social history of refugees and survivors of mass violence, particularly to the issues of bereavement, traumatic loss or disability of family members, especially spouses and children and because of the high prevalence of emotional distress in this population, they should include a mental status examination in their treatment plan.

It is documented that racial and ethnic minorities in the United States are less likely than whites to seek mental health treatment, which largely accounts for their under-representation in most mental health services (Vega and Rumbaut 1998; Zhang et al. 1998) and most refugees fall into this category. Hence, the development of culturally competent mental health services is essential to assist refugees address their mental health issues. Weine (2001) asserts that traditionally, mental health services tend to focus on treatments for individuals who are willing to present themselves as patients and even though many refugees suffer, only few refugees are willing to be patients. He advocates for a "Contact Perspective approach," which refers to a cross-cultural approach of exchange of ideas, negotiation, and interaction between refugees, their families, and professionals. The "contact perspective" insists that providers should examine professional ideology, service organizations, and refugees' attitudes to eliminate the pattern of under-utilization of mental health services by refugees (Weine 2001).

Miller (2007) asserts that the presence of trauma resulting from exposure to violence increases the need for contemporary psychological interventions and prevention strategies to meet the needs of human beings facing trauma in their lives. Moreno et al. (2001) advocate for health care professionals to be willing to work in multi-disciplinary teams, including attorneys and other non-health professionals, to provide effective care for these patients. According to them, refugees and asylees often struggle for years with language and cultural barriers, family reunification issues, and legal status problems in addition to health problems; hence, an integrated approach where advocates work together will ameliorate these problems for the refugees (Moreno et al. 2001).

Social workers should become familiar with the histories and socio-economic politics and issues of the global south as refugee conflicts have humanitarian and social justice implications for the core missions and ethical responsibilities of the social work profession. In addition, social workers should be involved in advocacy and culturally competent policies and programs for refugees' socio-economic development, education, and empowerment.

Conclusion

Refugees' life span begins with various types of emergencies, such as political upheavals, genocide, civil conflicts and wars, and ends with a durable solution in the form of voluntary repatriation, local integration, or resettlement in a third country. These life events and transitions contribute negatively or positively to the development of general health and the mental well-being of refugee's post-resettlement. Many of these life events can be modified by social, economic, and political factors and the goodwill of the global communities concerning their sustainable response to the plights of refugees. Refugees are not helpless people; however, they are a group of vulnerable, marginalized, displaced, and stateless people, who need humanitarian and sustainable assistance to become independent and self-sufficient. Therefore, it is important to affirm and celebrate their perseverance, survival, resilience, and self-determination as they transition into a more normal, stable, and safe environment.

References

Allwood, M. A., Bell-Dolan, D., & Husain, S. A. (2002). Children's trauma and adjustment reactions to violent and non-violent war experiences. *Journal of American Academy of Child Adolescent Psychiatry, 41,* 450–457.

Aroche, J. (1998). Therapy with children. Retrieved April 22, 2008 from http://www.startts.org.au/default.aspx?id=83.

Avega. (1999). *Survey on violence against women in Rwanda.* Kigali: AVEGA.

Baltes, P. B., Reese, H., & Lipsett, L. (1980). Lifespan development psychology. *Annual Review of Psychology, 31,* 65–110.

Berry, J. W. (2003). Conceptual approaches to acculturation. In K. M. Chun, P. Balls Organista & G. Marin (Eds.), *Acculturation advances in theory, measurement, and applied research.* Washington, DC: American Psychological Association.

Bhui, K., Abdi, A., Abdi, M., Pereira, S., Dualey, M., Robertson, D., et al. (2003). Traumatic events, migration characteristics and psychiatric symptoms among Somali refugees. *Social Psychiatry & Psychiatric Epidemiology, 38*(1), 35–43.

Birman, D. (1998). Biculturalism and perceived competence of Latino immigrant adolescents. *American Journal of Community Psychology, 26*(3), 335–354.

Birman, D., Trickett, E. J., & Vinokurov, A. (2002). Acculturation and adaptation of Soviet Jewish refugee adolescents: Predictors of adjustment across life domains. *American Journal of Community Psychology, 30*(5), 585–607.

Chen, G. (2004). *A global campaign to end refugee warehousing.* Boston: 2004 World Refugee Survey.

Connolly, M. A., Gayer, M., & Ottmani, S. (2007). Tuberculosis care and control in refugee and displaced populations: An interagency field manual. Retrieved April 21, 2008 from http://whqlibdoc.who.int/publications/2007/9789241595421_eng.pdf.

Cunningham, M. (1991). Torture and children. Paper presented at the 9th Annual Conference of the Australian Early Intervention Association Inc N.S.W in association with the Australian Association for Infant Mental Health Inc, University of Sydney.

Da Costa, R. (2006). The administration of justice in refugee camps: A study of practice. Geneva: UNHCR: Department of International Protection.

De Jong, J. T., Komproe, T. V. M., Ivan, H., Van Ommeren, M., El Masri, M., & Araya, M. (2001). Lifetime events and posttraumatic stress disorder in four post-conflict settings. *Journal of the American Medical Association, 286*, 555–562.

Delgado, M., Jones, K., & Rohani, M. (2005). *Social work practice with refugee and immigrant youth in the United States.* Boston, MA: Pearson Education, Inc.

Dybdahl, R. (2001). Children and mothers in war: An outcome study of a psychosocial intervention program. *Child Development, 72*, 1214–1230.

Farwell, N. (2001). 'Onward through strength': Coping and psychological support among refugee youth returning to Eritrea from Sudan. *Journal of Refugee Studies, 14*, 1–69.

Fazel, M., Wheeler, J., Danesh, J. (2005). Prevalence of serious mental disorder in 7000 refugees resettled in western countries: A systematic review, *The Lancet*, 365, (9467), 1309–1314.

Foster, R. P. (2001). When immigration is trauma: Guidelines for the individual and family clinician. *American Journal of Orthopsychiatry, 71*, 153–170.

Gonsalves, C. J. (1992). Psychological stages of the refugee process: A model for therapeutic interventions. *Professional Psychology: Research and Practice, 23*, 382–389.

Groves, B., Zuckerman, A., & Marans, S. (1993). Silent victims: Children who witness violence. *Journal of the American Medical Association, 2*, 262–265.

Gureje, O., & Alem, A. (2000). Mental Health policy development in Africa. *Bulletin of the World Health Organization, 78*(4), 475–482.

Harrell-Bond, B. (2000). Are refugee camps good for children? Working paper No. 29. Retrieved March 12, 2008 from http://www.unhcr.ch/refworld/pubs/pubon.htm.

Henderson, S. W. (2001). New approaches to health care for displaced populations. *Journal of American Medical Association, 285*(9), 1212.

Herz, M. (2007). *Refugee camps in Chad: Planning strategies and the architect's involvement in the humanitarian dilemma.* Geneva: UN Refugee Agency Policy Development and Evaluation Service.

Human Rights Watch. (2002). Sexual violence rampant: Unpunished in DR Congo war. *Retrieved January 10, 2007 from* http://www.hrw.org/doc.

Jastram, K., & Newland, K. (2003). Family unity and refugee protection. In E. Feller, V. Türk & F. Nicholson (Eds.), *Refugee protection in international law: UNHCR's global consultations on international protection.* Cambridge: Cambridge University Press.

Loescher, G. (2001). *The UNHCR and world politics: A perilous path.* Oxford: Oxford University Press.

Mehraby, N. (2000). Therapy with refugee children. Retrieved March 11, 2008 from http://www.swsahs.nsw.gov.au/areaser/Startts/article_2.htm.

Miller, T. W. (2007). Trauma, change, and psychological health in the 21st century, *American Psychologist*, 889–898.

Mollica, R. F., & Jeon, W. T. (2001). The magnitude of the refugee mental health problem: A worldwide survey. In W. T. Jeon, M. Yoshioka & R. F. Mollica (Eds.), *Science of refugee mental health: New concepts and methods*. Harvard: Center for Mental Health Services.

Mollica, R. F. (2001). Assessment of trauma in primary care. *Journal of American Medical Association, 285*(9), 1213.

Moreno, A., Piwowarczyk, L., & Grodin, M. A. (2001). Human rights violations and refugee health. *Journal of American Medical Association, 285*(9), 1215.

Moss, W. J., Ramakrishnan, M., Storms, D., Siegle, A. H., & Weiss, W. M. (2006). Child health in complex emergencies. *Bulletin of the World Health Organization, 84*(1), 58–64.

Murphy, H. B. M. (1955). The extent of the problem. In H. B. M. Murphy (Ed.), *Flight and resettlement*. Paris: UNESCO.

Office of Refugee Resettlement. (2007). *Unaccompanied refugee minors*. Washington, DC: Office of Refugee Resettlement.

O'Hara, R. (2006). 2005 statistical issue: 2005–2006 US refugee program. *USCRI Refugee Report, 27*(1), 1–20.

Papadopoulos, R. K. (2001). Refugee families: Issues of systemic supervision. *Journal of Family Therapy, 23*, 405–422.

Refugees International. (2004). Sexual exploitation in Liberia: Are the conditions ripe for another scandal? Retrieved January 20, 20007 from http://www.refugeesinternational.org/content/article/detail/957/?mission.

Rumbaut, R. G. (1991). The agony of exile: A study of the migration and adaptation of Indochinese refugee adults and children. In F. L. Ahearn & J. L. Athey (Eds.), *Refugee children: Theory research, and services*. Baltimore: The Johns Hopkins Press.

Secretary General's Bulletin. (2003). Special measures for protection from sexual exploitation and sexual abuse, *United Nations DocumentSGB/2003/13*.

SIPRI. (2004). *Armaments, disarmament and international security*. Sweden: SIPRI Yearbook.

Steel, Z., Silove, D., Phan, T., & Bauman, A. (2003). Long-term effect of psychological trauma on the mental health of Vietnamese refugees resettled in Australia: A population based study. *Lancet, 360*, 1056–62.

Sossou, M. A., Craig, C. D., Ogren, H., & Schnak, M. (2008). A Qualitative Study of Resilient Factors of Bosnian Refugee Women Resettled in the Southern United States, *Journal of Ethnic & Cultural Diversity in Social Work, 17*(04), 365–385.

The State of the World's Refugees. (2006). *Human displacement in the new millennium*. Oxford: Oxford University Press.

United Nations, (1951). The 1951 refugee convention. Geneva: UNHCR.

UNHCR, (1998). State of the World's Refugees, 1997–1998: A Humanitarian Agenda. Geneva: United Nations High Commissioner for Refugees.

UNHCR. (1999). Protecting Refugees: A field guide for NGOs. UNHCR: United Nations Publications Number GV.E.99.0.22.

UNHCR. (2002). UNHCR resettlement handbook. Geneva: UNHCR.

UNHCR. (2003a). Refugee youth: Building the future. Retrieved March 11, 2008 from http://www.unhcr.org/events.html.

UNHCR. (2003b). Framework for durable solutions for refugees and persons of concern. Geneva: UNHCR.

UNHCR. (2004). *Resettlement handbook*. Geneva: UNHCR Department of International Protection.

UNHCR. (2005). *2004 global refugee trends: Overview of refugee populations, new arrivals, durable solutions, asylum-seekers, stateless and other persons of concern to UNHCR.* Geneva: Population and Geographical Data Section Division of Operational Support.

UNHCR. (2006a). Refugees by numbers 2006 edition. Retrieved March 11, 2008 from http://www.unhcr.org/basics.html.

UNHCR. (2006b). *2005 global refugee trends: Statistical overview of populations of refugees, asylum-seekers, internally displaced persons, stateless persons, and other persons of concern to UNHCR.* Geneva: UNHCR field information and coordination support section & division of operational services.

UNHCR. (2007). *UNHCR statistical yearbook 2006: Trends in displacement, protection and solutions.* Geneva: UNHCR.

UNIFEM. (2005). The Impact of the Conflict on Congolese Women. Retrieved January 20, 2007 from http://www.womenwarpeace.org/drc/drc.htm.

USCRI. (2003). *World refugee survey 2003 Country Report.* Washington, DC: United States Committee for Refugees and Immigrants.

Vega, W. A., & Rumbaut, R. G. (1998). Ethnic minorities and mental health. *Annual Review of Sociology, 17*, 351–383.

Ward, C., Bochner, S., & Furnham, A. (2001). *The psychology of culture shock.* New York: Routledge.

Weine, S. (2001). From war zone to contact zone: Culture and refugee mental health services. *Journal of American Medical Association, 285*(9), 1214.

WHO. (2007). Health of migrants: Migration flows and the globalized world. WHO Report by the Secretariat, EB122/11. Retrieved April 20, 2008 from http://www.who.int/gb/ebwha/pdf_files/EB122/B122_11-en.pdf.

WHO. (2008). Health of migrants: Migration flows and the globalized world: WHO Report by the Secretariat A61/12. Retrieved April 20, 2008 from http://www.who.int/gb/ebwha/pdf_files/A61/A61_12-en.pdf.

Women's Commission for Refugee Women and Children. (2004). *Global survey on Education in Emergencies.* New York: Women's Commission for Refugee Women and Children.

World Refugee Survey. (2003). Country Report.

Zhang, A. Y., Snowden, L. R., & Sue, S. (1998). Differences between Asian and White-Americans' help-seeking and utilization patterns in the Los Angeles area. *Journal of Community Psychology, 26*, 317–326.

Chapter 25

Religious Worldviews and Stressful Encounters: Reciprocal Influence from a Meaning-Making Perspective

Crystal L. Park, Donald Edmondson, and Mary Alice Mills

The goal of this chapter is to explore religion and spirituality (R/S) in the context of stressful life events. In particular, we examine two primary issues: (1) how R/S influences people's appraisal of, and coping with, both normative transitions and unexpected crises, and (2) as part of the coping process, how life transitions and crises influence individuals' subsequent R/S. We begin with a description of the meaning-making framework of stress and coping (Park and Folkman 1997; Park 2005a) and describe how religiousness/spirituality is a central part of this framework for many people. We then use this framework to integrate theory and empirical literature on these two primary issues. The meaning-making framework is broad enough to encompass the coping challenges that are considered within both the stressful life events approach and the developmental or normative transition approach. This broader framework, therefore, includes positive events that may be stressful but that are sought after (e.g., college, marriage), as well as negative life events. While many have noted the role of religious beliefs in transforming the appraisal or interpretation of negative events (e.g., Pargament 1997), we propose that the interaction of R/S meaning systems and stressful life events is best conceptualized as an ongoing and recursive process of mutual influence (see Fig. 25-1). This chapter will examine the existing empirical research relevant to the recursivity hypothesis and conclude with suggestions for future research.

A Framework of Meaning-Making Coping

A meaning-making framework is a useful construction for integrating and further developing the research on coping with life stressors. This framework is based on a stress and coping model (Lazarus and Folkman 1984), but furthers the model in a number of ways. Like the stress and coping model, the meaning-making model relies heavily on the assumption that individuals' cognitive appraisal of stressors underlie and drive the process of coping. However, the meaning-making model provides a more sophisticated framework by explicitly

From: *Handbook of Stressful Transitions Across the Lifespan*,
Edited by: T.W. Miller, DOI 10.1007/978-1-4419-0748-6_25,
© Springer Science+Business Media, LLC 2010

Reciprocal Influences of R/S Meaning System and Traumatic Experiences

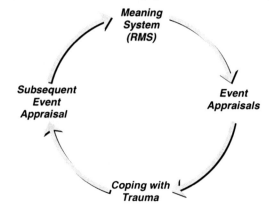

Fig. 25-1. Reciprocal influences of R/S meaning system and traumatic experiences

distinguishing between two levels of meaning, global meaning and the appraised meaning of specific events.

Global meaning refers to individuals' core beliefs and goals. Global *beliefs* are basic internal cognitive structures that individuals construct about the nature of the world. These core beliefs guide individuals throughout the lifespan by informing their ongoing construal of reality, including their under-standing of themselves, the world, and themselves in relation to the world (Silberman 2005). Global *goals* are basic internal representations of the over-arching desired ends toward which people strive. These global goals consist of goal hierarchies that encompass overarching ends and all of the intermediate goals that lead towards those ends (Emmons 2005; Park and Folkman 1997). Appraised *meanings* refer to meanings assigned to particular events, such as categorizing an event as a loss, threat, or challenge; determining the causes of the event's occurrence and assigning attributions (e.g., God's will, coinci-dence). These situational judgments follow from the global meaning system and determine the extent to which the event is discrepant with the global system of meaning. On the basis of these (often unconscious) calculations, individuals make decisions regarding appropriate cognitive, emotional, and functional responses to the event (i.e., choosing coping strategies).

According to this model, distress arises when an individual's appraised meaning of a particular event challenges or violates her global beliefs or goals. This perceived discrepancy between appraised and global meaning is an exceedingly uncomfortable state, one that people are highly motivated to reduce. To alleviate the attendant distress, the discrepancy between the appraised meaning of the event and the basic beliefs and goals that have been disrupted by it must be reduced (Park 2005a). The processes through which people reduce this discrepancy involve changing the appraised meaning of the situation, changing their global beliefs and goals, or both. Such changes of either the appraised meaning of situations or the global meaning facilitate integration of the appraised (or eventually reappraised) meaning of the event into the global meaning system (Parkes 1993; Klinger 1998). Such integration should lead to resolution of and adjustment to the event (e.g., McIntosh et al. 1993; Park et al. 1996).

Meaning-making coping is often characterized as attempting to see the event in a better light (e.g., Pearlin 1991) or as cognitively "working through" the event (e.g., Creamer et al. 1992). It may involve meaning-making mechanisms, such as reappraising events as more positive or creating more benign reattributions (i.e., finding more acceptable reasons why an event occurred and who or what is responsible for its occurrence (Baumeister 1991; Taylor 1983). Meaning making is the primary means by which individuals cope with major trauma and loss, since such events are highly discrepant with one's global beliefs and are not amenable to "problem solving" efforts. Through meaning-making coping, the individual is able to endure the negative event by either transforming its meaning so that it contains (at least somewhat) positive elements and can be assimilated, or transforming the meaning system itself to accommodate such an occurrence (Joseph and Linley 2005). It seems that the former strategy is more prevalent than the latter in most cases, as even slight changes to meaning systems impact on the entire system, thus becoming precarious.

Religion as a Primary Meaning System

Meaning systems are transmitted and maintained by culture, and as such reflect cultural beliefs and more. Although meaning systems are not necessarily constructed on religious or spiritual foundations, they often are (Park 2005a). This is particularly true in the U.S., which is among the most religious of the developed nations (Paul 2005). The General Social Survey conducted in 2004 found that 86% of Americans are affiliated with a religious faith and 78% pray at least once a week (Norris and Inglehart 2004). Another indication of religion's importance in the U.S. is the low opinion of most Americans regarding people without religious faith. Over half of the population reports an unfavorable opinion of atheists (54%) and people without religious faith (51%) (Pew 2002). Given the prominent role religion plays in American society as a whole, it is not surprising that for many people, religious beliefs and attitudes form the core of a global meaning system that informs their beliefs about the world, the self, and their interaction (Pargament et al. 2005b; McIntosh 1995).

Religion is often highly salient in times of highly stressful events, and some theorists have asserted that religion arose from humanity's need to understand the deepest problems of existence (Geertz 1966). Nietzsche wrote that "He who has a why to live for can bear almost any how" (1886). Religion is often referred to as the prime example of a belief system that shapes individuals' understanding of the world and makes the reality of suffering understandable and bearable (e.g., Pargament 1997). In this capacity, religious belief systems provide individuals with comprehensive and integrated frameworks of meaning that can explain events in highly satisfactory ways (Spilka et al. 2003). Such stable frameworks of meaning are particularly important in interpreting and responding to the most extraordinary and difficult aspects of life, such as suffering, death, tragedy, and injustice (e.g., Pargament 1997), but provide a way of understanding mundane occurrences as well (e.g., Geyer and Baumeister 2005; Spilka et al. 2003). Because of their roots in the sacred and supernatural, religious meaning systems can be highly comprehensive, fundamental, and unfalsifiable, creating a system that informs both situational and global beliefs, as well as personal goals with a high degree explanatory power and low-likelihood disconfirmation (Emmons et al. 1998; Emmons 2005).

In the same way that one's culture colors all facets of perception, including judgments of others (Miller 1984; Wojciszke et al. 1998), memory construction (Kunda 1990), and moral boundaries on cognition (Tetlock 2003), the religious meaning system influences information processing at a situational level. The ubiquity of religion's influence for the devout may be likened to the theory of chronic construct accessibility in cognition research. Chronic accessibility suggests that individuals are more likely to perceive new information as related to constructs that are self-relevant and have been employed frequently over a long period (Bargh 1984). In the case of religious meaning systems, individuals possess robust frameworks for stimulus interpretation that are frequently used, rarely falsifiable, and are usually reinforced by a community of like-minded stimuli interpreters (Baumeister 1991). As such, belief systems allow a measure of automaticity in perception, attribution, and decision-making; they, therefore, shape the experience of situational events as well as provide a sense of ultimate purpose (Becker 1962). Thus, the way that people interpret events and respond to them may be largely determined by the particulars of their religious faith, and events that may appear objectively neutral or value-free may be infused with religious meaning.

The influence of religion on global beliefs is far-reaching. In addition to explicit religious beliefs, such as the existence of God and the possibility of an afterlife, religion can inform and influence other global beliefs that are less explicitly religious, such as beliefs in fairness, control, coherence, benevolence of the world and other people, and vulnerability (Pargament 1997). For example, in describing the Just World Theory (Lerner 1980), Janoff-Bulman and Frantz (1997) note that "Theories of deservingness generally encompass many religious perspectives, which enable believers to perceive meaning through the expectations of rewards and punishments that may be considerably delayed, such as one's fate after death" (p. 93). When religion is incorporated into people's global meaning systems, their understanding of God (e.g., loving and benevolent, wrathful) is connected to beliefs about the nature of people (e.g., inherent goodness, sinful), of the self (e.g., chosen by God, unworthy of God), of this world (e.g., transient, illusion), and the next (e.g., Heaven, reincarnation) (McIntosh 1995; Silberman 2005).

Similar to its role in shaping beliefs, religion is central to the life purpose of many people (e.g., Baumeister 1991; Emmons 2005) and provides the ultimate motivation or goal for living as well as prescriptions and guidelines for selecting and achieving goals. In addition to supplying meaning for events, religion also provides a sense of control and order, standards by which one may judge one's actions, and a source of self-esteem based on the adherence to such standards. Perhaps because of its chronic accessibility and ubiquitous influence on individuals' perceptions of reality, R/S beliefs and their subjective importance are fairly constant across the lifespan. Some evidence suggests that the intensity of religiosity increases slightly as people age (see Park 2006, for a review) but there are also important, and often radical, individual differences (e.g., religious conversions) (Paloutzian 2005).

The meaning system that is primarily steeped in religious faith is more stable than most because of its cultural transmission, community and divine assent, and claims on eternity, though it is not immune to alteration or, in some cases, radical overhaul (Rambo 1993). Stressful life transitions often include taking on new roles and incorporating new ways of thinking, perceiving, and navigating in the natural or social world. Often, the new demands imposed by development cause individuals to reconsider certain modes of perceiving or understanding. While the initial system alterations may be small in the case of a transition, such as from high school to college (e.g., contact with new ways of thinking, new cosmologies), they may create incongruencies in the meaning system (e.g., evidence seems to support evolution). The meaning-making framework, similar to cognitive dissonance theory, posits that such discrepancies must be reconciled for psychological equanimity to be restored.

The possession of a culturally transmitted, community-supported, and unfalsifiable system for understanding the world and one's place in it is thought to be helpful for people undergoing stressful life transitions as well as encountering traumatic events (Emmons 2005; Pargament et al. 2005a). One of the characteristics of a religious meaning system that is unique in this regard is that religion usually claims to transcend time. Thus, while people usually understand transition periods to be circumscribed, the significance and possible benefits associated with those periods in light of eternity may help to make the temporary discomfort bearable (Baumeister 1991). While the notion that ascribing meaning to suffering is beneficial for people in the midst of hardship is not new (Kierkegaard 1843/1985; Nietzsche 1886; Frankl 1946, 1969), finer distinctions have recently been drawn that impose qualifications on such assertions when meaning is derived from religious systems. Empirical studies have shown that religious meaning systems are generally helpful in coping with stressful life events, but may also be harmful. Whether a particular individual will reap benefits from a religious meaning system in a given situation may be determined by a number of religious, personal, event-specific, temporal, and contextual factors (see Pargament 1997, for a review). For example, a number of studies of bereavement have shown that religious beliefs may initially be associated with more distress, more perceptions of violations of global meaning, and more cognitive processing (e.g., Park 2005a; McIntosh et al. 1993). These studies indicate that religiousness may eventually be helpful, following an extended period of meaning making. It also appears that some types of religious meaning systems can give rise to excessive self-blame or guilt, leading to poorer adjustment following stressful encounters (Exline and Rose 2005). The meaning system perspective attempts to explain the activation, impact, and outcome of religious coping from a transactional framework that allows for mutual influence between the meaning system and life events.

The transactional nature of religious meaning and life events becomes most visible in the case of traumatic events that temporarily overwhelm the entire meaning system. In some cases, such events create a dramatic and severe discrepancy between the religious meaning system and the initially incongruent appraisal of the event. In this situation, the individual becomes unmoored, as the implications of the discrepancy are sufficient to call into question the veracity of the entire meaning system. The individual's state in the aftermath of an event in which such a discrepancy is initiated has been called one of "shattered assumptions" (Janoff-Bulman 1992). Religion is not always implicated in such discrepancies, but the likelihood that religious meaning will be activated in response to a stressful event would likely correspond to the degree that religion is used as a coping strategy (i.e., its centrality in the individual's global meaning system). Therefore, for individuals for whom religious constructs are chronically accessible, it is highly likely that religious coping will be activated in response to a given stressor (Pargament 1997).

The impact of the religious meaning system in coping with life stressors is multi-faceted and far reaching. Because religion serves as the basis for the global beliefs and goals of many individuals, religious meaning often plays crucial roles throughout the coping process (Pargament 1997). In the following section, we describe the influences of religious global meaning systems in coping with stressful life events and transitions. One part of this process, the changing of global meaning in response to/as part of coping with, stressful life experiences is a particular focus because this component, although the subject of surprisingly little empirical study, holds the key to understanding an immensely influential aspect of the development and change in individuals' religious meaning over the life course.

Influence of Religious Meaning Systems on Coping with Life Stressors and Transitions

Religious meaning systems can influence the kinds of initial appraised meaning that people give to events, the extent to which this appraised meaning is discrepant with their global meaning, and the types of resources and coping strategies available to reduce their distress. The extent to which religion is involved in a given individual's coping with a particular event is largely predicated on the extent to which religion is part of his or her meaning system: Religion is far more likely to be used in the coping of those for whom religion is a highly salient aspect of their understanding of self and world than in the coping of those who are less devout (see Pargament 1997, for a review).

The nature of the event also determines the likelihood of religious involvement. For example, if the stressful event is one that is not amenable to being "repaired" (i.e., problem-solved), such as illness or death, meaning-making efforts become more central (Mattlin et al. 1990). It is in these situations that religion may have its greatest impact, by helping to restore beliefs that the world is safe, predictable, fair, and controllable, and that there is, perhaps, a benevolent God in charge of it all (Pargament 1997; Dull and Skokan 1995). Spilka et al. (1985) were some of the first researchers to offer an explicit theory of religion's role in the construction of meaning. Their attribution theory of religion focused on three circumstances in which people are likely to draw on religious beliefs as a means of understanding events. First, novel or unexpected events that challenge the individual's existing meaning system are likely to initiate religious attributional processes. Secondly, events that challenge individuals' sense of personal control or the predictability of events trigger similar searches. Thirdly, events that damage the individual's self-esteem may be transformed in an effort to restore a positive self-concept. The activation of religious explanation is a function of characteristics of the individual (e.g., the degree and character of the R/S held), the event (e.g., the degree of importance to the individual), and the context (e.g., whether the event occurred in a religious setting). Importantly, Spilka et al.'s (1985) attribution theory of religion proposes that the specific aspects of an individual's religious faith that will be activated to form attributions of stressful events will be those that are congruent with the individual's established meaning system, that restore controllability to events, and that enhance self-esteem.

Religion and Initial Appraised Meaning of Stressors

Research indicates that religion commonly influences the initial appraised meanings of stressors (Pargament 1997). For example, religion is often involved in causal attributions following traumatic events (Spilka et al. 1997). In their classic study of spinal cord injury victims, Bulman and Wortman (1977) found that over a third of the sample spontaneously mentioned God's will as the reason for their injury. Similarly, in a study of bereaved college students, most attributed the death at least partially to a loving or purposeful God (Park and Cohen 1993). Beyond that, the same event can be viewed quite differently depending on an individual's specific religious views. Some individuals may believe that God would not harm them or visit upon them more than they could handle, increasing their sense of coping efficacy, whereas others may believe that God is trying to communicate something important through the event, or that the event is a punishment from God (Exline and Rose 2005; Gall 2004). For example, a study of prostate cancer survivors found that the most common attributions were to a purposeful God, and that those who attributed their cancer to an angry God had poorer mental and social functioning and higher levels of self-blame (Gall 2004).

Religion and Meaning-Making Coping

If an event is determined to be discrepant with one's global beliefs and goals, attempts at meaning-making coping – the process of reappraising a situation and thinking through its implications – will follow. The eventual outcomes of this meaning-making coping are changes in appraised meaning of the stressful event and, sometimes, changes in global meaning. Because religious beliefs tend to be relatively stable, people confronting crises are more likely to reappraise their perceptions of situations to fit their pre-existing beliefs than to change their religious beliefs (Pargament 1997). Once meaning has been made (i.e., the event is integrated satisfactorily into one's global meaning system), the distress will be alleviated (Baumeister 1991; Janoff-Bulman and Frantz 1997). This pattern is well demonstrated by a study of parents who lost a child to Sudden Infant Death Syndrome (SIDS) (McIntosh et al. 1993). Results showed that parents who reported more religiousness engaged in more meaning-making coping (defined as thinking about the child and the death, which reflected attempts to integrate the death into existing schemas) 3 weeks after the death, and that meaning-making coping was related to more distress cross-sectionally. Longitudinally, however, meaning-making coping was related to less distress and higher levels of well-being. Further, religiousness was only indirectly related, through meaning-making coping, to overall adjustment.

Religion and Changes in Appraised Meaning

Religion can influence the specific coping options available to individuals confronted with difficult situations (Pargament 1997). In addition to prayer, individuals frequently report using a wide variety of other religious coping strategies, including benevolent religious reappraisals, "punishing God" reappraisals, religious forgiveness, seeking of religious support, and spiritual discontent (Pargament et al. 2000). Thus, it appears that making reappraisals is a major form of religious coping.

Pargament (1997) described the power of religion to transform the meaning of events: "When the sacred is seen working its will in life's events, what first seems random, nonsensical and tragic is changed into something else – an opportunity to appreciate life more fully, a chance to be with God, a challenge to help others grow, or a loving act meant to prevent something worse from taking place" (p. 223). While conceptually, these additional insights can be either positive or negative, research suggests that religion often facilitates more benign reattributions (Frazier et al. 2004; Kunst et al. 2000). Religion can be involved in changing the appraised meaning of a stressful situation by (a) providing a means to make more benign reattributions, (b) helping the individual to see the positive aspects of the stressful situation, and (c) facilitating perceptions of stress-related growth (Park 2005a).

Because religious beliefs, like other basic beliefs, tend to be relatively stable, people confronting crises are thought to more often change their perceptions of situations to fit their pre-existing beliefs than they are to change their religious beliefs (Joseph and Linley 2005; Pargament 1997). Religion can be involved in reappraisals, or changes in situational meaning, by offering additional possibilities for causal attributions and by illuminating other, potentially more positive, aspects of stressful situations including perceptions of growth from the stressor. While, theoretically, reappraisals can be either positive or negative, the motivation to reduce stress generally leads to placing stressful situations in more positive contexts by giving them a more acceptable meaning, one more consistent with global beliefs and goals. As reviewed below, numerous lines of research suggest that religion is often involved in these attempts to make more benign attributions and facilitating the perception of positive aspects of stressful situations and stress-related growth.

Religious Reattributions

In the context of significant stress or traumatic events, the, attributional process involves the development of an understanding of why an event occurred. Although initial attributions may be made following a trauma or crisis, a search for more acceptable reasons for the event's occurrence in the months following it is common (Davis et al. 1998). People often make reattributions that help to alleviate their initial distress (see Park and Folkman 1997). For example, people may initially feel that God neglected to care for them or even deliberately and unjustly caused their trauma. Over time, however, people often come to see the stressful event as the will of a loving or purposeful God, even if it is a God who is inscrutable and beyond human understanding (Spilka et al. 2003). Religion offers many avenues for making positive reattributions, and is frequently invoked in the search for a more acceptable reason why an event occurred than the cause originally identified, attributions that are more consistent with individuals' global beliefs and goals. For example, people can come to see the stressful event as a spiritual opportunity, as the result of a punishing God, or as the result of human sinfulness (Pargament 1997). Baumister (1991) described the "attributional blank check" that many religions offer, that possibility of believing that God may have higher purposes that humans cannot understand, so that one may remain convinced that events that seem highly aversive may, in fact, be serving desirable ends, even if one is unable to guess what these ends might be. Thus, religious explanations may allow religious individuals to trust that every event, regardless of its initial appearance and painfulness, is part of God's plan (Baumeister 1991).

Religion and Positive Reinterpretation

Positive reinterpretation involves identifying and focusing on the benefits or positive implications that may follow from stressful encounters. Positive reinterpretation is a very common, and generally very adaptive, coping response (Aldwin in press). Many religious traditions emphasize the necessity of, and possible positive outcomes of, enduring the difficulties in life (Aldwin in press). For example, Christian scripture states, "Not only so, but we also rejoice in our sufferings, because we know that suffering produces persever-ance; perseverance, character; and character, hope. And hope does not disap-point us, because God has poured out his love into our hearts by the Holy Spirit, whom he has given us" (Romans 5:3–5, NIV).

While few psychologists of religion have studied the concept of theodicy, this construct seems to hold great promise for understanding how people come to withstand life's difficulties, even severely traumatic events. Theodicy refers to the explanation for human suffering, "philosophical/theological attempts to reconcile the presence of evil and suffering in the world with the idea of an all-powerful and good creator God" (Hall and Johnson 2001, p. 5). Hall and Johnson (2001) discussed how individuals can hold only two of the following three propositions simultaneously: God is all-powerful, God is all good, and evil exists. They note that people struggle to find some way to believe that these three statements are not logically incompatible or defend the plausibil-ity of God's existence in the light of these seemingly contradictory proposi-tions. Such struggle to make meaning or hold onto one's beliefs in a powerful and loving God when one has personally experienced evil or severe negative trauma can be great (Pargament 1997; Kushner 1981).

Several solutions to this dilemma can be found, that avoid having to alter one's global meaning system. Hall and Johnson (2001) note that one influential Christian viewpoint holds that goodness can occur only in a world where evil also exists, particularly those virtues that an individual comes to practice only through suffering because of evil, such as patience, mercy, forgiveness, endurance, faith, courage, and compassion (Hall and Johnson 2001). Under this meaning system, one can come to see one's traumatic or stressful experience as an opportunity to grow through one's suffering (e.g., to build one's soul, to become more Christ-like, to grow in agape love; Hall and Johnson 2001). Another solution may be to view one's suffering as necessary for reaching future events, such as one's ultimate goal of salvation (Baumeister 1991).

Religion and Stress-Related Growth

In addition to reattributions and more positive or hopeful views of the stressful event, religious meaning systems may help individuals to identity the personal growth that often follows even the most highly stressful situations (Park 2006). This phenomenon of "stress-related growth" (Park et al. 1996) or "post-traumatic growth" (Tedeschi and Calhoun 1996) has garnered intensive research focus in the past 10 years (Park and Helgeson 2006); high proportions of individuals encountering even the most stressful of circumstances, including cancer, rape, natural disasters, and combat, often report experiencing benefits or growth from their stressful encounter. While the veridicality of these reports has yet to be validated, the fact that many people do identify positive changes and that these positive changes may help individuals adjust to stressful encounters, is established (Park and Helgeson 2006). Further, one of the most robust predictors of growth following stressful events is religiousness (see Joseph and Linley 2005, for a review).

Alterations in the appraised meaning of a crisis or trauma usually allow the individual to view the stressful situation in a less distressing way, and religion clearly commonly plays an important role in reappraisals of the meaning of the situation. Although religion commonly facilitates the making of more positive meanings, religious reinterpretations are not always positive. For example, people sometimes come to believe that God harmed them, either through deliberate action or through passivity and neglect. These negative results of the making-meaning process can lead to mistrust, anger, hurt, and disappointment towards God, or even doubt regarding God's existence (Exline and Rose 2005).

Religion and Changes in Global Meaning

Although less common than reappraisals of the particular stressor, traumatic events are sometimes so discrepant with global meaning that no amount of situational reappraisal will restore a sense of congruence with the individual's pre-existing global meaning. In such instances, individuals may reduce the discrepancy between their understanding of an event and their global meaning by changing their fundamental global beliefs or goals. Thus, following traumatic events, people sometimes dramatically alter their beliefs about God, themselves, and the world (McCullough et al. 2005). For example, sometimes those with faith may come to view God as less powerful (Kushner 1981), or cease to believe in God altogether. Others may come to believe that they are unable to comprehend everything that happens in the world or God's reasoning for it, while others may become convinced of their own sinful nature (Exline and Rose 2005; Pargament 1997). Individuals may also change or reprioritize their global goals (Emmons et al. 1998).

Such changes in global beliefs and goals may entail the development of new models for the world, the self, or their interaction. When people experience extreme stress and have difficulty coping, they may end up switching their congregations or denominations, or even undergoing a religious conversion – far more radical religious or spiritual transformation (Spilka et al. 2003; Paloutzian et al. 1999). Their new-found denomination or religion may provide alternative frameworks of meaning that help people answer their difficult questions and solve their life problems as well as a new system of purposes and goals (Pargament 1997; see Paloutzian 2005, for a review). One interesting outcome of a meaning system overhaul, such as religious conversion, is an increase in the convert's certainty of life's meaning and associated goals (Paloutzian 1981).

Religious Meaning-Making Coping and Adjustment

Research suggests that the adjustment outcomes of religious meaning-making coping are often positive (see Ano and Vasconcelles 2005, for a review). These relationships between religion, coping, and adjustment following stressful events are complex, however. Particularly in cases in which an individual must modify the meaning system to accommodate new information, an implied uncertainty about the system may persist (e.g., "if I was wrong before..."). Thus, there may be a decrement in well-being while the modified system is consolidated, with improvement occurring as the meaning system once again becomes automatic in providing a framework for events, a view of self, and a prescription for appropriate responses to future stimuli. Such a proposition has yet to be fully tested, although some prior studies provide preliminary support for this process (e.g., Park 2005b; McIntosh et al. 1993).

Lasting Impact of Stressful Life Events on Religious Meaning Systems

Many studies have demonstrated that religious strategies are among the most common forms of coping following stressful life events (e.g., Koenig et al. 1988), and, as reviewed above, religious coping often plays a central role in making meaning following stressful events. While much remains to be learned about many aspects of religion and the meaning-making process, one critical aspect remains virtually unexamined: what are the long-term effects of coping with traumatic or highly stressful events on one's religious meaning system? Can an individual experience the most challenging of life's events without some alteration, in one direction or another, in the religious meaning system? Theoretically, global beliefs, and in particular religious global beliefs, are robust and capable of absorbing the vast majority of events and information encountered. In a properly functioning meaning system, traumatic events should be reappraised to reduce the discrepancy between situational and global meanings in order to facilitate integration of new material into the pre-existing structure and avoid the long-term distress that accompanies a ruptured belief system (Park 2005a). As discussed earlier, religion may have some negative consequences at the initial stages of coping, when individuals are struggling to make meaning of negative events that seem to contradict their religiously oriented beliefs (Hall and Johnson 2001), yet religious systems also encourage the meaning making of negative events in benign ways that ultimately reduce distress and protect pre-existing global meaning.

Empirical work on this question is sparse, and results are contradictory (see Smith 2004). Some answers to the question are found in studies of conversion, which suggest that for some people encountering high levels of life stress, their entire religious meaning system may be discarded in favor of a newer and more emotionally satisfying one (see Paloutzian 2005, for a review). However, most individuals do not experience a conversion following highly stressful events. How do their meaning systems change, if at all, as a result of their stressful encounters? Studies addressing this issue have produced somewhat equivocal results, with some showing trauma appears to strengthen religious beliefs and behaviors (Emmons et al. 1998; Pargament 1997; Valentine and Feinauer 1993), and others showing it to be associated with more negative religious meaning systems (Finkelhor et al. 1989; Rossetti 1995). One rare prospective study of trauma and global beliefs (assessing beliefs prior to the experience of a trauma) found that beliefs in fatalism and justice were not significantly affected by a range of traumatic events, whereas self view and vulnerability were negatively impacted (Gluhoski and Wortman 1996). Interestingly, in the case of justice, individuals who experienced only one self-focused trauma demonstrated an increase in just world beliefs, an effect the authors suggest might be attributable to self-blame attributions, which would serve to preserve the existing meaning structure. Such an interpretation is consistent with the negative shift in self view that was observed following trauma. Another study of survivors of war trauma in the former Yugoslavia found that they had higher levels of religious faith than did a sample of matched controls (Basoglu et al. 2005).

A study focusing explicitly on religious belief change in individuals who had experienced at least one high magnitude stressor found that close to 30% reported some change in religious beliefs after their first or only traumatic event. Further, the experience of multiple victimizations was associated with higher levels of intrinsic religiosity (Falsetti et al. 2003). Using logistic regression, Falsetti and colleagues explored multiple potential predictors of belief change and found the post-traumatic stress disorder (PTSD) status to be the only significant indicator. That is, significantly more individuals with PTSD reported changes in beliefs than those without PTSD. The direction of the change was inconsistent, however, with 20% of individuals with PTSD becoming more religious after trauma (compared to 9% of the PTSD negative group) and 30% becoming less religious (compared to 6% of the PTSD negative group). Whether PTSD might result in part from a disruption to the religious meaning system, or whether PTSD may in part effect a disruption of beliefs is unclear. The process may in fact be transactional, with multiple individual, coping, and contextual factors contributing to and maintaining distress. Pargament (1997) points out that individuals use a system of both religious and non-religious beliefs and practices to manage stressful events, making it difficult to isolate effects. The term "religious coping" itself covers a broad array of strategies, some of which may be assimilative in nature (i.e., seeking to maintain one's belief system) and some of which may be more transformational (i.e., seeking new sources of meaning) (Pargament 1997). Though empirical data describing what might determine the use of one strategy over another is lacking, it is likely that individuals with more deeply held and chronically accessible religious meaning systems will engage more successfully in assimilation (ultimately fitting the event into pre-existing meaning structures) compared to those who attempt to access a religious meaning framework primarily in response to a challenging event. This may be partly due to the fact that religion assures the individual that everything will make sense at some point, a comforting belief that cannot be disconfirmed (Baumeister 1991).

Fortunately, life-shattering events are relatively rare occurrences, and it is possible that a religious meaning system might never be tested against the backdrop of severe trauma. However, given the generally high prevalence of high magnitude stressors, experiences of normative but stressful life transitions, and vicarious exposure to tragic world events, it is fair to assume that, for many individuals, religious meaning systems are continually tested and gradually modified across the lifespan. While some individuals experience a loss of faith in the face of extreme or cumulative stress, others may become strengthened in their current religious meaning system and develop an increasingly effective repertoire of coping skills based on that understanding. Still others may undergo more radical changes, converting their faith. Understanding the long-term impact of coping with stressful encounters on one's global meaning system of beliefs and goals, and particularly their religious meaning system, is a potential avenue not only for gaining a better understanding of human nature but also for developing interventions for individuals undergoing stressful experiences. Unfortunately, for now, the literature consists primarily of intriguing hypotheses and minimal solid empirical findings.

Directions for Future Research

In general, our review of the literature suggests that much remains to be understood about meaning systems in the processes of confronting stressful events, including the influences of meaning systems on appraising, coping with, and adjusting to stressors. Because so little is understood, many areas are ripe for sophisticated research; in particular, we think that the issues of theodicies, long-term changes in religious meaning systems, and individual differences in the meaning-making process are especially promising areas for future study.

This research must take a more sophisticated approach to the subject matter than much of the research to date has, first because meaning-making processes are, by definition, *processes*. Thus, the nuanced changes unfold over time. Therefore, longitudinal research is requisite, particularly research that involves multiple measurements of both meaning and adjustment constructs over time. Ideally, future studies would be prospective, assessing individuals' meaning systems prior to the stressful event under study as well as afterward. Unfortunately, prospective studies of stressful events are extremely difficult to conduct for logistic reasons, as most highly stressful experiences are not anticipated (which is part of the reason why they are perceived as all that stressful). Some possibilities for prospective studies include examining people about to embark on transitions that are considered generally positive, but that are still highly stressful (e.g., moving away from home or having a child). Another approach is longitudinal research with large samples, as such studies will eventually yield large enough numbers of individuals encountering stressful events (e.g., see prospective research on conjugal bereavement by Bonnano et al. 2004). If prospective research is not possible, then control groups as closely matched to the sample as possible should be employed.

Secondly, the issues of measurement are critical in examining the influence of religious and spiritual meaning and meaning making on the experience of and adjustment to stressful life events. These constructs are theoretically very rich, but the strategies for capturing them empirically have been heretofore relatively impoverished. In particular, it behooves researchers to carefully select assessment tools that closely match the constructs which they purport to measure (Park and Ai 2006). Unfortunately, good measures of most of the meaning-making constructs have not been developed. Qualitative research is still needed in this area, as is rigorous quantitative measurement development.

Another means by which to target specific aspects of meaning systems, most likely to be influenced by negative events, is through experimental manipulation. Work on the identification, creation, and maintenance of meaning in the face of physical or psychological threats has flourished over the past two decades (see Greenberg et al. 2004, for a review) and continues to yield promising findings and novel research methods (see Proulx and Heine in press, for a review).

In sum, we propose that the meaning-making framework is a useful way to organize the current literature regarding the role of religion on adjustment to stressful life encounters. Further, we believe that gaining a more comprehensive understanding of the recursive processes through which religious meaning systems shape the ways that individuals experience challenging events, and, in turn, how those events shape religious meaning systems will ultimately shed light on processes of faith development and maturation, as well as provide insight into one potential road to resilience and wisdom.

References

Aldwin, C. M. (2007). *Stress, coping, and development,* 2nd edn. New York: Guilford.

Ano, G. G., & Vasconcelles, E. B. (2005). Religious coping and psychological adjustment to stress: A meta-analysis. *Journal of Clinical Psychology, 61,* 461–480.

Bargh, J. A. (1984). Automatic and conscious processing of social information. *Handbook of social cognition,* vol 3. pp. 1–43.

Basoglu, M., Livanou, M., Crnobaric, C., Franciskovic, T., Suljic, E., Duric, D., et al. (2005). Psychiatric and cognitive effects of War in Former Yugoslavia: Association of lack of redress for trauma and posttraumatic stress reactions. *JAMA: Journal of the American Medical Association, 294,* 580–590.

Baumeister, R. F. (1991). *Meanings of life.* New York: Guilford.

Becker, E. (1962). *The birth and death of meaning, a perspective in psychiatry and anthropology.* New York: Free Press of Glencoe.

Bonnano, G. A., Wortman, C. B., & Nesse, R. M. (2004). Prospective patterns of resilience and maladjustment during widowhood. *Psychology and Aging, 19,* 260–271.

Bulman, R. J., & Wortman, C. B. (1977). Attributions of blame and coping in the "real world": Severe accident victims react to their lot. *Journal of Personality and Social Psychology, 35,* 351–363.

Creamer, M., Burgess, P., & Pattison, P. (1992). Reaction to trauma: A cognitive processing model. *Journal of Abnormal Psychology, 101,* 452–459.

Davis, C. G., Nolen-Hoeksema, S., & Larson, J. (1998). Making sense of loss and benefiting from the experience: Two construals of meaning. *Journal of Personality and Social Psychology, 75,* 561–574.

Dull, V. T., & Skokan, L. A. (1995). A cognitive model of religion's influence on health. *Journal of Social Issues, 51,* 49–64.

Emmons, R. A. (2005). Striving for the sacred: Personal goals, life meaning and religion. *Journal of Social Issues, 61,* 731–751.

Emmons, R. A., Colby, P. M., & Kaiser, H. A. (1998). When losses lead to gains Personal goals and the recovery of meaning. In P. T. P. Wong & P. S. Fry (Eds.), *The human quest for meaning* (pp. 163–178). Mahwah, NJ: Erlbaum.

Exline, J. J., & Rose, E. (2005). Religious and spiritual struggles. In R. F. Paloutzian & C. L. Park (Eds.), *Handbook of the psychology of religion and spirituality* (pp. 315–330). New York: Guilford.

Falsetti, S., Resick, P., & Davis, J. (2003). Changes in religious beliefs following trauma. *Journal of Traumatic Stress, 16,* 391–398.

Finkelhor, D., Hotaling, G. T., Lewis, I. A., & Smith, C. (1989). Sexual abuse and its relationship to later sexual satisfaction, marital status, religion, and attitudes. *Journal of Interpersonal Violence, 4,* 379–399.

Frankl, V. E. (1946). *Man's Search for Meaning: An introduction to logotherapy.* Washington, DC: Washington Square Press.

Frankl, V. E. (1969). *The will to meaning.* New York: New American Library.

Frazier, P., Tashiro, T., Berman, M., Steger, M., & Long, J. (2004). Correlates of levels and patterns of positive life changes following sexual assault. *Journal of Consulting and Clinical Psychology, 72,* 19–30.

Gall. (2004). The role of religious coping in adjustment to prostate cancer. *Cancer Nursing, 27,* 454–461.

Geertz, C. (1966). Religion as a cultural system. In M. Banton (Ed.), *Anthropological approaches to the study of religion* (pp. 1–46). London: Tavistock.

Geyer, A. L., & Baumeister, R. F. (2005). Religion, morality, and self control: Values, virtues, and vices. In R. F. Paloutzian & C. L. Park (Eds.), *Handbook of the psychology of religion and spirituality* (pp. 412–432). New York: Guilford.

Gluhoski, V. L., & Wortman, C. B. (1996). The impact of trauma on world views. *Journal of Social and Clinical Psychology, 15,* 417–29.

Greenberg, J., Koole, S. L., & Pyszczynski, T. A. (2004). *Handbook of experimental existential psychology.* New York: Guilford.

Hall, M. E. L., & Johnson, E. L. (2001). Theodicy and therapy: Philosophical/ethological contributions to the problem of suffering. *Journal of Psychology and Christianity, 20,* 5–17.

Janoff-Bulman, R. (1992). *Shattered assumptions: Towards a new psychology of trauma.* New York: Free Press.

Janoff-Bulman, R., & Frantz, C. M. (1997). The impact of trauma on meaning: From meaningless world to meaningful life. In M. Power & C. Brewin (Eds.), *The transformation of meaning in psychological therapies: Integrating theory and practice.* Sussex, England: Wiley & Sons.

Joseph, S., & Linley, P. A. (2005). Positive adjustment to threatening events: An organismic valuing theory of growth through adversity. *Review of General Psychology, 9,* 262–280.

Koenig, H. G., George, L. K., & Siegler, I. (1998). The use of religion and other emotion-regulating coping strategies among older adults. *The Gerontologist, 38,* 303–310.

Kierkegaard, S. (1843/1985). *Fear and trembling.* New York: Penguin Books.

Klinger, E. (1998). The search for meaning in evolutionary perspective and its clinical implications. In P. T. P. Wong & P. S. Fry (Eds.), *The human quest for meaning* (pp. 27–50). Mahwah, NJ: Erlbaum.

Kunda, Z. (1990). The case for motivated reasoning. *Psychological Bulletin, 108*(3), 480–498.

Kunst, J. L., Bjorck, J. P., & Tan, S. (2000). Causal attributions for uncontrollable negative events. *Journal of Psychology and Christianity, 19,* 47–60.

Kushner, H. S. (1981). *When bad things happen to good people.* New York: Avon Books.

Lazarus, R. S., & Folkman, S. (1984). *Stress and coping.* New York: Springer.

Lerner, M. J. (1980). *The belief in a just world: A fundamental delusion.* New York: Plenum Press.

Mattlin, J. A., Wethington, E., & Kessler, R. (1990). Situational determinants of coping and coping effectiveness. *Journal of Health and Social Behavior, 31,* 103–122.

McCullough, M. E., Bono, G., & Root, L. M. (2005). Religion and forgiveness. In R. F. Paloutzian & C. L. Park (Eds.), *Handbook of the psychology of religion* (pp. 394–411). New York: Guilford.

McIntosh, D. N. (1995). Religion as schema, with implications for the relation between religion and coping. *The International Journal for the Psychology of Religion, 5,* 1–16.

McIntosh, D. N., Silver, R. C., & Wortman, C. B. (1993). Religion's role in adjustment to a negative life event: Coping with the loss of a child. *Journal of Personality and Social Psychology, 65,* 812–821.

Miller, J. G. (1984). Culture and development of everyday social explanation. *Journal of Personality and Social Psychology, 46*(5), 961–978.

Nietzsche, F. (1886). *Beyond good and evil (W. Kaufmann, Trans.).* New York: Vintage.

Norris, P., & Inglehart, R. (2004). *Sacred and secular: Religion and politics worldwide.* Cambridge: Cambridge University Press.

Paloutzian, R. F. (1981). Purpose in life and value changes following conversion. *Journal of Personality and Social Psychology, 41,* 1153–1160.

Paloutzian, R. F., Richardson, J. T., & Rambo, L. R. (1999). Religious conversion and personality change. *Journal of Personality, 67,* 1047–1079.

Paloutzian, R. F. (2005). Religous conversion and spiritual transformation: A meaning-system analysis. In R. F. Paloutzian & C. L. Park (Eds.), *Handbook of the psychology of religion and spirituality* (pp. 331–347). New York: Guilford.

Pargament, K. I. (1997). *The psychology of religion and coping: Theory, research and practice.* New York: Guilford.

Pargament, K. I., Ano, G. G., & Wacholtz, A. B. (2005a). The religious dimension of coping: Advances in theory, research, and practice. In R. F. Paloutzian & C. L. Park (Eds.), *Handbook of the psychology of religion and spirituality* (pp. 479–495). New York: Guilford.

Pargament, K. I., Koenig, H. G., & Perez, L. M. (2000). The many methods of religious coping: Development and initial validation of the RCOPE. *Journal of Clinical Psychology, 56,* 519–543.

Pargament, K. I., Magyar, G. M., & Murray-Swank, N. (2005b). The sacred and the search for significance: Religion as a unique process. *Journal of Social Issues, 61,* 655–687.

Park, C. L. (2005a). Religion and meaning. In R. F. Paloutzian & C. L. Park (Eds.), *Handbook of the psychology of religion and spirituality* (pp. 295–314). New York: Guilford.

Park, C. L. (2005b). Religion as a meaning-making framework in coping with life stress. *Journal of Social Issues, 61,* 707–730.

Park, C. L. (2006). Religion, health, and aging. In C. M. Aldwin, C. L. Park & A. Spiro III (Eds.), *Handbook of health psychology and aging.* New York: Guilford.

Park, C. L., & Ai, A. L. (2006). Meaning-making and growth: New directions for research on survivors of trauma. *Journal of Loss and Trauma, 11,* 389–406.

Park, C. L., & Cohen, L. H. (1993). Religious and nonreligious coping with the death of a friend. *Cognitive Therapy and Research, 6,* 561–577.

Park, C. L., Cohen, L. H., & Murch, R. (1996). Assessment and prediction of stress-related growth. *Journal of Personality, 64,* 71–105.

Park, C. L., & Folkman, S. (1997). Meaning in the context of stress and coping. *General Review of Psychology, 1,* 115–144.

Park, C. L., & Helgeson, V. S. (2006). Growth following highly stressful life events: Current status and future directions. *Journal of Consulting and Clinical Psychology, 74,* 791–796.

Parkes, C. M. (1993). Bereavement as a psychosocial transition: Processes of adaptation to change. In M. S. Stroebe, W. Stroebe & R. Hansson (Eds.), *Handbook of Bereavement* (pp. 91–101). Cambridge, UK: Cambridge University Press.

Paul, G. S. (2005). Cross-national correlations of quantifiable societal health with popular religiosity and secularism in the prosperous democracies. *Journal of Religion and Society, 7,* http://moses.creighton.edu/JRS/2005/2005-11.html Retrieved 9/4/06.

Pearlin, L. I. (1991). The study of coping: An overview of problems and directions. In J. Eckenrode (Ed.), *The social context of coping* (pp. 261–276). New York: Plenum.

Pew Research Center for the People and the Press (2002). *Americans struggle with religion's role at home and abroad.* http://pewforum.org/publications/surveys/religion.pdf. Retrieved 9/4/06.

Proulx, T., & Heine, S. J. (2006). Death and black diamonds: Meaning, mortality, and the meaning maintenance model. *Psychological Inquiry, 17,* 309–318.

Rambo, L. R. (1993). *Understanding religious conversions.* New Haven, CT: Yale University Press.

Rossetti, S. (1995). The impact of child sexual abuse on attitudes toward God and the Catholic Church. *Child Abuse and Neglect, 19,* 1469–1481.

Silberman, I. (2005). Religion as a meaning system: Implications for the new millennium. *Journal of Social Issues, 61,* 641–663.

Smith, S. (2004). Exploring the interaction of trauma and spirituality. *Traumatology, 4,* 231–243.

Spilka, B., Hood, R. W., Jr., Hunsberger, B., & Gorsuch, R. (2003). *The psychology of religion: An empirical approach* (3rd ed.). New York: Guilford Press.

Spilka, B., Shaver, P., & Kirkpatrick, L. A. (1985). A general attribution theory for the psychology of religion. *Journal for the Scientific Study of Religion, 24,* 1–20.

Spilka, B., Shaver, P. P., & Kirkpatrick, L. A. (1997). A general attribution theory for the psychology of religion. In B. Spilka & D. N. McIntosh (Eds.), *The psychology of religion: Theoretical approaches* (pp. 153–170). Boulder, CO: Westview Press.

Taylor, S. E. (1983). Adjustment to threatening events: A theory of cognitive adaptation. *American Psychologist, 38,* 1161–1173.

Tedeschi, R. S., & Calhoun, L. (1996). The Posttraumatic Growth Inventory: Measuring the positive legacy of trauma. *Journal of Traumatic Stress, 9,* 455–471.

Tetlock, P. E. (2003). Thinking the unthinkable: Sacred values and taboo cognitions. *Trends in Cognitive Sciences, 7,* 320–324.

Valentine, L., & Feinauer, L. (1993). Resilience factors associated with female survivors of childhood sexual abuse. *The American Journal of Family Therapy, 21,* 216–224.

Wojciszke, B., Bazinska, R., & Jaworski, M. (1998). On the dominance of moral categories in impression formation. *Personality and Social Psychology Bulletin, 24,* 1251–1263.

Chapter 26

Life Stress Buffer: The Salubrious Role of African-Centered Spirituality

Evangeline A. Wheeler

Life Stress Buffer: The Salubrious Role of African-Centered Spirituality

Contemporary life is challenging enough for most of us with interminable to-do lists, multitasking, long work days and commutes, and struggles to meet simple goals like assembling the family for a traditional dinner around the kitchen table. But for a large proportion of the African American population, the simple stress of living is often magnified. Additional factors of entrenched poverty, chronic disease, juvenile crime and societal prejudice raise questions of how people cope under such circumstances. Many African Americans find that the negative consequences of blatant prejudice ultimately manifest in issues of mental and physical well-being (Carter 1994; Landrine and Klonoff 1996). People cope with life stress and transitions in the lifespan in myriad ways, but for many people identified with African American culture, a primary resource is an African-centered spiritual base.

The Need for an African-Centered Spiritual Perspective

Unlike ethnic immigrants from Europe or Asia who migrated voluntarily to the United States early in its history, African Americans were forced here by the economics of institutionalized slavery. For centuries now, concomitant with the growth of the United States itself, African Americans have lived with the legacy, in manifestations both subtle and overt, of origins as enslaved Americans. And even though the culture of this group has been the foundation of many national artistic and cultural trends, most notable recently in the twenty-first century global youth culture, the psychological legacy commonly reflects adjustments to centuries of systemic and systematic racial bias. Analysis of the historical effect is complex and multidisciplinary, not unlike an African worldview that emphasizes connectedness and Gestalt. Curry (1981) found that both African Americans and African-born Blacks perceive their relationship to their environment in terms of cooperative

From: *Handbook of Stressful Transitions Across the Lifespan,*
Edited by: T.W. Miller, DOI 10.1007/978-1-4419-0748-6_26,
© Springer Science+Business Media, LLC 2010

and interdependent social relations. Though the life experiences of African Americans are the focus, there is at all times the more general implicit reference to the psychological experiences of all people in the African diaspora whether they are living now in Europe, Africa, Asia, the Caribbean, Central America, or elsewhere.

Arguably, the effects of American slavery are indelibly imprinted in the psychological state of present day African Americans. Slavery itself was designed as an institution to destroy self-esteem and self-identity. For example, Guthrie (1998; original source: Cartwright 1851), in a discussion of how nineteenth century scientists interpreted the mental health of African people, explains that as enslaved Africans tried to cope with the dehumanizing aspects of slavery, they often attempted physical escape from bondage. Scientists of the day labeled this behavior draptomania, and defined it as a mental illness rather than as a coping strategy. It was said to afflict Africans with moods of sullenness, and the preventative way was to treat them like children. It is no wonder, then, that the lifespan development of African Americans might take a different trajectory, one which incorporates the realities of longstanding racial bias. The scientific literature holds many instances of how racism was officially codified and objectified.

In early nineteenth century Europe, several worldviews about human identity and difference competed for cultural and political authority, with consequences for how African Americans would later be viewed. Religious theories, for example, rivaled scientific ones for legitimacy, and potentially offered alternative worldviews for the representation of human variation. But, by the middle of the century, scientific theories, and particularly theories of stages of human development, had won in the contest for the most authoritative representation of the facts of nature. The eminence of scientific stage theories coincided not only with the popularity of Darwin's theory of evolution, but also with the nascent colonial imperialism of the time. Now stage theories could be used to justify ranking and categorizing cultures. European culture was typically at the top levels of the hierarchy. Stage theories produced by western culture/cultural scientists tended to judge people from other cultures and ethnic groups in terms of how closely their resemblances matched, placing themselves in a relatively superior level of development, a process that feminists scholars label as constructing the other. The German philosopher Hegel, for example, ranked all societies on a scale based on classification of religious beliefs, ranking at the top, Christianity, which later came to be used as a weapon of cultural and racial oppression. Eventually, colonized and enslaved African people were forbidden to practice their traditional spirituality and were offered the oppressor's religion instead.

Social scientists Morgan (1877) and Spencer (1876) proposed that humanity had progressed from savagery (African culture) to civilization (European culture) in a series of stages. Lévy-Bruhl's (1928) great divide theory separated the cognitive processes of western culture people and others, ranking that of the other as deficient. Thus, throughout history hierarchical theories provided academic justification for imposing western culture hegemony around the world, since it could be demonstrated with scientific methods that European culture was, by definitions and standards of the European theorists themselves, superior. The utility, then, of a traditional stage theory approach can be very dubious when used to account for the normal psychological development of the African people. Many people of Africa and the African diaspora harbor a tenacious distrust of scientific theory since history shows us that slavery and colonialism were perpetuated with the support of scientists.

There are several different critiques of scientific theorizing, as historically conceptualized, which have important implications for the psychological well-being and lifespan development of African Americans. Stage theories have been used not only to impose nonAfrican culture, and to rank people of African descent at the bottom of the heap, but they have been used as a tool of scientific oppression, and critiqued on the basis of being antithetical to African worldview elements of nonlinear progression, social collectivity, and the centrality of spirituality. A related problem with the application of stage theories is the implicit assumption that the culture being described places a high value on individual achievement. For instance, in Erikson's (1950) theory of psychosocial development, it is apparent that the successful progression through the eight stages results in the individual becoming increasingly autonomous, independent, industrious, and self-initiating. These stages embrace values of rugged individualism, and apply less to Africans' traditional cultural infrastructure, which tends to be firmly collectivist in orientation with an emphasis on interpersonal relations and community. Kelsey and Ransom (1983) found that African Americans are more communally oriented than are European Americans.

Instead, in African-centered psychology, the belief is that you can know who you are only after you have achieved intimacy, not independence. The importance of this is that community becomes a source of strength and serves as a cushion in terms of crisis. An individual is never alone and thus less likely to need help in the form of psychotherapy. The values associated with western culture are replaced in African culture by interdependence, self-sacrifice, and dedication to family and group members. Thus, the problem with stage theories, from the perspective of African-centered psychology, is that they were initially used to justify imperialism, and they usually assume that the individual is more vital than community.

Yet another problem with stage theories is in the conception of a linear progression through stages, moving forward in time from less developed to more developed psychological states. A more African-centered approach would view adult development in many dimensions with people passing through life events when the time is right, and perhaps in nonlinear fashion (Dahl 1995). Also, the flexible functioning of African Americans with regard to time is well known in African American communities.

It was also in the nineteenth century that scientists began measuring racial characteristics of African Americans in terms of hair texture, shades of skin color, thickness of lips, and shape of skulls (Gould 1993). Such enterprising anthropometric research could be dismissed as the work of scientists living in a racist milieu were it not for the strong connection between this early work and current twenty-first century issues of psychological development in blacks. Their findings helped to create ideas on ideal skin tone (Clark and Clark 1940) and hair texture that became precursors for current self-esteem issues among blacks. Spirituality plays a role in helping to overcome issues of negative self-esteem as African-descended people appeal to supernatural forces, God and gods to restore positive self-concepts eroded by the work of some scientists.

Historically, most of the canonical lifespan researchers and stage theorists like Erikson do not typically include any complete discussion of the role of spirituality in their theories of human psychological development. Piaget (1952) does not mention spirituality in cognitive development, nor does Kohlberg (1984) address it in moral development. According to Maslow's (1962) theory of self-actualization, people are motivated first to satisfy biological, safety and belongingness needs before tackling the highest goal of self-actualization. This hierarchy is in potential conflict with the African-centered emphasis on social harmony and spiritual interdependency as the highest attainment. In order to apply stage theories of the life span to people of Africa and the African diaspora, the interconnectedness of community and spirituality must be incorporated, and should occupy indeed a privileged place.

As a general critique, traditional lifespan theories raise an issue for groups of people outside the western cultural tradition on the grounds that theory devoid of spirituality as a primary focus cannot apply to a description of their developmental progress, for spirituality is an integral, indispensable constituent of daily lives. How, then can theories of lifespan development presume to apply universally? How can theories be instead revised to include psychological elements that affect a large majority of the world's people, and not just those primarily of western culture? Again, Erikson, who did incorporate a cross-cultural aspect in his work, wrote that all people go through eight stages of psychosocial development across the lifespan, resolving a predictable challenge at each one. The first challenge and crisis of adulthood, for example, is how to establish intimacy with other people. The last challenge of elder hood/the elderly is acceptance of one's life already lived, and of imminent death. This is an interesting order of challenges, since Erikson proposes that people in this final stage also achieve spiritual tranquility and acquiescence of their lives. From the point of view of African-centered psychological development, though, it seems that spiritual challenges in this last stage of adulthood might in fact occur earlier, since a measure of spiritual tranquility is often a necessary ingredient for successful transition through all adulthood stages, early to late. It is here that we arrive at one concrete example of the reasons that western culture theories cannot always be generalized to people of African descent. Erikson's theory, however, is still a useful frame of reference as an adjunct to life span theory infused with African-centered spiritual notions.

Most lifespan theories tend to group African American samples as part of the larger group of Americans, who are largely middle class and of European descent, but since the social and economic backgrounds of the American majority and the American minority are so drastically different, new developmental models need to account solely for the experiences of African Americans, in the manner of cross-cultural life span developmental psychology, as demonstrated by Baltes and Baltes (1990), who are sensitive to sociohistorical contexts. The lifespan literature now contains scholarship that acknowledges cultural differences and its influence on human development. Many researchers have tested the development of ethnic identity primarily in terms of stage models with their characteristic qualitatively distinct changes. However, given the concerns of the stage model to truly capture the dynamic nature of ethnic identity, other researchers examine the development of ethnic identity in terms of continuous growth as opposed to discrete changes in a particular stage. The traditional stage model may not capture subtle changes in ethnic identity over short periods of time, whereas a model of continuous growth will do so.

This maturing cultural perspective originated with the recognition that theoretical perspectives based principally on the observations of middle-class white European culture did not often seem applicable to people of Chinese, Indian, Middle-Eastern or African descent. Before this, most of developmental child psychology, for instance, concerned itself with the influence of parent–child relations and prenatal environment while largely omitting culture and race as significant variables in lifespan development. Most mainstream researchers believed that, for example, except for differences in phenotype and socioeconomic status, black children and white children progressed psychologically in not dissimilar ways. The consequence of theorizing with no assumed basis of difference is that the mental, psychological and physical developmental patterns of European middle-class children became the standard by which the development of all children was judged. But now, many developmental and social psychologists regard ethnic identity as one of many facets of an individual's social identity (Sellers et al. 1998), due in large part to the presence of ethnic researchers and the changing demographics of the nation. Bernal et al. (1990) used a cognitive developmental framework to examine the steps in the process of the acquisition of ethnic identity in preschool and elementary school-age children. Multiple models of ethnic identity development have been proposed for African Americans, Latino Americans, and European Americans. A more appropriate theoretical framework for discussing development,need to incorporate also the centrality of spirituality in the healthy life-span psychology of African Americans, explain the inadequacy of traditional psychology as a model of healthy psychological development for African Americans, and create a workable synthesis between traditional western approaches to stage theories of human development and the spirituality of African peoples. For people of African descent, spirituality pays attention to key moments in the life span of each individual as well as in the community.

If we understand the role of spirituality, it can help to counter prevalent notions of African Americans and other blacks as a people hopelessly and psychologically crippled by racism and economic disadvantages. Recurrent in the history of African American culture is a theme pertaining to the need for the salubrious effects of a spiritual orientation in order to maintain psychological health. The psychological character and behavior of African Americans whether labeled normal or abnormal can be comprehended only in terms of the historic power relations between privileged and oppressed groups here in the United States. Spirituality tinged with an acute awareness of social conditions is the uniqueness offered from the lived experiences of black people descended from Africa.

The Concept of African-Centered Spirituality

Spirituality is identified with experiencing a deep-seated sense of meaning and purpose in life, together with a sense of belonging. It is about acceptance, integration and wholeness. The centrality of spirituality for African Americans, and its modern manifestation in daily life, is a legacy of the treatment that enslaved and colonized Africans received worldwide beginning over four hundred years ago. This important spiritual factor is absent in most traditional Eurocentric explanations of life-span development relevant to African Americans. Spirituality concerns the age-old human quest to understand the inexplicable and to seek fulfillment and transcendence amidst the welter of human experience. In an African-centered framework, it is something that permeates all human activities and experiences, rather than being additional to them. It is a process of transformation and growth. By prioritizing, for African Americans, an African-centered spirituality in Western theories of human development, we gain a better appreciation for the enormous influence it has on cognitive, social, interpersonal, physical and emotional aspects of daily living. To theorize about how psychological development occurs throughout life, it is necessary to locate developing individuals within their spiritual milieu. Mainstream psychology textbook chapters on psychological development, typically discuss how we learn love and attachment, recognize human facial expressions, learn gender roles, make friends and face the crises of adulthood as we grow through life, but rarely is there mention of forming spiritual bonds. Even in many cross-cultural texts, the word "spirituality" cannot be found in the index.

Within the field of psychology, a number of definitions of spirituality have been offered (Jagers and Smith 1996; Elkins et al. 1988), although until recent decades, spirituality was considered by psychologists to be antithetical to scientific study. Since discussions of spirituality are oftentimes confused with talk of religions (see Mattis 2000 for a distinction), psychologists have had to be careful with operational definitions. Elkins et al. for example, synthesized a list of nine spirituality components as a part of their definition of spirituality from a humanistic perspective: transcendent dimension, meaning and purpose in life, mission in life, sacredness of life, material values, altruism, idealism, awareness of the tragic, and fruits of spirituality. Such definitions facilitate academic discussions of spirituality, but the problem with this and some other popular conceptions is that they developed out of the intellectual formulations of Western thinkers rather than out of the direct experiences and articulations of African-descended people. Definitions of the concept of spirituality for African Americans must involve the major influencing factor of racism and the fact that spirituality is an integral element of daily existence. In an African-centered framework, psychology and spirituality are not separate, the secular and the sacred are one, and psyche and spirit are united (Edwards 1994).

People of Africa and the African diaspora have come to express a similar spirituality in many different ways from each other given the singular influences from African, European, Islamic, and Native American cultures with which they have lived. They are alike in that all recognize the special priority of their African roots. Each spiritual tradition, in its development in varying cultural contexts, was presented with particular challenges to its fight for survival, which in turn shaped the development of its cultural heritage. The numerous spiritual traditions are alike in that each shares a long cultural history of enslavement both psychological and physical, and of severe racial discrimination. The various traditions all developed, to some extent, as a reaction against psychological oppression. Voudoun, candomblé, santeria, revival Zion (an Afro-Christian religious sect in Jamaica), the African-American Christian church, are examples.

For example, in North America, while scarcely one-ninth of antebellum Virginia's African people were free, the black church gained ascendance. In the republic of Haiti, Africans transformed their traditional religion into voudoun as the country achieved independence from France in 1804. In Brazil, where slavery was not outlawed until 1888, a different spiritual expression, candomblé, developed. Although originally confined to the slave population, banned by the Catholic church and even criminalized by some governments, candomblé thrived for over four centuries, and expanded considerably after the end of slavery in the late 1800s. In pre abolition Cuba free people of color made up nearly one-third of the colony's African population. The colonial period from the standpoint of African slaves may be defined as a time of perseverance when colonial laws criminalized their religion and their familiar ways of coping with the world. Paramount was a need to maintain survival under harsh plantation conditions. This was accomplished by maintaining, in secret, the essence of what today is called Santería. Santeria, a combination of African and Catholic traditions, developed among the displaced Africans in Cuba. Sandoval (1979) notes that, Santeria serves as a mental health system for many Afro-Cubans. Even today, there continues to be sociocultural influences on the varieties of contemporary African-American spiritual practices such as the Yoruba (a traditional African religion from Nigeria), the Akan (a traditional African religion from Ghana), the Moors, the Nation of Islam, and the Hebrew Israelites.

Each spiritual tradition became the focus for an extraordinary struggle against and triumphs over the local systems of brutal psychological and physical exploitation. They share an elevated sense of solidarity against injustice and a commitment to the protection and advancement of their communities. Many spiritual rituals of African people have certain elements in common. Most of them share rhythmic drumming, dancing, the use of trance as a catharsis, and call-response that encourages active participation in worship. Afrocentric scholars like Nobles (2006), Ani (1997), and Welsing (1991), while not developmental theorists, all include spirituality as consequential in their definitions of healthy psychological functioning throughout life. Collectively, they define spirituality as the vital life force that animates us and connects us to the rhythms of the universe, nature, the ancestors, and the community. A full realization and acceptance of the fact that our spiritual force is a primary drive leads to bonding with community in ways that alleviate psychological suffering caused by centuries of oppression.

African spirituality marks through ritual and ceremony many of the key moments in the life of the individual, particularly birth, initiation, marriage and death. Fully developed, general lifespan theories must describe rituals that people go through at each stage of life because psychologically, the ritual instills self confidence and courage to take on a new role in the community (Mbiti 1975). Spirituality tells the individual at these moments that she exists because of the community. Therefore the community celebrates these key points on the life journey of the person. In doing so the community is renewing its own life, and reliving the cycle of its existence. These important components of spirituality fit traditional stage theories in two interesting ways. The first is the way in which stage theories were used historically to aid in the psychological and political oppression of certain groups, and the second is the implicit cultural values of stage theories. Spirituality is a reaction to the culture's attempt at oppression.

It was Azibo (1991) who wrote that since African-centered psychology requires an understanding of the past, present and future that this worldview actually began with the ancient civilization of Kemet, where Africans had produced an organized system of knowledge. As a theoretical perspective, formulations of African-centered psychology developed within African Studies departments in the university in the 1970s, during a time of great societal attention to and activism on the issue of civil rights for African Americans. This particular point of view privileges the interpretations of reality as experienced by people of African descent. It determines which events are meaningful and which are not. Early theorists emphasized the differences between African centered and Eurocentric worldviews, and psychologists began to apply the approach to the understanding of African American psychology, including new diagnoses of culturally specific disorders and a delineation of the characteristics of an African personality, as an alternative to theories which had often cast African Americans in positions of deficiency and inferiority. Differences in the two worldviews lie principally among the dimensions of spirituality, interdependence, collectiveness, time orientation, death and immortality and kinship.

Many scholars now work to define a general cultural developmental framework relevant to African Americans, even though the population is widely diverse along a number of different dimensions. Several in the academic tradition of African-centered psychology have addressed the inadequacy of applying models of human functioning based on European-centered assumptions and standards to the behavior of people of African descent (Akbar 1981; Awanbor 1982; Azibo 1991; Baldwin 1985, 1986; Dixon 1976; Kambon 1998; Lambo 1974; Nobles 1976; White 1972). According to African-centered psychology, one cannot function as a self-assured, confident and productive adult in the community unless one has achieved, for instance, a measure of Erikson's last stage, first. But, of course, Erikson recognized cultural factors that might affect psychological development. That is, some societies make the transitions through life changes much easier with rites of passage, for instance, which serve to give the young person a definite sense of who she is and how she is relevant to the community, thereby attenuating the crisis of Erikson's fifth stage, identity versus role confusion. This sort of acknowledgement of cultural factors is just one example of how African-centered and Western theories can mesh.

Literature in Afrocentric psychology highlights the various limitations of traditional psychological approaches developed in a Western cultural context when applied to people of African descent (Toldson and Toldson 2001). Using a case study approach Atwell and Azibo (1991) compared clinical diagnoses of black clients using two distinct diagnostic systems, the DSM-III-R and the African centered Azibo Nosology. The importance of the comparison is that the standard used Eurocentric DSM-III-R is often challenged as inadequate regarding the diagnosis of personality disorder in people of African descent. Eighteen disorders peculiar to the African personality are found in the Azibo Nosology that have no precedent in the DSM-III-R. They conclude that the African centered diagnoses more accurately reflect the real-life conditions of Africans and recommend that therapists working with African American clients take note. Researchers propose that an African-centered perspective need be adopted, one that explains how the African perspective operates in the context of the diasporic family with regard to such psychological issues as identity development, mental health, self-esteem, and crisis intervention. It links the context of African peoples' lives to the traditions, values and spiritual essence of traditional African culture in an attempt to acknowledge the African, and generally, the nonWestern worldview.

One example of a framework for understanding an African centered approach is that of *sankofa* (Wheeler 2002), an Akan term that means, "We must go back and reclaim our past so we can move forward, so we understand why and how we came to be who we are today." Another very well-known model of African American psychological development from an African centered perspective is Cross's (1971) model of Nigrescence. It is a five-stage model (preencounter, encounter, immersion-emersion, internalization, internalization-commitment) for moving from self-hatred to self-love. Cross (1995) suggests that people in the first preencounter stage believe that one's race does not influence events and they rarely prioritize their racial group membership. Their group-esteem could be positive or negative, but their exploration is very low. A person in this stage might even think of European culture as superior. The second encounter stage follows the occurrence of a bewildering, often surprising, overtly racially, and perhaps personally experienced prejudiced event that startles a person from her original naïve view to one that recognizes racism. According to Cross, this critical encounter can be initiated from a series of many small, negative incidents which increase awareness of racism, as well an event of singular racial import. Many African Americans report daily small encounters with suspected racism, as experienced in impolite service in retail outlets, sub-optimum medical care, or lower grades in school. An individual might enter this stage as a result of witnessing a racial event happening to a close friend or family member. As a result of the encounter, the person now decides to fully embrace the concept of her ethnic identity, exploring the meaning of this and fully immerses herself into everything that is defined by the concept. This is an attempt to combat feelings of negative worth as an effect of the encounter.

Upon emerging from this third immersion-emersion stage, people enter the fourth internalization stage in which they are confident and proud of their identity as an ethnic Black person and have a positive group-esteem. Individuals in the fifth internalization-commitment stage take their confidence in and commitment to their race one step further and work actively toward elevating the status of African Americans and often engage in antiracism activist work. It is possible for individuals to stagnate at the immersion-emersion stage and not move on or to recycle back through the stages at later points in life after experiencing a new encounter (Parham 1989).

Theorists see the need even to formulate different, specific diagnoses of psychological dysfunction in African-descended people, diagnoses that are culturally biased and take into account the ramifications of the conditions of longtime cultural oppression (Azibo 1989; Baldwin 1984; Wilson 1993). Recent clinical research supporting such distinctions shows that interventions with women of African descent that result in increased endorsement of Afrocentric values and beliefs, particularly a belief in spiritual, nonmaterially based satisfaction, may lead to a reduction in psychological symptoms like depression, anxiety, and anger (Dubois 1999; also see Potts 1991). Spiritually based beliefs and practices provide strategies for finding solutions to life problems as well as peace of mind. African American folk beliefs and traditional healing practices provide coping strategies that are particularly important for psychological health and survival. Four elements of folk healing have been determined: spirituality, ritual, power of words and dreams (Parks 2007).

The primary factor to consider in the healthy psychological development and lifespan of African Americans is the effect of the longstanding history of worldwide oppression of African people and the chronic exposure to racially charged experiences. Spirituality holds a unique position in the psychology of African-descended people because of systematic political and social oppression around the world, so people of African descent and people of European descent experience life differently and thus could be expected to develop dramatically different psychological processes which allow them to cope. Given this difference in life experiences, it is not surprising that African-descended people have developed psychological strategies for making the transition through the various stages of life which may not be described by Western-culture inspired theories. These different experiences usually result in varying perspectives, contrasting worldviews, assumptions, expectations, levels of trust, issues of identity, coping styles, values and self-esteem.

Several empirical studies (Azibo 1983; Curry 1981; Fine et al. 1985; Kelsey and Ransom 1983) have noted beliefs and behaviors among African Americans that reflect of an African centered worldview. Azibo (1983) found that African Americans with higher levels of Black consciousness exhibited a more communal orientation than did African Americans with lower levels of Black consciousness. Fine et al. (1985) found that African Americans with an African centered worldview were more likely to be optimistic, holistic, and spiritual than were those who were not African centered. They were also more likely to possess intrinsic self-worth. Among youth, McMahon and Watts (2002) suggest that ethnic identity is an important component of development and is associated with a range of positive feelings and health-related outcomes, more active coping strategies, and lower levels of aggression.

How Spirituality Facilitates Transitions

Everybody encounters developmental milestones, but African Americans may go through uniquely characterized ones given the quotidian nature of perceived racism (Pinel 1999) to which most admit. Several studies suggest that spirituality as a factor is important for adjustment to many of life's challenges like dealing with chronic medical concerns of cancer or obesity, suicide, mental illness, general well-being, academic performance, self-actualization, coping with stress and sense of community.

General Health

At all levels of income, education and age, a spiritual focus or religious affiliation is a reliable predictor of self-reported senses of well-being, satisfaction with family life and subjective health. In fact, four out of every five Americans believe that spirituality promotes health (Matthews 1997). A study of African American women with breast cancer (Simon et al. 2007) suggests that while the women participants expressed varied methods of coping with breast cancer, overall spirituality was a key component in their coping process from diagnosis through recovery and on to survivorship. This finding might warrant a caveat, however, because sometimes people with strong spiritual beliefs may, to their detriment, delay seeking needed medical care or refuse procedures which could save their lives. Lannin et al. (1998) suggest that one reason the death rate from breast cancer is higher among African American women than among white women is because some cultural beliefs may lead to a delay in seeking appropriate care. African American women, for instance, are more likely to agree with the statement: "If a person prays about cancer, God will heal it without medical treatment."

In efforts to develop existing client resources and strengths, Hatch and Derthick (1992) explored the ways that Black churches may be incorporated in the promotion of health and wellness in African American communities. They recommend empowering Black churches to develop and implement prevention programs in health promotion and disease prevention. Church-based efforts focused on prevention and early intervention would reach a large subset of obese or overweight African American women who might not otherwise seek support or assistance with their eating problems or concerns about body image. Structured twelve-step approaches to treating overeating might be another useful approach because they complement thinking styles that reflect a belief or emphasis on the power of spiritual forces in the universe to influence everyday life, and they support the belief that functioning is optimal when in synchronicity with this spiritual life force (Davis et al. 1999).

Coping

African Americans of all ages use several different coping strategies such as spirituality, activism, cultural pride, and reliance on kinship ties and other forms of social support (Bryant-Davis 2005; Christian and Barbarin 2001; Spencer et al. 2003). Utsey et al. (2007) investigated the role of culture-specific coping in relation to resilient outcomes in African Americans from high-risk urban communities. Findings indicated that spiritual and collective coping were statistically significant predictors of the quality of life outcomes above and beyond the traditional predictive factors.

Religiosity is often reported as a crucial coping mechanism, but, a primary difference in the lifespan development for African Americans is that religion and spirituality have historically played such a large and salient role in the life cycle of most. They tend to attend church services more regularly than nonblacks and to engage more in religious behaviors like reading religious texts, praying in daily rituals or listening to gospel music. Jackson and Sears (1992) studied a sample of African American women and found that among those who experience low levels of emotional well-being, an African centered worldview may be especially helpful since many of their stressors are a result of oppression and other cultural factors. Therefore, counselors with an understanding of African centered worldview can assist in empowering African American women with an understanding of their behaviors and feelings from a culturally positive perspective.

Psychological Illness and Health

In the scientific literature on nursing, much new work examines the role of spiritual resources in the successful assessment and treatment of mental illnesses in African Americans. Positive outcomes associated with spiritual support (Newlin et al. 2002) are heightened interpersonal connectedness, emotional equilibrium and personal empowerment. An anthropologically oriented work by a Jungian analyst (Buhrmann 1987) has corroborated the pervasiveness of spiritual focus in traditional African therapy and healing, and has validated the richness of specific African healing traditions as a source of knowledge about human growth and healing. Buhrmann conducted an extensive study of the sophisticated training procedures required of the traditional healers of the Xhosa people of South Africa. The study uncovered parallels to the process of training Jungian analysts in the west, focusing on the discovery of self-knowledge by introspection. With regard to empirical examination of the link between spirituality and suicidal behavior, abused African American women who endorse high levels of spiritual well-being are at reduced risk for attempting suicide (Kaslow et al. 2002).

Alternatively, community-oriented clinical psychologists might actively cultivate relationships with Black church groups in order to develop independent nutrition-and-fitness and body-image programs within the church community that would shape specific goals and objectives according to the needs of the individuals and group. It is conceivable that differences between individual and social etiology and spiritual or religious beliefs could be interpreted by a mainstream therapist as an inclination to externalize, suggesting denial on the part of the client. Instead, externalizing may simply reflect a spiritual orientation rather than resistance to accept personal responsibility. Ultimately, to the extent that therapy is seen as a context for increasing or restoring personal control and efficacy in clients, certain adjustments are required when servicing highly spiritual clients.

Sense of Community

The African American church is a site of health lessons, community meetings and political activities aimed at improving the conditions of life. African American elders look to the church and their spiritual practice as a resource beyond the family for the inner strength to withstand daily stressors and physical ailments (Armstrong and Crowther 2002; Wallace and Bergeman 2002). Although there is evidence to believe that social networks are important determinants of religious practices in general, the expansive literature on African American religion provides strong theoretical bases for expecting their influence to be especially powerful among blacks (Lincoln and Mamiya 1990; Ellison and Sherkat 1990). Literature documents the historically prominent role of black churches in the community life of African Americans, making special note of the reinforcing relationship between religion and community cohesion. For example, studies have shown that religion plays an important role in the development and continuity of identity for many African Americans and contributes to a sense of social support and well-being (Walls and Zarit 1991). Walls and Zarit's (1991) research, examining the influence of informal support from African American churches on the well-being of its elderly members, suggests that social service agencies might work within the organizational structures of the churches to provide more services to elderly individuals living in African American communities, thereby enhancing medical and mental health care.

Due to the long history of racial oppression and the absence of strong secular organizations, African Americans have historically looked to their churches as the chief source of community cohesion. As early as the 1930s, researchers observed that rural black churches provided one of the only means for blacks to establish and sustain social contacts with their peers. Because of this, attendance at religious services and participation in other church activities became seen as normative.

Children and Young Adults

Elementary school children completed a battery of scales which measured spirituality along with racial attitudes and attitudes toward illicit drug use (Oler 1996) showing correlations with spirituality and altruistic behaviors, positive school performance, general satisfaction with life and negative attitudes toward drug use. Among youth, high levels of spirituality are associated with less violent behavior and greater self esteem (Walker 2000). Very little research has examined spirituality in young children, but ethnic identity studies (Phinney 1989; Yip et al. 2006) suggest that ethnic identity development is a facet of adolescence. Models of ethnic identity usually suggest that individuals begin in a state of unawareness or disinterest about what it means to be a member of their ethnic group. From this initial state, individuals move through a process of exploration into their ethnicity. Ideally, after this process, individuals are able to come to terms and are satisfied with their sense of self as a member of their ethnic group and have a positive group-esteem. Cross writes that there are some African Americans who have been socialized from childhood to have positive group-esteem and racial awareness and are not in need of Nigrescence. While ethnic identity models sometimes fail to specifically address spirituality, they do indicate cultural differences in psychological development.

Walker and Dixon (2002) examined spirituality and religious participation among African American and European American college students. Of particular interest was the relationship between these variables and academic performance. Findings were consistent with previous research suggesting that African Americans have higher levels of spiritual beliefs and religious participation than European Americans do. Correlation analyses suggested that spiritual beliefs and religious participation were positively related to academic performance for both groups; however, the pattern of the relationship was different.

Bowen-Reid and Harrell (2002) used college students to assess the effects of racism on health. They found that spirituality served as a significant moderator between racial stress and negative psychological health symptoms.

Art and Literature

Though few authors of textbooks in psychology are concerned with spirituality as a separate topic worthy of whole chapters, to many people, the complete psychological development of a person cannot happen without it. Many African American writers, on the other hand, have recognized the relationship between spirituality and psychological development and have presented several literary characters who have embarked on the journey to self realization only when these characters have embraced revised forms of spirituality.

Literary figures can offer a way to integrate African-centeredness into our theories. Many African-American adults face real-life crises stimulated by lost spiritual connections with themselves and their African cultural roots. A reconnection with spirituality can restore a proper inner balance, permitting a reorienting to outer life and a more enhanced sense of self.

Black women writers in the last few decades have offered mechanisms of spiritual healing through their works of fiction (Wheeler et al. 2002). Young (1999) argues that the ways that African-American spirituality resists racism is coded in a literary tradition with three compelling dimensions: the inner might to resist injustice, the powerful insight into one's virtue and the vices of one's oppressor, and the struggle against those who would disempower you.

Conclusion

The stages of lifespan development for typical African Americans are bedeviled by the legacy of hundreds of years of human slavery. In spite of this, the culture of this group is vibrant and highly influential to the current worldwide youth culture. The irony is that the youth may not realize their influence around the world, and people around the world absorb African culture while simultaneously, historically, despising the people who create it. Spirituality, as a reaction to cultural oppression, is deeply embedded in the healthy life-span development of people of Africa and the African diaspora. Spiritual issues do not wait to become pertinent in elder hood, as some theorists have suggested. Rather an awareness of the spirit is instilled from a very early age and reinforced through daily practices. This helps black folk to weather stressful times.

References

Akbar, N. (1981). Mental disorders among African Americans. *Black Books Bulletin, 7*(2), 18–25.

Ani, M. (1997). *Let the circle be unbroken: African spirituality in the diaspora.* New York: Nkonimfo Publications.

Armstrong, T., & Crowther, M. (2002). Spirituality among older African Americans. *Journal of Adult Development, 9*, 3–12.

Atwell, I., & Azibo, D. (1991). Diagnosing personality disorder in Africans (Blacks) using the Azibo nosology: Two case studies. *Journal of Black Psychology, 17*(2), 1–22.

Awanbor, D. (1982). The healing process in African psychotherapy. *American Journal of Psychotherapy, 36*(2), 206–213.

Azibo, D. (1983). Perceived attractiveness and Black personality: Black is beautiful when the psyche is Black. *The Western Journal of Black Studies, 7*, 229–238.

Azibo, D. (1989). African-centered theses on mental health and a nosology of Black/African personality disorder. *Journal of Black Psychology, 15*(2), 173–214.

Azibo, D. (1991). Towards a metatheory of African personality. *Journal of Black Psychology, 17*(2), 37–45.

Baldwin, J. A. (1984). African self-consciousness and the mental health of African Americans. *Journal of Black Studies, 15*(2), 177–194.

Baldwin, J. A. (1985). Psychological aspects of European cosmology in American society. *Western Journal of Black Studies, 9*(4), 216–223.

Baldwin, J. A. (1986). African (Black) psychology: Issues and synthesis. *Journal of Black Studies, 16*(3), 235–249.

Baltes, P. B., & Baltes, M. M. (eds). (1990). *Successful aging: Perspectives from the behavioral sciences.* Cambridge: Cambridge University Press.

Bernal, M.E., Knight, C.P., Garza, C.A., Ocampo, K.A., & Cota, M.K. (1990). The development of ethnic identity in Mexican American children. *Hispanic Journal of Behavioral Sciences, 12,* 3–24.

Bowen-Reid, T., & Harrell, J. (2002). Racist experiences and health outcomes: An examination of spirituality as a buffer. *Journal of Black Psychology, 28*(1), 18–36.

Bryant-Davis, T. (2005). Coping strategies of African American adult survivors of childhood violence. *Professional Psychology: Research and Practice, 36*(4), 409–414.

Buhrmann, M. V. (1987). *Living in two worlds: Communication between a white healer and her black counterparts.* Wilmette, IL: Chiron Publications.

Carter, J. (1994). Racism's impact on mental health. *Journal of the National Medical Association, 86,* 543–547.

Cartwright, S. A. (1851). Diseases and peculiarities of the Negro race. *New Orleans Medical and Surgical Journal, 7,* 691–715.

Christian, M., & Barbarin, O. (2001). Cultural resources and psychological adjustment of African American children: Effects of spirituality and racial attribution. *Journal of Black Psychology, 27,* 43–63.

Clark, K. B., & Clark, M. P. (1940). Skin color as a factor in racial identification of Negro pre-school children. *Journal of Social Psychology, 11,* 159–169.

Cross, W. E. (1971). The Negro to Black conversion experience: Towards a psychology of Black liberation. *Black World, 20*(9), 13–27.

Cross, W. E. (1995). The psychology of nigrescence: Revising the Cross model. In J. G. Ponterotto, J. M. Casas, L. A. Suzuki & C. M. Alexander (Eds.), *Handbook of multicultural counseling* (pp. 93–122). Thousand Oaks, CA: Sage.

Curry, A. (1981). An African worldview exploratory examination of traditional attitudes, values, and personality correlates of Black African people. *Dissertation Abstracts International, 42*(3), 1165B.

Dahl, O. (1995). When the future comes from behind: Malagasy and other time concepts and some consequences for communication. *International Journal for Intercultural Relations, 19,* 197–209.

Davis, N., Clance, P., & Gailis, A. (1999). Treatment approaches for obese and overweight African American women: A consideration of cultural dimensions. *Psychotherapy: Theory, Research, Practice, Training, 36*(1), 27–35.

Dixon, V. (1976). Worldviews and research methodology. In L. King (Ed.), *African philosophy: Assumptions and paradigms for research on Black persons.* Los Angeles: Fanon Research & Development Center.

Dubois, K. E. (1999). Racial identity, Afrocentric orientation and well-being among African-American women. *Dissertation Abstracts International, 59*(9-B), 5077.

Edwards, K. L. (1994). A cogno-spiritual model of psychotherapy. In R. Jones (Ed.), *Advances in Black psychology,* vol 1. Hampton, VA: Cobb & Henry.

Elkins, D., Hedstrom, L., Hughes, L., Leaf, J., & Saunders. (1988). Toward a humanistic-phenomenological spirituality: Definition, description and measurement. *Journal of Humanistic Psychology, 28,* 5–18.

Ellison, C., & Sherkat, D. (1990). Patterns of religious mobility among black Americans. *The Sociological Quarterly, 31,* 551–568.

Erikson, E. H. (1950). *Childhood and society.* New York: W. W. Norton.

Fine, M., Schwebel, A., & Myers, L. (1985). The effects of world view on adaptation to single parenthood among middle class adult women. *Journal of Family Stress, 6*(1), 107–127.

Gould, S. J. (1993). American polygeny and craniometry before Darwin. In S. Harding (Ed.), *The "racial" economy of science* (pp. 84–115). Indiana University Press: Bloomington.

Guthrie, R. V. (1998). *Even the rat was white: A historical view of psychology* (2nd ed.). Boston, MA: Allyn & Bacon.

Hatch, J., & Derthick, S. (1992). Empowering Black churches for health promotion. *Health Values, 16*(5), 3–8.

Jackson, A., & Sears, S. (1992). Implications of an African centered worldview in reducing stress for African American women. *Journal of Counseling and Development, 71*(2), 184–190.

Jagers, R. J., & Smith, P. (1996). Further examination of the spirituality scale. *Journal of Black Psychology, 22*, 429–442.

Kambon, K. K. (1998). *African/black psychology in the American context: An African-centered approach.* Tallahassee, Florida: Nubian Nation.

Kaslow, N. J., Thompson, M. P., Okun, A., Price, A., Young, S., Bender, M., et al. (2002). Risk and protective factors for suicidal behavior in abused African American women. *Journal of Consulting and Clinical Psychology, 70*, 311–319.

Kelsey, R., & Ransom, R. (1983). A comparison of African and European groups utilizing a worldview opinionnaire. Paper presented at the sixteenth annual meeting of the National Association of Black Psychologists, Washington, DC.

Kohlberg, L. (1984). *The psychology of moral development: The nature and validity of moral stages*, vol 2. New York: Harper & Row.

Lambo, T. A. (1974). Psychotherapy in Africa. *Psychotherapy & Psychosomatics, 24*, 311–326.

Landrine, H., & Klonoff, E. (1996). The Schedule of Racist Events: A measure of racial discrimination and a study of its negative physical and mental health consequences. *Journal of Black Psychology, 22*, 144–168.

Lannin, D., Mathews, H., Mitchell, J., Swanson, M., Swanson, F., & Edwards, M. (1998). Influence of socioeconomic and cultural factors on racial differences in late-stage presentation of breast cancer. *Journal of the American Medical Association, 279*, 1801–1807.

Lévy-Bruhl, L. (1928). *How natives think.* London: Allen & Unwin.

Lincoln, C., & Mamiya, L. (1990). *The black church in the African American experience.* Durham, NC: Duke University Press.

Maslow, A. H. (1962). *Toward a psychology of being.* Princeton, NJ: Van Nostrand.

Matthews, D. (1997). Religion and spirituality in primary care. *Mind/Body Medicine, 2*, 9–19.

Mattis, J. S. (2000). African American women's definitions of spirituality and religiosity. *Journal of Black Psychology, 26*(1), 101–122.

Mbiti, J. S. (1975). *Introduction to African religion.* Oxford: Heinemann.

McMahon, S. D., & Watts, R. J. (2002). Ethnic identity in urban African American youth: Exploring links with self-worth, aggression, and other psychosocial variables. *Journal of Community Psychology, 30*, 411–431.

Morgan, L. H. (1877). *Ancient society.* New York: Henry Holt.

Newlin, N., Knaft, K., & Melkus, G. (2002). African American spirituality: A concept analysis. *Advances in Nursing Science, 25*(2), 57–70.

Nobles, W. W. (2006). *Seeing the Sakhu: Foundational writings for an African psychology.* Chicago: Third World Press.

Nobles, W. (1976). Extended self: Re-thinking the so-called Negro self-concept. *Journal of Black Psychology, 2*(2), 15–24.

Oler, C. H. (1996). Spirituality, racial identity, and intentions to use alcohol and other drugs among African American youth. *Dissertations Abstracts International: Section B: The Sciences & Engineering, 56*(8-B), 4590. US: Univ. Microfilms International.

Parham, T. A. (1989). Cycles of psychological Nigresence. *The Counseling Psychologist, 17*, 187–226.

Parks, F. (2007). Working with narratives: Coping strategies in African American folk beliefs and traditional healing practices. *Journal of Human Behavior in the Social Environment, 15*(1), p135–p147.

Phinney, J. S. (1989). Stages of ethnic identity in minority group adolescents. *Journal of Early Adolescence, 9*, 34–49.

Piaget, J. (1952). *The origins of intelligence in children*. New York: International Universities Press.

Pinel, E. (1999). Stigma consciousness: The psychological legacy of social stereotypes. *Journal of Personality and Social Psychology, 76*, 114–128.

Potts, R. (1991). Spirits in the bottle: Spirituality and alcoholism treatment in African-American communities. *Journal of Training and Practice in Professional Psychology, 5*, 53–64.

Sandoval, M. (1979). Santeria as a mental health care system: An historical overview. *Social Science and Medicine, 13*, 139–151.

Sellers, R. M., Smith, M. A., Shelton, J. N., Rowley, S. A. J., & Chavous, T. M. (1998). Multidimensional model of racial identity: A reconceptualization of African American racial identity. *Personality and Social Psychology Review, 2*, 18–39.

Simon, C., Crowther, M., & Higgerson, H. (2007). The stage-specific role of spirituality among African American Christian women throughout the breast cancer experience. *Cultural Diversity & Ethnic Minority Psychology, 13*(1), 26–34.

Spencer, H. (1876). *Principles of sociology*. New York: D. Appleton.

Spencer, M., Fegley, S., & Harpalani, V. (2003). A theoretical and empirical examination of identity as coping: Linking coping resources to the self processes of African American Youth. *Applied Developmental Science, 7*, 181–188.

Toldson, I. A., & Toldson, I. L. (2001). Biomedical ethics: An African-centered psychological perspective. *Journal of Black Psychology, 27*(2), 57–70.

Utsey, S., Bolden, M., Lanier, Y., & Williams, O. (2007). Examining the role of culture-specific coping as a predictor of resilient outcomes in African Americans from high-risk urban communities. *Journal of Black Psychology, 33*(1), 75–93.

Walker, E.A. (2000). Spiritual support in relation to community violence exposure, aggressive outcomes, and psychological adjustment among inner-city young adolescents. *Dissertations Abstracts International: Section B: The Sciences & Engineering* (pp. 278–296), *6161*(6-B). US: Univ. Microfilms International.

Walker, K., & Dixon, V. (2002). Spirituality and academic performance among African American college students. *Journal of Black Psychology, 28*(2), 107–121.

Wallace, K. A., & Bergeman, C. S. (2002). Spirituality and religiousity in a sample of African American elders: A life story approach. *Journal of Adult Development, 9*, 141–154.

Walls, C. T., & Zarit, S. H. (1991). Informal support from Black churches and the well being of elderly Blacks. *The Gerontologist, 31*(4), 490–495.

Welsing, F. C. (1991). *The Isis papers: The keys to the colors*. Chicago: Third World Press.

Wheeler, E. (2002). "And, does it matter if he was racist?": Deconstructing concepts in psychology. *Race, Gender, & Class, 9*(4), 33–44.

Wheeler, E., Ampadu, L., & Wangari, E. (2002). Lifespan development revisited: Spirituality through an African-centered lens. *Journal of Adult Development, 9*(1), 71–78.

White, J. (1972). Toward a black psychology. In R. L. Jones (Ed.), *black psychology* (1st ed.). New York: Harper & Row.

Wilson, A. N. (1993). *The falsification of Afrikan consciousness*. New York: Afrikan World InfoSystems.

Yip, T., Seaton, E. K., & Sellers, R. M. (2006). African American racial identity across the lifespan: Identity status, identity content, and depressive symptoms. *Child Development, 77*(5), 1504–1517.

Young, J. (1999). Dogged strength within the veil: African-American spirituality as a literary tradition. *Journal of Religious Thought, 55/56*(2/1), 87. 21p.

Part VII

Directions and Interventions in Stressful Life Transitions

Chapter 27

Surviving and Thriving: How Transition Psychology May Apply to Mass Traumas and Changes

Dai Williams

History says, *Don't hope on this side of the grave.*
But then, once in a lifetime
the longed for tidal wave of justice can rise up,
and hope and history rhyme.
So hope for a great sea-change on the far side of revenge.
Believe that a farther shore is reachable from here...
Call miracle self-healing...
Seamus Heaney (Heaney 1990)

Introduction

The transition process has fascinated me since 1971 when a Peace Corps volunteer in northern Uganda described the hazards of *culture shock* for people adjusting to life in a new country. The remote community had its own traumas and changes from a recent cholera epidemic, and the early months of Idi Amin's regime. Since then they have suffered dictatorship, AIDS, drought, famine, and civil war. How do communities survive generations of wars, oppression, epidemics, and natural disasters? The fight and flight response is a recognized trait for surviving immediate threats. The task of successfully adapting to major life events, traumas, or changes is more complex. Surviving *and* thriving involves the remarkable self-healing and development process known as *transition*.

This article reviews the essential features of transitions for individuals and subsequently the hazards and opportunities of collective transitions for organizations and communities that experience mass traumas or changes. It reflects on transition theory and practice in individual and organizational settings since the 1970s, and in political and community settings since 1997. It builds on ideas exchanged with Peter Herriot, Ashley Weinberg, and Richard Plenty at a BPS symposium on *Transition Psychology – the waves of change* in 1999 (Herriot et al. 1999). It explores examples of other major events and potential mass transitions from 1999 to the latest political changes and economic crisis in 2009.

From: *Handbook of Stressful Transitions Across the Lifespan,*
Edited by: T.W. Miller, DOI 10.1007/978-1-4419-0748-6_27,
© Springer Science+Business Media, LLC 2010

Transition awareness and transition briefings are an essential part of my practitioner's tool kit as an Occupational Psychologist. Leonie Sugarman described this new field in her Master's course lectures on Life-Span Development in 1978 (Sugarman 1986). I worked in Personnel with Shell in the UK and Canada and used transitions in relocation briefings and crisis support for international staff, students, and recruits. In 1986, I set up Eos as an independent consultant specialising in career development, crisis, and change management. The practical situations faced by my clients test the utility of all the models and techniques I can offer them for personal and career development, and managing organizational change. Most people can recognize the transition process from their own experiences and then add it to their own career management skills. In return, their transitions have given me new insights.

Transition psychology is important to understanding individual processes of development and change. These offer wider insights for the management of trauma and change in organizations and communities. Shell recognized transition processes as strategic issues in the management of change in the 1990s (Plenty 1999). In the current international debate about economic crises and political changes, commentators refer to periods of transition, e.g. the US Presidential transition, and hopes for transformation to a new world order. But economic analysts and political commentators appear unaware of the psychological processes involved and the field of transition theory and practice.

This chapter explores the application of transition psychology to mass transitions in three parts:

1. Individual and group responses to trauma and change
2. Mass transitions: societal responses to trauma and change
3. Applying transition analysis to mass traumas and changes

Part 1 explains the basic principles of transition theory for individuals and groups with practical examples. Part 2 explores the potential dynamics of mass trauma or change in larger populations with some case study observations, forecasts, and reviews since 1997. These provide the basis for the transition analysis techniques in Part 3. These are offered for practitioners and researchers from different disciplines and cultures to test on past, current, and future events.

Part 1: Transitions: Individual and Group Responses to Trauma and Change

1.1 The origin of transition psychology
1.2 The evolutionary function of transitions
1.3 Psychological tasks and phases of transition
1.4 Moving from crisis to recovery during transitions
1.5 Groups in transition crisis
1.6 Transition management
1.7 The effects of multiple transitions
1.8 Opportunities in periods of transition
1.9 Terminal transitions

The origin of transition psychology

The concept of *transition* was originally identified in studies of families, depression, and bereavement in the 1960s (Kübler-Ross 1969) and early 1970s (Parkes 1971). The U.S. Peace Corps appeared to use the concept to prepare volunteers for culture shock in overseas assignments by 1970 (Guthrie & Zektick 1967). By 1976, researchers like Hopson and Adams (Adams et al. 1976) realized that the transition process applied to a wide range of life-events, good as well as bad. In the 1980s and 1990s organizational psychologists like Nigel Nicholson (Nicholson & West 1988) and Peter Herriot (Herriot 1992) applied the concept of transition to large groups when studying organizational change.

I have used the transition model since 1983 – initially for briefing international students and recruits about culture shock. I have used it with over 700 clients to analyze life histories and to manage life events and career crises or changes. Since 1997 I have explored the possibility of a post-election transition in the new UK Parliament and potential periods of transition in other political contexts.

Several different models or theories offer explanations for the transition process or *transition cycle*. Most use a time sequence ranging from Hopson's seven stages simplified to three by Bridges (Bridges 1991a). Schlossberg et al. developed a *4-S* model (Schlossberg et al. 1995) that describes a dynamic interaction between self, situation, strategies, and support. All describe human responses to change with similar phenomena. Some recognize transition as a fundamental aspect of human development. I use a variation of the Hopson model, adapted for positive and negative events, and alternative outcomes, based on transition incidents reported by clients. This Eos version of the transition cycle is shown in Fig. 27-1.

The evolutionary function of transitions

Two psychological processes are important survival resources: 1) *human responses to threat or stress – the fight and flight response,* and 2) *human responses to change – the transition process.* Both can be valuable assets.

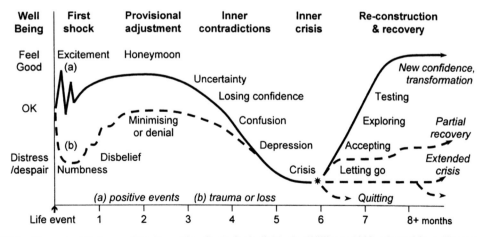

Fig. 27-1. Phases and features of the Transition Cycle for individuals (Williams 1999, adapted from Hopson et al.) (Williams 1999e)

But when they get out of control they can be hazardous, sometimes lethal. Understanding these processes may reduce the risks of strategic errors and aggression in political, military, and community contexts.

The transition process or transition cycle has several stages, see Fig. 27-1. It determines how humans respond and adapt to trauma and change over a period of time. This is crucial to understanding how individuals and organizations can adapt deeply held attitudes, beliefs, and behavior to new situations. These are the kind of changes needed to restore peace to communities in conflict, for new governments to stabilize, and for societies to adapt to new political regimes. But the process also includes a hazardous crisis period that can involve severe personal and group stress.

Humans appear to be remarkably adaptable, with the capability to learn and adjust day-to-day behaviors within days, e.g. when going on a holiday to a foreign country. However, the brain has powerful defences to protect deeply held values, beliefs, and expectations through processes like denial. These defences enable individuals and society to maintain continuity through temporary changes, but after 3–4 months contradictions with the new reality cause severe cognitive dissonance.

From time to time changes occur that violate deeply held beliefs or core values. Sooner or later, the individual has to come to terms with changes that render a past value, belief, or assumption obsolete. In order to function effectively in the new situation, these obsolete concepts have to be let go. Then we have to reconfigure many other assumptions and thought processes that were dependent on them. If these tasks are done successfully, our understanding of the world is transformed.

In simpler terms, human beings are like animals that have to shed their skins from time to time in order to grow. We grow psychologically through our changes – typically, through 10–20 life events in an average lifetime.

Not all changes cause transitions. If we have experienced a similar change and adapted our mind set appropriately (e.g. after bereavement) we may cope more easily with similar changes in the future. But a new job or relationship can be as psychologically disruptive as redundancy, separation, or bereavement.

Psychological tasks and phases of transition

The psychological tasks of transition are far more complex than the short-term responses to stress. So they operate over a longer timescale – typically, 6–12 months under favorable conditions. But individuals can be trapped in an extended crisis period for months or years if inner conflicts are not resolved.

The basic transition process works within each individual. Groups, organizations, or communities sharing the same trauma or change may have to make similar adjustments when obsolete concepts or beliefs were widely shared. This applies to organizations adjusting to new corporate values after a commercial merger or take-over, and to let go of hatred or prejudice in societies that have been in conflict.

The initial stages of the transition cycle enable individuals to cope with immediate, practical tasks required to adjust to the new situation. Learning is rapid, sometimes enhanced by the adrenaline associated with fight or flight. People cope. The mind shuts out the full implications of the new situation – apparently building its resources to prepare for the deeper issues to be resolved later.

However, after 3–4 months the mind cannot continue to defend deeply held beliefs against evidence of the new situation that is incompatible with them. Deep *inner contradictions* develop. A mother with her first child has to recognize that she has lost much of her freedom. A bereaved partner has lost lifelong support. A redundant employee may have to learn that loyalty was a naïve assumption. Newly elected politicians may have to learn that some election promises may not be viable against the harsh reality of limited budgets or the inertia of state administration or bureaucracy.

Once a deeply held belief, or valued assumption about the future, has been broken the individual's mind is in trouble. Contradictions develop between one's inner view of the world and external events. Many beliefs and behaviors are inter-linked: if one belief or assumption is broken then other thinking processes that depended on it will no longer function. This creates increased anxiety and affects any decision that was dependent on the obsolete assumption. People say that "their world is falling apart" and psychologically it is.

Over a period of weeks these inner doubts spread into many aspects of our lives and behavior. A change in our work or society may destabilize assumptions about our private lives or relationships and vice versa. This growing inner turmoil leads to the hazardous *transition crisis phase*. This is sometimes described as a "dark night of the soul" when individuals seem to face impossible choices, creating severe stress and potentially triggering the fight or flight reaction. However, since the stress is caused by an *inner crisis* its causes can be very hard for them or others to understand.

Individuals may feel a strong urge to escape these inner conflicts and may do so unwisely by escaping an outer role or responsibility. *Quitting* a job, relationship, or organization is a form of escape behavior typical of a transition crisis, e.g. the sudden departure of Finance minister La Fontaine from the new German Government in spring 1999, without even clearing his desk, just under 6 months after the election.

Individuals in transition crisis may become deeply withdrawn, or highly aggressive. Since the individual's judgement may be deeply impaired by inner contradictions they may make serious errors of judgement. These may be seen in "moments of madness" – untypical, dangerous, or unacceptable behavior in their work or personal lives.

This period of inner crisis and distress may cause *external conflicts* even with colleagues or friends, or direct aggression with enemies. These behaviors are partly explained by the operation of stress mechanisms described earlier and may be diagnosed medically as symptoms of stress or anxiety states.

Under extreme distress the individual may suffer nervous exhaustion, go into temporary collapse, complete breakdown, or quit life by suicide. Friends, colleagues, and medical practitioners tend to look to immediate circumstances to explain such behavior. If these are not obvious, they may assume that mental illness is the cause.

However, if a significant life event has occurred in recent months the underlying cause is more likely to be a transition crisis - a delayed reaction to trauma or change, sometimes better diagnosed as a temporary reactive depression, not to be confused with extended clinical depression.

In September 1998, the Norwegian Prime Minister took sick leave for reactive depression. This followed 4 months of extended crisis and unresolved policy conflicts in his new government, despite an early honeymoon phase.

Recognising his problem, he returned to work 4 weeks later and successfully resolved budget negotiations. Few other countries are as aware and tolerant of the *mental health pressures on senior politicians* as Norway. His temporary condition was respected, not exploited, by the Opposition and media.

For political and security reasons, most governments will cover up or deny periods when a national leader's mental condition is unstable. In the UK, Prime Minister Anthony Eden was seriously ill when he led the country into the Suez crisis. President Kennedy was reported to be using barbiturates during the Cuban crisis. President Reagan suffered the onset of Alzheimer's disease in his second term. President Brezhnev's alcohol problems were well known. These and other cases were described in Professor Hugh Freeman's study of *the mental state of world leaders in the 20th Century* published in the British Journal of Psychiatry in 1991 (Freeman 1991a).

From time to time national leaders display symptoms of mental illness, at great cost to their countries. Many, possibly all, are likely to suffer short periods of severe transition stress or trauma from visiting casualties after disasters or terrorist attacks. By civilian health and safety standards they would be regarded as unfit to pilot a passenger jet during these periods, and yet in the UK, USA, and other countries they are allowed to authorize military attacks overseas. Perhaps because of the principle of sovereign immunity the sanity of world leaders is a taboo subject in international affairs. There are obvious political pressures on the media not to report these conditions when suspected.

However, a distinction needs to be drawn between trauma, transition stress, and chronic mental illness. Few people realize that *high stress and temporary reactive depression are normal features of the crisis phase of transition*. Individuals may even need to undergo severe distress before they are willing to let go of obsolete beliefs and take a radically different approach to life - e.g. when politicians make a U turn on a key policy issue or manifesto promise that they have been deeply committed to before.

Moving From Crisis to Recovery During Transitions

In this most hazardous phase of transition, the obvious question is "how can individuals and their organizations or communities break out of crisis?"

The prime task of a work psychologist in professional practice is to help clients resolve their problems and make positive plans. Hundreds of clients described thousands of transitions, and most survived without professional help. This suggests that the transition process is an innate human coping mechanism that evolved with social support in extended families and integrated communities. Their reports, plus psychometric measures of stress (using the Occupational Stress Indicator) and interpersonal behavior (FIRO-B), helped to identify factors that appear to enable or inhibit successful recovery from a transition crisis. These are summarized in Tables 27-1 and 27-2.

Awareness of these enabling and inhibiting factors may add a new perspective to government policies, military tactics, and international initiatives needed to stabilize communities or regions in a transition crisis period.

Individuals can break out of the crisis by letting go of obsolete assumptions or beliefs. If this is done the crisis phase may last only 2–3 weeks. This allows the individual to reconstruct their thoughts in a way better adapted to the new reality. This process is remarkable but spontaneous, and can happen faster than the earlier deterioration - often within 1–2 months. The *optimum recovery* line

Table 27-1. Factors that ENABLE recovery during periods of transition.

- *Economic security* – surplus resources, no debt, stable income, own home, low commitments, multiple-income household

- *Emotional security* – supportive partner, stable childhood, support networks, openness on emotional and mental health issues

- *Health* – good physical fitness, prudent lifestyle, quality time for leisure

- *Prior transition skills* – positive transition experiences, clear goals

- *Supportive work environment* – high respect/low control culture, good team morale, clear role and contract terms, life-work boundaries respected

- *Transition support* - briefing, monitoring issues, practical support, life-career planning, tolerance, dignity, valuing the past, time off before illness, confidential counselling, freedom/recognition for new ideas

Positive outcomes: These enabling factors may minimize the severity of distress in the crisis phase, minimize risk of quitting or extended crisis and optimize recovery time for individuals and groups. They may also enable high innovation, personal transformation, heal old wounds and "rejuvenate" staff leading to high group morale and synergy and transforming the organization.

Table 27-2. Factors that INHIBIT recovery during periods of transition.

- *Economic insecurity* – low income, debt, high financial commitments, fear of job loss, temporary, ambiguous or onerous employment contract

- *Emotional insecurity* – no partner, few friends, dependent relatives, secret grief (lost lover or child), sense of guilt, unresolved issues or regrets, multiple transitions, anxiety over being diagnosed mentally ill

- *Health* – chronic or undiagnosed illness, low fitness, fatigue, unwise lifestyle

- *Hostile work environment* – work overload, unrealistic demands, insufficient resources, abuse of life-work boundaries, e.g. excessive working hours affecting relationships, leisure time and fitness. Low respect/high control culture. No time off except sickness absence. Discipline for absence. Scape-goating weaker members by stressed teams. Harassment or abuse by aggressive or stressed managers. Change of manager. Inflexible policies.

- *Poor transition management* – no support, no preparation for change, unrealistic timescales. No monitoring of key issues that may need change. No opportunity for fresh insights. Past achievements ignored or discounted.

Negative outcomes: These factors increase the risk of severe and extended crises, e.g. quitting, long-term sickness, breakdown or suicide. High risk of errors, e.g. accidents (at work or driving), indiscretions or strategic errors. Poor, broken, or abusing relationships. Poor team morale, turnover. Downgraded career prospects. Frustrated recovery – rebellious staff, unused insights, dissent, and conflict. Williams, D. (1999). *Life events and career change* www.eoslifework. co.uk/transprac.htm.

in Fig. 27-1 follows letting go of obsolete ideas and accepting the new reality. This can lead to new confidence and sometimes renewal or transformation – almost a human metamorphosis.

Groups in Transition Crisis

Groups in a transition crisis period may become highly unstable unless skilfully managed (Williams 1999a). Multiple conflicts can develop and scape-goating is typical. This situation is often reported by career clients in work organizations subject to recent traumas or changes. Examples included mergers or take-overs, the appointment of new leaders or senior managers, and the delayed impact of mass redundancies on the remaining workforce. In 1997, the new UK Parliament offered a classic case study.

In September 1997, I became suspicious of repeated claims about Tony Blair's *honeymoon* by the new UK Government following their landslide election victory in May. New job honeymoons may last 2–3 months (the first 100 days). Usually, the second 3-month period is when the full impact of the new situation begins to penetrate our psychological defences. Severe contradictions develop between expectations and the new reality for individuals and groups. Stress increases, relationships deteriorate, and individuals become accident prone or even quit. Stressed individuals make strategic errors. Severe personal and group crises may develop 5–6 months after the trauma or change, good or bad.

Do career transitions affect politicians and political parties - as they do in any other type of career or organization? This question was the basis for *After the Honeymoon* (Williams 1997a) – a transition briefing for MPs and parties warning of a possible transition crisis developing 5–6 months after the election.

Leaders in crisis may feel deeply insecure and become over-controlling, exacerbating the pressures on subordinates in a similar state. Or they may divert attention from these internal conflicts by targeting an external victim and projecting the group's anger and hostility outwards. Many leaders have used military action against external enemies or dissident groups to distract attention from internal political or military crises, e.g. Idi Amin's use of supposed invasions from Tanzania during army rebellions in 1971.

For groups in crisis, *the recovery phase is likely to take longer* to develop since a critical mass of members have to reach their breakthrough point before changes to collective beliefs are made. Unless skilful transition management skills are used the crisis period for groups and organizations may extend for at least 2–3 months. Figure 27-2 illustrates this *extended crisis* in *the post-election transition* for the UK Government after the 1997 election, based on events reported in the media:

The symptoms of political groups going through the transition crisis period (Fig. 27-2) are illustrated by press headlines for the period October 1997 to March 1998 - see extracts in Fig. 27-3.

The crisis was more dramatic, and lasted longer than expected in *After the Honeymoon*. I reviewed the exercises I use with clients to suggest practical ways for MPs and parties to move *from crisis to recovery*. These were added as Part 2 of the booklet *Parliament in Transition* (Williams 1997b) in December 1997.

The Opposition rebellion led to the notion of a *defining moment* mechanism when Individuals may lead the recovery process by putting their career on the line to challenge obsolete assumptions and assert their new vision.

"Few people appreciate the anger, pain or fear it takes to speak out in public to question your party, or to re-define your past beliefs or allegiances. You may be putting your career on the line. History suggests this is a hallmark of integrity. At some point you will have to make a crucial decision, privately or publicly, about what your new life has become - your defining action. When you act this is your defining moment." (ibid. pages 16–17)

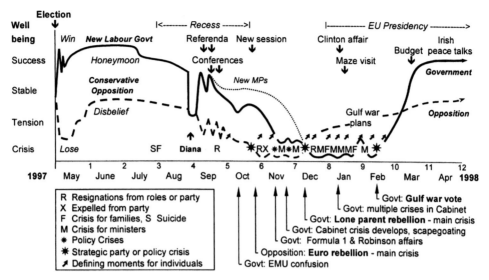

Fig. 27-2. Post-election transition events for the first year of the new UK Parliament 1997/98 (from review of Parliament in Transition, Jan 1999) (Williams 1999f)

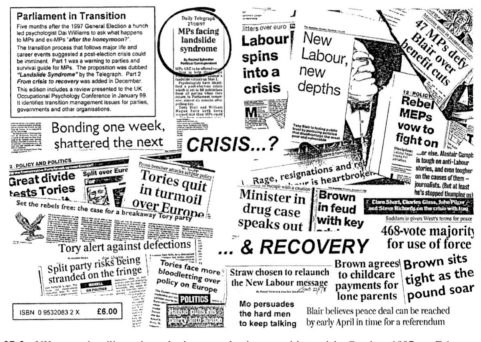

Fig. 27-3. UK press headlines through the post-election transition crisis October 1997 to February 2008 (Williams 1999f)

This action is politically hazardous, yet may be essential to enable a breakthrough in periods of crisis. Mo Mowlam's visit to The Maze prison in January 1999 to discuss peace prospects with prisoners opened up the Irish peace talks (see Fig. 27-2). David Trimble's decision in November 1999 to reverse his party's policy and agree to negotiate with Nationalists led to the restoration of the Northern Ireland Assembly six weeks later.

Defining moments can be crucial in community peace and reconciliation programmes. From my discussions with peace workers in Northern Ireland, many individuals in conflicting communities eventually reach a point where they turn against the traditional attitudes of prejudice and violence. This turning point can mark the recovery from a personal extended crisis that has lasted many years from earlier traumas. A new trauma or change may trigger recovery from an extended crisis. People with the courage to make this change can be "seeds of peace" in their communities. They may be the first to make links with others across traditional religious, or political divides as seen in South Africa and Northern Ireland (Williams 1999b) .

Like politicians these individuals may take grave personal risks in crossing their group's traditional boundaries. But many have already suffered such deep trauma or loss that they have nothing else to lose. At that point political and military or paramilitary intimidation and even torture becomes futile. In their recovery phase, their confidence and innovation inspires other to have the confidence to take initiatives for peace and reconciliation. These individual turning points are often transition-related but may appear random due to personal events (e.g. bereavement), unconnected with national transition cycles.

Figure 27-2 also illustrates *the risk that political leaders may seek to start wars in a period of crisis.* The proposal to attack Iraq in February 1998 was led by the UK Prime Minister, the U.S. President, and the UK Foreign Secretary. All three were likely to be in personal as well as political crises due to broken relationships or bereavement in July and August 1997.

In spring 2000, the UK Government was going through another crisis phase – despite their policy achievements in 1999 and the miraculous disappearance of the dreaded Y2K computer threat. In *Accidents waiting to happen?* (Williams 2000a) I analyzed the likely fluctuations in Government confidence on six different policy areas each month from summer 1998 and forecast to summer 2000. The aggregate scores for each month gave the chart in Fig 27-4.

During post-election transitions, governments and political parties need to be open to *revising their election manifestos,* budgets, and other commitments, just as employers may need to review business plans in the aftermath of mergers or take-overs. The challenge of the crisis period is a good test of core principles that can be reaffirmed and those that must be changed. Rigid adherence to pre-transition plans and commitments may fly in the face of the new reality created by their election and changing circumstances.

The recovery phase of transition brings new confidence and optimism, with new energy and insights for individuals and enhanced morale and co-operation in groups. This final phase is the most positive *window of opportunity* for initiating major changes that are well adapted to the new environment. Figure 27.2 illustrated the *amazing speed of recovery* in psychological climate, confidence, and effectiveness of the new UK Government in spring 1998, immediately after their 3-month post-election transition crisis.

The final defining moment for the Prime Minister and the Cabinet appears to have been the vote by Parliament to approve a war with Iraq. Fortunately, this action was pre-empted by Kofi Annan's UN peace initiative. Soon after the war vote, Chancellor Gordon Brown produced a restrained budget that increased business confidence in the new government. At the same time Prime Minister Tony Blair conducted peace talks with parties in Northern Ireland and the Irish Government. These led to the Good Friday peace agreement in April 98,

11 months after the election. This was a major achievement and amazing recovery from the Government's 3 month post-election transition crisis.

From these observations, the transition recovery phase can offer a new era of greater confidence and effectiveness for communities, organizations, and governments. When new governments reach this phase they are likely to stabilize and flourish. But how long does this take?

Transition Management

A key issue for national leaders and political organizations during periods of transition is *how to minimize the crisis period, and how to optimize recovery* to reach the potential transformations they are committed to. The enabling and inhibiting factors in Tables 27.1 and 27.2 provide a starting point for transition management strategies for individuals and communities.

The *Parliament in transition* project involved daily monitoring of media reports over a 4-month period, including reports of personal and domestic crises as well as political events and controversies. It was reported on BBC TV in October and on BBC news on the day of the Government's deepest crisis and rebellion 10 December 1997, see Fig.27-2. The project tried to offer practical advice for Party Leaders, Ministers, and MPs about the potential effects of a post-election transition crisis and ways to manage them from *a career management perspective* – available to MPs of all parties from a non-partisan position.

The project was reviewed several months later in another study for the transition symposium in January 1999. This identified *11 practical issues for transition management* - see Table 27-3. Although these were based on transitions in the UK Parliament they may be relevant to the management of trauma or change in any large organization or community.

Table 27-3. Practical issues for Transition Management in organizations.

1. The 1997 UK Election transition illustrates that *winners as well as losers, survivors as well as redundant staff, and senior managers as well as staff* are susceptible to the transition process after major change events.

2. *Unmanaged transitions* in organizations *risk many hazards in the crisis period and miss opportunities for transformation* during recovery.

3. *Differing vulnerability* of individuals affects the severity, timing, and duration of crisis periods. Factors include multiple transitions (work and personal events), job insecurity, and group support or hostility.

4. *Transition management awareness and skills* are essential to optimize individual and group adjustment to major changes in organizations.

5. *Strategic management decisions may be seriously impaired* during the crisis phase. Leaders need to monitor their own transitions, sharing workload and responsibility. Loyalty tests endanger the organization.

6. *Leaders and managers may be vulnerable to predatory influences*, which offer support during the crisis phase. Highly stressed teams or groups need to *support each other against scape-goating or dismissal.*

7. *Individual expectations and corporate agendas* for change (e.g. manifestos) cannot fully anticipate the new reality. They need to be continuously *monitored and open to review* during the crisis and recovery phases of transition.

(continued)

Table 27-3. (continued)

8. *Management style needs to adapt* at each stage of a mass transition process to minimize the crisis phase and harness the recovery phase. Over-control reduces confidence, trust, participation and wastes talent through resignations.

9. *Disciplinary and dismissal procedures should be used with extreme caution during transitions.* Key staff may quit, be disciplined, demoted or dismissed when they are about to become most valuable to the organization. Rebels may have a more accurate perception of the new environment and defective agendas than leaders or managers in crisis.

10. *Individual transitions affect total identity and transcend life-work boundaries.* Organization and career changes affect personal and family life and vice versa. Families and ex-employees may also go through transition. Personal life and time boundaries must be respected.

11. *Mental and organizational health are strategic issues for organization performance, especially during periods of rapid change.* Denial of the transition process in the UK Parliament reflected strong taboos about emotions and mental health in UK culture and organizations. Emotional literacy (awareness of factors for positive mental health) is a strategic issue for governments, organizations, and communities responsible for managing periods of trauma and change.

The Effects of Multiple Transitions

National politics and international relations are subject to increasingly frequent crises and changes. *Multiple traumas and changes* (political and personal) may lead to overlapping transition cycles. In ideal conditions, recovery from one change cycle may alleviate the crisis phase of another following it. In practice, a new transition crisis period may inhibit recovery from another already in progress. Both Israel and the USA went through multiple transitions in 2001.

Multiple political transitions affected the UK Government through 1999 and 2000. Transitions started by the Balkans War and Devolution were followed by other changes in Parliament and Northern Ireland. The separate and combined effects of transitions in different policy areas were charted in *Accidents Waiting to Happen and new opportunities to follow* published in March 2000 (Williams 2000b). These indicated an extended crisis period for the Government from November 99 - May 2000, temporarily eased when the global Millennium Bug threat did not materialize. The Government's recovery in 2000 began with a new agreement in Northern Ireland in May, and stabilized in mid July.

Opportunities in Periods of Transition

Although these notes contain many cautions about the hazards of transitions – for individuals, communities, governments, and national leaders – *the medium-term effect of transition periods are potentially highly beneficial for organizations and societies.* In national and international contexts, transition recovery periods may create the greatest opportunities for radical changes in attitudes and co-operation. Individuals rarely change deeply held beliefs except after periods of transition.

Within nations, the transition process creates *windows of opportunity for constructive action by political and community leaders in all sections of society.*

Terminal Transitions

William Bridges (1991b) uses a three-stage model to describe the transition process. Though we provide different interpretations for the transition phases, we describe the same developmental task for individuals and organizations. One special feature of this approach is to remind us that "every transition begins with an ending". This is especially relevant in the declining phase of political rule by leaders or governments.

"Terminal" transitions are more difficult to track because they may not be a clear starting event. Leaders may lose energy and credibility gradually. Some may continue in power for years after it becomes obvious that they are no longer mentally capable of running a state. Somehow they retain power - by charisma and by the loyalty of close supporters including the military whose future may rely on extending a failed regime as long as possible.

But at some point it becomes inevitable that the regime will fail, or that a politician will not survive his/her next election. One analogy is bereavement. Sudden death provides an obvious trauma for relatives and is likely to start the stages of grief or transition first identified by Elizabeth Kubler-Ross (Kübler-Ross, 1969). But death through terminal illness may involve a form of pre-bereavement transition for relatives - a slow but remorseless challenge to face the coming loss. The same process may affect political organizations who realize they will probably lose the next election. This is likely to have a progressive effect on morale and hopelessness.

Another analogy is redundancy: sometimes this can be anticipated. But in unskilful organizations, managers or staff are terminated with as little as one hour's notice - an equivalent of a sudden death trauma for the individual, family, and colleagues. This has a devastating psychological effect causing severe trauma and leading to months or years of severe mental distress or extended crisis. Such treatment is a clear signal to other staff that no employee is safe and that the organization cannot be trusted. This often results in a wave of "survivor syndrome" - a collective transition crisis manifested in a collapse of morale over the usual 6-month time period and followed by resignations of other key personnel the organization could not afford to lose.

In better managed organizations, staff are made aware of the possibility of redundancy, given time to prepare, and supported throughout the process.

"Leaving with dignity" is a hallmark of high quality change management that I recommend to employers planning redundancy programmes or staff redeployment. The objective is to minimize trauma for the individuals concerned, their families, and surviving staff, and retaining the commitment and performance of departing staff up to the day they leave.

In political transitions it is important to consider the effects of "terminal transitions" on departing leaders, ministers, MPs, and their support organizations. How well the "ending" period is planned and managed will have a great effect on individual and organization performance, and the ability to recruit and retain talented people in the future.

The ending of political power – for parties that lose an election, their leaders and elected politicians who lose their place in Parliament – will usually start a "loss" transition period following the general cycle shown in Figs. 27-3. Parties would be wise to support their "losers" for up to a year. Without sufficient support they may become dangerously distressed or vindictive in the transition crisis period that follows, potentially causing political scandals even though they are no longer in power (Fig 27-4).

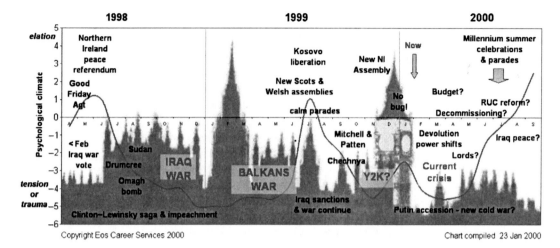

Fig. 27-4. Combined effects of six policy areas on the psychological climate in the UK Government from April 1998 to January 2000, and projected to September 2000 (from Accidents waiting to happen? (Williams 2000b)

If the loss of power or influence affects military or paramilitary organizations they may become extremely dangerous for months or years. This can be seen by the continued violence of paramilitary organizations in Northern Ireland and the Balkans after "peace" has been officially declared. The transition period for losers needs to be included in forecasts of political change or hoped for peace programmes after conflict. Far more work has to be done on the effects of loss transitions for losers – the hazards involved and potential opportunities for recovery.

In the best case, losers who make successful transitions to come to terms with their loss can become catalysts for the new order, e.g. prisoners in Northern Ireland who played a key role in opening peace talks. In the worst case ex-military or paramilitary personnel with unresolved transitions may turn to organized crime or plan political coups d'états. (See *Many Paths to Peace* (Williams 1999b)).

In some cases, depending on the ethical conduct of governments in power, losers may resort to continued political violence in a liberation war. Whether this is considered terrorism or freedom fighting depends on the methods they use, the targets they choose, the political history of their country, and the political and other beliefs of the observer.

Whatever the political context, governments and international organizations concerned with peacekeeping and peacemaking must pay attention to the psychological aftermath of political conflicts or change for losers as well as winners. In Part 2, this becomes a key issue when developing scenarios for the psychological aftermath of major conflicts and other mass traumas, e.g. the Balkans War in 1999 and the 9–11 attacks in the USA in 2001.

Part 2: Mass Transitions: Societal Responses to Trauma and Change

2.1 Effects of mass stress: fear and violence in stressed populations
2.2 Trauma and change: transitions and terrorism
2.3 Wider implications of social and political transitions

From 1997 to February 2001, my enquiries mainly followed the potential application of transition psychology to the behavior of national leaders, governments, and other political groups or organizations. However, events for political leaders frequently included *threats or traumas that affected whole communities, regions or nations,* e.g. wars and terrorist attacks. So my transition studies included the possibility that transition effects might affect much larger populations. If mass transitions do occur then the possibility of collective crisis periods could represent serious hazards for community health and national or international stability. On the positive side, if transitions have the potential to transform the lives of individuals and groups then mass traumas may even have longer term cathartic, peace-building potential, e.g. in Northern Ireland and in parts of the Balkans.

Many *mass trauma events* occur every year (see Table 27-4) – from wars to natural disasters – that can be used to test hypotheses and propositions about the dynamics of mass trauma and change. But it is important to consider *transition effects in the context with other psycho-social processes and cultural contexts.* My investigations start with individual psychological processes and resources that I have seen in the experiences of my clients and multi-cultural staff since I learned about transitions in 1978. Comprehensive assessments need to consider work roles and organizational settings, plus personal life-roles, family, and community settings. Both domains – work and personal life – involve identity, relationships, boundaries, values, beliefs, and expectations. These are mediated by personality, heritage, culture, faith, and personal geographical and historical context.

Effects of Mass Stress:
Fear and Violence in Stressed Populations

With so many variables for each individual how can we generalize the behavior of groups, communities, or nations? When societies are given time and space to evolve they develop diverse cultures. But certain dynamics appear similar in individual and group behavior across cultures – particularly, the *survival responses needed in times of trauma or change.* Sect 1.2 highlighted the evolutionary importance of *human responses to stress (fight and flight)* and *human responses to change (transitions).* These processes are connected but different in timing, process, and effects.

Discussion of stress in western countries recognizes the discomfort suffered by individuals under the increased pressures of life in relatively affluent cultures. Cumulative stress can have severe long-term effects on health and family breakdown plus traumatic stress from accidents or crime. Severe stress does occur in some contexts, e.g. poverty or extreme work expectations with violent results.

But western, largely lifestyle induced, stresses rarely compare with the acute life threatening stress of wars or natural disasters, or the chronic stress of military, economic, or ethnic oppression – situations that may unleash the extreme, primitive potential of the fight and flight response.

Table 27-4. Events that may have started strategic change or mass transition periods, 1998–2009.

Year	Political events	Economic events	Wars	Unrest or terror	Natural disasters
1998	UK: Northern Ireland Peace Agreement, April. German Election, September	Asian financial crises 1997-99, e.g. Indonesia – crisis January & riots in May. Also Thailand	Congo War, Aug 1998 to 2003. US strikes: –Afghanistan & Sudan, August –Iraq, November	US Embassies bombed in East Africa, August. Omagh bomb, N. Ireland, Aug	Earthquakes: Afghanistan, May Papua New Guinea, July
1999	Russia: New Prime Minister Putin & Government in Russia, August. UK: new Northern Ireland Assembly, November	Crises in Asia & south America. Fears of Y2K global computer crash	Balkans War & refugee exodus, March–July. Russian strikes & 2nd Chechen War. Sept +	Moscow bombs, September	Earthquakes: Colombia, January Turkey , August
2000	Millennium hope. U.S. election crisis, November–Dec	January: No Y2K crash. Dot Com boom peak Feb. US markets slide August on	Second Intifada Israel/Palestine, Sept–Dec	Sierra Leone rebellion, May–Sept.	UK: Foot & mouth disease, Aug–Dec Sri Lanka cyclone, Dec
2001	New U.S. President Bush, February, New Prime Minister Sharon, Israel, March UK Election, June	Enron scandal, US market slide, August–Sept. Argentine crisis, Dec.	US War on Terror, Sept War on Afghanistan, Oct+	Suicide bombs, Israel, Mar Nepal royal deaths, June 9-11 attacks, USA, Sept	India: Gujarat earthquake, January
2002	German Election, September	Argentine peso devaluation. US Market slide low July-Dec	Afghanistan war ongoing	Bali bombing, Oct	Afghan earthquakes, March
2003	Argentine Elections, Congo Transitional Government, July	US Market low Jan-Mar Argentine GDP recovery.	Darfur rebellion, Feb, Gulf War 2, March-April	Iraq, Afghanistan	Iran earthquake, December
2004	Arafat death, November. U.S. Election, November	EU expansion + 10 countries, May. Economic migration.	Iraq; Fallujah attacks, March, November	Spain: Madrid bombing, March Russia: Beslan massacre, Sept	Indonesian earthquake & Indian Ocean Tsunami, Dec

Year	Politics / Elections	Economy / Finance	Conflicts	Terrorism / Unrest	Natural Disasters
2005	UK Election, May. German Election, September & New Coalition, October. Sri Lanka Election, November		Escalating refugee crises in Africa, e.g. Sudan, eastern Congo. Chad civil war, Nov.	7-7 bombing London, July Bali bombs, October	Japan earthquake, March Hurricane Katrina, USA. Aug Kashmir earthquake, Oct
2006	Israel: Prime Minister Sharon stroke, January. Interim Prime Minister Ehud Olmert, Election, May		US more strikes Afghanistan, May Israel-Lebanon war , July-Aug	Lebanon protests December	Java earthquake, May
2007	UK new Prime Minister, June. Gaza Election Hamas, June. Israel New President, July. Georgia new Prime Minister, November.	EU +2 countries. US sub-prime mortgage crises July, UK August Rising global oil & food prices.	Conflicts in Sudan, Chad, Congo continue. Israel blockade Gaza, June on.	India unrest over rising food prices Pakistan: Dec, Benazir Bhutto assassinated	India floods June, Orissa, W Bengal. Japan earthquake. July. Cyclone Sidr, Bangladesh. Nov.
2008	New Presidents in: Georgia, January. Russia. March Lebanon. May. Pakistan, July Israel PM resigns, Sep Georgia PM. Nov. US Elections, Nov	Bear Stearns bank fails, US, March. Global food crisis, April. Oil $148, July Global Finance crisis & markets Crash, October. Multiple bank crises e.g. Iceland financial crash.	Chad crisis, Feb. Georgia/ South Ossetia/Russia conflict, August. Congo violence escalates Oct. Israel/Gaza conflict, Dec 07-Jan 08.	Feb to April: food riots –Africa, Haiti Bangladesh. Pakistan Marriott hotel bomb, Sept. India: Mumbai Hotel attack. Nov. Africa ongoing conflicts	Myanmar cyclone, May China: Sichuan earthquake, May Caribbean hurricanes, Aug. Haiti storm disasters, Sept.
2009	New U.S. President Obama, Jan Israeli election, Feb & coalition Government crises Pakistan,	Global recession: multiple financial crises. Rising unemployment. G20 summit, UK. March.	Ongoing conflicts in Africa, Middle East, Pakistan, and Sri Lanka. U.S. surge Afghanistan.	Suicide bombs in Iraq and Pakistan. Madagascar coup. March. Protests in Thailand. April.	Climate change: heat wave & wild fires. Australia. February Severe winter in US. Europe.

In March and April 1999, the mass exodus of Albanian refugees from Kosovo "was unusually large and swift – half a million people arrived in neighboring areas in the course of about two weeks, and a few weeks later the total was over 850,000" (UNHCR, Feb 2000). At the same time reported atrocities suggested that individuals had lost any trace of restraint or compassion. These events led me to question a possible connection between individual fight and flight responses, and the mass crisis behavior in populations exposed to chronic or acute stresses. At the limits of survival, individuals and groups may revert to primitive behavior with extreme fight or flight responses – violent attacks, atrocities, genocide, or refugee exodus. This shift is suggested in Fig. 27-5. When normal populations (a) are stressed anxiety increases and more individuals resort to violence (b). At a critical level, tensions may flash (sometimes in minutes) into open conflict or war. This flashpoint has dramatic effects on mental health and behavior where individuals may run, freeze, or fight (c).

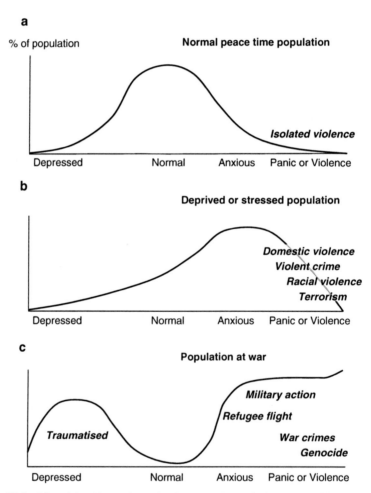

Fig. 27-5. Mental health and behavior in stressed populations: the shift to fear and violence from Fear and violence in stressed populations, Williams (1999, 2009) (Williams 1999g)

The shift to mass crisis behavior (c) may be triggered by trauma, e.g. military or terrorist attacks, or a natural disaster. It may start a mass post-trauma transition period. And in some cases it may be an expression of collective stress in a transition crisis period – typically, 6 months after an earlier event. The potential connections between mass stress in communities and genocide are explored by other researchers like Ervin Staub (2001), together with their complex cultural and historical contexts.

In late 2000, two events seemed likely to start major transition periods: the new Intifada conflict between communities in Palestine and Israel and the controversy over voting results in the U.S. Presidential election. These events were followed by the inauguration of the new U.S. President George Bush in January 2001 and Arial Sharon's election as the new Prime Minister of Israel in February. These four events had the potential to mark the start of major transition periods in both countries – with predictable hazards and opportunities. They became the focus for my next transition analysis exercise *the Eos Power or Peace project* (Williams 2001a) and forecasts in February 2001.

The wider context for the new leadership transitions in the USA and Israel for the Bush and Sharon administrations included the recent traumas in both countries. So the forecasts in the *Power or Peace project* also considered possible transition effects in wider groups – opposition parties and traumatized communities. Some of the effects anticipated in my February 2001 analysis are noted below. But actual events in September 2001 had far wider consequences than expected. In 2009, the latest conflict between Israel and Gaza, plus new governments in the USA and Israel, may trigger new transition periods, see Part 3.

Trauma and Change: Transitions and Terrorism

Transition forecasts highlight potentially vulnerable periods for governments that may have security implications. Personal and collective crisis behaviors in governments and other political organizations (e.g. Fig. 27-2) are obvious to media and political opponents when they arise. Are some terrorist attacks more likely when governments appear weak – e.g. the Al Qaeda bomb attacks on U.S. embassies in Kenya and Tanzania in August 1998 after the prolonged Lewinsky hearings?

Sometimes terrorist actions, especially random acts by individuals and small groups, may indicate that they and the groups they represent are in a period of internal crisis. This seems likely in highly stressed communities (see Figs. 27.5 and 27.6) or if the community is in a transition crisis period.

Terrorist violence by paramilitary groups in transition crisis may include brutal internal repression (e.g. punishment beatings in Northern Ireland) as well as external aggression. In 1998 paramilitaries in Northern Ireland faced an extended crisis during the transition period after the peace referendum because their former power and political justification to the communities they used represent was much reduced. In effect former fighters face a redundancy transition unless peace plans include provisions to give them an alternative role in society. Some dissident groups may continue violence after major conflicts appear to have been resolved, e.g. the Omagh bomb in Northern Ireland in August 1998. This problem occurs in fighting groups left over from past conflicts in many countries, e.g. in the Congo, Uganda, Indonesia, Thailand, UK, Spain. No group must be overlooked in transition planning.

The severity of violent attacks may increase during transition crisis periods 5–6+ months after key events. The *Power or Peace* observations and transition forecasts were written in February 2001. They were the basis for a letter sent to the Israel Prime Minister Arial Sharon on March 19 warning that social unrest in traumatized Palestinian communities might increase the potential post-trauma transition crisis period 6 months after heavy casualties in October 2000. (Williams 2001b) Based on the factors in Table 27-2 such unrest was likely to be increased, not suppressed by oppressive security operations. *"In highly stressed and traumatized communities this could be a psychological time-bomb with highly unpredictable consequences that no-one can control. Use of force is like spraying water on a petrol fire."* A long campaign of suicide bomb attacks started in March and June 2001.

Wider Implications of Social and Political Transitions

These propositions about the potential effects of transitions on psychological climate in governments and communities can be tested by monitoring signs of distress, crisis, or unrest 6–8 months after a trauma or change. This could have significant implications on the timing and nature of international support and peace interventions for countries involved in wars or internal conflicts.

They suggest that the first priority for communities in periods of psychological crisis is to stabilize short-term conditions and urge restraint by leaders and governments in crisis. Practical humanitarian support is likely to be more effective than military action in reducing violence – by reducing short-term stress in communities and creating better conditions for psychological recovery.

Temporary truces, independent observers, and peace-keeping resources may be important to improve psychological security, reduce fear and the increased risk of atrocities by any armed personnel who has suffered recent trauma. If these are rejected then human rights abuses and atrocities are to be expected. The effects of stress in communities in the Balkans in 1999 seemed relevant to understanding the refugee exodus and reported atrocities (Williams 1999c).

Attempts to seek long-term agreements in periods of crisis are unlikely to have much effect. But there may be major opportunities for new agreements if and when both groups move into a potential transition recovery period. These would be more effective if they allow participation from all levels of society, not just relying on high profile political leaders (see *Many paths to peace* (Williams 1999b)).

Transition theory offers the possibility that even the most tragic events – wars and disasters – may start periods of transition that will open opportunities to a new, more positive era for the populations concerned. If the transition process serves the evolutionary purposes suggested here then societies will eventually adapt through periods of change. External interventions may enable this process, or may inhibit it if political or commercial self-interest overrides humanitarian priorities, e.g. indiscriminate economic sanctions or military support to intensify conflicts.

A basic humanitarian question for societies in periods of trauma or change is *"How to minimize the level and duration of distress in extended crisis periods?"* This could reduce psychological casualties and maximize prospects for collective psychological recovery.

There have been major advances in psycho-traumatology, as part of emergency response capabilities in many countries since 9–11. The effects of PTSD (post-traumatic stress disorder) are widely recognized but medical research and practice rarely mentions the natural adaption process of transition. This has major implications for public mental health, economic performance, and long-term social stability. These implications are important to local communities, governments, and the long-term reputation of national leaders. They are likely to apply to many countries, for example in the trauma and post-conflict aftermath of the war in the Balkans from March–July 1999. In *Balkans Aftermath: The post-war transition – denial, crisis & world peace* (Williams 1999d) I explored the possibility of a post-conflict transition period for all communities through 2000, applying the transition template with variations for winners and losers (see Fig. 27-6). Expectations reversed due to NATO intervention: initial aggressors became losers, while some victim communities were reestablished. All communities were severely disrupted.

In addition to the refugee exodus in Kosovo during the conflict there were widespread population movements within the region and emigration after the war – escape or quitting behavior? An epidemic of depression (implying extended crisis symptoms) was reported in the Balkans in 2000. Earlier studies, e.g. Flogel and Lauc (Flögel & Lauc 2000), indicated a wide range of war-stress related mental health problems in the former Yugoslavia in the 1990s. In 2002, a survey indicated extensive mental health problems continuing over 2 years after the 1999 war. Almost half the people surveyed had symptoms of depression, 13% had symptoms of PTSD (Zimonjic 2002).

Forecasts and Reality: Mass Traumas in the USA on 9-11, 2001

In February 2001, the *Power or Peace project* had included similar forecasts (Fig. 27-6) for the post-election transition periods in the USA and Israel, and how these could be relevant to UK election date options. Prime Minister Blair chose an early election in May 2001 instead of stabilising international

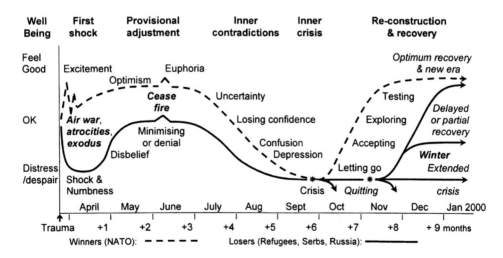

Fig. 27-6. Psychological stages of transition from the start of the Balkans war in 1999. Crisis and recovery scenarios forecast on 1 August 1999 (Williams 1999d)

relations - just as tensions in Israel and Palestine deteriorated into the predicted post-trauma crisis (Fig. 27-7). The Downside risk scenario forecast in this February chart was greatly exceeded by extended crisis in Israel, the 9-11 attacks in September 2001 in the USA, and the War on Terror.

The horrors of the attacks on 9-11 started a new mass trauma cycle in the USA with global consequences. Four weeks later, the War on Terror started with the war on Afghanistan. I updated my earlier scenarios for the new U.S. Administration in November 2001 in Fig. 27-8.

The psychological impacts of 9-11 across the United States were explored cautiously in my paper *Psychological aftermath of September 11th- Is there a 9-11 Transition?* (Williams 2002) July 2002.

Some aftermaths of the 9-11 attacks in New York and Washington were immediately obvious. The awesome clearing and recovery operation in New York illustrated the amazing resilience of human beings to trauma. The energy and support – psychological as well as technical – given to support the most traumatized areas of Manhattan, bereaved relatives, and displaced workers was immense for many weeks. This resilience was partly reflected in the temporary revival of NASDAQ share prices in the first three months after the trauma (see Fig. 27-9). But the challenges to residents and workers were not a single, brief shock. Workers from large corporations like Amex were relocated for up to 6 months miles away in New Jersey and many were made redundant. For these people, organizations, and communities the disruption continued at least until they could return to their offices.

In these situations the basic timescale of transition has to be extended at least as long as it takes to return to some form of normal living and working. The mental health consequences of this were likely to be as significant in New York and the Pentagon neighborhood as they were in the Balkans for at least a year after the 1999 war, i.e. widespread anxiety problems, reactive depression, and PTSD for bereaved families, emergency services, and local workers and communities. However, communities in New York may have had more security and emotional support (Table 27-1).

The Tsunami Effect of Delayed Shocks From 9-11 and Other Mass Traumas

The regional, national, and international effects of 9-11 involved complex human responses far beyond the scope of this chapter. But the basic transition model and its typical stages for individual life events may be a primary survival pathway for people directly and deeply affected by any major trauma. Most bereaved relatives, friends, and colleagues of 9-11 casualties were immediately affected and traumatized by an irreversible loss. Many people across the USA (and other countries) were shocked at the TV reports of the several 9-11 attacks and twin towers collapse as a vicarious, second-hand trauma. These images were a likely source of fear or anger, not yet an immediate personal loss, but for many a major violation of American national identity and invulnerability. The wider impacts became more personal from economic trauma - unemployment, restrictions on travel, fear, and a call to war. These effects spread across the wider community in New York – *Beyond Ground Zero* (Comprehensive Study Finds Problems Mount For "Indirect Victims" of WTC Attacks 2002) – and across the USA in a chain of cascading

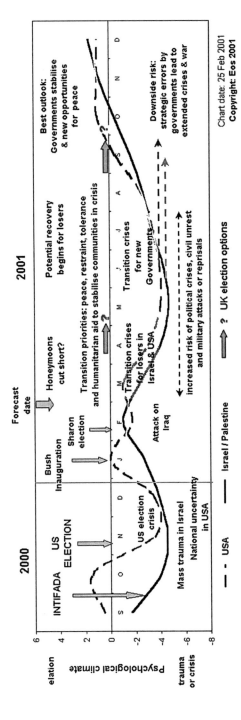

Fig. 27-7. Outlook for new governments in the USA and Israel in 2001 and UK election options (from Power or Peace?) (Williams 2001)

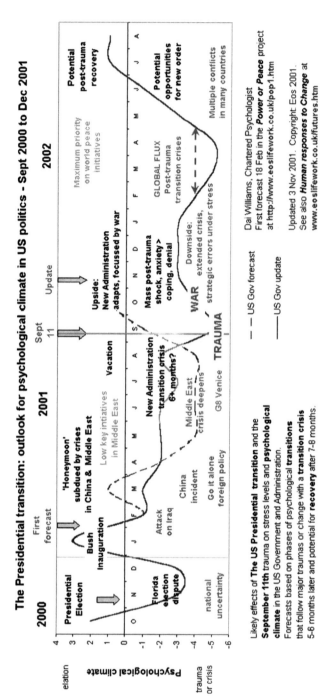

Fig. 27-8. The Presidential transition: outlook for psychological climate in U.S. politics, September 2000 to December 2001, updated for the potential impact of mass traumas on 9-11 to August 2002. (from *Psychological aftermath of September 11th Is there a 9-11 Transition?*) (Williams 2002)

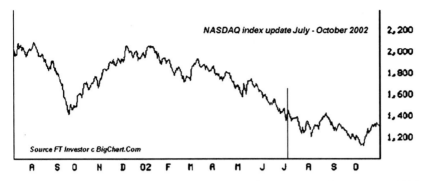

Fig. 27-9. The U.S. NASDAQ stock market prices from August 2001 to October 2002 (Chart from the Financial Times www.ft.com and BigChart.com)

consequences, e.g. severe cuts in commercial aviation hit workers in Seattle when Boeing reduced 27,000 jobs over the next 3 years.

The full economic and psychological impacts of mass traumas, like 9-11, will spread over several weeks and months – like the ripples from throwing a brick into a pool of water, or more ominously like the shock waves from an undersea earthquake that become tsunami when they finally reach the land. The *tsunami metaphor* is useful to warn of delayed psychological effects of major events – e.g. wars or natural disasters. Depending on the type of event its psychological, economical, political or other effects may be delayed by geographic distance and/or by time delays.

Ironically, the tsunami metaphor for the propagation of mass transition effects from an initial trauma became a grim reality on December 26, 2004 when an earthquake off the coast of Indonesia triggered *the Indian Ocean Tsunami* – waves that devastated coastal locations in 11 countries killing 225,000 people. The psychological, economic, and political consequences of this event can be analyzed with the techniques in Part 3. Levels of support to traumatized communities and human consequences varied widely between countries. Some had reforms (Aceh, Maldives), others had conflict and extended crises (Sri Lanka), and some had more disasters (cyclone Nargis in Myanmar).

One crucial feature of a physical tsunami is the combined effect of a high energy event that may pass almost unnoticed in a deep ocean, but which multiplies rapidly when it encounters a limiting condition (like shallow water or a beach). Then its effects may be devastating and sometimes unexpected because of time or distance from the original event. This offers a metaphor for wider or delayed economic, psychological and health impacts of mass transitions after a major trauma or change. This is relevant for planning emergency and transition support for communities, organizations, or nations from a major event, e.g. the effects of financial market collapse on businesses like banks and insurance companies, and on vulnerable economies, e.g. Iceland in 2008.

Possible Indicators of Mass Transitions

Whether the attacks of 9-11 caused the war on terror, or served to justify major military operations against Afghanistan and Iraq, they certainly had massive national and international consequences. Some of these operations were directly under the control of key decision makers whose strategic judgement may have been severely impaired both by trauma (shock) and more deeply by the stress and uncertainty involved in responding to major personal, work, or national life events.

Stressed or bizarre behavior and strategic errors are fairly obvious for high-profile public leaders. But mass traumas or changes should have observable indicators in the affected populations. Where available there should be direct indicators of distressed, depressed, or crisis behavior from mental health statistics, or sickness and absence statistics for organizations. Stock markets data give real-time indicators of the economic confidence of decision makers in many countries (Fig. 27-9).

The US NASDAQ market prices for 14 months from August 2001 (Fig. 27-9) reflected the immediate trauma of 9-11 and remarkable resilience for the next three months. But this was followed by a progressive decline. Brief increases, possibly from oil price increases in response to more war rumors, delayed the slide by two months but did not alter the downward trend of market confidence. The potential post-trauma recovery and new order scenarios forecast for the USA (Fig. 27-8) for mid-year 2002 did not happen. The downside scenario, *multiple conflicts in different countries,* became War on Terror interventions in many countries and plans for Gulf War 2 in 2003.

Other Reflections on the 9-11 Transition Proposition

The possibility of a large scale 9-11 transition in the USA raised several issues:

Transition is a Different Process From PTSD
The transition cycle has not been widely used by psychologists except in some aspects of counselling and organizational change. It is rarely referred to in medical settings or guidance in the UK except by some occupational health professionals.

The concept of PTSD is widely used by medical personnel, counsellors, and therapists for relatives and communities directly affected by trauma and loss, though less than 1 in 5 people involved may report intrusive symptoms requiring medical support. But many more people whose lives or work have been deeply affected by a major trauma or change are likely to experience transition effects as a normal, and possibly necessary, response that usually enables people to adapt to their new reality.

PTSD appears to be a dysfunctional response to trauma. But transition appears to be a natural adaptation process with potential for positive outcomes (Adler 1975), though with a hazardous crisis phase that can deteriorate into long-term problems (anxiety or depression) needing mental health support.

Continuing research into the psychological aftermath of 9-11 might include transition analysis and awareness for traumatized populations. Ideally this would be done by analysts in the USA with direct knowledge of the U.S. economy, and of diverse communities and local social systems.

Organizational symptoms of transition can be recognized by anyone familiar with the process, e.g. managers, human resources, and occupational health professionals - not just the psychologists. Economic and political analyses need to consider psychological dimensions of trauma and change in the USA, and a timeframe that extends at least 1–2 years before and after September 11, 2001.

Regular community health statistics (e.g. for anxiety and reactive depression) could be valuable indicators of mass transition effects in a community. But in

New York most of the internet health statistics after 9-11 were quarterly or annual, and published a year later. Weekly or monthly statistics published as soon as possible could be important indicators in recently traumatized communities. However, many local health studies started in the aftermath of the 9-11 attacks may have more relevant indicators.

Reflections for Transition Management Strategies

If a post-trauma 9-11 transition period did occur then to what extent did organizations and communities use, or develop their own transition management strategies spontaneously? How many people have worked through their personal 9-11 experiences themselves, or with mutual help and encouragement from family or friends? Transition awareness, or exceptional empathy and other social skills are important to maintain trust and cohesion within organizations in periods of rapid or severe change (Herriot et al. 1998). Managers and Human Resource professionals for corporations based in or near the World Trade Centre – Ground Zero for the 9-11 attacks - faced major challenges to maintain operations through loss of staff and facilities, temporary relocation, then redundancies and return while relying on many traumatized but committed staff. How did commercial, city, and community organizations manage through the 9-11 transition? How did they survive? How did they adapt, change, or thrive? Prior learning from their challenging transition experiences after 9-11 may increase the resilience of many New York organizations through potential transition periods in 2009.

Differing Vulnerability in Periods of Transition

The transition model is subject to individual differences. Some individuals may have been more vulnerable than others, e.g. if they had experienced a major life event in the year before 9-11, due to varying social and economic circumstances, or to personality differences. Community mental health research into the psychological effects of 9-11 may have considered vulnerable groups like children. How were ethnic minority communities affected by harassment or many internments from security operations searching for suspected Al Qaeda networks?

Delayed Effects of Trauma and Change

The impact of major traumas on larger organizations and national populations, like the USA, may be concealed or delayed depending on how directly people were affected at the time – the Tsunami effect mentioned in Sect. 2.5 above. The propagation of psychological trauma may be delayed by weeks or months until individual's lives, wealth, or work are directly affected, e.g. by redundancy or loss of investments. If such patterns were identified in the USA after 2001, these may be relevant in forecasting the propagation effects of the global Credit Crunch and Crash in 2008/9.

Gold in the Ashes?

What did *not* emerge from the 9-11 post-trauma transition period was a national upturn in confidence, optimism, creativity, and harmony within 9–12 months as expected in my U.S. transition forecasts updated in November 2001 (Fig. 27-8). The individual transition cycle indicates potential recovery and growth for individuals in the third 3-month period after major traumas or changes. This can happen even after devastating loss. The essence of the transition process appears to be to enable us to survive *and* thrive – to find *gold in the ashes* of life traumas.

I did find positive attitudes in New York itself one year after 9-11. By the first anniversary in September 2002 the sense of community, confidence, and optimism in central New York was impressive. A group of bereaved relatives founded *Peaceful Tomorrows* and built links with families in Afghanistan bereaved from the retaliation bombing 7–8 months after their loss.

William McDonough was the CEO of the Federal Reserve Bank of New York. His address at Trinity Church on the first anniversary of 9-11 questioned the ethics of excessive executive pay (McDonough 2002). This was a courageous issue to raise and an insightful warning 5 years before the global financial crisis developed in 2007. His statement had *defining moment* qualities (see 1.5) like those I observed among some UK politicians in 1997/98 (Fig. 27-2).

Seen from Europe, reactions to 9-11 in Washington seemed different from the resilience in New York. The USA was at war with elusive enemies in the Middle East – mainly, Afghanistan and later Iraq. National and international air travel suffered widespread anxiety and severe airline security restrictions (Williams 2004). Civil aviation responded with determination and vigilance. But the War on Terror became a mission of great passion for the Governments in the U.S. and UK. Was the mystery about alleged WMD's (weapons of mass destruction) in Iraq a classic example of the Groupthink syndrome (Janis 1982a) identified by Irving Janis after the Bay of Pigs fiasco? If so, there was a risk that strategic errors and collective delusions would be used to justify escalating the conflict with Iraq. Were these signs of cohesion and inspiration, or chronic stress verging on obsession; of transition recovery or of extended crisis? The psychological health of heads of state and senior statesmen influenced national and international events, and appeared to influence levels of national confidence or paranoia.

History suggests that mass transitions can occur for large populations, but much more slowly than for individuals. Two major examples of mass traumas leading to mass transitions and societal transformation were the rebuilding of Japan and Germany after World War 2. Both populations largely rejected the militaristic values and international aggression that led to their defeat. Both countries channelled their reconstruction to build two of the strongest economies and innovative technological infrastructures in the world for the next 50 years. But at the national level, these recoveries took at least 9 years, not 9 months, to build momentum and to produce *gold from the ashes* of their war time experiences in 1939–45.

In 1997–98, the transition crisis period in the UK Government continued for four months until several senior ministers had reached personal turning points or defining moments accepting their new reality and responsibilities. Once this critical mass was reached the Government's collective morale and recovery appeared to gather momentum with considerable speed and synergy (Fig. 27-2).

The prospect of communities and nations finding gold in the ashes of major conflicts or disasters should be possible if the transition process is an evolutionary survival trait among humans of all races. This was discussed in a seminar about psycho-history in York (UK) in March 2002. If further research finds evidence of this (see Part 3), then transition theory may offer a basis for hope and long-term optimism for communities in periods of extended crisis or chaos, e.g. in Africa and the Middle East, or facing human or natural disasters, e.g. from wars or climate change.

Part 3: Applying Transition Analysis
to Recent and Future Mass Traumas

Events that May Trigger Mass Transitions

Terrorist attacks and wars have many human dimensions in their causes and effects. The impact of natural disasters on communities may have contributory human factors. Whatever their origin, mass traumas or changes have the potential to start periods of mass transition for individuals and groups.

Table 27-4 offers a list of major events that may have started mass transition periods and responses in communities, nations, or regions from 1998 to 2009. It includes political and economic changes, unrest, wars, and natural disasters. Such events are analyzed by the media, politicians, and national and international institutions for economic, security and political implications, and for humanitarian support issues. Some consider mental health indicators of mass distress, depression, or despair (Paton & Long 1996).

Transition psychology offers another perspective for analysis of individual and collective responses to trauma and change. *Transition analysis* can be applied at community, national, and regional levels. It may be a useful tool for aid organizations and disaster response planners. It may be important for strategic decision makers to be alert for *unexpected psychological hazards*, e.g. delayed or extended crises, and to be alert for exciting *opportunities* for innovation, change, and sometimes reconciliation or other cultural transformation following mass traumas or changes.

As a practitioner in work and community psychology I am looking for ways of harnessing these observations and propositions to add to the growing *"toolkit"* of applied psychology. Each of my explorations into the use of transition analysis to topical events has been an opportunity to test and build on earlier hunches and techniques. Where possible I have suggested priorities and techniques for individuals and organizations who manage, respond to, or research trauma or change.

Between 1997 and 2001 I developed two *transition tracking* techniques while observing and analysing the events with political or mass transition potential reported in Parts 1 and 2:

(a) *Eos Transition Tracking Timeline charts* – for pre-cursor events and outlook scenarios
(b) *The Eos Transition Tracking Checklist* – factors, issues, and stages for analysis and response

Either or both methods can be tested as a basis for analysing any major trauma or change for its transition potential. Some events listed in Table 27-4 were key political changes. Some were brief traumas, while others involved extended periods of trauma or crisis.

Eos Transition Tracking Timeline Charts

Many of the events listed in Table 27-4 were likely to start *individual transitions* for people directly involved – from casualties, troops, or bereaved relatives to newly elected political leaders. Personal *life-line exercises* (Williams 2008) help individuals to recognize key life events and their personal experiences of transitions. Personal awareness of transitions (Part 1) is helpful for practitioners and researchers to appreciate the potential stages, indicators, and effects of transitions for other people.

I use a similar timeline format for *transition tracking* in groups or *organizations*. Key events and reported incidents are used as indicators of collective psychological climate or morale (e.g. the UK press headlines in Fig. 27-3). I used this for forecasting the potential post-election transition in the UK Parliament in 1997, and reviewing actual events through the first year of the new UK Government through 1997-98 (Fig. 27-2). I used a more structured method for *Accidents Waiting to Happen* in 2000 (Williams 2000c) (Fig. 27-4), with monthly ratings charted on several themes using a ± 5 point scale on Excel. Social anthropologists have long used critical incidents to monitor group and community processes. Transition tracking also looks for psychological indicators of individual and group behavior associated with stages of transition, e.g. from quitting to defining moments for individuals, and from scape-goating to innovative and collaborative achievements in groups (Fig. 27-2).

The *Eos Transition Tracking Timeline* chart in Fig. 27-9 was developed in 2001 as a quick diagnostic diagram for major traumas or unexpected crisis events, considering recent past, present, and near future. The first stage *reflects* the *recent events* in the 6–9+ month *"transition window"* period prior to a dramatic event of human origin. This may indicate personal or collective triggers for extreme crisis behavior, e.g. prior to the Royal family massacre in Nepal (June 2001) or sudden terrorist or military attacks (Beslan 2004, Georgia 2008). In natural disasters, the prior period may indicate the psychological state or resilience of affected communities and key decision makers managing disaster response.

The second stage of the transition tracking chart invites forward projection of the *outlook* and *scenarios* for typical phases of transition and change over 3, 6, and 9 months. These include coping (honeymoon or denial), potential delayed shock or crisis behavior, and potential for recovery, growth, or transformation (see also Fig. 27-1). The crisis period for individuals and groups is typically 6 months after a trigger event, plus or minus 3–4 weeks. The period from crisis to recovery may happen quickly for individuals - within days or weeks of a crisis point. But it may be much slower for groups, organizations, and communities (weeks, months, or years). Recovery may be totally blocked for months or years by repressive conditions, resulting in extended crisis scenarios. A longer timescale is needed to map extended crises, and potential delayed impacts with secondary transition periods where the key event is very large, triggering *tsunami-type* human or economic effects that propagate over time (see 2.5).

Specific outcomes after the transition crisis phase are hard to predict. Key agencies may have desired outcomes, or seek to impose change. In the 1970s Shell moved to scenario planning for complex futures. I look for at least two or three different *scenarios* following the crisis phase, e.g. optimum recovery, delayed recovery, and extended crisis periods (see Fig. 27-10). Unpredicted shifts may emerge during major transition periods, e.g. transformation to new economic models, political structures, or migrations. The concept of recovery

This chart can be used to develop a timeline for analysing key events related to a period of trauma, crisis or change. It is intended for use with the *Eos Transition Tracking Checklist*. It may be used to track perceived changes in psychological climate i.e. well-being or distress for one or more groups directly affected by the key event. This may give clues to periods of transition* prior to, or following the key event.

Instructions

a) Use the date of the key event as month 0, write months on the date line.
b) Note positive events above the centre line and negative ones below it. Mark an **x** for each event to indicate its likely severity or benefit at the time.
c) Draw a line like a temperature chart to reflect the level of well-being or distress for each group affected throughout the analysis period.
d) If several groups are affected in different ways use separate charts.

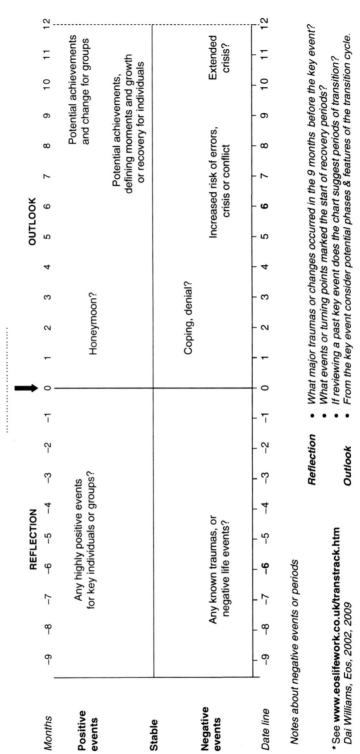

Key event or crisis

Notes about positive events or periods

Notes about negative events or periods

Reflection
- What major traumas or changes occurred in the 9 months before the key event?
- What events or turning points marked the start of recovery periods?

Outlook
- If reviewing a past key event does the chart suggest periods of transition?
- From the key event consider potential phases & features of the transition cycle.

* See **www.eoslifework.co.uk/transtrack.htm**
  Dai Williams, Eos, 2002, 2009

Fig. 27-10. Transition tracking timeline: Key event date or start (return to past norms or ideologies) may obscure more radical shifts in values or alliances that were unthinkable before the trauma or change.

The Eos Transition Tracking Checklist

Transition tracking timeline charts are useful to illustrate stages of change based on a systematic investigation of the event, the population involved, their context, and likely processes. Mass transitions may develop as a consequence of several types of mass trauma or change events (see Chart 4). Many governments, international organizations, and businesses have sophisticated security or emergency response procedures. Many will have some change management specialists. But *transition management* is rarely reported. The *Eos Transition Tracking Checklist* in Table 27-5 is designed for evaluating significant traumas

Table 27-5. The Eos transition tracking checklist

1. Identify key events
   (a) *Description* – Positive or negative? Expected or unexpected? Obvious causes?
   (b) *Timing* – When? Single event (e.g. an election or earthquake) or a series of related incidents/events over a period of time (e.g. an epidemic or period of conflict?).
   (c) *Transition potential* – Permanent changes to the life of individuals, groups or communities affected? Potential source of transition?
   (d) *Other key events* Have people concerned had other major events or changes recently? Could the crisis be a symptom of recent trauma or change?

2. People or groups affected
   (a) *Primary impacts* – Who is directly affected - individuals, groups? How, why and when?
   (b) *Secondary impacts* Who else may be indirectly affected? How and why?
   (c) *External groups or organizations*
What positive forces may be available – allies, resources?
What negative forces may affect the situation – hostile or predatory forces?
   (d) *Participation & ongoing monitoring* – Who is involved in transition analysis?
Who provides ongoing data about effects, needs, support, coping, health, welfare?

3. Context appraisal
   (a) *Assessment* – of economic, environmental, social, cultural, religious, political, and security context for people or groups involved in the event – past, present, and near future.
   (b) *Inter-disciplinary dialogue* with other specialists for different perspectives and exchange transition awareness for their interpretation of events, outcomes, and strategic priorities.

4. *Transition analysis*
   (a) *Transition tracking timeline* (see chart) for a period at least 6–9 months before the key event and continuing for 12+ months afterwards.
   (b) *Other time-related factors?* For example, seasons, religious, political or cultural events that have occurred recently or are expected in the next year.
   (c) *Potential hazards* Likely consequences of the trauma or change without intervention. Use transition cycle template to identify potentially crisis periods (typically 5–6 months, possibly extended, longer timescales for groups) and transition crisis behaviour – anxiety, depression, errors, conflict, quitting etc
   (d) *Potential opportunities* for people to adapt successfully to trauma and change. Positive periods:
      (i) 1–3 months: honeymoon or denial phase,
      (ii) 7–9+ months: potential recovery.

Table 27-5. (continued)

5. Develop scenarios

   (a) *Several options,* e.g. minimum change, positive change, and negative change.

   (b) *Probability* of each without intervention – low, medium or high? Potential severity?

   (c) *Plan* for high probability scenarios. Consider unusual or unthinkable options.

   (d) *Contingency plans* for low probability/high impact scenarios.

6. *Transition management options*

   (a) *Transition awareness* – Existing levels for each group? How can this be increased?

   (b) *Identify* key agencies – Sources of power or influence for transition management support?

   (c) Hazard analysis – What enabling and inhibiting factors exist? (Tables 27.1 and 27.2).

Identify potential transition crisis periods for leaders and communities.

   (d) Opportunity analysis

Optimum timing for strategic interventions, projects or initiatives?

   (e) Identify options for transition management interventions.

   (f) Evaluate options. Assess positive and negative aspects for each option.

   (g) Update scenarios

Transition management interventions may alter the initial scenarios

7. Dissemination and implementation

   (a) *Participation, communication* – Link transition scenarios and transition management issues with other assessments. Strategic briefings and action.

   (b) *Promote community readiness* for delayed crises, secondary effects, new traumas.

   (c) *Ongoing review* - Monitoring, update assessments, scenarios and policy advice.

8. *Post-transition follow-up*

   (a) *Check points - monthly for first year, quarterly for 2-3+ years to identify:*

      (i)   successful individuals/groups,

      (ii) casualties?

      (iii) People in extended crisis.

9. *Long-term transitions*

   (a) *Major societal traumas or changes* (e.g. wars, economic recession, and natural disasters) may involve multiple transitions over longer periods. Transition monitoring and analysis of a strategic management theme and priority for practitioners in community, education, and medical support projects.

   (b) *Continuing trauma and slow onset transitions* (e.g. wars, refugees, climate change, slow onset health epidemics, migration) have major potential to cause individual and mass transitions. Similar transition analysis can be applied for community support and strategic planning and research but with much longer timescales.

or change events as potential causes or symptoms of periods of transition. It also provides a framework for using *transition analysis* to develop change scenarios and opportunities for applying transition management techniques.

Not all events cause transitions. Not all crises are due to transitions. So part of this analysis involves sorting out whether an obvious crisis situation is the start of a new potential transition cycle, or a delayed reaction to a recent trauma or change event – i.e. a transition crisis (also included in the chart in Fig. 27-9). Natural disasters may be totally unexpected (earthquakes, tsunamis) or seasonal hazards (storms, floods, droughts). Human crises (war, other violence, economic, or political turbulence) may be symptoms of a response to a recent trauma or political or economic change.

Although the transition process may affect large groups, organizations, or communities it operates within the mind of each individual affected. Group or mass transitions are fundamentally the sum of these individual experiences of adapting to a shared trauma or mass change event. However, the combined effects of stress and other factors will involve additional group dynamic processes. Thus, potential mass transition trigger events need to be analyzed for their possible effects on individuals and groups, and in their wider context.

This checklist is primarily designed for *recent or current events*. But the same framework can be applied to *historic events* where there is sufficient data about the time period approximately one year before and after the key event, e.g. from personal diaries and other contemporary reports.

Leaders and facilitators need to be adaptable in periods of mass trauma or change. The early tasks may be obvious (e.g. survival needs) but priorities and outcomes may evolve in unexpected directions as people and organizations through stages of adapting to the new situation. The checklist indicates stages of a learning process in which users with different roles can contribute to the evolving responses needed for mass trauma or change. These can be repeated and updated.

Every life event that affects an individual is an opportunity for personal growth, development, and change. Societal changes are the sum of individual transitions in response to shared traumas or changes. Large-scale transition management programmes must be aware of the remarkable ability of individuals to adapt to trauma and change, and facilitate these wherever possible. Attempts to dominate or control personal transitions by governments or other agencies may impede recovery.

One key to successful group transitions and community transformation may be the diversity of visionary insights from the unique outcomes of individual transitions, whether from inspired individuals or visionary groups. The amazing pace of technological development in times of war, and strategic community initiatives in some post-conflict periods, may be indicators of significant personal, group, and community transitions. Historians and biographers might test this proposition.

Research Challenges: Peace, Political, and Community Psychology

The human and natural events with mass transition potential explored in this paper – from elections to wars, and from large-scale economic or financial disasters - are recognized as strategic issues in many disciplines and professions. These issues are the subject of extensive economic, political and military research, analysis and funding. This research may have humanitarian objectives, e.g. disaster relief or it may be focussed on social control, economic exploitation, or political domination.

Until recently, there have been relatively few psychological inputs to strategic political or financial behavior. A rare exception was Professor Hugh Freeman's paper *The Human Brain and Political Behaviour* (Freeman 1991b) in 1991 (see 1.3). There is a thriving international network of trauma support practitioners and researchers (ISTSS), e.g. psycho-traumatology therapies particularly the use of CBT for PTSD. I am not a therapist but a range of normal human and organizational behavior principles (e.g. for managing stress and change) should be relevant to political events and wars or natural disasters. Other organizational behavior techniques and models may also be relevant to disaster planning, emergency response, and strategic political, economic, and military decision-making.

These explorations of potential mass transition events and periods highlight the need for multi-disciplinary analysis of large-scale trauma and change. Psychologists have much to exchange with historians, biographers, and many other professionals from national and international organizations with direct experience of mass transitions. Experienced practitioners often have multiple career perspectives, e.g. ex-military personnel in peace negotiations and scientists in relief operations.

Psychologists seek evidence-based analysis and interpretation. I am a practitioner with tendencies of a researcher. I look for new insights and tools that I can offer to my clients to help them manage their lives and organizations in a turbulent world. They need comprehensive, workable models that they can apply and adapt themselves in the light of their experiences, and so do I. These enquiries have drawn a mix of action research from clients and events, the work of the life span development and transition psychology pioneers in the 1970s plus elements of personal construct psychology, open systems, chaos theory, and participant observation from social anthropologists.

To verify or refine these propositions about mass transitions on a national and international scale will take a decade of research, combining the talents of several disciplines and professions, and from many cultural perspectives. The effects of trauma stress and change will need correlating with other psychological, social, and organizational processes and with medical and epidemiological research.

Transition psychology may enable medical professionals to review the boundaries of predictable fluctuations in mental health, e.g. anxiety, distress, and depression from more severe conditions. Short periods of distress after recent life events is not just normal but may be a necessary stage of psychological adjustment after major life events. Situational factors in organizations, families, or communities are critical in enabling or inhibiting healthy adaptation to individual or collective loss or trauma. Initially, these aspects of mass trauma transitions are as much community empowerment (Orford 1992) as occupational health awareness issues, freeing therapeutic support for acute crises or prolonged conditions, e.g. PTSD and clinical depression, with sensitivity for cultural and religious differences and community support. Community psychology is an emerging resource.

A major research priority for traumatized populations may be the *thresholds of extreme fight and flight behavior*. The insights of psychiatrists and clinical and forensic psychologists are essential to understand the danger zones where ordinary people flash over to extreme violence under chronic or acute threat or duress (Fig. 27-5). Are some of these episodes triggered or exacerbated by transition crisis situations, as well as by extreme stress or severe ideological domination?

The economic, political, and environmental challenges of the 21st century require greater insights into how individuals, communities, and countries can survive, co-exist, and thrive in adverse and rapidly changing conditions.

In the last two years the twin threats of global financial collapse and climate change make *the dynamics of mass transitions* an increasingly urgent area for well-coordinated research and professional practice.

If a fraction of the research funding invested in studying the psychology of military pilots was spent on studying the behavior and performance of politicians and the organizational behavior of governments, the results might enable a more stable world. In the last 20 years, the arms industry has diversified into global security and surveillance. The civil and military security sectors are primary sponsors for psychological research into trauma, stress, and change. These are important for combat performance, trauma support, civil order, and counter terror operations. Understanding mass trauma transitions may be relevant in many conflict situations. However, researchers and practitioners need to be vigilant and accountable for where and how psychology is applied.

Strategic Issues in the Psychology of Government and World Order

A quest that started from an exchange of culture shock survival tips between young travellers in a remote desert has become a mission with wider applications than I realized – certainly relevant to individual and corporate change and development programmes. Since transition management has become recognized as a strategic human resources issue in a multi-national corporation, aspects may be transferable to other complex institutions like governments and international programmes for economic development and support.

This chapter suggests that transition management and related psychosocial processes (e.g. normal and dysfunctional effects, stress, and trauma from PTSD, groupthink (Janis 1982b) and scape-goating to extreme violence) may be particularly relevant to understanding the impact of trauma or large-scale change on governments and communities. Regional, national, and international events observed since 1997 suggest that these factors are as relevant in political careers, governments, and organizations as they are in most other occupations and commercial organizations. They indicate several *strategic issues:*

- Need for *transition awareness* in governments and communities
- Opportunities to recognize and encourage *transition management skills* in politics
- Importance of *reducing stress and fear* to stabilize organizations and communities in crisis
- *Timing and priorities* for international support for communities in crisis
- *Vigilance for strategic errors* by key individuals and organizations in crisis
- *Timing of strategic decisions or initiatives*, e.g. elections, peace agreements

My studies on political transitions over the last 10 years have tried to be politically balanced and my analyses written to be relevant and available to all parties in the UK and via the Internet. Politicians and political leaders, like senior executives, are still human. They experience the ups and downs of life, periods of personal and career transitions, like most other people. They can be inspired at times, and lethal at others.

Some aspects of the psychology of stress and change outlined in this chapter already give us and them a much sharper idea of when and why these hazards and opportunities are likely to occur. If we can give a problem a name we are half-way into solving it. Transition psychology offers another technique for professional analysts, planners, and decision makers to understand why and when political, commercial or other leaders and groups may be safe, dangerous or inspired. Media commentators and the public need to be aware of the hazards and opportunities of transitions too – for our personal survival and to understand those who seek to enhance or dominate our world.

Awareness of these insights is equally important to political analysts, politicians, and political parties to understand how best to manage the immense responsibilities of government. One possibility is that politicians may become more aware of when to take extra care in relationships with leaders, allies, colleagues, or specialist advisors that they rely on for strategic advice or decisions, or when to understand the motivation and intentions of political or military opponents.

2009 and beyond: applying transition psychology in a turbulent world

In April 2009, the world may be in the eye of a storm between the 2008 global financial crash and a period of increasing economic and political turbulence as traditional institutions are unable to adapt to new conditions. The G20 Summit in London was well timed to encourage global dialogue at a potentially critical time for psychological as well as economic reasons. Initial reports were positive indicating some consensus about the need for international cooperation, in response to the global crisis. Was this enough to stop the developing Recession in many countries? Time will tell. For now planners and leaders need to consider *multiple scenarios* until economic conditions stabilize.

If the transition process enables individuals to survive and thrive in good times and bad then it could be valuable in times of mass trauma or change. Readers can test this themselves by applying the *Transition Tracking Checklist and Transition Tracking Timeline charts* to the turbulent events of the global financial crisis from 2007–2009 and the next few years.

In Fig. 27-10 – *the Financial Crash and US Presidential transitions, October 2008 & January 2009* - the transition tracking chart is used to monitor two distinct, but related transition periods.

The chart invites readers to reflect on significant events in the year before the financial crash in October 2008. Two years would be even better, e.g. starting with the *sub-prime lending crisis in July 2007*. Was this a sufficient trauma or revelation to start a *first transition period* for key economic decision makers? If yes, did the *Bear-Sterns collapse* and reports of panic in world markets in *March 2008* indicate a mass transition crisis response in many financial institutions? Did fear of global financial collapse then start a *second transition cycle* for crucial decision makers – from national leaders to individual traders? If so, were senior executives coping with the financial crises in *Lehman Brothers, AIG*, and *Meryl-Lynch* in *September 2008*, losing strategic control in another crisis phase, or continuation of an extended crisis from March? Or was the whole financial system in collapse?

Who was directly and immediately affected by these financial traumas? What deeply held beliefs, values or assumptions may have been broken, or became obsolete, for individuals, corporations, and governments? How were crucial political and economic decisions affected by the psychological

560   D. Williams

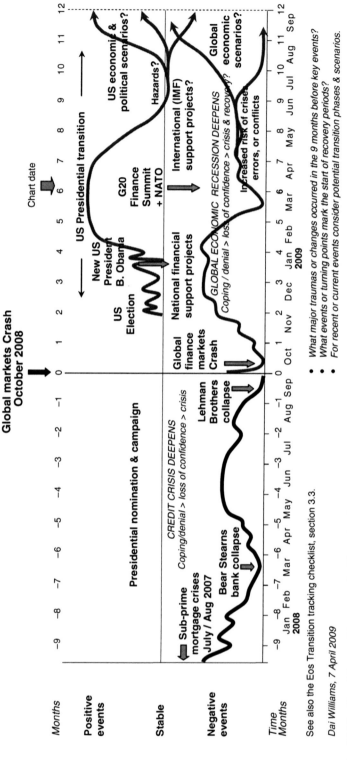

Fig. 27-11. Transition tracking example: Financial Crash & U.S. Presidential transitions, October 2008 & January 2009 (Williams, 2009)

pressures on individuals and groups? What strategic errors occurred during this period? Were some of them indicators of 6+ months delayed transition crisis behavior?

Occasionally individuals go down *a "staircase" of transitions* when panic decisions in one period of personal crisis can create new traumas and transitions – *out of the frying pan into the fire*. For example, an individual may quit his/her job 6 months after bereavement, and then quit their relationship 6 months after leaving his/her job. Have the psychological confidence and core principles of international banking and finance been destabilized by a series of mass trauma transition crises?

If so did another economic trauma transition start in October 2008 with a crisis phase in March or April 2009? Did markets truly bottom out in early March rising to the G20 and beyond? If so, G20 was an inspired transition management event ("something to look forward to" in the crisis phase). Or will they collapse again in the second quarter 2009? Figure 27.10 offers both scenarios though many separate scenarios are needed for different sectors and nations, plus variations for other events.

Studies of the first three years of the Tony Blair Government in the UK (Figs. 27.2 and 27.4) highlighted the hazards of leaders and governments making difficult strategic decisions under severe stress. Strategic decision-making may be fundamentally flawed when previous principles, manifesto pledges or assumptions no longer apply in the new conditions.

Individuals and groups may have to go through a crisis phase before they are willing to let go obsolete concepts or expectations and update personal or shared world views for the new reality.

Had the G20 planners and leaders discovered their personal and collective "new realities" when they set their priorities for action in March? Or will some very different economic shift or sea-change emerge from the current turbulence on the edge of chaos? Stabilization and consolidation may be more important than bold new plans in the uncertain crisis phase of transition. Perhaps the G20 offered a common meeting place for leaders in a time of crisis? That may have created a safe space for leaders to begin "to think the unthinkable" – to consider previously inconceivable new directions, options or alliances. But reflecting on the earlier observations of the UK, U.S. and other governments I think it unlikely that any political leaders or their advisors have discovered their personal new reality in response to the Global Crash in October 1998. This could be a significant test of the healing potential of the transition process.

An essential message in transition psychology is its evolutionary value – enabling individuals and groups to survive and thrive. The crisis phase of a transition can be a springboard to new insights and appropriate creativity – the darkest hour is just before dawn (or can be) in transitions. That encourages me to look for optimistic scenarios and to look for pathfinders of the new era. These *new catalysts* may already be working through their personal Credit Crunch and Crash transitions, or will do soon. They will come up with new, innovative but sound strategies that are far more tuned to the new global financial realities of 2009 and the 21st century.

There are many other potential mass transitions in process around the world in 2009. Another double war/election transition in Israel and Gaza parallels the *Power or Peace* analysis I did in February 2001. A more severe mass trauma transition started in December 2008 for Gaza and politicians and troops in Israel. The Israeli election led to a new coalition in March starting a new government transition. As in 2001, these twin transitions may have a crisis potential 6+ months after each event, i.e. between June and September 2009. After Arial Sharon's stroke in January 2006 the new government chose war on Lebanon in response to a border incident in July. Political crisis developed in both countries 6 months after the war, partially stabilising 1–2 years later. Were transition cycles a factor in these events?

Local analysts will have a deeper understanding of these and other complex, fast moving events in the Middle East. *Ideally mass transition tracking is done by people who know the cultures, personalities, and organizations affected by political or economic changes or mass traumas very well, and can recognize significant transition behaviors within the local context.*

Mass traumas for *impoverished communities* living in continuous fear (e.g. tsunamis, cyclones, floods, or drought) combined with political oppression (e.g. some south Asian and many African communities) seem most likely to be trapped in extended crisis periods for months or years, with increasingly distressed, dysfunctional, or violent behavior.

But in *communities where there is good emotional and economic support* (e.g. Manhattan after the 9-11 attacks, Aceh after the earthquake and tsunami, and southern Lebanon in 2006), there can be resilient reconstruction in weeks, renewed community cohesion and significant recovery, growth or constructive political engagement within 1–2 years.

Consequently, transition psychology suggests that analysts exploring post-conflict scenarios in many countries can include positive scenarios with opportunities for peace and reconciliation between warring communities – if both sides are encouraged with *stabilising transition support,* i.e. economic aid and a commitment to minimize or stop threats and violence (see Table 27-1). By contrast, violent repression will prevent transition recovery (Table 27-2) and may provoke continuing or increased violence – possibly a factor in ongoing conflicts on several continents.

Transition tracking forecasts can be done for many countries and regions in 2009 to anticipate social and economic hazards and opportunities, e.g. in Georgia, China, Pakistan, India, Madagascar, Iceland, and many other countries that experienced major traumas in 2008.

One of the most optimistic transition tracking opportunities in 2009 may be for *the new Presidential Transition for Barack Obama* and team in the United States despite obvious economic challenges. In Washington the Presidential Transition officially runs from election results to inauguration. As in 2001, the U.S. election may start a significant cycle particularly for the party that lost in November. But the main psychological transition for the new President is more likely to have launched on the Inauguration Day in January 2009. American readers can improve on the brief outline in Fig. 27-10 with your own transition tracking forecasts, including periods of potential crisis and opportunity for President Obama, combined with seasonal (e.g. summer vacation) and institutional factors.

The Presidential transition applies to the whole new Administration – mostly in new jobs in a new organizational transition period – with honeymoon, crisis, and recovery potential through the year. One special feature of President Obama's transition is that his honeymoon period is due to peak in

April – usefully counter-cyclical to the potential global financial transition crisis 6 months after the global crash last October. His optimism was an asset to the G20 meeting when many world leaders were under potentially greater psychological stress than any time in the last two years. Perhaps leaders from other countries who recover early from the crash transition can offer President Obama and the USA reciprocal support in the third quarter? This may be useful as the new Administration works through its own organizational transition, as well as managing the ongoing challenges of economic crises, recovery, and their long-term election goals for transformation. The outgoing President George Bush, his staff, and party may also go through a *loss of power transition* in the same period, possibly balanced with relief in view of global events?

Lessons Learned?

1. *Does transition psychology really have valid applications to strategic change management and mass transitions?* These propositions need wider testing and development. The examples given illustrate scenarios based on the transition process as a possible model for exploring major periods of trauma and change. The process of *transition analysis* using *transition tracking timelines* and *transition tracking checklist* can be tested by a wide range of practitioners and researchers. Readers with different perspectives may find more accurate or quite different interpretations.

2. *The transition process can be important for all of us at critical times in our lives.* It warns of potentially difficult periods when we were expecting things to get easier. And it gives vital hope that the darkest hour is often just before dawn where transition crisis periods occur.

3. *The effects of mass traumas and the process of mass economic transitions* may be important in many countries in 2009 as *the global economic crash transition* works around the world. Many *social, economic, and political consequences* will take several years to stabilize in some regions, e.g. mass unemployment and mass migrations of people seeking work. Table 27-4 reminds us of the variety of human and natural challenges or disasters some countries cope with almost every year.

4. *Major planned change projects* will be needed as *industrial and agricultural production is rationalized or redistributed nationally and internationally* in new economic conditions, e.g. in the U.S. and global automobile industry. *Transition management* is a strategic issue and technique in the growing toolkit of applied psychology resources for change management, personal, career, and community development developed in the last 30 years.

5. The *developmental and evolutionary significance of the transition process is rarely recognized* in academic or applied psychology, or in related fields like medicine. Even within psychology almost parallel research into the features of *culture shock* and of *transition psychology* contains no cross references – apparently, unaware that they are clearly studying the same process. Much research has been focussed on specific contexts, e.g. international migration, mental health consequences of traumatic life events, occupational effects of job change or redundancy, and collective effects of organizational change. In mass transition events all these perspectives

are important. *Culture shock research has a goldmine of insights into cross-cultural migration* that may be vital to managing mass transitions for new waves of refugees and economic migrants.

6. The *complex cognitive processes for individuals involved in transition are another important research area.* Personal Construct Psychology may partly explain how the human mind can deconstruct and reconstruct our personal understanding of ourselves and our world after a major event invalidates a core construct or deeply held belief. Systems theory explains the importance of delaying feedback to maintain stable systems – the utility of the denial phase. Analytical psychology may go much further to explain survival processes. Can Gestalt explain the miracle of reconstructing disrupted cognitive structures spontaneously in weeks? Schlossberg et al. explore the interaction of internal and situational variables as coping resources. Other chapters in this book may offer new approaches and more detailed insights from recent research and practice.

7. *Transitions appear to be an innate evolutionary mechanism.* If so they may happen spontaneously anyway for individuals and communities whenever challenged to change. In some cases, they may work most effectively with minimum intervention. How smoothly and quickly they flow may be subject to the enabling or inhibiting factors listed earlier, and how these are helped or hindered by governments, corporations, and other powerful institutions. Social anthropologists and humanitarian organizations may have observed and compared communities that have responded to mass trauma or change successfully or unsuccessfully. Their conclusions may already be in place in disaster response or post-conflict support in UN and other relief agencies.

8. Most transition research in occupational psychology has been focussed on adults. My practice suggests that a person's identity and values are largely determined before the age of 10. Thirty percent of the world's population are children under 15. Much of northern Uganda, where I first learned about culture shock and transition, is now controlled by the Lord's Resistance Army (LRA) with thousands of abducted child soldiers trapped between brutality, starvation, and fear. Transition theory gives hope that some will survive and thrive to become a new generation more like Nelson Mandela than Idi Amin. But without hope and security children in many countries who are traumatized by disasters, war or oppression are likely to become new generations of fighters. *One of the highest priorities for transition psychology should be how to stabilize the effects of mass trauma transitions on children in all continents.*

9. Large-scale humanitarian programmes (UN, Oxfam etc) recognize the need to build local capacity, *empowering communities, and traumatized governments* in disaster response. Small scale centres are developing pioneering treatment, training, and reconciliation programmes for traumatized communities, e.g. the *Trauma and Transition* programme in South Africa and the *Northern Ireland Centre for Trauma and Transformation.* This review suggests that *insights from helping individuals to rebuild lives after trauma or change* using natural psychological processes like transitions *may offer basic design principles (fractals) for understanding large-scale events* – mass traumas, changes, and transition periods - and empowering the communities involved, e.g. by valuing the past.

Rates of change and opportunities for transformation in current and future mass transitions are likely to be much slower in large populations. Initial impacts may be acute in local regions, e.g. after the 9-11 attacks in 2001, or the Sichuan earthquake in central China in May 2008. But secondary economic consequences may take months or years to impact distant communities and may not be anticipated until secondary crises develop, e.g. as mass migrations or major conflicts.

Nevertheless, the transition process can enable most individuals to adapt our minds and lives to profound trauma or loss within a year or two. This is the miracle of self-healing that has been crucial to human survival and evolution. Transition is the only innate psychological process I know of with the power to enable large populations to abandon past lifestyles or prejudices for a new order with individual dignity and confidence, and without therapy, education or coercion. Transition psychology may hold an alternative path to societal change in a densely populated planet; a path to peaceful co-existence and away from the mutually assured destruction of violence and revenge.

We can help, ignore or hinder communities in transition. Transition awareness may provide societies facing mass trauma or change more options to harness their natural healing processes and to reduce individual distress, enable recovery, and evolve sustainable social and economic systems.

"You cannot change what's over - but only where you go" (Enya 2000).

References

Adams, J., Hayes, J., & Hopson, B. (1976). *Transition – understanding and managing personal change*. London: Martin Robertson.

Adler, P.S. (1975). *The transitional experience: an alternative view of culture shock*. Journal of Humanistic Psychology, 15, 13–23. Extract in Furnham, A. & Bochner, S (1986). *Culture Shock.*(pp.130–131).

Bridges, W. (1991). *Managing Transitions: Making the Most of Change*. Perseus Books Group. Cambridge, MA.

Comprehensive Study Finds Problems Mount For "Indirect Victims" of WTC Attacks. United Way of New York City, April 23 2002. Press release summarising *Beyond Ground Zero*. UWNYC. Retrieved from http://www.appleseedinc.com/reports/UWNYCGroundZero.pdf

Enya (2000). *Pilgrim*. From the CD *A Day without Rain*. Warner Music.

Flögel, M. and Lauc, G. (2000). War stress in the former Yugoslavia in G.Fink (ed) *Encyclopaedia of Stress A-D*, Academic Press. San Diego. (pp. 678–683).

Freeman, H. (1991). The Human Brain and Political Behaviour. *British Journal of Psychiatry, 159*, 19–32.

Guthrie, G. M., & Zektick, I. N. (1967). Predicting performance in the Peace Corps. *Journal of Social Psychology, 71*, 11–21.

Heaney, S. (1990). *The Cure at Troy*. Faber and Faber. Extract from Across the Bridge of Hope, White Records –a tribute CD for victims of the Omagh bomb, August 1998

Herriot, P. (1992). *The Career Management Challenge*. London: Sage. & Herriot, P., Hirsch, W., Riley, P.D., & Bevan, S. (1998) *Trust and Transition*. Cambridge University Press.

Herriot, P., Hirsch, W., Riley, P.D., & Bevan, S. (1998) *Trust and Transition*. Cambridge University Press

Herriot, P., Plenty, R., Weinberg, A., and Williams, D. Symposium papers in *Proceedings of the UK BPS Occupational Psychology Conference*, January 1999, (pp. 282-303). Summary: Williams, D. (1999) Human responses to change, *Futures*, 31 (6) (pp. 609-616). doi: 10.1016/S0016-3287(99)00017-8

Janis, I.L. (1982). *Groupthink*. Houghton Mifflin Company. (pp. 174–177).

Janis, I.L. (1982). *Groupthink – Psychological Studies of Policy Decisions and Fiascoes*. Houghton Mifflin Company. Key points retrieved from www.cedu.niu.edu/~fulmer/groupthink.htm

Kübler-Ross, E. (1969). *On Death and Dying*. Simon & Schuster/Touchstone.

McDonough, W.J. (2002) *CEO Calls for End to Excessive Executive Pay*. Retrieved September 11, 2002 from http://www.trinitywallstreet.org/news/alert_197.shtml

Nicholson, N. & West, M.A., (1988). *Managerial Job Change: Men & Women in Transition.*Cambridge University Press.

Orford, J. (1992). *Community Psychology Theory and Practice* (pp. 252–255). Chichester: Wiley.

Parkes, C. M. (1971). Psycho-social transitions: a field for study. *Social Science & Medicine, 5,* 101–115.

Paton, D., & Long, N. (1996). *Psychological aspects of disasters: impact, coping and intervention*. NZ: The Dunsmore Press.

Plenty, R. (1999) Transition Strategies in Shell. *BPS Occupational Psychology Conference, Blackpool. Proceedings* (pp. 286–7).

Schlossberg, N.K., Waters, E.B., and Goodman, J. (1995). *Counselling Adults in Transition*. Springer Publishing Company.

Staub, E. (2001). Genocide and mass killing: their roots and prevention. Ch 6 in Peace, Conflict and Violence: Peace Psychology for the 21st Century. Englewood Cliffs, New Jersey: Prentice Hall.

Sugarman, L. (1986). *Life-Span Development* (pp. 131–165). London: Methuen.

Williams, D. (1997). *After the Honeymoon – potential effects of the post-election transition on the health of UK Members of Parliament*. Eos. Retrieved from www.eoslifework.co.uk/pit1.htm . Later Part 1 of *Parliament in Transition*. Retrieved from www.eoslifework.co.uk/pitintro.htm .

Williams, D. (1997). *After the Honeymoon – potential effects of the post-election transition on the health of UK Members of Parliament*. www.eoslifework.co.uk/pit2.htm

Williams, D. (1999a). *Transitions: managing personal and organisational change*. Eos, In ACDM, April 1999. Retrieved from http://www.eoslifework.co.uk/transmgt1.htm

Williams, D. (1999b). *Many paths to peace – Opportunities for the Peace Process in Northern Ireland*. Eos. Retrieved from www.eoslifework.co.uk/mptp1.htm

Williams, D. (1999c). *Fear and violence in stressed populations*. Eos. Retrieved from www.eoslifework.co.uk/gturmap.htm

Williams, D. (1999d). *Balkans Aftermath: the post-war transition – denial, crisis & world peace*. Eos. Retrieved from www.eoslifework.co.uk/balkaft.htm

Williams, D. (1999e). Life events and career change: transition psychology in practice. *BPS Occupational Psychology Conference Proceedings*. (pp. 296–303). Online: www.eoslifework.co.uk/transprac.htm

Williams, D. (1999f). *Parliament in transition – effects of the 1997 UK election landslide*. UK BPS Occupational Psychology Conference Proceedings (pp. 296–303). Figure 3 from the Review edition, 1999.

Williams, D. (1999g). *Fear and violence in stressed populations*. Eos. Retrieved from: www.eoslifework.co.uk/gturmap.htm and in a presentation to the *CRS Symposium on Psychology of Peace & Conflict*, March 2009, Goldsmiths College, London.

Williams, D. (2000a). *Accidents waiting to happen? Political events and psychological climate for the UK Government 1998–2000*. Eos. Retrieved from www.eoslifework.co.uk/govtran2k.htm

Williams, D. (2000b). *Accidents waiting to happen? Political events and psychological climate for the UK Government 1998–2000*. Eos. Retrieved from www.eoslifework.co.uk/govtran2k.htm

Williams, D. (2000c). *Accidents waiting to happen?* Retrieved from www.eoslifework. co.uk/govtran2k.htm

Williams, D. (2001). *The Power or Peace Project.* Eos. Retrieved from: www.eoslife-work.co.uk/pop1.htm

Williams, D. (2001). An open letter to Prime Minister Sharon. *International Bulletin of Political Psychology.* 10 (14). April 20 2001. Retrieved from http://security.pr.erau. edu or at http://miniurl.org/Iip

Williams, D. (2002). *Psychological aftermath of September 11th – Is there a 9–11 Transition?* Eos. Retrieved from www.eoslifework.co.uk/pdfs/911transition23J.pdf

Williams, D. (2004). *Managing stress, trauma and change in the airline industry: some human and psychological factors.* Presentation to the IATA Aviation Security Conference AVSEC 2004, Vancouver. Retrieved from www.eoslifework.co.uk/pdfs/ AVSECeospaper5.pdf

Williams, D. (2008). *Eos Life-Line Exercise.* Retrieved from www.eoslifework.co.uk/ pdfs/lifeline.pdf

Zimonjic, V.P. (2002) *Extensive depression reported in Serbia.* Retrieved from www. ipsnews.net/interna.asp?/idnews=24086

ISTSS – International Society for Traumatic Stress Studies. Retrieved from http:// www.istss.org

Trauma and Transition Programme. CSVR. Retrieved from www.csvr.org.za/wits/ projects/ttp.htm

Northern Ireland Centre for Trauma and Transformation. Omagh. Retrieved from www.nictt.co.uk

Chart from the Financial Times www.ft.com and BigChart.com

Chapter 28

Posttraumatic Growth: A Positive Consequence of Trauma

Cassie M. Lindstrom and Kelli N. Triplett

You gain strength, courage and confidence by every experience in which you really stop to look fear in the face. You are able to say to yourself, 'I lived through this horror. I can take the next thing that comes along'…You must do the thing you think you cannot do. – Eleanor Roosevelt

Life in the fast-paced 21st century includes a multitude of stressors. Interactions with loved ones, pressures at work, and failing health are stressors faced by thousands of adults each day. Traumatic events, as defined by the DSM-IV-TR, are extremely stressful events causing a fear of death, helplessness, or horror (American Psychiatric Association 2000). Unfortunately, traumatic events are rather common (Norris and Sloane 2007) and most trauma research has focused on the development of problems due to traumatic experiences (Joseph et al. 2005). However, despite emotional and physical strain caused by traumatic experiences, some trauma survivors report positive changes in their lives due to their struggle to cope with the aftermath of these events. The idea that traumatic events can lead to positive personal change, referred to here as posttraumatic growth (PTG) (Calhoun and Tedeschi 1999, 2004, 2006; Tedeschi and Calhoun 1995, 1996, 2004), is not a new concept. Since their inception, the religions of Buddhism, Christianity, Hinduism, Islam, and Judaism have all recognized positive changes as an outcome of traumatic events (Joseph and Linley 2005).

In the past few decades, trauma research has shifted from focusing solely on negative outcomes of trauma to incorporating positive consequences of traumatic experiences. Furthermore, research regarding posttraumatic growth has increased dramatically in recent years. Growth following a traumatic experience has been referred to as benefit-finding (Davis et al. 1998), stress-related growth (Park et al. 1996; Park 1998), and adversarial growth (Joseph and Linley 2004; Linley and Joseph 2004). However, the model of posttraumatic growth (PTG) has been referred to as the most comprehensive model of growth due to adversity (Joseph and Linley 2005). It is important to note that PTG does not suggest that negative consequences of traumatic experiences are nonexistent. Instead, PTG offers a more complete understanding of trauma

From: *Handbook of Stressful Transitions Across the Lifespan,*
Edited by: T.W. Miller, DOI 10.1007/978-1-4419-0748-6_28,
© Springer Science+Business Media, LLC 2010

outcomes by focusing on positive consequences while acknowledging that negative outcomes do occur. Further, it appears possible for each survivor to find both negative and positive aspects of their experience (Janoff-Bulman and Yopyk 2004); negative and positive consequences of the same traumatic event are not mutually exclusive. Before discussing PTG in detail, a general overview of trauma is offered.

Trauma: A Brief Overview

It is important to clarify the definition of trauma before embarking on a discussion of trauma and its consequences. For our purposes, trauma is defined as it is in the DSM-IV-TR (Diagnostic and Statistical Manual of Mental Disorders, Fourth Edition, Text Revision, American Psychiatric Association 2000):

> An extreme traumatic stress or involving direct personal experience of an event that involves actual or threatened death or serious injury, or other threat to one's physical integrity or witnessing an event that involves death, injury, or a threat to the physical integrity of another person; or learning about unexpected or violent death, serious harm, or threat of death or injury experienced by a family member or other close associate (p. 463).

Though trauma has been a part of life throughout the ages, it appears that people today are exposed to more stressful events than at any other time in history (O'Brien 1998). In the United States, where natural disasters and murder are all too common, the likelihood that people will experience trauma is quite high. In addition to widespread events, people often experience trauma on a more personal level. Most people have had trauma in their own families or close social circles, including death of a loved one, serious injury or illness, and other losses. Technology is partly responsible for the increased exposure to negative and even traumatic events. Information on tragedies is readily available and even to some extent unavoidable, due to technological advances, including television and more saliently, the Internet.

Findings from a nationwide probability sample of American adults, a survey of 5,800 men and women ranging in age from 15 to 54, suggest that 61% of men and 51% of women have experienced a traumatic event in their lives (Kessler et al. 1995). Moreover, people were likely to report multiple traumatic events, of which the most common were witnessing the death or injury of another person (36% of men, 15% of women), involvement in a life-threatening incident (25% of men, 14% of women), and involvement in a natural disaster or fire (19% of men, 15% of women). These findings were based on the DSM-III criteria for a traumatic event, which were more stringent than the criteria in the DMS-IV-TR. Thus, these statistics likely underestimate the prevalence of traumatic events when using the current DSM's criteria for a traumatic event, which are more inclusive than those of the DSM-III (American Psychiatric Association 1980).

Use of the DSM-IV-TR criteria may be partly responsible for the higher prevalence rates found in the Detroit Area Survey, which suggest that 90% of adults between 18 and 45 years of age have been exposed to at least one traumatic event. On average, people who had been exposed to at least one traumatic event had actually experienced five traumatic events in their lifetime. The most common event, experienced by 60% of the sample, was sudden, unexpected death of a loved one. Women were more likely to report sexual assault, but men were approximately twice as likely as women to report that they had experienced violent physical assault, including shootings and stabbings. In addition to gender differences, findings suggest the incidence of violent trauma also varies according to race, with non-Caucasians having twice the likelihood of experiencing violent trauma (e.g., muggings, stabbings,and beatings) than Caucasians. Further, individuals with higher income and educational level (i.e., college graduates with income of $75,000+) were approximately half as likely to have experienced such trauma than those with less education and lower income (i.e., those that had not completed high school and earned less than $25,000/year) (Breslau et al. 1998).

Risk for exposure to trauma also appears to vary across the lifespan. Findings from the Detroit Area Survey indicate that risk is highest for people between 16 and 20 years old. However, upon further examination, it appears that certain types of traumatic events are more likely to occur during certain age ranges. As would be expected, risk for violent traumatic events decreases after age 20 and continues to do so over the years. Other types of trauma also decrease after age 20, but then remain relatively stable over time. This is true of the likelihood of the sudden loss of a loved one, which peaks between 41 and 45 years of age (Breslau et al. 1998). In sum, by adulthood, 25% of Americans will have experienced a traumatic event and the majority of people will have had such an experience by their mid-forties (Norris and Sloane 2007).

Studies of trauma in children are less common than those of adults, possibly due to the erroneous idea that children are unaffected by stress and/or too young to understand or remember traumatic events (Osofsky 1995). However, findings suggest that children are all too often exposed to traumatic events with estimates around 26% for girls and 44% for boys (Boney-McCoy and Finkelhor 1995). It is estimated that overall, at least 25% of children and adolescents experience a traumatic event by the time they turn 16 (Costello et al. 2002). The consequences of traumatic experiences will be discussed next.

Consequences of Trauma

It is clear that traumatic events are common in this day and age. Thus, the consequences of trauma become a pertinent issue. Perhaps the most well known reaction to trauma is Posttraumatic Stress Disorder, which was first officially listed in the DSM-III in 1980 (Friedman et al. 2007). Posttraumatic Stress Disorder (PTSD) is defined as a reaction to trauma that includes re-experiencing the trauma, avoiding stimuli related to the trauma, increased arousal, and distress or impairment for more than one month. Although it appears that most people are exposed to at least one traumatic event in their lifetime and often more than one, most people do not develop PTSD (American Psychiatric Association 2000).

Estimates suggest that the lifetime prevalence for PTSD is approximately 8% for American adults (American Psychiatric Association 2000). Further, evidence suggests that the likelihood of developing PTSD varies according to the type of trauma experienced. Findings from the Detroit Area Survey indicate that people who were exposed to violent assault were most likely to develop PTSD, with a prevalence rate of about 20% (Breslau et al. 1998). Corroborating evidence is found in the National Comorbidity Survey, where violent personal events, such as combat, physical assault, and molestation, were more likely to be associated with subsequent PTSD. Rape is the type of trauma most strongly associated with PTSD, with 65% of male rape victims and 46% of female rape victims meeting criteria for diagnosis (Kessler et al. 1995). Even when controlling for type of event, women are more likely to have PTSD than men, with estimates at 8% for men and 20% for women who have experienced a trauma (Schnurr et al. 2002).

Despite most trauma research focusing on adults, several studies regarding the prevalence of PTSD in children and adolescents have been conducted. In a community sample of adolescents, 6% had a lifetime prevalence of PTSD (Giaconia et al. 1995) and 10% of adolescents in the National Comorbidity Survey study met criteria for PTSD (Kessler et al. 1995). A recent longitudinal study of children from ages 9–16 found exposure to traumatic events to be common (30.8% of participants exposed to at least 1 traumatic event), but also found PTSD to be rare with only 0.5% of participants meeting the DSM-IV-TR criteria (Copeland et al. 2007). Even so, subclinical levels of PTSD were reported by 13.4% of participants. These studies suggest that children and adolescents experience posttraumatic stress symptoms similar to adults.

In addition to the type of traumatic event, gender, and age, another variable that affects the development of PTSD is the severity of the trauma. Severity of trauma is based on the duration of the trauma, the number of times the event happened, and the degree to which one's life or physical integrity was threatened. Those who experienced severe trauma appear to be more likely to develop PTSD (Schnurr et al. 2002).

One of the particularly troubling aspects of PTSD is the persistence of the disorder. Findings from the National Comorbidity Survey suggest that individuals who received treatment for PTSD had a median remission time of 3 years post-onset, while those that did not seek treatment had a median remission time of more than 5 years post-onset of symptoms. PTSD persisted over many years for approximately one-third of the individuals in the National Comorbidity Survey, including people who did not seek treatment and those that did (Kessler et al. 1995).

While it is true that the majority of people do not develop PTSD in the aftermath of trauma, most people still experience distress. Individuals may not experience significant distress that meets the criteria for PTSD, but still experience negative emotions such as fear, anxiety, and sadness. For example, school-aged children exposed to violence often display depressive symptoms (Hammack et al. 2004), anxiety, and sleep disturbances such as nightmares (Pynoos 1993). The death of a parent in adolescence has been linked to tearfulness, school phobias, rebelliousness (substance abuse) and declining schoolwork (Wenar and Kerig 2000). Although such reactions do not meet the criteria for PTSD, clearly the lives of even young trauma survivors can be impacted in a negative manner.

It is necessary to reiterate at this point that distress and growth are not mutually exclusive reactions to trauma. Although it is clear that experiencing traumatic events often results in negative outcomes, our discussion turns now to the positive consequences of the struggle with trauma.

Posttraumatic Growth

As previously mentioned, PTG refers to the positive changes experienced in the aftermath of struggle with traumatic events (Calhoun and Tedeschi 1999, 2004, 2006; Tedeschi and Calhoun 1996, 2004). Calhoun and Tedeschi (2006) note several publications in the 1990s that focused on growth or thriving in response to trauma or challenging events (Schaefer and Moos 1992; O'Leary and Ickovics 1995; Park et al. 1996; Tedeschi and Calhoun 1995). These works clearly encouraged others to research and write about growth – hundreds of documents on the subject now exist (Calhoun and Tedeschi 2006). Various traumatic experiences have been investigated in relation to PTG, including cancer (Barakat et al. 2006; Curbow et al. 1993; Sabiston et al. 2007; Thornton and Perez 2006; Weiss 2004), motor vehicle accidents (Harms and Talbot 2007; Rabe 2006; Salter and Stallard 2004), terrorist attacks (Hobfoll 2007; Val 2006), combat (Dekel 2007; Solomon et al. 1999), natural disasters (Cryder et al. 2006), HIV/AIDS (Siegel and Schrimshaw 2000), bereavement (Calhoun and Tedeschi 1989/1990), house fires (Thompson 1985), domestic violence (Cobb et al. 2006), and rape (Burt and Katz 1987), among others.

In most research on posttraumatic growth, a traumatic event is defined as an experience in which survivors' assumptions about themselves, other people, and the world, referred to as their "assumptive world," are shattered (Janoff-Bulman 1992). Individuals' assumptions or schemas about the world often include beliefs that the world is benevolent, life is fair, and the individual is deserving of good things. Following a trauma, such assumptions do not seem quite as true to many people and survivors' assumptions may "shatter." Once assumptions are shattered, individuals often search for meaning and are forced to rebuild their pre-existing schemas or develop new schemas regarding the self, others, and what the world is like (Janoff-Bulman 1992).

PTG is multidimensional with five identified domains on which growth often occurs (Tedeschi and Calhoun 1996). People often note changes in *personal strength* in that although they may feel more "vulnerable," they often feel "stronger" or more capable of handling other stressful events (Calhoun and Tedeschi 2006). Survivors who experience growth in this way may view the world as dangerous, but realize they are more capable of handling adversity than they had previously believed. In the words of one cancer survivor, "…somebody said to me well you know you could die…and I thought…I've seen other people do it, I can do this. I may not want to, but if I have to, I can," (Sabiston et al. 2007, p. 430).

Similarly, people often report *new possibilities* as a result of experiencing trauma. These new possibilities can include new interests, life paths, or activities (Calhoun and Tedeschi 2006). Further, survivors may experience things or meet people they would not have otherwise due to the traumatic experience. One individual who had a visible impairment from chronic illness or injury said the following in a qualitative study by Salick and Auerbach (2006):

> I feel like I'm a better person. I like myself better now. I just feel like, as horrible as it is, and I wouldn't wish it upon anyone, suffering does make you grow. It gives you a certain depth and maturity and adds another element to your personality that wasn't there before. You become more creative. Deeper you just access other parts of yourself so that your self is bigger than it was before (p. 1032).

Trauma survivors may also notice positive changes in the way they *relate to others* (Calhoun and Tedeschi 2006). For instance, many survivors find that they have more compassion for others than they did pre-trauma. Others have reported a greater connection to people in general. The traumatic experience may also improve relationships with friends and family.

Some trauma survivors note a greater *appreciation of life* and may have a shift in their priorities, i.e., spending more time with family and less time at work (Calhoun and Tedeschi 2006). This may be due to the realization that they have a second chance at life and want to live life to the fullest. Life may be thought of as precious and special or as a gift after surviving a trauma (Janoff-Bulman and Yopyk 2004). In the words of one trauma survivor, "But my priorities are better. I'm a better husband now; spend more time with my wife and my family. I prioritize what's important now," (Salick and Auerbach 2006, p. 1033).

One final area of growth often noted in survivors is that of *spiritual change*. Many survivors find that they have a closer relationship with God or a strengthening in faith post-trauma (Calhoun and Tedeschi 2006). In addition, some survivors report feeling a greater sense of purpose in life, greater sense of meaning, greater life satisfaction, and a feeling that existential questions are answered (Calhoun and Tedeschi 2006). As one survivor of the September 11th terrorist attacks noted: "It has reaffirmed, possibly confirmed for the first time, a sense of faith – actually faith, belief in something I cannot see, touch, feel, or hear," (Ai et al. 2005, pp. 538–539).

Factors Related to the Process of Growth

The general model of PTG proposed by Tedeschi and Calhoun (1995, 1996, 2004) is complex and includes multiple components (Fig. 28-1). The process of growth includes characteristics of the person pretrauma, characteristics of the traumatic event, social and cultural factors, rumination, and self-disclosure. While the model offers a general illustration of the process through which growth is theorized to occur, it is important to note that this process is likely somewhat different for each individual who experiences growth. Relevant factors and their role in the process of growth will now be discussed.

Characteristics of the Survivor Pre-trauma

Characteristics of the trauma survivor such as gender, age, education, and personality characteristics appear to be related to growth. Researchers have found gender to be related to growth with women tending to report more growth than men (Joseph et al. 2005), but some studies found no difference in amount of growth between women and men (Ho et al. 2004; Rieck et al. 2005). A recent meta-analysis of 70 studies measuring PTG found women to report significantly more PTG than men (g =.27, 95% CI = .21 – .32; Vishnevsky, Cann, Calhoun, Tedeschi, & Demakis, under review). The meta-analysis results revealed a small to moderate gender difference even when data from unpublished studies were included, suggesting it is likely that women do experience more growth than men.

Age appears to be related to growth with younger persons reporting more growth (Cordova et al. 2001). Several studies have found a relationship between age and growth with older individuals tending to report lower levels of growth (e.g., Lechner et al. 2003; Milam 2004; Widows et al. 2005).

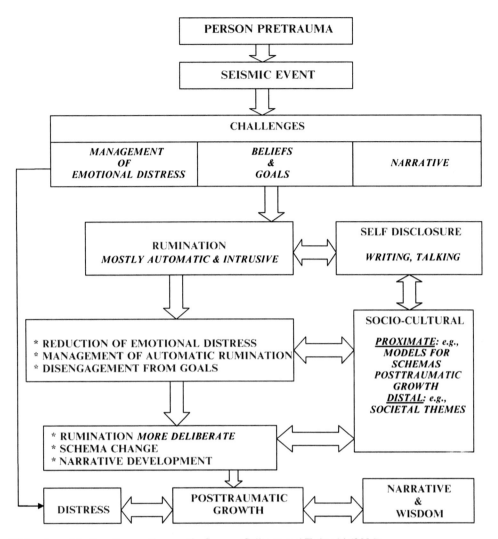

Fig. 28-1. A model of posttraumatic growth. *Source*: Calhoun and Tedeschi (2006)

The age difference may be due to older individuals having experienced previous traumas where their assumptions were challenged and revised at a younger age.

The education of the survivor may also be related to growth. Several studies found less education to be correlated with more growth (Cordova et al. 2001; Thornton and Perez 2006). For instance, in a study of growth in partners of cancer patients, partners who did not graduate from college reported more growth (Thornton and Perez 2006). Reasons for a relationship between lower levels of education and growth remain unclear.

Finally, personality characteristics such as optimism and extraversion appear to be related to growth. In several studies, optimism was found to be associated with more growth (Updegraff 2005; Urcuyo et al. 2005). Extraversion was also found to be related to growth with higher levels of extraversion predicting higher levels of growth (Linley and Joseph 2004). These results are not surprising considering both extraversion and optimism are linked to positive affect and growth requires the survivor to put a positive spin on their circumstances.

Characteristics of the Traumatic Event

Characteristics of the traumatic event such as the severity of the event, the amount of distress the event causes, and time since the event also appear to be related to growth. Appraisal of the event as more severe is related to more growth in cancer patients (Cordova et al. 2001). Other studies have found subjective appraisal of severity or greater life threat related to growth while objective risk (doctor's opinion, clinical rating) not necessarily related to growth (Barakat et al. 2006; Sears 2003; Rieck et al. 2005; Updegraff 2005). Rieck et al. (2005) found that objective severity was related to growth but the relationship between subjective severity and PTG was stronger ($r = 0.36$ vs. $r = 0.14$). Thus, it appears that the perception of severity influences growth more so than objective measures of severity. In other words, it is not actually how severe the event is, but how severe the survivor perceives the event to be that promotes growth.

It has been hypothesized that some amount of time must pass for cognitive processing to occur and lead to growth. In one study, the amount of time since diagnosis of cancer was inversely correlated with growth so that the more time passed, the less growth was reported (Weiss 2004). Several other studies also found time since the event unrelated to growth (Joseph et al. 2005; Rieck et al. 2005; Urcuyo et al. 2005). However, a study of breast cancer survivors found time since diagnosis to be positively correlated with growth (Cordova et al. 2001). Results might be consistent with a curvilinear relationship such that PTG peaks around 1 year and then decreases (Calhoun and Tedeschi 1999). Overall, the findings related to time and growth remain unclear and more research in this area is needed.

Emotional Distress

Research examining the level of distress and PTG has found higher levels of arousal (PTSD) related to higher levels of growth (Lev-Weisel and Amir 2003). Levl-Wiesel et al. (2005) also found PTSD correlated with PTG ($r = 0.53$, $p < 0.001$). These findings have led Calhoun and Tedeschi to note that while "a minimal level of exposure is necessary, extremely high levels of exposure may not result in any increase in experienced growth" (Calhoun and Tedeschi 2006).

Core Beliefs

As previously discussed, the model of posttraumatic growth (Calhoun and Tedeschi 2006) posits that a traumatic event challenges a survivor's assumptions of how the world works. Recent studies suggest that the extent to which one's core beliefs are challenged is a key element to the growth process. In a study with college undergraduates, challenges to core beliefs explained 23% of the variance in posttraumatic growth, with more core belief challenge being associated with more growth (Lindstrom and Triplett 2008). This finding suggests that individuals whose core beliefs are challenged experience more growth than those that are challenged to a lesser extent. Individuals whose core beliefs are shaken by a traumatic event may be plagued with intrusive thoughts about the event than those whose core beliefs are less challenged, or not challenged at all. These individuals may be motivated to engage in deliberate rumination and this entire process may result in more posttraumatic growth.

Rumination

The shattering of assumptions leads to cognitive processing, or rumination. Rumination, as it is often defined in the literature, has a negative connotation and refers to intrusive, distressing thoughts that might be likened to brooding (Calhoun and Tedeschi 2006). However, rumination can also refer to a more productive and deliberate processing of information (Martin and Tesser 1996). Although the trauma survivor may experience nightmares and intrusive thoughts, the attempts to understand and cope involve ruminations that can lead to a revision of the assumptive world (Tedeschi and Calhoun 2004). In a recent study with traumatized undergraduates, rumination about the traumatic event explained 15% of the variance in PTG, suggesting that the degree to which one engages in rumination, both intrusive and deliberate, is a key factor in how much growth is experienced (Lindstrom and Triplett 2008). A lot more information is needed in the area of rumination to better understand the process of growth.

Sociocultural Influences

Social and cultural factors can be divided into proximate and distal categories and they can be key elements of growth following a trauma (Calhoun and Tedeschi 2006). The proximate cultural environment includes a person's primary reference groups which are the family, friends, and neighbors that interact with a person most often. Whether or not growth occurs may depend partly on a survivors' primary reference group and their beliefs that growth is a possibility. For example, having friends or family members who found benefits from a traumatic experience may influence the survivor to find benefits from their experience.

Distal cultural elements include themes in the society or geographic area of a survivor (Calhoun and Tedeschi 2004). How a survivor's society expects people to react and cope with traumatic events may influence whether or not the survivor grows from the experience. For example, Calhoun and Tedeschi (2006) note that Americans may be more likely to create personal narratives based on religious and optimistic themes than Europeans. If a model of growth is present in society (such as a general belief that trauma survivors find benefits), a survivor will be more likely to find growth.

Disclosure of the Traumatic Event

Self-disclosure of the trauma to members of the primary reference groups and the consequences of disclosure may play key roles in the development of PTG. Actual disclosure and reactions to disclosure may be particularly important in determining whether or not people experience growth. Social constraint, however, may cause people to feel they cannot speak to loved ones about the trauma, or, more specifically, growth themes, and so they may be less likely to report PTG. Assuming that survivors do disclose, responses to the disclosure may influence whether growth occurs. Survivors whose friends and family respond in a caring manner to disclosures that include growth themes may experience more growth than survivors met with unfavorable reactions to their disclosures. Responses to growth themes may be particularly crucial. If a person is considering some positive consequences of the struggle with a traumatic experience and is met with supportive reactions, the person may experience more growth than if his or her loved ones are not open to the idea that positive things can come from struggling with a traumatic event. Though research on the role of disclosure in PTG is limited, some findings with undergraduates indicate that people who receive or predict they will receive more supportive reactions to trauma and growth disclosures, report more growth than those who do not (Lindstrom and Triplett 2008).

PTG and Children

Very few studies of PTG in children and adolescents exist (Kilmer 2006). One reason for the lack of literature focusing specifically on PTG in children is that noticing growth in oneself requires cognitive maturity that children may not possess. For example, several studies by Harter have demonstrated that children differ by age group in their ability to note the co-occurrence of polar opposite emotions (Harter 1986). Although older children ($M = 11.43$ years) could identify the same event as evoking polar opposite emotions, younger children could not. This calls into question whether younger children are capable of perceiving a traumatic event as both negative and positive.

Despite concerns about children's ability to recognize growth, the model of PTG in children is similar to that of adults and includes the child's pre-trauma beliefs, characteristics of the traumatic event, ruminative thinking, social support, and competency beliefs. Studies of PTG in children reveal that children as young as 6 years old have reported growth following a traumatic event and results suggest that the more supportive the environment of the child, the more growth occurs in children (Cryder et al. 2006). In other studies, 42% of children involved in traffic accidents reported growth (Salter and Stallard 2004) and 59% of children and adolescents diagnosed with cancer reported at least a small degree of growth (Yaskowich 2003). Existing studies demonstrate that children do possess the ability to experience growth and suggest this is a promising area for further investigation.

Applications to Clinical Work

Questions remain regarding the outcomes of growth. The current model posits that growth can lead to wisdom, greater well-being, and satisfaction in life. However, further studies are necessary to determine whether these outcomes actually do occur and whether long-term benefits exist.

If research indicates benefits to PTG exist, implications also exist for clinical work. For one, clinicians may attempt to foster growth in clients. Because clients often enter the therapeutic relationship when they are distressed, it is likely that PTG often occurs in therapy. To help promote PTG in trauma survivors, clinicians should focus not only on distress and negative consequences of the trauma, but also establish an atmosphere which allows the client to explore the possibility of growth (Zoellner and Maercker 2006). As authors of the current chapter, it is our hope that any trauma survivors reading this chapter feel optimistic that they may eventually view some aspects of their experience as positive just as other trauma survivors have.

Conclusions

Despite many years of extensive research on the positive consequences of trauma, many questions remain. For one, the overall process by which growth occurs remains unclear. However, it is the opinion of the authors that the above-mentioned model is the "best guess" at this time. The complexity of the process as well as differences across individuals lead to a healthy skepticism about this process, but the model originally proposed by Tedeschi and Calhoun has changed little over the years, and thus far, this model has held up under investigation. The role of core beliefs and rumination in particular has been supported through research. Less empirical support exists for the role of self-disclosure but this is a result of a lack of research exploring this "piece" of the model, not due to evidence suggesting that the theorized process is inaccurate. Future research should explore the role of self-disclosure with particular attention to the contribution of discussing positive consequences of trauma vs. the importance of discussing its negative consequences. In addition, it is theorized that reactions to disclosures by important others in the discloser's life are highly important but it is not yet known what reactions are most facilitative of growth. Growth is theorized to occur through the shaking of the core beliefs followed by rumination, which is more intrusive earlier after the trauma, but in order for growth to occur, must become more deliberate and healthy as time passes. In addition, as a post-trauma person is ruminating, they are believed to be disclosing negative, but more importantly, positive consequences of their trauma. Supportive reactions to these disclosures are believed to be needed in order for the experience of PTG to be maximized.

Whether growth changes over time and if so, how the specific factors related to growth change are additional questions that remain. For instance, while the evidence suggests that rumination and the shaking of core beliefs are acting in the way the model of growth predicts, less is known about some of the other factors, particularly self-disclosure. Questions also remain regarding outcomes of growth: do people who experience growth garner wisdom, life satisfaction, and meaning in life from their experience? Future research should continue to address the aforementioned questions. Specifically, longitudinal studies are needed to determine how factors and growth in general may change over time. The current belief is that growth takes some time to develop as is implied by the complexity of the process by which growth occurs. In theory, growth would increase as time since event increases but only to a certain point.

Another question for future exploration is whether there is a ceiling as to how much growth a given person can experience in a lifetime (i.e., if one's core beliefs are shaken by a traumatic event early in life and growth occurs, it may be that the next traumatic event does not shake their world as much, if at all, which would then be unlikely to result in additional growth). If early experiences teach a person that the world is not safe, for example, then the subsequent traumatic events may not challenge their beliefs (Tedeschi et al. 2007). In other words, a person who expects the worst from the world will not examine or ruminate on a traumatic event when it happens – it will simply confirm the person's beliefs that the world is a bad place making growth unlikely.

The negative consequences of trauma are well-documented, and people who experience such events would likely opt out of these experiences if given the choice. These are not issues that these authors are interested in challenging nor are the discussions of positive consequences of trauma meant to downplay the very real pain that people experience in such circumstances. However, perhaps the knowledge that positive things can come from the struggle with difficult experiences can offer some hope to trauma survivors.

Acknowledgements: The authors would like to thank Lawrence Calhoun, Ph.D., Arnie Cann, Ph.D., and Richard Tedeschi, Ph.D. for their invaluable support and guidance throughout the development of this chapter.

References

Ai, A. L., Cascio, T., & Santangelo, L. K. (2005). Hope, meaning, and growth following the September 11, 2001, terrorist attacks. *Journal of Interpersonal Violence, 20*, 523–548.

American Psychiatric Association. (1980). *Diagnostic and statistical manual of mental disorders* (3rd ed.). Washington, DC: American Psychiatric Association

American Psychiatric Association. (2000). *Diagnostic and statistical manual of mental disorders* (4th ed.). Text Revision. Washington, DC: American Psychiatric Association

Barakat, L., Alderfer, M. & Kazak, A. (2006). Posttraumatic growth in adolescent cancer survivors and their mothers and fathers. *Journal of Pediatric Psychology*, 31(4), 413–419.

Boney-McCoy, S., & Finkelhor, D. (1995). Psychosocial sequelae of violent victimization in a national youth sample. *Journal of Consulting and Clinical Psychology, 63*, 726–736.

Breslau, N., Kessler, R. C., Chilcoat, H. D., Schultz, L. R., Davis, G. C., & Andreski, P. (1998). Trauma and posttraumatic stress disorder in the community: The 1996 Detroit Area Survey of Trauma. *Archives of General Psychiatry, 55*, 626–632.

Burt, M. & Katz, B. (1987). Dimensions of recovery from rape: Focus on growth outcomes. *Journal of Interpersonal Violence*, 2(1), 57–81.

Calhoun, L. G., & Tedeschi, R. G. (1999). *Facilitating posttraumatic growth: A clinician's guide*. Mahwah, NJ: Lawrence Erlbaum Associates.

Calhoun, L. G., & Tedeschi, R. G. (2004). The foundations of posttraumatic growth: New considerations. *Psychological Inquiry, 15*, 93–102.

Calhoun, L. G., & Tedeschi, R. G. (2006). *Handbook of posttraumatic growth: Research and practice*. Mahwah, NJ: Lawrence Erlbaum Associates.

Cobb, A. R., Tedeschi, R. G., Calhoun, L. G., & Cann, A. (2006). Correlates of posttraumatic growth in survivors of intimate partner abuse. *Journal of Traumatic Stress, 19*(6), 895–903.

Copeland, W., Keeler, G., Angold, A., & Costello, J. (2007). Traumatic events and posttraumatic stress in childhood. *Archives of General Psychiatry, 64*, 577–584.

Cordova, M., Cunningham, L., Carlson, C., & Andrykowski, M. (2001). Posttraumatic growth following breast cancer: A controlled comparison study. *Health Psychology, 20*, 176–185.

Costello, E. J., Erkanli, A., Fairbank, J., & Angold, A. (2002). The prevalence of potentially traumatic events in childhood and adolescence. *Journal of Traumatic Stress, 15*, 99–112.

Cryder, C., Kilmer, R., Tedeschi, R., & Calhoun, L. (2006). An exploratory study of posttraumatic growth in children following a natural disaster. *American Journal of Orthopsychiatry, 76*, 65–69.

Curbow, B., Legro, M., Baker, F., Wingard, J., & Somerfield, M. (1993). Loss and recovery themes of long-term survivors of bone marrow transplant. *Journal of Psychosocial Oncology*, 10(4), 1–20.

Davis, C., Nolen-Hoeksema, S., & Larson, J. (1998). Making sense of loss and benefiting from the experience: Two construals of meaning. *Journal of Personality and Social Psychology, 75*, 561–574.

Dekel, R. (2007). Posttraumatic distress and growth among prisoners of war: The contribution of husbands' posttraumatic stress disorder and wives' own attachment. *American Journal of Orthopsychiatry, 77*(3), 419–426.

Friedman, M. J., Resick, P. A., & Keane, T. M. (2007). PTSD: Twenty-five years of progress and challenges. In M. J. Friedman, P. A. Resick & T. M. Keane (Eds.), *Handbook of PTSD* (pp. 3–18). New York, NY: The Guilford Press.

Giaconia, R. M., Reinherz, H. Z., Silverman, A. B., Pakiz, B., Frost, A. K., & Cohen, E. (1995). Traumas and posttraumatic stress disorder in a community population of older adolescents. *Journal of the American Academy of Child and Adolescent Psychiatry, 34*, 1369–1380.

Hammack, P., Richards, M., Luo, Z., Edlynn, E., & Roy, K. (2004). Social support factors as moderators of community violence exposure among inner-city African American young adolescents. *Journal of Clinical Child and Adolescent Psychology, 33*, 450–462.

Harms & Talbot. (2007). The aftermath of road trauma: survivors' perception of trauma and growth. *Health and Social Work, 32*, 129–137.

Harter, S. (1986). Cognitive-development processes in the integration of concepts about emotions and the self. *Social Cognition, 4*, 119–151.

Ho, S. M. Y., Chan, C. L. W., & Ho, R. T. H. (2004). Posttraumatic growth in Chinese cancer survivors. *Psycho-Oncology, 13*, 377–389.

Hobfoll, S., Hall, B., Canetti-Nisim, D., Galea, S., Johnson, R., & Palmieri, P. (2007). Refining our understanding of traumatic growth in the face of terrorism: Moving from meaning cognitions to doing what is meaningful. *Applied Psychology: An International Review, 56*, 345–366.

Janoff-Bulman, R. (1992). *Shattered assumptions: Towards a new psychology of trauma*. New York: Free Press.

Janoff-Bulman, R., & Yopyk, D. (2004). Random outcomes and valued commitments: Existential dilemmas and the paradox of meaning. In J. Greenberg, S. Koole, & T. Pyszczynski (Eds.), *Handbook of experimental and existential psychology*. New York, NY: Guilford Press

Joseph, S., & Linley, P. A. (2004). Adversarial growth and positive change following trauma: Theory, research, and practice. *Psychological Research, 27*, 2004.

Joseph, S., & Linley, A. (2005). Positive adjustment to threatening events: An organismic valuing theory of growth through adversity. *Review of General Psychology, 9*(3), 262–280.

Joseph, S., Linley, A., & Harris, G. (2005). Understanding positive change following trauma and adversity: Structural clarification. *Journal of Loss and Trauma, 10*, 83–96.

Kessler, R. C., Sonnega, A., Bromet, E., Hughes, M., & Nelson, C. B. (1995). Posttraumatic stress disorder in the National Comorbidity Survey. *Archives of General Psychiatry, 52*, 1048–1060.

Kilmer, R. (2006). *Resilience and posttraumatic growth in children. From Handbook of posttraumatic growth: Research and practice*. Mahwah, NJ: Lawrence Erlbaum Associates.

Lechner, S.C., Zakowski, S.G., Antoni, M.H., Greenhawt, M., Block, K., & Block, P. (2003). Do sociodemographic and disease-related variables influence benefit-finding in cancer patients? Preview *Psycho-Oncology, 12*, 491–499.

Lev-Weisel, R. & Amir, M. (2003). Posttraumatic growth among Holocaust child survivors. *Journal of Loss and Trauma, 8*, 229–237.

Levl-Wiesel, R., Amir, M., & Besser, A. (2005). Posttraumatic growth among female survivors of childhood sexual abuse in relation to the perpetrator identity. *Journal of Loss and Trauma, 10*, 7–17.

Lindstrom, C.M., & Triplett, K. (2008). *Factors involved in the process of posttraumatic growth*. Poster presentation at Southeastern Psychological Association Conference, Charlotte, NC 3/08

Linley, P. A., & Joseph, S. (2004). Positive change following trauma and adversity: A review. *Journal of Traumatic Stress, 17*, 11–21.

Martin, L. L., & Tesser, A. (1996). Clarifying our thoughts. In R. S. Wyer Jr. (Ed.), *Ruminative thoughts* (pp. 189–208). Hillsdale, NJ: Lawrence Erlbaum Associates, Inc.

Milam, J.E. (2004). Posttraumatic growth among HIV/AIDS patients. *Journal of Applied Social Psychology, 34*, 2353–2376.

Norris, F. H., & Sloane, L. B. (2007). The epidemiology of trauma and PTSD. In M. J. Friedman, P. A. Resick & T. M. Keane (Eds.), *Handbook of PTSD* (pp. 3–18). New York, NY: The Guilford Press.

O'Brien, L. S. (1998). *Traumatic events and mental health.* Cambridge, UK: Cambridge University Press.

O'Leary, V. E., & Ickovics, J. R. (1995). Resilience and thriving in response to challenge: An opportunity for a paradigm shift in women's health. *Women's Health: Research on Gender, Behavior, and Policy, 1*, 21–142.

Osofsky, J. D. (1995). The effects of exposure to violence on young children. *American Psychologist, 50*, 782–788.

Park, C. L. (1998). Stress-related growth and thriving through coping: The roles of personality and cognitive processes. *Journal of Social Issues, 54*, 267–277.

Park, C. L., Cohen, L. H., & Murch, R. L. (1996). Assessment and prediction of stress-related growth. *Journal of Personality, 64*, 71–105.

Pynoos, R. S. (1993). Traumatic stress and development psychopathology in children and adolescents. In J. M. Oldham, M. B. Riba, & A. Tasman (Eds.), *American psychiatric press review of psychiatry* (Vol. 12). Washington, DC: American Psychiatric Press

Rabe, S., Zollner, T., Maercker, A., & Karl, A. (2006). Neural correlates of posttraumatic growth after severe motor vehicle accidents. *Journal of Consulting and Clinical Psychology, 74*, 880–886.

Rieck, M., Shakespeare-Finch, J., Morris, B., & Newbery, J. (2005). A mixed-method analysis of posttrauma outcomes: Trauma severity and social support from a psychotherapeutic perspective. *Canadian Journal of Counselling, 39*, 86–100.

Sabiston, C. M., McDonough, M. H., & Crocker, P. R. E. (2007). Psychosocial experiences of breast cancer survivors involved in a dragon boat program: Exploring links to positive psychological growth. *Journal of Sport and Exercise Psychology, 29*, 419–438.

Salick, E. C., & Auerbach, C. F. (2006). From devastation to integration: Adjusting to and growing from medical trauma. *Qualitative Health Research, 16*, 1021–1037.

Salter, E., & Stallard, P. (2004). Posttraumatic growth in child survivors of a road traffic accident. *Journal of Traumatic Stress, 17*, 335–340.

Schaefer, J. A., & Moos, R. H. (1992). Life crisis and personal growth. In B. N. Carpenter (Ed.), *Personal coping: Theory, research, and application* (pp. 149–170). Westport, CT: Praeger.

Schnurr, P. P., Friedman, M. J., & Bernardy, N. C. (2002). Research on posttraumatic stress disorder: Epidemiology, pathophysiology, and assessment. *Journal of Clinical Psychology, 58*, 877–889.

Sears, S.R., Stanton, A.L., & Danoff-Burg, S. (2003). The yellow brick road and the emerald city: Benefit finding, positive reappraisal coping and posttraumatic growth in women with early-stage breast cancer. *Health Psychology, 22*, 487–497.

Siegel, K. & Schrimshaw, E.W. (2000). Perceiving benefits in adversity: Stress-related growth in women living with HIV/AIDS. *Social Science and Medicine, 51*(10), 1543-1554.

Solomon, Z., Waysman, M.A., Neria, Y., Ohry, A., Schwarzwald, J., & Wiener, M. (1999). Positive and negative changes in the lives of Israeli former prisoners of war. *Journal of Social & Clinical Psychology, 18*(4), 419–435.

Taku, K., Calhoun, L. G., & Cann, A. (2008). The role of rumination in the loexistence of distress and posttraumatic growth among bereaved Japanese university students. *Death Studies, 32*, 428–444.

Tedeschi, R. G., & Calhoun, L. G. (1995). *Trauma and transformation: Growing in the aftermath of suffering*. Thousand Oaks, CA: Sage.

Tedeschi, R. G., & Calhoun, L. G. (1996). The posttraumatic growth inventory: Measuring the positive legacy of trauma. *Journal of Traumatic Stress, 9*, 455–471.

Tedeschi, R. G., & Calhoun, L. G. (2004). The foundations of posttraumatic growth: New considerations. *Psychological Inquiry, 15*, 1–18.

Tedeschi, R. G., Calhoun, L. G., & Cann, A. (2007). Evaluating resource gain: Understanding and *misunderstanding* posttraumatic growth. *Applied Psychology: An International Review, 56*, 396–406.

Thompson, S. (1985). Finding positive meaning in a stressful event and coping. *Basic and Applied Social Psychology, 6*(4), 279–295.

Urcuyo, K., Boyers, A., Carver, C., & Antoni, M. (2005). Finding benefit in breast cancer: Relations with personality, coping, and concurrent well-being. *Psychology and Health, 20*, 175–192.

Updegraff, J.A., & Marshall, G.N. (2005). Predictors of perceived growth following direct exposure to community violence. Preview. *Journal of Social & Clinical Psychology, 24*, 538–560.

Val, E., & Linley, P. (2006). Posttraumatic growth, positive changes, and negative changes in Madrid residents following the March 11th, 2004, Madrid train bombings. *Journal of Loss and Trauma, 11*(5), 409–424.

Vishnevsky, T., Cann, A., Calhoun, L.G., Tedeschi, R.G., & Demakis, G.J. (under review). Gender differences in Posttraumatic Growth: A meta-analysis.

Weiss, T. (2004). Correlates of posttraumatic growth in husbands of breast cancer survivors. *Psycho-Oncology, 13*, 260–268.

Wenar, C., & Kerig, P. (2000). *Developmental psychopathology: From infancy through adolescence* (4th ed.). New York: McGraw-Hill.

Widows, M.R., Jacobsen, P.B., Booth-Jones, M., & Fields, K.K. (2005). Predictors of posttraumatic growth following bone marrow transplantation for cancer. Preview. Health Psychology, 24, 266–273.

Yaskowich, K. (2003). Posttraumatic growth in children and adolescents with cancer. *Dissertational Abstracts International: Section B: The Sciences and Engineering, 63*, 3948.

Zoellner, T., & Maercker, A. (2006). *Posttraumatic growth and psychotherapy. From Handbook of posttraumatic growth: Research and practice*. Mahwah, NJ: Lawrence Erlbaum Associates.

Chapter 29

Psychological Impact of Genetic Testing

Introduction

News reports about how our genes affect many aspects of our life and health are increasing in both frequency and complexity. The last several years have seen amazing progress in our understanding of human genetics. The completion of the Human Genome Project in 2003 brought this issue into the mainstream more than any other single event (Collins et al 2003). Perhaps contrary to expectations, this milestone created more questions than it answered. Certainly, knowledge of the human genome sequence has increased the pace of genetic discovery for many diseases, but translating discoveries into patient care applications is not always straightforward.

One way that genetic disease information can be harnessed in clinical medicine is through genetic testing. In the coming years, information about our genes will lead to the routine use of diagnostic testing, based on genetic markers for common diseases such as asthma, coronary artery disease, and diabetes. Genetic tests for these diseases may lead to substantive changes in medical management depending on the results. However, many of the genetic changes associated with these disorders have only a small risk effect, and a person may need to inherit several of these "small effect" genes to develop the condition. These are called complex genetic diseases, and the reader is referred to recent reviews that discuss how to understand and apply the information from such studies in clinical care (Attia et al. 2009a, 2009b, 2009c; Fontanarosa et al. 2008).

There are also many possibilities for genetic information to influence treatment of human diseases. The possibilities extend beyond the concept of "gene therapy" to replace a missing gene. Genetic testing is now available to influence decisions about the dose of a medication based on a genetic predisposition to metabolize the drug faster or slower than usual, but that discussion is beyond the scope of this chapter.

Currently, most clinically available genetic tests are for genes that have a very strong effect, meaning that one genetic change is sufficient to lead to that condition. There are hundreds of genetic tests available for these types of diseases, also

From: *Handbook of Stressful Transitions Across the Lifespan,*
Edited by: T.W. Miller, DOI 10.1007/978-1-4419-0748-6_29,
© Springer Science+Business Media, LLC 2010

585

called "single gene" disorders, meaning that a change in just one gene causes the disease. The increased availability of genetic tests, coupled with efforts to advertise this testing to the public through "direct-to-consumer" marketing of tests has created an increased awareness among the public about how genetics contributes to disease risk. At the same time, the number and complexity of genetic tests with clinical applications often confuse individuals about the options. This potential for confusion has led to recommendations about the best process for making sure that individuals who have a genetic test understand the results and know how to apply them ("Control of direct-to-consumer genetic testing" 2008; Kuehn 2008).

Genetic knowledge is applicable to essentially all medical specialties, but judicious application of such knowledge presents many challenges (Guttmacher and Collins 2002). While society anxiously awaits applications such as gene therapy, the ability to diagnose genetic changes is a current reality. Moreover, the menu of available genetic tests will continue to expand (Amos and Patnaik 2002).

In many cases, the availability of genetic testing outpaces our ability to understand how best to apply such tests. Who are the appropriate candidates for genetic testing? Who will offer the tests and be available to counsel patients about potentially unexpected and anxiety-provoking results? Individuals making the transition from suspecting the presence of a genetic predisposition to a disease to actually *knowing* that they carry such a predisposition are faced with a uniquely stressful situation. In order to clarify the context of the problem, a brief overview of genetic testing will precede a discussion of its psychosocial impact.

Genetic Testing Basics

A genetic test may be defined as "the analysis of human DNA, RNA, chromosomes, proteins, and certain metabolites in order to detect heritable disease-related genotypes, mutations, phenotypes, or karyotypes for clinical purposes" (Burke 2002). For the purposes of this chapter, only testing of deoxyribonucleic acid (DNA) will be discussed. DNA is the chemical format for storing all of the instructions necessary to make a person. Genes are composed of DNA, and each gene contains the instructions for making a protein. Proteins have many different functions, and are needed by every cell in the body. Alterations (mutations) in DNA may result in production of a deficient protein, possibly leading to a disease. Genetic testing can detect DNA mutations even *before* a person gets a disease.

Genetic tests can look at genes and chromosomes in different ways. For example, a common type of genetic test is called gene sequencing to look for tiny changes in the genetic code. Another type of genetic testing looks for changes in gene copy number. Normally, there are two copies of every gene. Missing or extra copies of a gene can also cause disease. For the purposes of this chapter, a "positive" genetic test result implies that a person carries a mutation predisposing to that disease; a "negative" test result implies that a person carries no mutation, and "inconclusive" would mean that some ambiguity remains after the test is complete.

Categories of Genetic Testing

People may have different reasons for seeking a genetic test. Essentially, three broad categories encompass the majority of genetic testing. First, diagnostic genetic testing would look for a genetic change in a gene known to cause a disease for the purpose of verifying a diagnosis in a patient who already has symptoms of that disease. Second, predictive testing would look for a genetic change that causes a disease in a person who currently has no symptoms of that disease. A predictive test may be able to describe the likelihood that a person will develop a disease. Third, carrier screening would look for the presence of a genetic change in a person who does not have the disease (a carrier), but who could pass along a genetic change that might affect the children of the carrier.

Diagnostic Genetic Testing

Diagnostic testing is used to confirm or establish a clinical diagnosis of a particular disorder. Often, the diagnosis will be suspected prior to testing, although the clinician may order a test because they are unable to determine a diagnosis. In either of these types of cases, the patient is typically already affected by the disorder at the time of testing.

Box 1. *Case Example – Diagnostic Testing for a Symptomatic Patient*

A newborn baby's hearing is tested prior to leaving the hospital. The screening test identifies a mild-to-moderate hearing loss. Upon examining the child, no other medical problems are found. The pediatrician knows that approximately 50% of nonsyndromic hearing loss is associated with mutations in the connexin-26 gene, and orders a DNA test to determine the specific cause of hearing loss in this patient. The test shows a mutation in both copies of the patient's connexin-26 gene.

This is one example of diagnostic genetic testing. In this case, the person is already affected by the disorder prior to testing. The genetic test provides information about the cause of the patient's illness. In this case, the test results have additional utility for the parents because they will be told that they are both carriers for this mutation and have a 25% chance for each subsequent offspring to inherit two mutated copies of the gene. This may help the parents with family planning issues, but those decisions will certainly not evolve without some degree of psychological turmoil.

Diagnostic genetic testing can also be performed on pre-symptomatic individuals, meaning the person has no symptoms at the time of testing. Such is the case in testing for some adult-onset neurological disorders and familial cancer syndromes. This application of genetic testing may be accompanied by the greatest emotional impact to an individual because the diseases are so devastating and the genetic effects so strong that presence of the genetic change makes it almost certain that the person will develop the disease.

Carrier Genetic Testing

Sometimes the purpose of a genetic test is to determine a person's carrier status for a genetic trait. In the case of recessively inherited disorders, a person could have one normal copy of a gene and one copy bearing a disease-causing mutation. In most recessively inherited disorders this person would be an unaffected carrier, but if they had a child with another carrier then one in four of their children would receive two copies bearing a mutation and thus be affected by the disease.

Box 2. *Case Example*

An example of the role of this type of testing would be carrier screening for cystic fibrosis. The American College of Obstetricians and Gynecologists (ACOG) currently recommends that all people intending to have children be offered DNA testing to identify mutations in the gene causing cystic fibrosis ("ACOG Committee Opinion. Number 325, December 2005. An update on carrier screening for cystic fibrosis", 2005). Ideally, these types of tests are performed prior to conception or early in pregnancy so that the information can be used in making reproductive decisions.

Carrier screening can present unique psychological challenges as compared to the other types of testing. For example, the carrier is not generally burdened with the thought they might develop the disease (there are some exceptions to this rule, but generally a carrier is either not affected or only mildly affected). Rather, the carrier must confront the possibility that inherited disease could affect his or her offspring. This presents the potential for feelings of anxiety and guilt.

Carrier testing may be applicable to a variety of disorders. The ability to test for disorders must be tempered by concern for the impact of the information on the person being tested. For example, screening for a disorder with a significant impact on one's health and well being would not be appropriate if some type of intervention is not available to the patient and/or the patient's family. A full review of the topic is beyond the scope of this chapter. The relevant issues have been summarized elsewhere (Khoury et al. 2003).

Although it is easy to see how carrier screening could result in stressful circumstances, there are also scenarios in which it could lessen psychological stress. A parent who already has a child challenged by a disease such as cystic fibrosis may not be able to contemplate having another similarly affected child. Prenatal testing, by providing them the opportunity to have an unaffected child, may be able to alleviate some of their stress.

Predictive Genetic Testing

Predicting that an apparently healthy person will develop a potentially fatal disease leads to the potential for psychological distress for the patient. Genetic testing for inherited forms of breast, ovarian, and colon cancer is now offered routinely. Benefits of predictive genetic testing may include: early or more frequent surveillance for signs and symptoms of disease; early detection of disease through enhanced surveillance; and early treatment leading to improved chance for cure or survival. One "cost" that offsets this benefit is the potential for psychological distress. Genetic testing for Huntington disease, an inherited and ultimately fatal neurodegenerative disorder, is also widely available. However, most people with a family history do not elect to have genetic testing (Oster et al. 2008).

In order to minimize potential psychological stress, predictive genetic testing is typically offered through specialized clinics staffed by professionals attuned to the sensitivities of those being tested. The genetic counseling process involves at least two, and often three, visits by the patient. Visit 1 involves pretest counseling with a goal of identifying patients with difficult social situations, poor coping mechanisms, or a predisposing psychiatric condition which may inhibit the person's ability to deal effectively with test results. This evaluation does not typically incorporate formal psychological testing, but through a formal interview may elicit features suggestive of a vulnerable patient such as symptoms of depression, potential to attempt suicide, and life stressors (Fox et al. 1989). Patients known to engage in maladaptive coping responses, such as substance abuse, may also be vulnerable. In addition, the pretest counseling session can be used to identify sources of social support available to the patient.

Once a patient has determined their desire to obtain a predictive genetic test, the test might be sent off at the end of this first visit. The second visit would occur after the results of the test become available. The process of revealing the test results to the patient is referred to as disclosure. This is a time when the patient is perhaps most vulnerable and in need of psychological support from the genetic professional and family members of friends. Ideally, a third visit would occur some weeks after disclosure to assess the patient's success in coping with the test results. This type of visit would benefit the patient who receives a positive test result in obvious ways. It is important to remember that patients who learn they are not a carrier still may have stressful issues such as so called "survivor's guilt".

Predictive genetic testing is designed to assess the risk of developing a genetic disease. For the individual, knowledge of this increased risk impacts psychological well being. Genetic information also has implications for other family members, including dependent children. Knowledge of genetic susceptibility influences many important life decisions, including: reproductive decisions; financial planning; lifestyle modifications; and career planning. Knowledge of genetic susceptibility may cause overreaction to physical symptoms that would otherwise be ignored. The goal of genetic counseling (reviewed elsewhere in this volume) is to assure that participants in genetic testing are well informed about the implications of their genetic test results to facilitate appropriate decision making.

In spite of genetic counselors' best efforts, predictive genetic testing can create significant psychological turmoil for the patient, especially when testing for untreatable or incurable disorders. In the case of Huntington's disease, a positive test result indicates that the person will definitely develop a debilitating and fatal disease that has no treatment. In the case of most hereditary cancer syndromes, the certainty that a person with a positive genetic test will develop a disease may be much less than 100% but is much higher than a person with a negative genetic test.

Regardless of the predictive power of a genetic test, several aspects of predictive genetic testing can result in increased stress for the participants. Obviously, it would be stressful to learn that you are going to develop a terrible illness. One might assume that stress is primarily associated with learning of a positive test result. In fact, receiving a negative test result is also a source of stress for many people. In addition, because these tests deal with heritable disorders, the test results have implications for other family members and can have profound impact on family dynamics.

Psychological Stress in Predictive Genetic Testing

Predictive Testing for a Disease that has no Treatment

Testing for Huntington's disease (HD) provides an example of a predictive genetic test for a disease that is fatal and incurable. HD, a progressive degenerative neurological disorder, is inherited in a dominant pattern, meaning that a person only needs one copy of the altered gene to be affected. It is also a fully penetrant disease, meaning that a person who has the genetic change will develop the disease 100% of the time. Onset of symptoms occurs at approximately 40 y of age, after the typical reproductive years. The disease is universally fatal within approximately 15 y.

The identification of the HD locus (Gusella et al. 1983) allowed unaffected people with a family history of HD to be tested. Thus, HD was the first adult onset disease for which unaffected persons could be tested. Genetic testing can determine if a person will develop HD, even before symptoms become apparent. A person with a family history of HD may want to be tested prior to having children. If such persons were shown to carry the HD gene, they would have a 100% chance of developing HD and a 50% chance of transmitting the gene to each child they might conceive. Even if testing helped such a person make reproductive decisions, the knowledge of their genetic potential could be psychologically traumatic.

Operating under the assumption that an asymptomatic person who learns that he or she will develop HD would be exposed to psychological stress, a number of prospective studies have sought to characterize the psychological effects of predictive genetic testing for HD. Case reports are certainly available to document increased stress in patients who learn that they will develop HD. It is important to determine, however, if these negative outcomes apply to a significant number of persons tested.

Wiggins et al. (1992) studied patients at risk of developing HD (Wiggins et al. 1992). In their study the term "at risk" referred to the presence of a positive family history; the people involved did not know their carrier status and thus had a 50% statistical risk based on family history alone. The authors actually found that patients at risk of developing HD manifested less psychological stress 12 months after discovering they were carriers than did a group of patients at risk who were not tested and therefore unsure of their carrier status.

Tibben et al. (1997) attempted to identify the criteria to predict the likelihood of a negative response to testing. Hopelessness, intrusive thoughts, and avoidance behaviors functioned as measures of psychological stress in participants of an HD testing program. They found that post-test levels of these variables were most reflective of pre-test levels of the same variables. However, they also found increased depressive symptoms among patients receiving a positive test result (Tibben et al. 1997).

Codori et al. (1997) also examined pretest variables that might be linked to post-test psychological stress in neurologically asymptomatic persons being tested for HD carrier status (Codori et al. 1997). They included a more extensive list of potential predictors of stress: genetic status, gender, marital status, perception of risk for HD, and estimated years to onset of the disease. These variables were also assessed at various post-test intervals to determine the temporal pattern of stress response/adjustment. Their measures of adjustment were the Beck Depression Inventory and the Beck Hopelessness Scale. Their assessment measures for psychological status were the Schedule for Affective Disorders and Schizophrenia-Lifetime Version. Similar to Tibben et al. (1997), Codori et al. (1997) found that post-test levels of depression and hopelessness were strongly correlated with pre-test levels of the same variables. Overall, they found that significant predictors of increased post-test hopelessness among participants included: increased pretest hopelessness, positive genetic status, being married, how recently they received the results, having children, and sooner likelihood of disease onset.

These findings may be helpful indicators of post-test psychological stress, and the authors proposed conclusions for their unexpected results. The increased stress among married persons was unexpected because married persons have been generally found to be more stable psychologically. They theorized that the affected person may feel anxious about the increased burden that their illness will place upon their spouse. The same reasoning may apply to the increased stress among affected persons who have children. This study is important because it identifies variables which may lead to poor adjustment after predictive genetic testing.

A more recent study of 121 individuals (52 noncarriers, 54 gene carriers, and 15 gene carriers with symptoms of HD) showed four variables predicting increased depression and low mental quality of life among non-carriers, including: (1) low perceived social support; (2) no intimate relationship; (3) female gender; (4) younger age (Licklederer et al. 2008). As in earlier studies, this study suggests that consideration of the patient's social support network is an extremely important aspect of genetic counseling for presymptomatic genetic testing for Huntington's disease.

Predictive Genetic Testing for a Disease where Intervention is Possible

---

Box 3. *Case Example: Breast Cancer*

A 54 y old woman is being seen in a high risk breast cancer clinic which specializes in families with a strong history of breast cancer. In addition, her sister developed breast cancer at the age of 47 followed by ovarian cancer at the age of 56 and her father's brother was diagnosed with breast cancer at the age of 59. This man with breast cancer has two daughters in their thirties; both are healthy.

This family history of breast cancer prior to age 55, breast and ovarian cancer in the same person, and a case of breast cancer in a male is highly suggestive of the presence of genetic predisposition to cancer in this family. Specifically, these characteristics are associated with mutations in the first of the two genes known to be involved in familial breast cancer, *BRCA1* and *BRCA2* (Couch et al. 1997)

Box 3. (continued)

The oncologist recommends testing for mutations in the *BRCA1* gene. When the results show that our patient has a mutation in that gene, she is counseled that she has a significantly increased risk of developing breast and ovarian cancer. She may wish to consider prophylactically having her breast and ovaries removed. This type of surgery creates several psychological challenges.

In addition, the patient is very anxious about telling her relatives. It would appear that the mutation was passed down through her father's side of the family, so her uncle's two daughters are also at risk of carrying the mutation.

The National Cancer Institute estimates that 126 out of every 100,000 US women developed breast cancer each year from 2001–2005 (http://seer.cancer.gov/statfacts/html/breast.html; accessed 1/25/09). For a U.S. population of 300 million, this would equate to approximately 396,000 new cases of breast cancer each year. One of every nine women is predicted to develop breast cancer in her lifetime, or approximately 11%. Although family history is a strong predictor for the likelihood of developing any type of cancer, less than 5% of breast cancer occurs in patients with ta known family history (Malone et al. 2006).

Mutations in one of the two genes, *BRCA1* or *BRCA2*, confers a lifetime risk of developing breast cancer in the range of 55% to 85% (Easton et al. 1995; Ford et al. 1994; Ford et al. 1998; Struewing et al. 1997) Although the *BRCA1* and *BRCA2* genes account for only a minority of all cases of breast cancer, they are thought to be responsible for the majority of cases of hereditary breast cancer (Ford et al. 1998).

Knowing that a family member has a *BRCA1* or *BRCA2* mutation creates a potentially stressful situation. Studies have documented the presence of persistent psychological stress among women with a positive family history of breast cancer (Kash et al. 1992; Lerman et al. 1993). The stress was manifested as intrusive thoughts and feelings, sleep disturbance, and impairment in daily activities (Kash et al. 1992).

Not all psychological effects of genetic testing for hereditary breast cancer are necessarily negative. Schwartz et al. (2002) studied the psychological impact of genetic testing for mutations in *BRCA1* and *BRCA2* among 279 high risk women and their family members. They assessed these subjects prior to testing and six months after disclosure of test results. At both points in time, they measured the perceived risk for breast cancer, cancer-specific distress, and general distress. Their measure for cancer-specific distress was the Impact of Event Scale (Horowitz et al. 1979; Weiss and Marmar 1996), and for general distress they used the short form of the Hopkins Symptom Checklist (HSCL-25; (Hesbacher et al. 1980). They found no effect of test results among the 279 high risk women. Among unaffected relatives who received negative test results they found significant reductions in perceived risk and distress as compared to those relatives who received positive test results. Also, unaffected relatives who received positive test results did not demonstrate a significant increase in distress. In summary, they found reduced distress among participants receiving negative results and no increase in distress among those receiving positive results.

Ironically, receiving a negative test result for genetic testing in breast cancer does not remove the threat of developing breast cancer. The negative result removes the additional risk of a mutation in one of the genes predisposing to breast cancer, but the patient would still be faced with at least the population risk as well as any additional empiric risk based on family history. In the case of patients with a strong family history but a negative genetic test, this could conceivably create more psychological distress because the information available does not indicate a clear course of action. In fact, some patients find relief in a positive genetic test because they can proceed with a more clear idea of the risks they face.

Stress Associated with Predictive Testing

Neurodegenerative disorders, such as HD, and adult cancer syndromes, such as breast cancer, are both late-onset disorders. The outcome in both cases is a severe illness often resulting in premature death. The psychological impact of these disorders may differ among different patients but may also differ within the same patient depending on the diagnosis.

Dudodke-Wit (DudokdeWit et al. 1998) assessed patients having a 50% risk for HD ($n=41$), hereditary cerebral hemorrhage with amyloidosis ($n=9$), familial adenomatous polyposis coli ($n=45$), and hereditary breast and ovarian cancer ($n=24$). Participants were assessed for pretest intrusion and avoidance by the Impact of Event Scale (Weiss and Marmar 1996), anxiety and depression (Hospital Anxiety and Depression Scale (Zigmond and Snaith 1983)), feelings of hopelessness by the Beck Hopelessness Scale (Beck and Steer 1988), and psychological complaints by the Symptom Checklist (Derogatis 1994).

Higher anxiety and depression scores as well as increased psychological symptoms were found among patients at risk for neurodegenerative disorders as compared to those at risk for cancer syndromes. The reason for this discrepancy is unclear, but one could speculate that the patients perceive the threat of neurodegenerative disorders differently. In fact, the two types of disorders may not be comparable. In the case of HD, a positive genetic test confers essentially a 100% likelihood to develop the disease. Although the relative risks for familial cancer syndromes are quite high relative to the general population, a cancer geneticist or genetic counselor would never quote someone a 100% risk of developing cancer.

Additionally, they found that participants reporting increased scores for intrusion and avoidance also had higher anxiety and depression scores and increased psychological complaints. This increased intrusion and avoidance did not necessarily indicate a negative response since the authors found that patients with higher intrusion and avoidance scores were more reflective about their emotional responses. The authors suggest that low stress scores may merely reflect a failure to confront the issue at hand.

Disclosure to Family Members Represents a Difficult Transition

Regardless of how well an individual is able to process the stress of a genetic test result, there are additional challenges. Genetic information affects not only the individual, but potentially the entire family. Some genetic conditions are sporadic, meaning that they appear for the first time in a particular individual. Sporadic genetic disorders could be passed on to any children of the affected person, but would not affect their siblings. In comparison, when an individual is diagnosed with HD that person's siblings and children are instantly at 50% risk of carrying the affected gene. This creates an unusual family dynamic where one person's illness presents others in the family with the possibility that they may also become ill in the future. The complexities of this situation are optimally addressed through close follow-up between family members and the medical professionals offering the testing.

A Model for Genetic Testing as a Stressful Life Event

Clearly there are different challenges of predictive genetic testing for HD versus breast cancer, and each disease and its associated test will likely create unique challenges to those involved. A framework for understanding the relevant issues should facilitate the best adjustment of the individual undergoing this difficult transition. Baum et al. (1997) have described a model to conceptualize the impact of psychological stressors on patients receiving genetic testing (Baum et al. 1997). In their model, stressor characteristics include the nature of the result (positive is risk enhancing, negative is risk reducing, and inconclusive has unclear implications) and the disease characteristics. The extent to which these results create psychological stress depend on other variables, such as: the availability of surveillance measures, treatments, or other interventions for a positive test result. Additional personal variables include: the individual's coping skills, preparation for the test, and perception about the severity of the disease and risk that the disease will result in death.

To the extent that test results are viewed as a stressor, there may be associated psychological, emotional, and cognitive effects on the person being tested. In their model, the psychological stress is viewed as a function of: the test results; characteristics of the disease; uncertainty remaining after testing; the degree of uncertainty reduction; coping factors; and personal factors, including social support structure.

The issue of uncertainty is clearly important in the clinical setting. The degree to which the test result is correlated with a particular outcome is quite variable in genetic testing. In some diseases, a negative test result means that a person will almost certainly not develop a disease (e.g., HD). In other diseases, a negative test result may decrease the risk but not eliminate it entirely (e.g., breast cancer).

The individual's perception of the genetic test can vary from that expected by the medical community. For example, in a survey of 246 women considering breast cancer screening, Press et al. (2001) found that women were much less interested in genetic screening for breast cancer once they discovered that the test was not highly predictive (Press et al. 2001). These women had expected that the test would give them a clear answer about their risk of breast cancer, followed by very specific and effective noninvasive intervention. In fact, the test is neither able to predict an exact level or risk nor is the intervention noninvasive.

Returning to the model of Baum et al. (1997), uncertainty and uncertainty reductions are thought to be very important indicators of subsequent distress. In other words, uncertainty can create negative emotional distress. On the other hand, uncertainty also leaves open the hope of a positive outcome. In this way, uncertainty may decrease distress. The authors propose that personal factors will influence the orientation of the individual with respect to the distress caused by uncertainty. The term "uncertainty reduction" refers to the ability of the test to rule out the possibility of the disease; this is better in the case of HD than breast cancer.

Baum et al. (1997) correctly point out that family history of a serious illness can create uncertainty among other family members. This represents another opportunity for genetic testing to facilitate uncertainty reduction. However, this uncertainty reduction does not eliminate the possibility of psychological stress. Even in the case of negative results indicating a decreased risk to the patient, the result can be stressful (Lerman et al. 1991; Lynch et al. 1999). This increased stress can result from feelings of guilt about not being affected as compared to a family member (Biesecker et al. 1993). In general, noncarriers will tend to show less distress as the time passes (Lerman et al. 1996)

In summary, this model takes a comprehensive view of the many personal factors associated with the response to genetic test results. In general, the main variables being modified by the test results are uncertainty and uncertainty reduction. The degree to which the variables will be affected will be different from person to person. Although reduction of uncertainty can be helpful in easing the transition which occurs through learning one's genetic potential, it will not guarantee psychological adjustment.

Should Children Receive Predictive Genetic Testing?

Genetic tests are routinely used in the diagnosis of childhood disorders. This question is directed more at predictive genetic tests on asymptomatic children. In general, the consensus among genetic professionals dictates that predictive genetic testing is not acceptable in children (ASHG/ACMG 1995; Borry et al. 2006). This policy is a direct extension of the belief that patients seeking predictive genetic testing must give informed consent. Children are not considered capable of understanding the complexities involved in predictive genetic testing and therefore not eligible for predictive genetic testing for diseases with onset in adulthood.

There are, however, exceptions to the moratorium on predictive genetic testing of children. If a genetic test could identify the risk of the disease in a child and if that risk could be reduced through some type of intervention, then a genetic test may be acceptable (Lwiwski et al. 2008). This will be covered in the next section.

In terms of the practical impact of predictive genetic testing on children and their families, knowledge of genetic susceptibility to a disorder may alter the family relationships in a harmful way. Children bearing a genetic predisposition may be treated, knowingly or not, as vulnerable. This could impede their psychosocial development. The vulnerable child syndrome is a well described entity that pertains to situations not necessarily limited to genetics. It has been described in children suffering from chronic illness, as well as siblings of children who have a chronic illness or have died of an illness (Green 1986; Thomasgard and Metz 1995)

Guilt over transmission of a genetic predisposition is an important psychological consideration. Even though parents may wait until their children have reached an age of maturity before they participate in predictive genetic testing, a parent may feel responsible for their child's positive test result. This is, of course, especially true for the similarly affected parent, but may also be true for the nonaffected parent. Parents of children with disabilities may experience psychological stress in the form of guilt that they somehow have contributed to the disability (Eden-Piercy et al. 1986; Gardner 1969)

Regardless of the prohibition on testing children for disorders of adult onset, persons with a strong family history of a disorder should be offered testing once they reach adulthood, preferably prior to making reproductive decisions.

Will Predictive Genetic Testing of Children Produce Negative Psychological Effects?

Familial adenomatous polyposis (FAP) is a dominantly inherited colorectal cancer syndrome. This type of cancer is caused by inheritance of a mutation in the adenomatous polyposis coli (APC) gene. Any person inheriting the mutated gene will almost certainly develop colon cancer (Groden et al. 1991; Kinzler et al. 1991; Petersen et al. 1993; Powell et al. 1993). The development of colon cancer is preceded by the appearance of polyps in the colon. Since this type of cancer can start at a young age, persons with a known genetic risk are advised to begin annual screening by colonoscopy during childhood (Herrera et al. 1989).

The American Gastroenterological Association (2001) recommends genetic counseling to consider genetic testing in individuals at risk for FAP. Although the community of genetics professionals does not generally recommend genetic testing on children, they agree that it is ethically appropriate in the case of FAP (ASHG/ACMG 1995). Although testing children places them at a risk for anxiety related to the identification of risk, this liability is offset by the benefit of identifying patients who should have annual colonoscopy to detect colon cancer before it becomes advanced. Although one goal of genetic testing is to identify patients who should have colonoscopy, another benefit is that it identifies persons who do not require colonoscopy, sparing them repeated invasive procedures.

One could argue that the anxiety caused by knowing the genetic risk for FAP is worse than any benefit it provides. Of course, the validity of this argument may vary from person to person and objective measures of the anxiety induced in this scenario are only now becoming available. Codori et al. (2003) attempted to assess the psychological impact of genetic testing for hereditary colorectal cancer in children (Codori et al. 2003). They studied 48 children and their parents before genetic testing for FAP and three times post-testing. Their measures included the Children's Depression Inventory (Kovacs 1985) for the younger children and the Reynold's Adolescent Depression Scale (RADS; Reynolds, 1996).

Of forty-eight children tested, twenty-two tested positive. Perhaps surprisingly, there were no clinically significant differences between the children who tested positive and those who tested negative when assessed at 3, 12, and 23–55 months after disclosure. The only significant increase in depression symptoms was among the children who tested positive and also had a sibling who was positive. In these cases, the depression symptoms were subclinical. Also of note, several children who tested negative had significant increases in anxiety thought to be related to the fact that a sibling had tested positive. Ultimately, their data showed that the majority of children can be tested for FAP risk without suffering a detectable level of psychological stress in the early post-test period. This should not imply that testing should be undertaken casually. Their results also underscore the need for careful attention to the potential psychological impact of such testing on some patients. As it is impossible to predict which children will have negative responses to testing, all should be followed cautiously for signs of psychological stress.

Decision Support

Can Positive Genetic Tests Relieve Psychological Stress?

One might suppose that a person's anxiety about genetic testing would be inversely proportional to their likelihood of having a positive test result. Anecdotally, many parents with familial adenomatous polyposis are relieved when they test positive for the affected gene. This seemingly counterintuitive response is related to their concern for others in their family. In the case of FAP, the diagnosis can be made on clinical grounds, for example: the age of onset for colon cancer; the number of polyps in the colon; and other features. Only about 80% of people with the clinical symptoms of FAP will test positive with the currently available genetic test. A patient with FAP will require the same treatment regardless of their genetic test result. If their test result is negative, family members cannot be tested. When the patient's test is positive, however, that information can be used to screen family members (see Case Example). If a person with FAP had children, those children would need to begin annual colonoscopy at age 12–14 due to the 50% risk of having inherited the disease-causing gene. With a negative genetic test, a child of an affected parent could be spared annual invasive procedures, with obvious medical, psychological, and financial benefits.

Box 4. *Case Example: Testing Unaffected Children for Genetic Diseases*

JS is an 8-year-old girl. Her mother, TS, is known to have Familial Adenomatous Polyposis (FAP). TS was fortunate to have known about her family history and received annual screening colonoscopy in her early teenage years. When several colon polyps were detected, TS had her colon surgically removed to decrease her risk of developing colon cancer. TS has sought genetic counseling to determine the appropriate management of her daughter.

After taking a family history, the genetic counselor reviews the options. JS is offered a genetic test to look for mutations in the gene which causes FAP. After her mother signs the informed consent, JS

Box 4. (continued)

has her blood drawn and sent to a DNA diagnostic lab in another state. Before leaving the office, another appointment is scheduled for JS in six weeks. After five anxiety-provoking weeks, TS receives a call from the genetic counselor instructing the family to return to the clinic next week to discuss the results. Although TS would like to know the answers right away, she understands that it is not appropriate to disclose this sensitive information over the phone.

Upon returning to the genetic counselor's office, JS and her family are told that no mutations in the *APC* gene were found. TS is reassured that her daughter will not have to undergo the multiple medical procedures that she did in her youth. Although JS is an only child, the genetic counselor reminds TS that the risk of passing on the gene for FAP would be 50% in any future pregnancy.

Are Negative Responses to Genetic Testing Predictable?

Certainly not everyone who receives positive genetic test results will suffer undue psychological stress. It would, nevertheless, be clinically useful to be able to predict negative outcomes and target additional psychosocial support to psychologically vulnerable patients. To a certain extent, patients who know they are incapable of coping with positive genetic test results may self select against participation in genetic testing. In spite of this bias, potentially significant numbers of patients will choose to undergo genetic testing and suffer unanticipated psychological stress.

As discussed in the section on HD, Tibben et al. (1993) and Codori et al. (1993) found that post-test levels of depression and hopelessness were strongly correlated with pretest levels of the same variables. In a subsequent study involving patients being tested for HD as well as familial adenomatous polyposis and hereditary breast and ovarian cancer, DudodkeWit et al. used the Impact of Event Scale to measure intrusion and avoidance as indicators of stress both before and after presymptomatic genetic testing (DudokdeWit et al. 1998). They found that symptoms of depression prior to testing were predictive of more distress after testing, whereas pre-test symptoms of anxiety correlated with less post-test distress. Other patient characteristics predicting higher post-test stress included: female gender; having children; and pre-test intrusion symptoms. They concluded that the test result itself does not generate psychological stress and that the stressful responses are more a function of the individual. This suggests that some type of psychological screening would be beneficial prior to initiating genetic testing.

Perhaps Stress is a Good Thing

In a study designed to assess the stress response to predictive genetic testing, DudokeWit et al. again used the Impact of Event Scale to measure intrusion and avoidance as indicators of stress both before and after presymptomatic genetic testing (DudokdeWit et al. 1998). Their sample population included patients being tested for HD and hereditary cancer syndromes. One focus of their study was the hypothesis that low intrusion and avoidance scores among patients receiving genetic test results may be a reflection of denial of the results rather than that learning of the results was not stressful. Their study measured differences in the reported levels of anxiety, depression, hopelessness, and psychological complaints. They compared patients' self report of stressful feelings (by a survey) with an observer's assessment of the patient's response to test results (by an independent judgment of interview texts).

Similar to previous studies, they found that patients with high intrusion and avoidance scores had higher scores on scales for anxiety and depression and more psychological complaints than those with low intrusion and avoidance scores. The independent assessment of the interview text suggested that the patients reporting higher intrusion and avoidance scores were more carefully examining their own emotions whereas those reporting low scores may have been avoiding confrontation with the difficult news of a genetic test result. Long-term follow-up may have been able to address the utility of the different coping styles.

Genomic Profiling as a Predictive Genetic Test

Recently, predictive genetic tests are being offered as direct-to-consumer "genome scans" by commercial testing laboratory companies. These genomic profiles test a large number of genetic markers called single nucleotide polymorphisms (SNPs). Humans have about ten million SNPs in the genome where the letters of DNA in the genetic code are different from one person to another. Some of these changes may increase the likelihood to develop a disease. Rapid technological advances now make it possible for diagnostic laboratories to rapidly check thousands of SNPs from a single patient for a few hundred dollars.

However, these genome scans are still not being used in doctor's offices because the significance of many of these genetic changes is unclear, or the risks may be very small and therefore it would not be clear if some specific treatment or intervention would be warranted. The increased risk is often no larger than the risk from other known risk factors such as smoking or high cholesterol. Such risk factors increase the chances of developing heart disease, but they do not make it inevitable. Genetic tests that scan the entire genome are not as predictive as tests for HD or familial breast and colon cancer syndromes. A person who carries the HD mutation has a 100% chance of developing that disease, and a person with a *BRCA1* or *BRCA2* mutation has approximately 80% lifetime risk of breast cancer.

Demographic Differences in Patients' Perspectives on Genetic Testing

Ethnicity may influence utilization of genetic testing. In a case-control study, African-American women with a family history of breast or ovarian cancer were less likely than Caucasian women to seek genetic testing, even after adjustment for socioeconomic status, risk perception, and level of anxiety (Armstrong et al. 2005). Other studies have demonstrated similar levels of anxiety about genetic risk for breast cancer among African-American and Caucasian women (Halbert et al. 2005), yet there are significant differences in the utilization of genetic testing. These differences could arise from historical mistrust of the healthcare community among African–Americans (Corbie-Smith et al. 2002; Rose et al. 2004). Addressing this question will require further studies.

Another example of cross-cultural differences relating to genetic testing was found among members of a Native American Navajo tribe. In this case, there was a Navajo family with a high incidence of colorectal cancer, a disease that normally occurs infrequently among Native Americans. Members of the affected family received genetic testing for one of the genes involved in Hereditary Nonpolyposis Colorectal Cancer (Lynch et al. 1996). Several members of the family, some of whom had already developed cancer and others who were asymptomatic, were identified as having the mutation. All of the participants received similar genetic counseling. Some members of the family were able to accept the information, but others took the information as an implication that the family had been cursed. Previous knowledge of these potentially unanticipated and culturally rooted responses will help genetics professionals ease the transitions involved with the disclosure of genetic testing results.

Communities of individuals with certain medical conditions may have unique ideas about genetic testing. People with hearing loss can be considered as part of a distinct cultural group. Many deaf people come from families where one or both of the parents are deaf. These families may associate primarily with other deaf families because communication may be easier within such a group as compared to communication with their non-deaf peers. Children of such families may attend a school for deaf children. Although modern technologies, such as cochlear implants, are changing this scenario for some deaf people, many still feel more comfortable around others who share the same physical challenge.

In a survey conducted in the United Kingdom (Middleton et al. 1998), 87 deaf adults were asked about their opinions related to genetic testing for hereditary deafness. Of those sampled, 55% thought genetic testing would do more harm than good, 46% thought that its use would devalue deaf people. With regard to prenatal testing, 16% of those surveyed said they would consider prenatal testing. Of these, 29% said they would prefer to have deaf children. The last point is perhaps the most crucial. Deaf persons, or persons with other genetic conditions, may not view their condition as a disability in the way that a non-affected person might.

Privacy and Insurance Issues

There are other potential non-medical stresses associated with genetic testing. In 2008, the Genetic Information Nondiscrimination Act (GINA) was passed by the US Congress and signed into law. GINA protects Americans against discrimination for employment or health insurance based on their genetic information. It does not protect against discrimination for life insurance. Therefore, predictive testing for a disease that could cause early death, such as HD or familial cancer, could affect one's ability to obtain life insurance.

Concluding Remarks and Future Directions

Genetic testing is one of many rapidly advancing medical technologies. Like any technology, it has the potential to provide great benefits tempered by the potential for negative impact, either incidentally or through misuse. In keeping with the Hippocratic Oath, the benefits of any medical intervention must always be considered in the context of the potential to cause harm to the patient. It remains the duty of the clinician offering the genetic test to assess the patient's psychological well being both before and after testing and to facilitate appropriate psychosocial supports.

Special attention to the psychological state of each patient will be essential. Although little formal information is yet available regarding cross-cultural issues and genetic testing, it is likely that different reactions to genetic testing results will reflect unique aspects of disparate cultural and religious norms. Those from more closed societies may be less likely to take advantage of potentially advantageous genetic testing due to privacy issues. Genetic professionals must be sensitive to these concerns. At the same time, people wary of revealing their genetic information to relatives must realize that genetic information has implications extending beyond the individual. The concern for privacy must be weighed against the responsibility of informing relatives who might be impacted by positive, or negative, test results.

The studies reviewed in this chapter certainly demonstrate that genetic testing can create psychological stress for the individual. In spite of that, it is clear that the information gained through such tests provides health-related information that can have a profound positive impact for the patient and/or the patient's family. Even in cases where patients are confronted with positive test results indicating they may develop a terrible disease, most patients do not manifest lasting negative effects. In addition, these patients are often able to assimilate this information and use it to their benefit and the benefit of the family members.

References

ACOG Committee Opinion. Number 325, December 2005. Update on carrier screening for cystic fibrosis. (2005). *Obstet Gynecol, 106*(6), 1465–1468.

Amos, J., & Patnaik, M. (2002). Commercial molecular diagnostics in the US The Human Genome Project to the clinical laboratory. *Human Mutation, 19*(4), 324–333.

Armstrong, K., Micco, E., Carney, A., Stopfer, J., & Putt, M. (2005). Racial differences in the use of BRCA1/2 testing among women with a family history of breast or ovarian cancer. *JAMA, 293*(14), 1729–1736.

ASHG/ACMG. (1995). Points to consider: ethical, legal, and psychosocial implications of genetic testing in children and adolescents. American Society of Human Genetics Board of Directors, American College of Medical Genetics Board of Directors. *American Journal of Human Genetics, 57*(5), 1233–1241.

Attia, J., Ioannidis, J. P., Thakkinstian, A., McEvoy, M., Scott, R. J., Minelli, C., et al. (2009a). How to use an article about genetic association: A: Background concepts. *JAMA, 301*(1), 74–81.

Attia, J., Ioannidis, J. P., Thakkinstian, A., McEvoy, M., Scott, R. J., Minelli, C., et al. (2009b). How to use an article about genetic association: B: Are the results of the study valid? *JAMA, 301*(2), 191–197.

Attia, J., Ioannidis, J. P., Thakkinstian, A., McEvoy, M., Scott, R. J., Minelli, C., et al. (2009c). How to use an article about genetic association: C: What are the results and will they help me in caring for my patients? *JAMA, 301*(3), 304–308.

Baum, A., Friedman, A. L., & Zakowski, S. G. (1997). Stress and genetic testing for disease risk. *Health Psychology, 16*(1), 8–19.

Beck, A. T., & Steer, R. A. (1988). *Manual for the Beck Hopelessness Scale.* San Antonio, TX: Psychological Corporation.

Biesecker, B. B., Boehnke, M., Calzone, K., Markel, D. S., Garber, J. E., Collins, F. S., et al. (1993). Genetic counseling for families with inherited susceptibility to breast and ovarian cancer. *JAMA, 269*(15), 1970–1974.

Borry, P., Stultiens, L., Nys, H., Cassiman, J. J., & Dierickx, K. (2006). Presymptomatic and predictive genetic testing in minors: a systematic review of guidelines and position papers. *Clinical Genetics, 70*(5), 374–381.

Burke, W. (2002). Genetic testing. *New England Journal of Medicine, 347*(23), 1867–1875.

Codori, A. M., Slavney, P. R., Young, C., Miglioretti, D. L., & Brandt, J. (1997). Predictors of psychological adjustment to genetic testing for Huntington's disease. *Health Psychology, 16*(1), 36–50.

Codori, A. M., Zawacki, K. L., Petersen, G. M., Miglioretti, D. L., Bacon, J. A., Trimbath, J. D., et al. (2003). Genetic testing for hereditary colorectal cancer in children: long-term psychological effects. *American Journal of Medical Genetics, 116*(2), 117–128.

Collins, F. S., Green, E. D., Guttmacher, A. E., & Guyer, M. S. (2003). A vision for the future of genomics research. *Nature, 422*(6934), 835–847.

Control of direct-to-consumer genetic testing. (2008). *Lancet, 372*(9647), 1360.

Corbie-Smith, G., Thomas, S. B., & St George, D. M. (2002). Distrust, race, and research. *Archives of Internal Medicine, 162*(21), 2458–2463.

Couch, F. J., DeShano, M. L., Blackwood, M. A., Calzone, K., Stopfer, J., Campeau, L., et al. (1997). BRCA1 mutations in women attending clinics that evaluate the risk of breast cancer. *New England Journal of Medicine, 336*(20), 1409–1415.

Derogatis, L. R. (1994). *Symptom Checklist-90-R Administration, Scoring and procedures manual.* Minneapolis, MN: National Computer Systems.

DudokdeWit, A. C., Tibben, A., Duivenvoorden, H. J., Niermeijer, M. F., & Passchier, J. (1998). Predicting adaptation to presymptomatic DNA testing for late onset disorders: who will experience distress? Rotterdam Leiden Genetics Workgroup. *Journal of Medical Genetics, 35*(9), 745–754.

Easton, D. F., Ford, D., & Bishop, D. T. (1995). Breast and ovarian cancer incidence in BRCA1-mutation carriers. Breast Cancer Linkage Consortium. *American Journal of Human Genetics, 56*(1), 265–271.

Eden-Piercy, G. V., Blacher, J. B., & Eyman, R. K. (1986). Exploring parents' reactions to their young child with severe handicaps. *Mental Retardation, 24*(5), 285–291.

Fontanarosa, P. B., Pasche, B., & DeAngelis, C. D. (2008). Genetics and genomics for clinicians. *JAMA, 299*(11), 1364–1365.

Ford, D., Easton, D. F., Bishop, D. T., Narod, S. A., & Goldgar, D. E. (1994). Risks of cancer in BRCA1-mutation carriers. Breast Cancer Linkage Consortium. *Lancet, 343*(8899), 692–695.

Ford, D., Easton, D. F., Stratton, M., Narod, S., Goldgar, D., Devilee, P., et al. (1998). Genetic heterogeneity and penetrance analysis of the BRCA1 and BRCA2 genes in breast cancer families. The Breast Cancer Linkage Consortium. *American Journal of Human Genetics, 62*(3), 676–689.

Fox, S., Bloch, M., Fahy, M., & Hayden, M. R. (1989). Predictive testing for Huntington disease: I. Description of a pilot project in British Columbia. *American Journal of Medical Genetics, 32*(2), 211–216.

Gardner, R. A. (1969). The guilt reaction of parents of children with severe physical disease. *American Journal of Psychiatry, 126*(5), 636–644.

Green, M. (1986). Vulnerable child syndrome and its variants. *Pediatrics in Review, 8*(3), 75–80.

Groden, J., Thliveris, A., Samowitz, W., Carlson, M., Gelbert, L., Albertsen, H., et al. (1991). Identification and characterization of the familial adenomatous polyposis coli gene. *Cell, 66*(3), 589–600.

Gusella, J. F., Wexler, N. S., Conneally, P. M., Naylor, S. L., Anderson, M. A., Tanzi, R. E., et al. (1983). A polymorphic DNA marker genetically linked to Huntington's disease. *Nature, 306*(5940), 234–238.

Guttmacher, A. E., & Collins, F. S. (2002). Genomic medicine–a primer. *New England Journal of Medicine, 347*(19), 1512–1520.

Halbert, C., Kessler, L., Collier, A., Paul Wileyto, E., Brewster, K., & Weathers, B. (2005). Psychological functioning in African American women at an increased risk of hereditary breast and ovarian cancer. *Clinical Genetics, 68*(3), 222–227.

Herrera, L., Carrel, A., Rao, U., Castillo, N., & Petrelli, N. (1989). Familial adenomatous polyposis in association with thyroiditis. Report of two cases. *Diseases of the Colon and Rectum, 32*(10), 893–896.

Hesbacher, P. T., Rickels, K., Morris, R. J., Newman, H., & Rosenfeld, H. (1980). Psychiatric illness in family practice. *Journal of Clinical Psychiatry, 41*(1), 6–10.

Horowitz, M., Wilner, N., & Alvarez, W. (1979). Impact of Event Scale: A measure of subjective stress. *Psychosomatic Medicine, 41*(3), 209–218.

Kash, K. M., Holland, J. C., Halper, M. S., & Miller, D. G. (1992). Psychological distress and surveillance behaviors of women with a family history of breast cancer. *Journal of the National Cancer Institute, 84*(1), 24–30.

Khoury, M. J., McCabe, L. L., & McCabe, E. R. (2003). Population screening in the age of genomic medicine. *New England Journal of Medicine, 348*(1), 50–58.

Kinzler, K. W., Nilbert, M. C., Su, L. K., Vogelstein, B., Bryan, T. M., Levy, D. B., et al. (1991). Identification of FAP locus genes from chromosome 5q21. *Science, 253*(5020), 661–665.

Kovacs, M. (1985). The Children's Depression, Inventory (CDI). *Psychopharmacology Bulletin, 21*(4), 995–998.

Kuehn, B. M. (2008). Risks and benefits of direct-to-consumer genetic testing remain unclear. *JAMA, 300*(13), 1503–1505.

Lerman, C., Daly, M., Sands, C., Balshem, A., Lustbader, E., Heggan, T., et al. (1993). Mammography adherence and psychological distress among women at risk for breast cancer. *Journal of the National Cancer Institute, 85*(13), 1074–1080.

Lerman, C., Narod, S., Schulman, K., Hughes, C., Gomez-Caminero, A., Bonney, G., et al. (1996). BRCA1 testing in families with hereditary breast-ovarian cancer. A prospective study of patient decision making and outcomes. *JAMA, 275*(24), 1885–1892.

Lerman, C., Trock, B., Rimer, B. K., Jepson, C., Brody, D., & Boyce, A. (1991). Psychological side effects of breast cancer screening. *Health Psychology, 10*(4), 259–267.

Licklederer, C., Wolff, G., & Barth, J. (2008). Mental health and quality of life after genetic testing for Huntington disease: a long-term effect study in Germany. *American Journal of Medical Genetics, 146A*(16), 2078–2085.

Lwiwski, N., Greenberg, C. R., & Mhanni, A. A. (2008). Genetic testing of children at risk for adult onset conditions: when is testing indicated? *Journal of genetic counseling, 17*(6), 523–525.

Lynch, H. T., Drouhard, T., Vasen, H. F., Cavalieri, J., Lynch, J., Nord, S., et al. (1996). Genetic counseling in a Navajo hereditary nonpolyposis colorectal cancer kindred. *Cancer, 77*(1), 30–35.

Lynch, H. T., Watson, P., Tinley, S., Snyder, C., Durham, C., Lynch, J., et al. (1999). An update on DNA-based BRCA1/BRCA2 genetic counseling in hereditary breast cancer. *Cancer Genetics and Cytogenetics, 109*(2), 91–98.

Malone, K. E., Daling, J. R., Doody, D. R., Hsu, L., Bernstein, L., et al. (2006). Prevalence and predictors of BRCA1 and BRCA2 mutations in a population-based study of breast cancer in white and black American women ages 35 to 64 years. *Cancer Research 66*, 8297–8308.

Middleton, A., Hewison, J., & Mueller, R. F. (1998). Attitudes of deaf adults toward genetic testing for hereditary deafness. *American Journal of Human Genetics, 63*(4), 1175–1180.

Oster, E., Dorsey, E. R., Bausch, J., Shinaman, A., Kayson, E., Oakes, D., et al. (2008). Fear of health insurance loss among individuals at risk for Huntington disease. *American Journal of Medical Genetics, 146A*(16), 2070–2077.

Petersen, G. M., Francomano, C., Kinzler, K., & Nakamura, Y. (1993). Presymptomatic direct detection of adenomatous polyposis coli (APC) gene mutations in familial adenomatous polyposis. *Human Genetics, 91*(4), 307–311.

Powell, S. M., Petersen, G. M., Krush, A. J., Booker, S., Jen, J., Giardiello, F. M., et al. (1993). Molecular diagnosis of familial adenomatous polyposis. *New England Journal of Medicine, 329*(27), 1982–1987.

Press, N. A., Yasui, Y., Reynolds, S., Durfy, S. J., & Burke, W. (2001). Women's interest in genetic testing for breast cancer susceptibility may be based on unrealistic expectations. *American Journal of Medical Genetics, 99*(2), 99–110.

Rose, A., Peters, N., Shea, J. A., & Armstrong, K. (2004). Development and testing of the health care system distrust scale. *Journal of General Internal Medicine, 19*(1), 57–63.

Schwartz, M. D., Peshkin, B. N., Hughes, C., Main, D., Isaacs, C., & Lerman, C. (2002). Impact of BRCA1/BRCA2 mutation testing on psychologic distress in a clinic-based sample. *Journal of Clinical Oncology, 20*(2), 514–520.

Struewing, J. P., Hartge, P., Wacholder, S., Baker, S. M., Berlin, M., McAdams, M., et al. (1997). The risk of cancer associated with specific mutations of BRCA1 and BRCA2 among Ashkenazi Jews. *New England Journal of Medicine, 336*(20), 1401–1408.

Thomasgard, M., & Metz, W. P. (1995). The vulnerable child syndrome revisited. *Journal of Developmental and Behavioral Pediatrics, 16*(1), 47–53.

Tibben, A., Timman, R., Bannink, E. C., & Duivenvoorden, H. J. (1997). Three-year follow-up after presymptomatic testing for Huntington's disease in tested individuals and partners. *Health Psychology, 16*(1), 20–35.

Weiss, D. S., & Marmar, C. R. (1996). *The Impact of Event Scale – Revised.* New York: Guilford.

Wiggins, S., Whyte, P., Huggins, M., Adam, S., Theilmann, J., Bloch, M., et al. (1992). The psychological consequences of predictive testing for Huntington's disease. Canadian Collaborative Study of Predictive Testing. *New England Journal of Medicine, 327*(20), 1401–1405.

Zigmond, A. S., & Snaith, R. P. (1983). The Hospital Anxiety And Depression Scale. *Acta Psychiatrica Scandinavica, 67*, 361–370.

Chapter 30

Functional Fitness, Life Stress, and Transitions Across the Life Span

John Nyland and James D. Abbott

Function refers to activities identified by a client as being essential to support physical, social, and psychological wellbeing and to create a personal sense of a meaningful life (Physical Therapist Guide to Practice 2000; Brody 2002). Maintaining functional fitness across the lifespan is essential both to independent living and to the overall quality of life. Functional fitness is the presence of adequate cognitive, neuromuscular, cardiovascular and pulmonary, musculoskeletal, and integumentary system function to enable participation in activities of daily living considered to be vital to one's quality of life (Nyland 2007).

The goals of rehabilitation generally focus on returning a client to functional activities such as those associated with their vocation, daily activities, sports, or recreational pursuits. Functional rehabilitation and conditioning relies on exercise activities to simulate the weight-bearing and nonweight-bearing components of daily activities in a manner that replicates three-dimensional function within joint ranges and velocities that facilitate the desired physiological responses (Nyland et al. 2005) (Fig. 30-1). With activation of large lower extremity muscle groups creating movement across the hip, knee, and ankle joint, clients can positively influence cognitive, neuromuscular, cardiovascular and pulmonary, musculoskeletal, vestibular, and integumentary system function throughout the lifespan (American College of Sports Medicine Position Stand 1998).

Multisystem evidence supports the need for exercise and activity and the need to avoid prolonged bed rest, immobility, and inactivity as we age (Krasnoff and Painter 1999). Inactivity and aging contribute to decreased femoral artery diameter (De Groot et al. 2006), increased risk of sustaining an upper respiratory infection (Nieman 1994), and decreased total muscle mass (Thompson 2002). After 30 years of age the cross-sectional muscle area decreases and intramuscular fat increases tending to slow body metabolism (Thompson 2002). Thompson (2002) reported that total body muscle mass decreases by approximately 50% between 20 and 90 years of age. Between 50 and 70 years of age there is a 30% strength loss and a 15% reduction in

From: *Handbook of Stressful Transitions Across the Lifespan*,
Edited by: T.W. Miller, DOI 10.1007/978-1-4419-0748-6_30,
© Springer Science+Business Media, LLC 2010

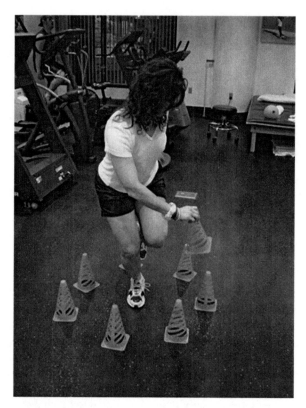

Fig. 30-1. Functional exercises blend strength, balance, coordination, proprioception, and cognition challenges

fat-free body mass. After 70 years of age there is a 30% strength loss for each additional decade of life.

The benefits of regular participation in weight-bearing and progressive resistance exercises for muscle function (Deley et al. 2007; Candow 2008; Johnston et al. 2008; Suetta et al. 2008), bone tissue properties (Lanyon 1992; Sparling et al. 1998; Rubin et al. 1996; Layne and Nelson 1999), and joint health (Bijlsma and Knahr 2007; Hanna et al. 2007; Hinman et al. 2007; Koster et al. 2008b) have been widely reported, as have been the negative influence of smoking (Marks and McQueen 2002), excessive alcohol intake (O'Keefe et al. 2007), and poorly regulated hormonal and dietary changes (Jackson and Shidham 2007; Campbell 2008).

Many clients may not be aware of the long-term, possibly systemic effects of a seemingly minor joint injury that is sustained early in their lives. Ligamentous or meniscal knee injury, for example occurring early in one's life, can create bone mineral density deficiencies throughout the lower extremity and spine that never return to premorbid levels (Leppala et al. 1999; Reiman et al. 2006). Regardless of whether or not a ligament is repaired or reconstructed, some level of permanent damage has been done to the joint. Knowing and understanding this important fact is essential to the health behavior decisions that clients are likely to make throughout their life.

With normal aging, growing deficiencies in neuromuscular, musculoskeletal, balance-vestibular, cardiovascular and pulmonary, vision, and auditory system function occur. The percentage of older adults who experience impaired vision and hearing increases steadily from 65 to 74, 75 to 84, and >85 years of age (Meisami 1992). Connective tissues such as ligaments and tendons also tend to have lower ultimate strength with aging (Woo et al. 1991). Bone mass and bone mineral density tend to decrease with advancing age, particularly among women (Riggs and Melton 1983). These changes, however, may not be as strongly linked to chronological age as was once believed. Lifestyle choices and behaviors and regular participation in healthy functional exercises and activities may reduce the magnitude or delay the onset of these changes (Ross and Huttlinger 2006).

A significant percentage of older adults will be affected by chronic diseases such as arthritis (men=49.5%, women=63.8%), high blood pressure (men=40.5%, women=48%), heart disease (men=24.7%, women=19.2%), cancer (men=23.4%, women=16.7%), diabetes (men=12.9%, women=11.5%), and stroke (men=10.4%, women=7.5%). Being overweight or obese is related to the onset and exacerbates the effects of many chronic diseases (USA Center for Disease Control, 2003). The percentage of American adults >20 years of age who are overweight or obese increased by 23% between 1988 and 1994, while also increasing by 11% for children and adolescents between 6 and 19 years of age (United States Department of Health and Human Services 2000).

The issue of being overweight or obese has many contributing factors, but a particularly strong component relates to energy intake versus energy expenditure. Excessive energy intake can be due to large food portion size, selection of high energy density foods or those with a high glycemic index, soft drinks and "junk food", added sugar, easy and often food access, low cost, variety, convenience, great taste, and the constant bombardment of advertisements related to food or eating. Poor energy expenditure in combination with excessive energy intake creates a strong negative feedback cycle. Energy expenditure issues are also related to sedentary workplaces and schools, the lack of organized physical education or sports programs in schools (organized health education in addition to free "gym time"), activity "unfriendly community designs", automobiles, drive-through conveniences, elevators/escalators, remote controls, sedentary entertainment, and labor-saving devices including computers and cell phones (Peters 2006).

A linear relationship has been reported between the body mass index (BMI) of 11,728 health care and university employees and the number of workers' compensation claims (Ostbye et al. 2007). Employees with BMI$\geq$40 had 11.65 claims/100 FTEs compared to employees with the recommended BMI (5.8 claims/100 FTEs). Employees with a BMI>40 also had more lost workdays, more medical claims costs, and more indemnity claims costs. On the basis of this finding, a client who has excessive body weight may also be more likely to sustain an injury.

The BMI is equal to a client's weight in pounds divided by his/her height in inches squared, multiplied by 703: Underweight BMI=<18.5, normal weight BMI=18.5–24.9, overweight BMI=25–29.9, and obesity BMI=$\geq$30. A high waist circumference measurement is associated with an increased risk for type 2 diabetes, dyslipidemia, hypertension, and cardiovascular disease when combined with a BMI that is between 25 and 34.9 (Lorenzo et al. 2007; World Health Organization Website 2008). Waist circumference correlates closely with BMI and the ratio of waist-to-hip circumference is an approximate index of intraabdominal fat mass and total body fat (Sanches et al. 2008). There is an increased risk of metabolic diseases such as cardiovascular disease for older men with a waist circumference of ≥ 102 cm and for older women with a waist circumference of ≥ 88 cm (Koster et al. 2008a, b). Simple measurements such as these provide clients with a simple "rule of thumb" with a fair discriminatory power to approximate their general health status and chronic disease onset risk (with consideration for multiple other variables including genetic predisposition) (Heinrich et al. 2008).

Personal psychosocial factors such as self-efficacy have been reported to contribute to >45% of the performance variance of men and women with medial knee joint osteoarthritis during walking, stair climbing, or transferring, while mechanical factors including obesity, quadriceps femoris muscle group strength, and hamstring muscle group strength contributed only 10–15% (Maly et al. 2005). Clients' preoperative perceived self-efficacy of knee function is an important predictor of whether or not they eventually return to acceptable physical activity levels, with reduced symptoms and improved function at one year after anterior cruciate ligament (ACL) reconstruction (Thomee et al. 2008) and with knee osteoarthritis (Maly et al. 2007). Clients who have a more internal health locus of control also reportedly have lower perceived physical function deficits following ACL injury (Nyland et al. 2002) and superior perceived function following ACL reconstruction than patients who have a more external health locus of control (Nyland et al. 2006). There is a strong relationship between a client's psychological state and how well they "navigate" through the injury recovery process (Prochaska et al. 1994; Livneh and Antonak 1997).

Who counsels the client regarding the significance of a lower extremity joint injury, an upcoming surgery, or the need for psychobehavioral changes? If orthopedic surgery is performed without the client completely understanding the prognosis, or how the health behaviors that they select may positively or negatively influence all aspects of their health, the likelihood of a successful long-term outcome is poor.

Synovial joints represent the "transmissions" through which the neuromuscular and skeletal systems create movement. Unfortunately, osteoarthritis has reached epidemic proportions in the USA with the diagnosis by examination rate increasing from 4% to 8.9% for men and women between 40 and 59 years of age to 20.3% and 40.8% for clients who are over 60 years of age (USA Center for Disease Control 2008). Although genetic endowment is essential to prevent "tissue sabotage", maintaining the needed levels of flexibility, strength, balance, coordination, and power in addition to preserving native joint anatomical architecture and alignment is essential (Dye 1996; Sparrow 2001). Compared to walking, jogging on an unyielding concrete surface increases knee joint reaction forces 3–5 times potentially contributing to joint degeneration (Andriacchi et al. 2000). Articular hyaline cartilage and meniscal fibrocartilage serve as the "fire wall" between a healthy knee joint and osteoarthritis; therefore their functional preservation across the lifespan is a high priority (Lewis et al. 2006).

In many ways the knee joint formed by the mechanical "long bone" intersection of the lever arms of the thigh ending in the distal femur and of the leg beginning at the proximal tibia is at particular risk for sustaining torsional injury. Because of this precarious arrangement knee joint health also provides a reasonable indicator of a client's capacity for acquiring, maintaining, or improving general health. Dye (1996) described the knee joint as a biological transmission in that it accepts, transfers, and dissipates loads. In this conceptualization ligaments serve as sensate adaptive linkages, articular cartilage serves as immobile insensate bearings, menisci serve as mobile sensate bearings, and muscles serve as living engines (concentric action), and brakes or dampening (eccentric action) systems that are under complex neurological control. Knee joint homeostasis is maintained when load magnitude and frequencies occur within the "envelope of function" (Dye 1996). The upper limit of the envelope of function is the threshold between homeostatic loading and loading which initiates a biologic cascade of trauma induced inflammation and repair. Knee joint pain, tenderness to touch, giving way, swelling, or warmth may express this cascade. The potentially healing attributes of the normal biologic inflammatory cascade are unavailable to articular hyaline cartilage which is avascular, relying instead on diffusion for nutrition. Without vascular channels, reparative mesenchymal stem cells cannot reach the area of damaged cartilage. Mueller and Maluf (2002) described a Physical Stress Theory based on how differing tissues respond to loads with consideration for magnitude, time (duration, repetition, rate), and direction (tension, compression, shear, torsion). Other factors that influence the effects of loading included movement and alignment variables such as posture, physical activity, and tissue extensibility; extrinsic factors such as footwear selection, orthosis or assistive device use, and gravitational forces. Physiological factors such as age, medication use, systemic pathology, and obesity; and psychosocial factors such as self-efficacy and empowerment also influence tissue responses.

The multifactorial nature of joint health and its relationship to general health necessitates comprehensive problem solving during the physical examination. When an exercise plan is prescribed Morris (2000) listed several factors that clinicians should consider including having a thorough understanding of the existing movement disorder, whether or not cognitive impairments exist, the specific needs of a given client or their caregiver, the presence of any secondary adaptive changes, the effects of aging and concurrent pathologies, medication history, their environment, and activity of daily living task requirements.

Emotional stress as it relates to bodily pain has cognitive, sensory, and affective dimensions. While pain may not be the primary factor that drives functional exercise program adjustments, it should not be ignored. The key to client care is to ascertain to what extent these stress dimensions combine to negatively influence behavior and functional level. Are they channeled into an adaptive stress response where survival and homeostasis is restored, or into a maladaptive, ongoing stress response where health is likely to decrease (Gifford 1998)? When designing a functional exercise program, client expectations, education level, perceived barriers, and other potential compliance issues should be considered in addition to age, quality of life values, and medications (Mancuso et al. 2001; Mahomed et al. 2002; Dorr and Chao 2007).

Both younger (Gerber et al. 2007) and older (LaStayo et al. 2003, 2007) clients can benefit from the negative work provided by progressive eccentric exercise. Older clients who used the cycling type apparatus that induced negative work also had a reduced fall risk (LaStayo et al. 2003). To adequately maintain or improve function and reduce falling risk in older clients, it is also important to create "sensory rich environments" that train appropriate internal representations, anticipatory and adaptive mechanisms, sensory strategies, neuromuscular synergies, and ultimately postural control (Shumway-Cook and Woollacott 1995; van Praag et al. 2000; Kempermann et al. 2000; van Praag 2008). Low-impact exercise activities like Tai Chi have been shown to decrease the incidence of lower extremity osteoarthritis, increase flexibility, lower resting blood pressure, improve postexercise blood pressure recovery, and improve behavioral test outcomes of subjects >60 years of age (Wolf et al. 2003).

Dynamic trunk stability is the capacity to control intervertebral and global trunk movements and to contribute to the control of distal segment movements and loading forces via coordinated muscle recruitment in response to expected or unexpected perturbations such that an equilibrium position (static stability) or intended trajectory (dynamic stability) can be maintained. Given that the trunk interfaces with both upper and lower extremity movements (Vleeming et al. 1995; Hodges et al. 2000), setting a goal of developing dynamic trunk stability is useful for individuals of all ages (Zazulak et al. 2007a, b). Innovative upright rotational exercise devices may help efficiently improve dynamic trunk stability by incorporating weight bearing, controlled, multisegmental eccentric exercise, and standing weight shifting-balancing simultaneously (Nyland and Shapiro 2002) (Fig. 30-2).

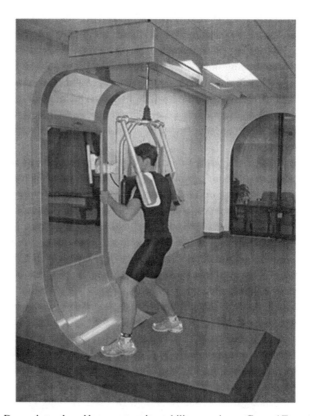

Fig. 30-2. Dynamic trunk and lower extremity stability exercise on Ground Force 360 device. Webb's Machine Design, Clearwater, FL, USA) http://www.webbsmachinedesign.com/

Multitasking and cognitive challenges during locomotion are becoming more commonplace as we live in the "cell phone, instant text messaging, and paging era". Simultaneous cognitive and locomotion challenges are known to increase fall risk in older individuals (Barra et al. 2006). In the future, technologies like cell phones may provide an effective way to progressively infuse cognitive challenges at specific instances during exercise. Random cell-phone tone or vibration settings could be used to cue movement or pace changes in addition to monitoring or measuring client metabolic information during exercise. Cell phones may be developed with power supplies that require a particular distance walked or exercise volume to be performed to maintain operational status or to garner "free" or reduced charge calling minutes. Greater effort must be placed on capturing that part of any new technology that enables the client to live a higher quality reality, not a higher quality "virtual" or simulated reality. Sitting in front of a computer for prolonged periods of time for example is a poor use of the technology if this substitutes completely for being outside doing activities that are both physically and cognitively challenging.

Varying the environment, and surface characteristics (hard pavement, soft cinder or rubberized tracks, inclines, declines, steps, and undulating trails and paths, etc.) upon which exercise activities are performed can be useful for modulating lower extremity joint load magnitude, loading rate, and movement velocity, etc. In addition to postural support and movement functions, the musculoskeletal system provides important mechano-transduction signals that stimulate tissue remodeling closely following the "blue print" drawn over time by accumulated lower extremity loading force vectors (Garcia-Castellano et al. 2000; Jones et al. 2004). Swimming or other aquatic therapy activities performed at a community center or motel swimming pool, as well as local lakes/reservoirs provide another excellent method of improving general health and functional fitness in a "joint friendly" environment (Hinman et al. 2007).

Optimizing the quality of life of an older client should include maximizing the yield from that part of the day that they dedicate to health, wellness, and functional fitness activities. Combining a walk, jog, run, or other health activity pursuit with esthetically appealing natural terrain along a lake or river, in a city or suburban park or golf course, or across a rolling field or hillside can enable the participant to combine exercise, spirituality, and social activities in a manner that best suits their needs and desires. Group activities also provide a useful environment for health information exchange, new advances in care, etc. Group activities also provide an excellent method for positive peer pressure and developing behavioral contracts (Miller et al. 2006). Sunshine, light rain or snow, and wind all contribute to the multisensory experience. Sunshine helps stimulate vitamin D production, which is essential to bone health. New technologies like cell phones and global positioning systems provide at least a minimal "safety net" should problems arise.

The primary reason for participation in exercise tends to change across the lifespan. Preadolescent experiences largely address neuromuscular coordination and kinesthetic awareness as well as the musculoskeletal changes associated with growth. During adolescence, strength, power, and body building-type appearance goals often manifest themselves (Fig. 30-3). Beginning in the late second or early third decade of life, however, exercise goals often shift more toward maintaining existing strength or power levels and appearance, while placing a greater priority on exercise as a health form. Unfortunately between the preadolescent years

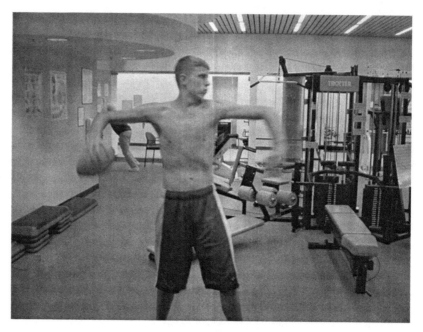

Fig. 30-3. Preparing to be a high school football quarterback

and later life, children and parents alike seldom are aware of the potential ramifications of an early lower extremity joint injury on long-term health and quality
of life. Having earlier and matter-of-fact knowledge of these potential ramifications prior to injury and certainly after injury may influence health decisions
and behaviors.

As we age, maintaining our zone of independent safe function becomes
a priority. This includes tasks like independently rising from a chair and
navigating stairs, ramps, inclines, declines, uneven surfaces, steps, and curbs.
Additionally, being comfortable navigating surfaces with characteristics ranging from the hardness of concrete to the softness of low density foam rubber
mats, and the slipperiness of ice is also important. Without compromising
safety, clinicians need to instill challenges to clients on a regular basis through
functional exercise programs that blend innovative technologies with physical
structure and impediments that are confronted on a regular basis. To accomplish this we need to vary the experience of load magnitude, rate, frequency,
and the environment in which the loads are experienced. Joint loads within
these activities should be "collagen and bone cell friendly" (Lane 2008) with
the client being encouraged to listen to their body, to understand the significance of musculoskeletal and joint symptoms, and to make the necessary program corrections in activity, load, loading rate, or frequency.

When screening potential players for their draft, the National Football
League (NFL) evaluates 40 yard dash, repeated bench press with 225 pounds,
vertical jump, broad jump, 3-cone agility drill, 20-yard shuttle run, and a
60-yard shuttle run in addition to position-specific drills, cognitive and
psychological tests (National Football League Combine Website 2008). This
type of screening is performed so that potential employers can base their
interest and the large sum of money that they will invest in a given prospect

on standardized test information in addition to past performance. Effectiveness in professional football is largely based on the power, endurance, agility-quickness, and psychobehavioral profiles that can be assessed by these tests. What if NFL stood for "non-impaired functional level"? Clients and clinicians need to contemplate what functional characteristics should be profiled with appropriate tests based on the frequency, importance, and quality of life relevance of a given task set.

Georges Hebert (2008) a French physical educator is credited with developing a natural method of fitness training composed of exercises from ten foundational groups: walking, running, jumping, quadrupedal movement, climbing, balancing, throwing, lifting, defending, and swimming. To accomplish this training session, he used an outdoor environment in which these tasks were performed either in a natural or spontaneous way on an unspecified route through the countryside, or within a specially designed environment with each session lasting 20–60 min. Hebert is considered to be one of the earliest proponents of the "parcours" or obstacle course form of physical training.

Only a few select individuals are potential NFL candidates. What the natural method of fitness training, parcourses, and the NFL combine have in common is functional fitness, providing the client and interested others with some idea of how they will likely survive and hopefully thrive in daily activities. Natural fitness training and parcourses in the USA, however, have largely been considered the domain of younger to middle-aged individuals considered by many to be "fitness fanatics". While these practices are certainly of value, consideration needs to be given to expanding their conceptual use, and their practical significance in terms of lifetime functional fitness, quality of life, and maintaining independent living. This is particularly true given the aging USA population and the increasing average lifespan of that population.

Health maintenance and independent living are directly related concepts and perceived and real environmental barriers may have tremendous implications on both. One simple daily living example is crossing a busy street intersection. Minimum safe crossing times vary from 30 to 120 s, with longer times generally allotted for busier intersections (Van Houten et al. 2007). Improved connectivity provided by pedestrian networks that increase neighborhood "walkability" and pedestrian access points should be an essential part of residential planning (Chin et al. 2008). Existing standards and regulations for ramp, curb, step, and handrail, etc. dimensions provide useful information in planning urbanized parcourses where clients can train and evaluate their ability to navigate physical barriers (The American Institute of Architects, 2001). Directional lines, lights, and audio signals can be included with timing feedback so both young and older clients have knowledge of both successful performance and for time-related safety issues. Clients can compare their performance with age-matched mean performance times. These courses should be multisensory experiences with terrain and surface diversity. Development of functional obstacle courses in urban and suburban settings (F.O.C.U.S.) would also provide clinicians with the opportunity to assign supplemental movement experiences to clients in the home therapeutic exercise programs that they routinely prescribe.

Since lower extremity health is vital to locomotion, general health, quality of life, and functional independence, we will present four knee joint injury cases and discuss how the concepts we present might influence each client.

The first client is an 81-year-old man with severe degenerative changes in the medial compartment of his left knee (Fig. 30-4a), while the lateral compartment is pristine (Fig. 30-4b). The second client is a 21-year-old man with a 2-year history of left knee ACL insufficiency and then failed ACL reconstructive surgery. At the time of initial consult he was 5 years status-post the index injury. His medial meniscus which is a secondary stabilizer to the ACL in controlling compressive, translational, and rotational knee joint loads is now degenerated to the point of being dysfunctional, requiring meniscal transplantation in addition to double bundle ACL reconstruction (Fig. 30-5). The third client is a 19-year-old woman who runs for a small college cross country team. She was an all state runner in high school and never sustained an injury. When she increased her training mileage as a college runner she began to experience right knee pain. With the exception of a tripartite patella (Fig. 30-6), which is a normal variant from birth, radiographs and clinical examination revealed no other signs of skeletal abnormality. Approximately 6 months following initial examination and conservative treatment failure she underwent partial patellar excision. Seven months postsurgery she still has not been able to return to competitive running.

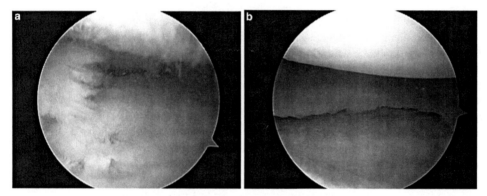

Fig. 30-4. a. Arthroscopic view of severe left knee medial compartment degeneration. b. Arthroscopic view of a healthy appearing left knee lateral compartment

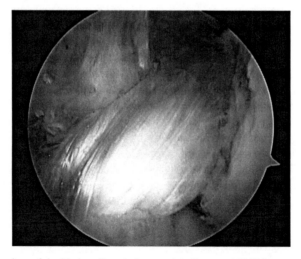

Fig. 30-5. Arthroscopic view of double bundle anterior cruciate ligament (ACL) reconstruction

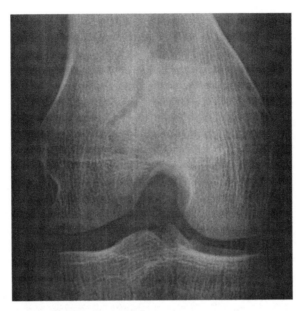

Fig. 30-6. Radiographic evidence of a tripartite patella at the right knee

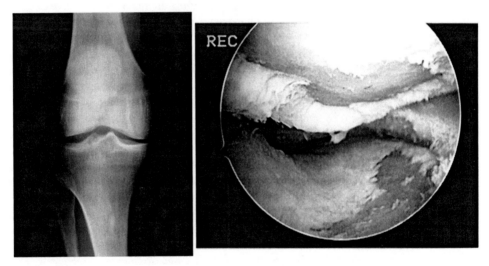

Fig. 30-7. a. Radiograph suggests minimal right knee medial compartment degeneration. b. Arthroscopic evaluation reveals severe right knee medial compartment degeneration

The fourth client is a 65-year-old man with minimal radiographic evidence of right knee medial compartment degenerative changes (Fig. 30-7a). Arthroscopic evaluation however revealed severe articular cartilage degeneration at the medial femoral condyle (Fig. 30-7b).

The medial knee joint compartment is the primary site of weight bearing, while the lateral compartment serves a greater transverse plane rotational function. While the first client certainly would qualify for undergoing medial unicompartmental knee arthroplasty, given his age, it is conceivable that he might decide to forego surgery with the understanding that certain weight-bearing activities should be restricted, and that aquatic therapy intervention might provide an excellent substitute for cardiovascular and pulmonary system fitness as well as active knee joint mobility exercises. Conceivably specific behavioral changes including orthosis use, and appropriate activity modification as knee symptoms dictate may enable a reasonable level of functional independence. Knee joint injection with hyaluronic acid (Caborn et al. 2004) and glucosamine or glucosamine-chondroitin sulfate supplementation (Gregory et al. 2008) may also help alleviate symptoms.

The second client provides an excellent example of how continued stresses applied to a knee that is functionally unstable leads to further damage. The index injury in combination with a poorly positioned ACL graft led to continued instability that led to medial meniscus degeneration. The combination of double bundle ACL reconstruction (Caborn and Chang 2005) and medial meniscal allograft transplantation (Rueff et al. 2006) largely restored knee stability; however, as mentioned earlier the index injury and all ensuing injuries and surgical interventions have contributed to the lower extremity "trauma" that has accumulated over time. Even though this client is only 21 years of age, he also should consider behavior modifications including less frequent impact loading, activities that focus on restoring dynamic knee joint stability, and limited or non–weight-bearing aerobic exercise via cycling, walking, or aquatic therapy interventions.

The third client represents an interesting dilemma. Prior to increasing running mileage she never experienced any knee pain over her four years of running in high school, despite having a tripartite patella. This case demonstrates how in many cases what is observed on radiographs or other diagnostic imaging tests does not carry nearly the same weight of evidence as the pain and other symptoms, or lack thereof that the client has experienced. Diagnostic imaging tests serve their greatest value in confirming or ruling out what the treating physician has identified as potentially being the factor or factors that contribute to joint dysfunction via a comprehensive clinical examination. In this client's case the decision was made to excise part of the patella. This surgical procedure in combination with postoperative rehabilitation and a gradual return to running progression should have been successful. However at 7 months postsurgery she was still experiencing the same knee pain when attempting to run. What other factors may have contributed to this outcome? Does she have a more external health locus of control? Did she experience a late growth spurt between her senior year of high school and freshman year of college that changed her lower extremity alignment in such as way that the previously latent tripartite patella now became a source of irritation? Had she never exceeded her envelope of function until her training mileage increased as a college runner? Did she continue to use a worn out pair of running shoes for too long? Was she having second thoughts about continuing competitive running and was looking for a justifiable reason to drop out and move on to other things? We do not know the answer to any of these questions. However, the possibility of different psychobehavioral issues is compelling. Had she not been a competitive runner, it is unlikely that she would have ever started to experience any symptoms despite having an obvious radiographic abnormality. At this point in time, having undergone surgery, she is not able to run even recreationally. What role does running truly play in her quality of life values? Activities with reduced impact loads such as a walk–jog interval progression, cycling, aquatic therapy, or similar reduced weight-bearing activities may be useful as substitutes to augment aerobic fitness while eliminating potentially injurious joint loads. Over time she may be able to return to recreational running with reduced pace, mileage, and frequency.

The fourth client confirms the importance of symptoms and comprehensive clinical knee joint examination. Radiographs of his right knee revealed only minimal evidence of osteoarthritis with some sclerotic changes near the tibial surface of the medial joint compartment. Changes observed on radiographs did not correlate with the pain, effusion, and joint warmth symptoms that the client was experiencing after activity. Arthroscopic evaluation revealed severe (grade IV) articular cartilage damage at the medial femoral condyle. Had he continued his prolonged nonsteroidal anti-inflammatory medication use, he could reduce symptom effects; however, degenerative changes would progress more leading to even more advanced osteoarthritis at a young age. Additional prolonged use of oral nonsteroidal anti-inflammatory medication would also have long-term detrimental effects to liver and gastrointestinal system. Surgical intervention was performed using a micro-fracture technique to induce type III collagen deposition at the injury site. Postsurgery the client limited weight bearing for 8–12 weeks in association with progressive physical therapy. For this intervention to be effective however long-term changes are needed in general health, activity, and exercise behaviors. Reduced body weight, healthy eating habits, cessation of smoking, determining and then regularly complying with functional fitness activities that stay well within his new envelope of function are essential. Additionally, he and the other clients should be instructed how to palpate key knee joint structures and how to interpret the functional significance of tenderness, pain, effusion, or warmth. Although hip and knee arthroplasty techniques (Mason 2008) have improved dramatically over recent years and client postoperative function may include participation in sports such as cycling, golf, tennis, and occasionally jogging and skiing, conserving one's own biological tissue for as long as possible prior to undergoing any arthroplasty procedure is highly advantageous.

Like many things in life taking a simple, basic approach often works best. Howard Baker is a 91-year old man who has always eaten food grown from his garden. After returning from World War II, during which he served in the Marine Corp, he spent a large part of his life working for the State of Kentucky as a Forest Ranger, in addition to being an avid sportsman. He lives in a house that does not have air conditioning, he regularly attends Sunday school, he never drank alcoholic beverages, and he only smoked cigarettes for a brief part of his life. Howard's wife passed away when he was 56 years of age leaving him and his 73-year-old mother to raise three children and eventually put all the three through college. Over the course of his life, he has undergone coronary bypass surgery, experienced a torn rotator cuff at his left shoulder, and suffered a stroke. Howard continues to live independently, tends to his garden, drives to Sunday school, and engages in most all activities that he values. He has never had a weight problem, he has never belonged to a health club, and he has never followed a fad diet or exercise program (Fig. 30-8).

Perhaps we as a society need to better determine how many innovative technological advances truly impact our lives. With proper reflection we will be better prepared to truly capture that part of these technological advances that improve our lives rather than substitute for and often replace simple "low tech" tools and physical tasks that are of equal or greater value. We need to make

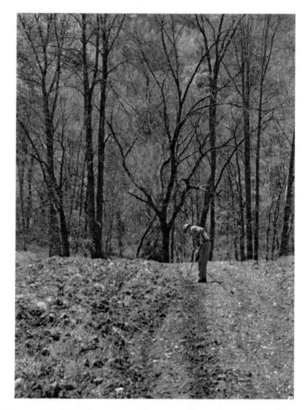

Fig. 30-8. Howard Baker of rural southeastern Kentucky tending his garden at 91 years of age

better decisions regarding technological advances to truly harvest the specific characteristic of the technology that we want while not damaging or marginalizing other more positive health behaviors. When we effectively blend innovative technological advances with high-quality real-life experiences, rather than as a virtual or "fantasy" substitute for real-life experiences, clients will more effectively reap significant health benefits.

References

American College of Sports Medicine Position Stand. (1998). Exercise and physical activity for older adults. *Medicine and Science in Sports and Exercise, 30*(6), 992–1008.

Andriacchi, T. P., Hurwitz, D. E., Bush-Joseph, C. A., & Bach, B. R. (2000). Functional adaptations in patients with ACL-deficient knees. In S. M. Lephart & F. H. Fu (Eds.), *Proprioception and neuromuscular control in joint stability* (pp. 181–188). Champaign, IL: Human Kinetics.

Architectural Graphic Standards. (2000). *Architect's handbook of professional practice* (13th ed.). New York: John Wiley & Sons.

Barra, J., Bray, A., Sahni, V., Golding, J. F., & Gresty, M. A. (2006). Increasing cognitive load with increasing balance challenge: Recipe for catastrophe. *Experimental Brain Research, 174*(4), 734–745.

Bijlsma, J. W., & Knahr, K. (2007). Strategies for the prevention and management of osteoarthritis of the hip and knee. *Best Practice and Research Clinical Rheumatology, 21*(1), 59–76.

Brody, E. B. (2002). Mental health. In C. E. Koop, C. E. Pearson & M. R. Schwarz (Eds.), *Critical issues in global health* (pp. 127–134). San Francisco: Jossey-Bass.

Caborn, D. N., & Chang, H. C. (2005). Single femoral socket double-bundle anterior cruciate ligament reconstruction using tibialis anterior tendon: description of a new technique. *Arthroscopy, 21*(10), 1273e1–1273e8.

Caborn, D., Rush, J., Lanzer, W., Parenti, D., Murray, C., & Synvisc 901 Study Group. (2004). A randomized, single-blind comparison of the efficacy and tolerability of hylan G-F 20 and triamcinolone hexacetonide in patients with osteoarthritis of the knee. *Journal of Rheumatology, 31*(2), 333–343.

Campbell, B. J. (2008). Osteoporosis: The basics and case-based advanced treatment update from the orthopaedic surgeon. *Instructional Course Lectures, 57*, 595–636.

Candow, D. G. (2008). The impact of nutritional and exercise strategies for aging bone and muscle. *Applied Physiology, Nutrition, and Metabolism, 33*(1), 181–183.

Center for Disease Control. (2008). Healthy aging: Preventing disease and improving quality of life among older Americans at a glance. http://www.cdc.gov/, Retrieved from the worldwide web April 12, 2008.

Chin, G. K. W., Van Niel, K. P., Giles-Corti, B., & Knuiman, M. (2008). Accessibility and connectivity in physical activity studies: The impact of missing pedestrian data. *Preventive Medicine, 46*, 41–45.

De Groot, P. C. E., Bleeker, M. W. P., & Hopman, M. T. E. (2006). Magnitude and time course of arterial vascular adaptations to inactivity in humans. *Exercise and Sport Sciences Reviews, 34*, 65–71.

Deley, G., Kervio, G., Van Hoecke, J., Verges, B., Grassi, B., & Casillas, J. M. (2007). Effects of one-year exercise training program in adults over 70 years old: A study with a control group. *Aging Clinical and Experimental Research, 19*(4), 310–315.

Dorr, L. D., & Chao, L. (2007). The emotional state of the patient after total hip and knee arthroplasty. *Clinical Orthopaedics and Related Research, 463*, 7–12.

Dye, S. F. (1996). The knee as a biological transmission with an envelope of function: A theory. *Clinical Orthopaedics and Related Research, 325*, 10–18.

Garcia-Castellano, J. M., Diaz-Herrera, P., & Morcuende, J. A. (2000). Is bone a target-tissue for he nervous system? New advances on the understanding of their interactions. *Iowa Orthopaedic Journal, 20*, 49–58.

Gerber, J. P., Marcus, R. L., Dibble, L. E., Greis, P. E., Burks, R. T., & LaStayo, P. C. (2007). Safety, feasibility, and efficacy of negative work exercise via eccentric muscle activity following anterior cruciate ligament reconstruction. *Journal of Orthopaedic and Sports Physical Therapy, 37*(1), 10–18.

Gifford, L. (1998). Pain. In J. Pitt-Brooke, H. Reid, J. Lockwood & K. Kerr (Eds.), *Rehabilitation of movement: Theoretical basis of clinical practice* (pp. 196–232). London: W.B. Saunders.

Gregory, P. J., Sperry, M., & Wilson, A. F. (2008). Dietary supplements for osteoarthritis. *American Family Physician, 77*(2), 177–184.

Hanna, F., Teichtahl, A. J., Bell, R., Davis, S. R., Wluka, A. E., O'Sullivan, R., et al. (2007). The cross-sectional relationship between fortnightly exercise and knee cartilage properties in healthy adult women in midlife. *Menopause, 14*(5), 830–834.

Hebert, G. (2008). Biography. http://en.wikipedia.org/wiki/Georges_H%C3%A9bert. Retrieved from the worldwide web on April 30, 2008.

Heinrich, K. M., Jitnarin, N., Suminski, R. R., Berkel, L., Hunter, C. M., Alvarez, L., et al. (2008). Obesity classification in military personnel: A comparison of body fat, waist circumference, and body mass index measurements. *Military Medicine, 173*(1), 67–73.

Hinman, R. S., Heywood, S. E., & Day, A. R. (2007). Aquatic physical therapy for hip and knee osteoarthritis: Results of a single-blind randomized controlled trial. *Physical Therapy, 87*(1), 32–43.

Hodges, P. W., Cresswell, A. G., Daggfeldt, K., & Thorstensson, A. (2000). Three dimensional preparatory trunk motion precedes asymmetrical upper limb movement. *Gait Posture, 11*(2), 92–101.

Jackson, R. D., & Shidham, S. (2007). The role of hormone therapy and calcium plus vitamin D for reduction of bone loss and risk for fractures: Lessons learned from the Women's Health Initiative. *Current Osteoporosis Reports, 5*(4), 153–159.

Johnston, A. P., De Lisio, M., & Parise, G. (2008). Resistance training, sarcopenia, and the mitochondrial theory of aging. *Applied Physiology, Nutrition, and Metabolism, 33*(1), 191–199.

Jones, K. B., Mollano, A. V., Morcuende, J. A., Cooper, R. R., & Saltzman, C. L. (2004). Bone and brain: A review of neural, hormonal, and musculoskeletal connections. *Iowa Orthopaedic Journal, 24*, 123–132.

Kempermann, G., van Praag, H., & Gage, F. H. (2000). Activity-dependent regulation of neuronal plasticity and self repair. *Progress in Brain Research, 127*, 35–48.

Koster, A., Leitzmann, M. F., Schatzkin, A., Mouw, T., Adams, K. F., van Eijk, J. T., et al. (2008a). Waist circumference and mortality. *American Journal of Epidemiology, 167*, 1465–1475.

Koster, A., Patel, K. V., Visser, M., van Eijk, J. T., Kanaya, A. M., de Rekeneire, N., et al. (2008b). Joint effects of adiposity and physical activity on incident mobility limitation in older adults. *Journal of the American Geriatric Society, 56*(4), 636–643.

Krasnoff, J., & Painter, P. (1999). The physiological consequences of bed rest and inactivity. *Advances in Renal Replacement Therapy, 6*(2), 124–132.

Lane, J.M. (2008). *Stem cell research in orthopaedics.* Presented at University of Louisville Department of Orthopaedic Surgery Grand Rounds, April 15, 2008.

Lanyon, L. E. (1992). Control of bone architecture by functional load bearing. *Journal of Bone and Mineral Research, 7*, S369–S375.

LaStayo, P. C., Ewy, G. A., Pierotti, D. D., Johns, R. K., & Lindstedt, S. (2003). The positive effects of negative work: increased muscle strength and decreased fall risk in a frail elderly population. *The Journals of Gerontology Series A: Biological Sciences and Medical Sciences, 58*, 419–424.

LaStayo, P., McDonagh, P., Lipovic, D., Napoles, P., Bartholomew, A., Esser, K., et al. (2007). Elderly patients and high force resistance exercise – a descriptive report: Can an anabolic, muscle growth response occur without muscle damage or inflammation. *Journal of Geriatric Physical Therapy, 30*, 128–134.

Layne, J. E., & Nelson, M. E. (1999). The effects of progressive resistance training on bone density: A review. *Medicine and Science in Sports and Exercise, 31*, 25–30.

Leppala, J., Kannus, P., Natri, A., Pasanen, M., Sievanen, H., Vuori, I., et al. (1999). Effect of anterior cruciate ligament injury of the knee on bone mineral density of the spine and affected lower extremity: A prospective one-year follow-up study. *Calcified Tissue International, 64*, 357–363.

Lewis, P. B., McCarty, L. P., Kang, R. W., & Cole, B. J. (2006). Basic science and treatment options for articular cartilage injuries. *Journal of Orthopaedic and Sports Physical Therapy, 36*(10), 717–727.

Livneh, H., & Antonak, R. F. (1997). *Psychosocial adaptation to chronic illness and disability.* Gaithersburg, MD: Aspen Publishers Inc.

Lorenzo, C., Serrano-Rios, M., Martinez-Larrad, M. T., Gonzalez-Villalpando, C., Williams, K., Gabriel, R., et al. (2007). Which obesity index best explains prevalence differences in type 2 diabetes mellitus? *Obesity (Silver Spring), 15*(5), 1294–1301.

Mahomed, N. N., Liang, M. H., Cook, E. F., Daltroy, L. H., Fortin, P. R., Fossel, A. H., et al. (2002). The importance of patient expectations in predicting functional outcomes after total joint arthroplasty. *Journal of Rheumatology, 29*(6), 1273–1279.

Maly, M. R., Costigan, P. A., & Olney, S. J. (2005). Contribution of psychosocial and mechanical variables to physical performance measures in knee osteoarthritis. *Physical Therapy, 85*, 1318–1328.

Maly, M. R., Costigan, P. A., & Olney, S. J. (2007). Self-efficacy mediates walking performance in older adults with knee osteoarthritis. *The Journals of Gerontology Series A, Biological Sciences and Medical Sciences, 62*(10), 1142–1146.

Mancuso, C. A., Sculco, T. P., Wickiewicz, T. L., Jones, E. C., Robbins, L., Warren, R. F., et al. (2001). Patients' expectations of knee surgery. *Journal of Bone and Joint Surgery, 83A*(7), 1005–1012.

Marks, J. S., & McQueen, D. V. (2002). Chronic disease. In C. E. Koop, C. E. Pearson & M. R. Schwarz (Eds.), *Critical issues in global health* (pp. 117–126). San Francisco: Jossey-Bass.

Mason, J. B. (2008). The new demands by patients in the modern era of total joint arthroplasty: A point of view. *Clinical Orthpaedics and Related Research, 466*(1), 146–152.

Meisami, E. (1992). Aging of the sensory systems. In P. S. Timiras (Ed.), *Physiological basis of aging and geriatrics* (2nd ed., pp. 115–132). London: CRC Press Inc.

Miller, T. W., Nyland, J., & Wormal, W. (2006). Therapeutic exercise program design considerations: Putting it all together. In J. Nyland (Ed.), *Clinical decisions in therapeutic exercise: Planning and implementation* (Upper Saddle River, pp. 451–500). Prentice Hall: NJ.

Morris, M. E. (2000). Movement disorders in people with Parkinson disease: A model for physical therapy. *Physical Therapy, 80*, 578–597.

Mueller, M. J., & Maluf, K. S. (2002). Tissue adaptation to physical stress: a proposed "Physical Stress Theory" to guide physical therapist practice, education, and research. *Physical Therapy, 82*, 383–403.

National Football League Combine. http://www.nfl.com/combine , Retrieved from the worldwide web on April 30, 2008.

Nieman, D. (1994). Exercise, upper respiratory tract infection, and the immune system. *Medicine and Science in Sports and Exercise, 26*, 128–139.

Nyland, J. (2007). *What is functional fitness and how does it affect joint preservation?* Presented at: Functional fitness and the science of joint preservation. University of Louisville School of Medicine, Louisville, KY, April 27, 2007.

Nyland, J., Cottrell, B., Harreld, K., & Caborn, D. N. (2006). Self-reported outcomes after anterior cruciate ligament reconstruction: an internal health locus of control score comparison. *Arthroscopy, 22*(11), 1225–1232.

Nyland, J., Johnson, D. L., Caborn, D. N., & Brindle, T. (2002). Internal health status belief and lower perceived functional deficit are related among anterior cruciate ligament-deficient patients. *Arthroscopy, 18*(5), 515–518.

Nyland, J., Lachman, N., Kocabey, Y., Brosky, J., Altun, R., & Caborn, D. (2005). Anatomy, function, and rehabilitation of the popliteus musculotendinous complex. *Journal of Orthopaedic and Sports Physical Therapy, 35*, 165–179.

Nyland, J., & Shapiro, R (2002). Development of a closed kinetic chain training device for the hip rotators. In: *Proceedings of the 49th Annual Meeting of the American College of Sports Medicine*, St. Louis, MO.

O'Keefe, J. H., Bybee, K. A., & Lavie, C. J. (2007). Alcohol and cardiovascular health: The razor-sharp double-edged sword. *Journal of the American College of Cardiology, 50*(11), 1009–1014.

Ostbye, T., Dement, J. M., & Krause, K. M. (2007). Obesity and workers' compensation: Results from the Duke Health and Safety Surveillance System. *Archives of Internal Medicine, 167*, 766–773.

Peters, J. C. (2006). Obesity prevention and social change: What will it take? *Exercise and Sport Sciences Reviews, 34*, 4–9.

Physical Therapist Guide to Practice. (2000). Alexandria, VA, American Physical Therapy Association.

Prochaska, J. O., Norcross, J. C., & Diclemente, C. C. (1994). *Changing for the good.* New York: HarperCollins.

Reiman, M. P., Rogers, M. E., & Manske, R. C. (2006). Interlimb differences in lower extremity bone mineral density following anterior cruciate ligament reconstruction. *Journal of Orthopaedic and Sports Physical Therapy, 36*(11), 837–844.

Riggs, B. L., & Melton, L. J. I. I. I. (1983). Evidence for two distinct syndromes of envolutional osteoporosis. *American Journal of Sports Medicine, 75,* 899–901.

Ross, R., & Huttlinger, K. (2006). Health promotion in the twenty-first century: Throughout the life span and throughout the world. In C. L. Edelman & C. L. Mandle (Eds.), *Health promotion throughout the lifespan. Chap. 25* (pp. 601–617). St.Louis: Elsevier Mosby.

Rubin, C., Gross, T., Qin, Y. X., Fritton, S., Guilak, F., & McLeod, K. (1996). Differentiation of the bone-tissue remodeling response to axial and torsional loading in the turkey ulna. *Journal of Bone and Joint Surgery, 78A,* 1523–1533.

Rueff, D., Nyland, J., Kocabey, Y., Chang, H. C., & Caborn, D. N. (2006). Self-reported patient outcomes at a minimum of 5 years after allograft anterior cruciate ligament reconstruction with or without medial meniscus transplantation: an age-, sex-, and activity level-matched comparison in patients aged approximately 50 years. *Arthroscopy, 22*(10), 1053–1062.

Sanches, F.M., Avesani, C.M., Kamimura, M.A., Lemos, M.M., Axelsson, J., Vasselai, P., et al. (2008). Waist circumference and visceral fat in CKD: A cross-sectional study. *American Journal of Kidney Disease, 52*(1), 66–73.

Shumway-Cook, A., & Woollacott, M. (1995). *Motor control theory and practical applications.* Baltimore: Williams & Wilkins.

Sparling, P. B., Snow, T. K., Rosskopf, L. B., O'Donnell, E. M., Freedson, P. S., & Byrnes, W. C. (1998). Bone mineral density and body composition of the United States Olympic women's field hockey team. *British Journal of Sports Medicine, 32,* 315–318.

Sparrow, J. (2001). Overuse injuries in gymnastics. In N. Maffulli, K. M. Chan, R. Macdonald, R. M. Malina & A. W. Parker (Eds.), *Sports medicine for specific ages and abilities* (pp. 119–130). Edinburgh: Churchill Livingstone.

Suetta, C., Andersen, J.L., Dalgas, U., Berget, J., Koskinen, S.O., Aagaard, P., et al. (2008). Resistance training induces qualitative changes in muscle morphology, muscle architecture and muscle function in elderly postoperative patients. *Journal of Applied Physiology, 105*(1), 180–186.

Thomee, P., Wahrborg, P., Borjesson, M., Thomee, R., Eriksson, B. I., & Karlsson, J. (2008). Self-efficacy of knee function as a pre-operative predictor of outcome 1 year after anterior cruciate ligament reconstruction. *Knee Surgery Sports Traumatology Arthroscopy, 16*(2), 118–127.

Thompson, L. V. (2002). Skeletal muscle adaptations with age, inactivity, and therapeutic exercise. *Journal of Orthopaedic and Sports Physical Therapy, 32,* 44–57.

United States Department of Health and Human Services. (2000). *Healthy people 2010 [Conference Edition].* Washington, DC: US Government Printing Office.

Van Houten, R., Ellis, R., & Kim, J.L. (2007). Effects of various minimum green times on percentage of pedestrians waiting for midblock "walk" signal. *Transportation Research Record,* ISSN: 0361-1981, pp 78–83.

van Praag, H. (2008). Neurogenesis and exercise: Past and future directions. *Neuromolecular Medicine,* [epub ahead of print].

van Praag, H., Kempermann, G., & Gage, F. H. (2000). Neural consequences of environmental enrichment. *Nature Reviews Neuroscience, 1,* 191–198.

Vleeming, A., Pool-Goudzwaard, A. L., Stoeckart, R., van Wingerden, J. P., & Snijders, C. J. (1995). The posterior layer of the thoracolumbar fascia. Its function in load transfer from spine to legs. *Spine, 20*(7), 753–758.

Wolf, S. L., Barnhart, H. X., Kutner, N. G., McNeely, E., Coogler, C., Xu, T., et al. (2003). Reducing frailty and falls in older persons: An investigation of tai chi and computerized balance training. *Journal of the American Geriatric Society, 51*(12), 1794–1803.

Woo, S. L.-Y., Hollis, J. M., Adams, D. J., Lyon, R. M., & Takai, S. (1991). Tensile properties of the human femur-anterior cruciate ligament-tibia complex. The effects of specimen age and orientation. *American Journal of Sports Medicine, 19,* 217–225.

World Health Organization Website. http://www.who.int/nutrition/topics/5_population_
nutrient/en/index5.html, Retrieved from the worldwide web on April 29, 2008.

Zazulak, B. T., Hewett, T. E., Reeves, N. P., Goldberg, B., & Cholewicki, J. (2007a).
Deficits in neuromuscular control of the trunk predict knee injury risk. *American
Journal of Sports Medicine, 35*(7), 1123–1130.

Zazulak, B. T., Hewett, T. E., Reeves, N. P., Goldberg, B., & Cholewicki, J. (2007b).
(2007) The effects of core proprioception on knee injury. A prospective biomechan-
ical-epidemiological study. *American Journal of Sports Medicine, 35*(3), 368–373.

Chapter 31

Nutrition Through the Life Span: Needs and Health Concerns in Critical Periods

Jasminka Z. Ilich and Rhonda A. Brownbill

Introduction

The focus of this chapter is to discuss the nutritional requirements of individuals in different periods of life, spanning from infancy and childhood to old age. We start with the pregnancy and maternal nutritional needs, which ultimately determine fetal growth and development. We continue by addressing the main issues in infancy, childhood, and adolescence, focusing on the critical nutrients in each period, dietary patterns and behaviors, and most common disorders associated with food intake in those periods. Adult period focuses on the balanced nutrition and lifestyle conducive to disease prevention and maintenance of healthy state. The section on older adults addresses some of the most critical nutrients for that period, as well as some chronic conditions and the ways to avoid or alleviate them.

Fetal and Maternal Nutrition

Nutritional Needs During Pregnancy

Pregnancy is a period demanding energy and most of the nutrients. The total energy cost of pregnancy is about 80,000 kcal, which breaks down to approximately a need for 2,500 kcal/day for an average woman in the second and third trimester of pregnancy, or 200–500 extra kcal/day, depending on her activity level. Most healthy women of normal weight should gain about 11–16 kg during pregnancy. Less than half of the weight gain is due to the weight of the fetus, placenta, and amniotic fluid, with the remainder of the weight from maternal reproductive tissues, fluid, blood, and stored body fat. Underweight women are advised to gain slightly more, 13–18 kg, and overweight women slightly less, 7–11 kg. Excessive weight gain is linked to greater risk for the development of hypertension and the need for a cesarean delivery.

During pregnancy, the current recommendations noted in the Dietary Reference Intake (DRI) for energy are 340 additional kcal during the second trimester and 452 additional kcal during the third trimester with

From: *Handbook of Stressful Transitions Across the Lifespan,*
Edited by: T.W. Miller, DOI 10.1007/978-1-4419-0748-6_31,
© Springer Science+Business Media, LLC 2010

~130 g carbohydrate/day, and ~1.1 g protein/kg body weight a day (2002). The requirement for fat is the same as for nonpregnant women and that is 20–35% of total energy intake (2002). Several nutrients are of particular concern during pregnancy. Folic acid is necessary for preventing neural tube defects and is an important nutrient involved in cell division. The current DRI for folate during pregnancy is 600 µg/day (1998). It is recommended that 400 µg of folic acid from supplements should be consumed in addition to foods rich in folic acid (orange juice, leafy green vegetables) by all women capable of becoming pregnant (1998). During pregnancy, the need for iron almost doubles and ranges from 18 to 27 mg/day, due to a 50% increase in the mother's blood volume (2001). For the majority of women whose iron stores are insufficient, a daily supplement of 30 mg of iron is recommended during the second and third trimesters of pregnancy. The best food sources of iron are liver and red meat, and good sources include fortified breads and cereals (due to iron fortification of grains), and dried fruit

During pregnancy, an adequate supply of long-chain polyunsaturated fatty acids, especially docosahexaenoic acid (DHA), is necessary for the fetal brain growth and visual development. A recent research shows that mothers with higher blood levels of DHA have infants born with more mature patterns of sleep and wake states, which indicate more mature central nervous systems (Cheruku et al. 2002). The International Society for the Study of Fatty Acids and Lipids recommends that pregnant women consume 300 mg/day of DHA (Simopoulos et al. 1999). Good sources of DHA include flax seeds, eggs, and fatty fish (salmon, anchovies, tuna, sardines). However, in consuming the latter, one needs to be aware of the potential contamination with heavy metals that can be detrimental to fetal development (see the following section).

Maternal Malnutrition

In the first trimester "morning sickness", characterized by nausea and/or vomiting experienced at any time of the day, may make it difficult for the expectant mother to consume a well-balanced diet. It is not quite elucidated what causes morning sickness, although at least partially, it is thought to be related to the changes in maternal hormones. Eating small frequent meals and consuming beverages between meals, may help to alleviate nausea. A reduced nutritional intake in early pregnancy is unlikely to affect the growth of the embryo, since its nutritional needs are small, although severe malnutrition could have adverse affects on the embryo. Malnutrition after the third month of pregnancy could interfere with fetal growth. In the last trimester of pregnancy, even a mild restriction in caloric and/or protein intake could negatively impact on the fetus, resulting in a low birth-weight baby, a small head circumference, poorly developed muscles, and/or reduced subcutaneous fat.

Food to Limit or Avoid

There are several foods that need to be either avoided or limited during pregnancy to prevent damage to the fetus. These include certain types of fish, meat and cheeses, artificial sweeteners, and trans fatty acids.

Fish contaminated with high levels of mercury (swordfish, shark, tile-fish, and king mackerel) should be avoided by pregnant women to prevent damage to the developing fetal nervous system. All types of fish may contain at least trace levels of mercury, so it is recommended that pregnant and lactating women limit their overall fish consumption to no more than 360 g per week. Paradoxically, fish is the best source of docosahexaenoic acid (DHA) as well as protein, and therefore, it is recommended in pregnancy. However, choosing the fish devoid of contaminants might be a challenge in the modern world.

Pregnant women should not eat undercooked meat, fish, eggs, or soft cheeses to avoid possible bacterial contamination. Caution should also be taken in consuming deli meats, since they may contain bacteria (listeria) that can cause food poisoning. To minimize this risk, it is best to cook deli meats before consuming them. Liver (although needed for iron) should be consumed in moderation, since it contains high levels of vitamin A, which is linked to birth defects (Rothman et al. 1995). Women who are, or might become, pregnant are advised to avoid consuming vitamin supplements containing more than 8,000 IU of vitamin A.

Artificial sweeteners such as aspartame (Nutra Sweet), saccharin, acesulfame-K (Sunett), and sucralose (Splenda) have not been shown to cause birth defects. Aspartame does not readily cross the placenta though it is not known what effect the heavy aspartame use may have on the fetus or even less so on possibility of the brain tumors in mothers. Therefore, it is recommended that "diet" drinks with aspartame could be consumed in moderation (about two cans diet soda a day) during pregnancy. Saccharin should also be consumed in moderation since it crosses the placenta into the fetus' bloodstream and it has been linked to bladder cancer in rats. The Food and Drug Administration considers sucralose to be safe for all populations, including pregnant and lactating women since it does not pass the placenta and does not accumulate in the body.

Consumption of trans polyunsaturated fatty acids, found in foods containing partially hydrogenated oils, is not recommended in pregnancy. Studies showed that the presence of trans fats in cord tissue is associated with reduced birth weights and smaller head circumference (Hornstra 2000). In general, individuals, whether pregnant or not, should choose foods that are made with vegetable oils or butter rather than shortening or margarine which contains trans fatty acids.

Caffeine, Alcohol, Drug-abuse, Smoking

The consumption of caffeine and alcohol during pregnancy has been well studied, however, due to inconsistent results, the threshold for the harmful amount of caffeine and alcohol on fetus is still unknown. Research suggests a high intake of caffeine (>900 mg/day – 2 dL of coffee contains ~103 mg caffeine) prior to pregnancy is associated with an increased risk of spontaneous abortion (Nehlig and Debry 1994), while intakes greater or equal to 300 mg/ day during the first trimester might increase the risk of spontaneous abortion (Tolstrup et al. 2003). In rats, maternal exposure to caffeine was shown to have long-term deleterious consequences on sleep, locomotion, learning abilities, and anxiety in the offspring (Wen et al. 2001). In humans, more studies are needed to determine long-term effects of caffeine ingestion during pregnancy on offsprings. Moderate caffeine intake during the second and third trimesters of pregnancy does not appear to be harmful to the human fetus when intake is spread throughout the day, though caffeine potentates the teratogenic effect of other substances such as tobacco and alcohol (Wen et al. 2001).

A low-to-moderate alcohol intake prior to pregnancy (1–13 drinks/week) does not appear to influence risk of miscarriage (Nehlig and Debry 1994), though excessive alcohol consumption during pregnancy is linked to the development of the fetal alcohol syndrome (FAS). FAS is characterized by anomalies of the eyes, nose, heart, and central nervous system that are accompanied by growth retardation, small head circumference, and mental retardation. FAS infants have poor rates of weight gain and are characterized with failure to thrive. Even moderate alcohol consumption may lead to "fetal alcohol effects" or infants showing more subtle features of FAS. Moderate drinkers also have higher rates of spontaneous abortion and low birth weights. Cigarette smoking is also linked to low birth weights, due to the effects of carbon monoxide and nicotine on placental perfusion and oxygen transport to the developing fetus.

Most of the illegal drugs also cross the placenta. Marijuana use during pregnancy may be linked to behavioral problems in the offspring. Cocaine use is linked to premature detachment of the placenta and premature birth, high blood pressure, and stillbirth. Drug use can also cause withdrawal and drug dependency in the newborn as well as growth retardation of the fetus. Drug use during the first trimester of pregnancy can cause severe birth defects, and damage the functioning of organ and central nervous systems in the second and third trimesters of pregnancy causing heart defects or mental retardation.

Infancy

Lactation

During the first few days after birth, a mother secretes colostrum or foremilk (2–10 ml per feeding), a thin yellowish liquid (due to high carotene content) rich in immune factors, protein, and minerals and lower in sugar and fat than mature milk. About a week after birth, a rapid increase in milk production occurs, though establishment of lactation may take several weeks. Adequate sucking stimulation from an infant or a breast pump is needed to maintain lactation. Mature breast milk at the start of a feeding session is lower in fat. At the end of a feeding session, the fat content in milk triples. The fatty acid composition of breast milk is very different from that of cow's milk. Breast milk contains more linoleic acid as well as the omega-3 fatty acids, DHA, and eicosapentanoic acid (EPA) that both seem to be involved in central nervous system development of infant. The content of DHA and EPA in breast milk will vary considerably based on the mothers' diet. Milk production will gradually decrease after several months as the infant is introduced to either formula or solid foods, and demands less breast milk.

Other than the fat and vitamin content, the nutrient composition of breast milk is not adversely affected by the mother's diet unless severe malnutrition is present. Maternal malnutrition, however, can affect the content of immunologic substances (including immunogloblulins and host resistance factors) in breast milk. American Academy of Pediatrics recommends that infants be breast fed for at least one year. If breast milk is unavailable, formula should be used until the child reaches one year of age. After their first birthday, children can be given cow's milk. Cow's milk contains about 30% less carbohydrates compared to human milk and a higher level of several amino acids that could be detrimental to infant. Breast milk has a higher level of the amino acid taurine which is needed for bile acid conjugation. Breast milk is also higher in fat, supplying 50% of energy from fat. Cow's milk has much higher levels of calcium, phosphorous, and sodium making it difficult for an infant to digest. While the mineral content of breast milk is not dependent on the mother's mineral intake, the vitamin intake (especially water soluble vitamins) is highly dependent on the mother's diet. The iron in cow's milk is poorly absorbed compared to iron from breast milk. Infants can receive enough iron from breast milk until they are 5–6 months old, and then iron fortified foods such as rice or oat cereals need to be introduced into the diet to prevent anemia.

Almost all substances ingested by a lactating woman, including drugs, caffeine, alcohol, food allergens, pesticides, and environmental pollutants will enter the breast milk, though most will not pose risk to the infant if consumed in moderate amounts. Overall, about 1–2% of drugs taken by the mother will end up in the breast milk. Some drugs may be harmful to the infant such as sedatives, antidepressants, antibiotics, illegal drugs, alcohol, caffeine, and nicotine. Although less than 1% of caffeine ingested by the mother is transported to the milk, caffeine can accumulate in the infant over time leading to wakefulness and irritability (Institute of Medicine 1991). One to two caffeinated drinks per day consumed by mother appear safe for the infant (Institute of Medicine 1991). Alcohol, however, enters human milk in a similar concentration to that in the mother's blood. Large amounts of alcohol during lactation can result in the development of Cushing's syndrome which is characterized by large fat deposits on the face, neck, and trunk as well as delayed psychomotor development (Institute of Medicine 1991). Drugs that are safe for pregnancy are generally safe during lactation, though it is best to avoid taking long-acting drugs and to take the drug immediately after breastfeeding to minimize the dose given to the infant.

Nutritional Needs of a Lactating Mother

A lactating mother will require about 640 additional kcal a day to produce breast milk (Institute of Medicine 1991). During pregnancy most women gain an additional 2–5 kg of stored body fat, which can be mobilized to supply a portion (200–300 kcal/day) of the additional energy requirement for lactation. The current energy requirement (DRI) for lactating women is additional 330 kcal/day for the first 6 months, or additional 400 kcal/day for the second 6 months (2002), which allows for a gradual weight loss during lactation. A lactating woman also has increased needs for protein (71 g/day) and for omega-3 and omega-6 fatty acids.

Breastfeeding has many advantages for both the baby and mother. Breast milk is bacteria-safe, contains many different immunological factors, and is less allergenic than infant formula. Breastfeeding also facilitates proper jaw and tooth development and promotes mother–child bonding. Some women experience anxiety over whether they are producing enough milk for their infant, though this is rarely a problem since the milk supply will almost always meet the demand. During the first month of life the infant should gain about 1/3 to 1/2 pound a week, and have at least six wet diapers a day. It is recommended that infants be breastfed for 1 year, though in many parts of the world children are breast fed successfully for 2–3 years.

Formula Fed Infant

There are several types of infant formula on the market, including ready to use cans and bottles, and concentrated liquid and powder forms which can be mixed with water. Formulas could be cow's milk-based, soy-based, lactose free, hypoallergenic and thickened with rice starch for babies with reflux. Several companies now have formulas that contain fatty acids DHA and EPA for vision and mental development. Infants generally feed every 2–4 h with 75 ml of formula for every pound of body weight. Formula should provide the majority of energy to an infant until it reaches one year, and then cow's milk can be introduced. To prevent tooth decay or "nursing bottle syndrome", an infant should not be allowed to fall asleep with a bottle.

Introduction of Solid Foods

Solid foods should not be introduced until about 4–6 months or after 6 months if the infant is at risk of food allergies. Infants are ready for solid food when they can control their head, sit with support, move food from the front of their mouth to the back, and have doubled their birth weight. At first, only a few tablespoons of iron fortified rice or barley cereal should be given, with breast milk or formula supplying the majority of their nutritional needs. Pureed fruits, vegetables, and fruit juice should be subsequently introduced, with no more than one new food every three days (Butte et al. 2004). At about eight months, pureed meat should be introduced as well as the table food that can dissolve easily in the mouth such as teething biscuits, infant crackers and cookies, and cheerios. By 12 months the child can be given cow's milk, either whole or 2% and soft table foods cut in small pieces such as pasta, cheese, cooked vegetables, and soft fruits. Juice consumption should be limited to about 4–6 oz a day. In children with a strong family history of food allergies, cow's milk, wheat, soy, tree nuts, and fish should be avoided until well after their first birthday. Generally for most children, eggs should be avoided until age 2, and peanuts and shellfish until age 3 (Butte et al. 2004).

Between 12 and 24 months of age a child will slowly learn how to eat with utensils, though finger foods will often be preferred. Foods need to be in small enough pieces to prevent choking. Foods that are associated with choking and should be avoided include hot dogs, popcorn, hard candy, nuts, and whole grapes. Most toddlers will eat frequently throughout the day with an average of 5–7 times per day. A young child's likes and dislikes may change day to day. Introducing a child to a variety of flavors and textures during the first year of its life may increase its acceptance of a wider variety of foods in later childhood and may increase its readiness of trying new foods (Butte et al. 2004).

Childhood

Physical Growth and Nutrient Needs

After the first year, the rate of growth is slowed compared to infancy, with a weight gain of about 4–6 lbs per year. Children will gain about 3 inches of height per year between ages 1 and 8, and 2 inches per year until puberty. As a child gains weight, muscle mass will make up a greater percentage of its body weight. Between the ages of 1 and 3 the DRI for protein is 13 g/day, which increases to 19 g/day for children 4–8 year old (2002). The DRI for carbohydrates is 130 g/day for children of all ages, and fat should be 25–35% of total energy intake for children 4–18 years (2002). Intakes of all nutrients gradually increase as a child grows from a young toddler to an adolescent. A child ages 1–3 needs about 1–2 servings of dairy a day to meet the DRI for calcium of 500 mg/day, and a child ages 4–8 needs about 2–3 servings of dairy a day to meet the DRI for calcium of 800 mg/day (1997). Due to the fortification of many foods with B vitamins, vitamin C, iron, and zinc, it is unlikely that a child would be deficient in these nutrients as long as a variety of foods is consumed.

Factors Influencing Food Choices

Environmental influences that affect eating behavior include advertising, marketing, food prices, and food availability. The types of foods consumed by children are affected by a variety of factors. If both parents work, the family may be consuming mainly convenience and prepared foods. Fast food outlets are becoming increasingly available. School aged children receiving lunch from school may be receiving foods or meals that are high in fat, sugar, and sodium and/or low in fruits and vegetables. Schools differ in method of food delivery to children that is due to increasing costs of maintaining a school lunch programs and decreases in government involvement (St-Onge et al. 2003). A study in Maryland found 20% of fourth-grade students skipped breakfast and/or lunch at least 3 times per week (Gross et al. 2004). Skipping breakfast is associated with decreased nutrient intake, poor school performance, and increased behavioral problems (Gross et al. 2004).

Overweight

About 13–16% of children ages 6–11 are estimated to be overweight and an additional 14% are at risk of becoming overweight (St-Onge et al. 2003; Ogden et al. 2002), putting them at higher risk for developing hyperinsulinemia associated with adverse cardiovascular risk factors (Sullivan et al. 2004). Overweight children have higher blood pressure, fasting insulin, and cholesterol levels than normal-weight children (St-Onge et al. 2003). The high rates of obesity in children may be related to changes in food consumption patterns. In the past several decades, food consumed from restaurants and fast food outlets by children has tripled, and the prevalence of snacking has increased (St-Onge et al. 2003). Soft drink consumption by children has also increased, providing almost 200 calories a day (St-Onge et al. 2003), and leading to a decrease in milk intakes. As children age, fast food consumption is found to increase leading to a decrease intake of more nutritious foods.

Prevention of Nutritional and Health Problems in Children

Obesity

Parents have the ability to influence their child's energy consumption/expenditure through diet and exercise. Parents control what food is available and influence their children's acceptance of food. Parents need to create opportunities for physical activity for their children to increase their energy expenditure and they need to provide a healthy eating environment. Parents need to be role models for healthy eating and exercise habits. Children should never be forced to eat food, but rather have them determine when they are full. Food should never be used as rewards or as a way to discipline children. Parents need to prevent food from being linked to emotions, such as eating candy when happy or depressed or eating junk foods when feeling stressed. Parents need to learn how to respond to their children's hunger and satiety cues by offering snacks between meals or smaller frequent meals if necessary.

Heart Disease

Major risk factors associated with the development of arteriosclerosis and subsequent heart disease are obesity, family history, sedentary life style, and elevated blood pressure and serum lipids. Evidence suggests that the athero-sclerotic process begins in early childhood and is linked to eating a diet high in total fat, saturated fat, and cholesterol. It is recommended that starting at age 2 the diet should be less than 30% of total energy from fat, 10% of total energy from saturated fat, and cholesterol limited to 300 mg/day. After age 2, low fat or reduced fat milk instead of whole milk should be used unless the child is underweight. Children should have cholesterol screening if they have a family history of heart disease.

Cavities

Children of all ages suffer dental caries caused by plaque build-up. Different types of carbohydrates, most notably sucrose, contribute to plaque formation. Snacking at bedtime and snacking throughout the day on foods high in sucrose is associated with increased formation of dental caries due to the decrease in saliva flow. By two years of age children should be brushing their teeth with fluoride-containing toothpaste. If the child cannot spit out all the toothpaste, no more than a pea-sized amount at least twice a day should be used. Before age 2 a safe-to-swallow toddler toothpaste can be used. Parents should always help young children with brushing their teeth to insure all teeth are adequately brushed. Around age 3 children should have their first dentist appointment to assess their dental health.

Behavioral Problems

Attention-deficit hyperactivity disorder (ADHD) has been related to various nutritional factors including food additives such as artificial flavors, colors and preservatives, refined sugars, food sensitivities/allergies, and fatty acid deficiencies (Schnoll et al. 2003). Current evidence suggests that children with behavioral problems are sensitive to at least one food component that affects their behavior (Schnoll et al. 2003). Each child with ADHD should have a treatment plan that includes an individually tailored modified diet.

Adolescence

Physiological and Psychosocial Growth

During adolescence (age 8–17) a child will gain about 20% of adult height and 50% of adult weight, and most of the body organs will double in size. Girls generally grow in height earlier than boys, though boys will tend to have a faster rate of growth. This period of growth will be characterized by five stages of sexual maturation and changes in body composition. Females will gain about 10% more body fat than males. Once a female starts menstruation, the longitudinal growth slows down. During adolescence, males will gain twice as much muscle mass and more bone mass compared to females. Males, therefore, will have higher requirements than females for protein, iron, zinc, and calcium. Acne is seen in almost all adolescences during this stage of growth and is caused by changes in hormones and stress, but has not shown to be related to any nutritional factors.

In addition to changes in the body, the adolescents will also go through stages of emotional, social, and intellectual development. The adolescent will learn to develop ideas, use abstract thinking, and learn to organize. However, adolescents are heavily influenced by their peers, and strive to be like them or like cultural icons. The media often reinforce the image that the ideal person should be tall, slim, muscular, and like, which could lead adolescents to think they are inferior because they do not conform to the society's ideal images. Teenagers will see unrealistic figures in magazines, driving them to weight loss diets and/or excessive exercise as they try to reach the "ideal" figure.

Nutritional Needs

The current DRIs provide recommendations for males and females for two age groups during adolescence, 9–13 years and 14–18 years. The DRI for protein for a male during both these age periods is 56 g a day and for a female 46 g a day (2002). A healthy male between the ages of 9–13 years and weighing 79 lbs will require 2,279 kcal a day, and a male between the ages of 14–18 years and weighing 134 lbs will require 3,152 kcal a day (2002). A healthy female between the ages of 9–13 years and weighing 81 lbs will require 2,071 kcal a day, and a female between the ages of 14–18 years and weighing 119 lbs will require 2,368 kcal a day (2002). Fat should contribute 30% or less of total energy, with saturated fat contributing less than 10% of total energy and dietary cholesterol less than 300 mg a day. Most of the adult skeleton is accrued during the adolescent period. For maximum peak bone mass to be reached, males and females between the ages of 9–18 years both require 1,300 mg calcium a day and 200 IU of vitamin D a day (1997). Males and females both have high requirements for iron. Males and females 9–13 years require 8 mg of iron a day (2001). Males 14–18 years require 11 mg/day while females 14–18 years require 15 mg/day (2001). Males need additional iron during adolescence for build-up of muscle mass and females need additional iron to replenish lost stores during menstruation.

Eating Behavior

Many factors influence an adolescents eating behavior such as family, peers, television, magazines, their nutrition knowledge, food fads, and personal experiences with food. A common nutritional concern seen in adolescents is irregular meal patterns. Teenagers often miss breakfast or lunch either because of time constraints or as an effort to lose weight. Skipping meals often lead to over consumption of food in the evening and subsequent weight gain. As adolescents gain more independence they start to eat more meals away from the home which may not be nutritionally balanced especially if they are fast foods or snack foods.

Eating Disorders

The cause of eating disorders is probably related to a combination of factors including psychological, biological, family, genetic, environmental, and social. Stressful life events can trigger the onset of anorexia. According to the Center for Disease Control, 15% of adolescents are considered obese and over 30% are considered overweight. Anorexia is much less prevalent affecting less than 1% of adolescents and mainly females, though it can develop in males or females at any age. Ballet dancers and gymnasts have the highest prevalence of eating disorders, 2–22% (Ravaldi et al. 2003). Anorexia usually develops between the ages of 13 and 20. Patients with anorexia are subclassified into either a *restrictive type* in which the person loses weight through dieting, fasting, or excessive exercise or as *binge/purger* in which the person loses weight through self-induced vomiting or abuse of laxatives, diuretics, or enemas. Anorexia is diagnosed as a refusal to maintain body weight at the minimum for height or 15% below ideal body weight, fear of gaining weight, disturbance in body image, and absence of three consecutive menstrual cycles (Diagnostic and Statistical Manual of Mental Disorders 1994). A person with anorexia often is obsessed about food most of the day, and often only eats foods he or she considers "safe" such as fat-free and/or sugar-free foods. Nutritional problems include muscle wasting, osteoporosis, loss of fat stores, and dehydration. Treatment includes taking the focus off of food and dealing with psychological problems. Using cognitive behavior therapy is shown to be significantly more effective than nutritional counseling in improving outcome and preventing relapse (Pike et al. 2003). Diet therapy involves teaching proper eating habits and encouraging the intake of high protein, high complex carbohydrate, and low fat foods on a gradual basis.

Bulimia nervosa is more prevalent, affecting 2–4% of college females and is characterized by consumption of large amounts of food in a short period of time followed by purging either by self-induced vomiting or laxative abuse at least twice a week for three months (Diagnostic and Statistical Manual of Mental Disorders 1994). It is also characterized by a lack of control over the binges, and an over-concern with body image and weight. These individuals are usually either normal or slightly overweight, and may have an irregular menstrual cycle. Physical symptoms include damaged teeth and throat, swollen glands, broken blood vessels in the face, dehydration, electrolyte imbalance, and possible damage to the GI tract and kidneys. Therapy deals with treating the psychological issues surrounding the disorder and education about the negative effects of binging and purging and developing a more realistic weight goal.

Prevention of Nutritional and Health Problems in Adolescents

If an adolescent has a strong family history of hypertension or hyperlipidemia or suffers from these conditions, a diet controlled in total energy, sodium, and fat will be a life-long goal. All adolescents should be advised to limit foods high in sodium, saturated fat, trans fatty acids, and cholesterol since they are all linked with cardiovascular disease. Exercise should also be strongly encouraged and should be stressed every day as part of weight management and disease prevention. Adolescents should be advised to make exercise part of their everyday routines by using stairs whenever possible, go for walks, ride a bike, play outside, and get involved in sport activities versus watching television or playing video games. The prevalence of obesity is lowest among children aged 8–16 who watch 1 or fewer hours of television a day, and highest among those who watch 4 or more hours a day (Crespo et al. 2001).

Adolescents often love to snack on refined carbohydrates putting themselves at risk of developing dental caries. About 80% of a person's total number of cavities occur during the teenage years. Adolescents often drink sugar containing beverages which decrease the buffering capacity of the oral environment. Sucrose is considered the most cariogenic carbohydrate. Sticky foods such as candy, eaten between meals and foods eaten before bedtime contribute to the incidence of dental caries. Optimum dental health involves frequent brushing and dental exams twice a year.

Adults

Components of a Healthy Lifestyle

Proper nutrition and a healthy life-style, which includes exercise, stress management, avoidance of tobacco, and excessive use of alcohol, are important for maintaining health and wellness.

Physical Activity

Regular physical activity provides many health benefits including weight maintenance, prevention of disease, improved sleep, and psychological health. The 2002 DRIs recommend a minimum of 30 min of moderate intensity physical activity (such as brisk walking, aerobics) most days of the week; however, to prevent weight gain and to accrue additional health benefits, 60 min of moderate intensity physical activity every day is recommended (2002). Benefits of exercise include improved sleep, decreased body fat, increased lean tissue, enhanced immune function, and improved cardiovascular efficiency and serum lipid levels. Sedentary adults, regardless of their age, should consult a physician before starting an exercise program. To prevent injuries while exercising, there should be a gradual progression in both duration and intensity. To achieve cardiovascular fitness, one should exercise at an intensity of 60–85% of his or her maximum heart rate (220 minus age), though this goal should be achieved gradually.

Tobacco Use

According to the Center for Disease Control, quitting cigarette smoking is the single most preventable cause of premature death in the United States (U.S. Department of Health and Human Services 2004). According to the American Heart Association, smoking kills over 440,000 Americans per year, and second-hand smoke kills almost 40,000 Americans. Cancer is the second leading cause of death and was among the first diseases to be linked to smoking (U.S. Department of Health and Human Services 2004). Lung cancer is the leading cause of cancer death, and cigarette smoking causes most of the cases (U.S. Department of Health and Human Services 2004). Additionally, smokers have a higher risk of developing heart disease and several types of cancer. Smoking increases blood pressure, decreases exercise tolerance, and increases the tendency for blood to clot. Smoking also increases the risks arising from alcohol abuse, high blood pressure, and diabetes. Smoking is found to reduce bone mineral density and increase the risk of hip fracture in men and women (U.S. Department of Health and Human Services 2004). Smokers are also found to have 2–3 times the risk of developing cataracts compared to nonsmokers (U.S. Department of Health and Human Services 2004).

Alcohol Use

Alcohol abuse increases the risk of chronic disease, including heart and liver disease and cancer of the oral cavity and esophagus. Excessive alcohol intake can reduce the absorption of many nutrients including, folic acid, vitamin B_{12}, vitamin B_6, and zinc. Alcohol adds empty calories to the diet, and further reduces the intake of important nutrients such as calcium, magnesium, zinc. and iron. However, alcohol, in moderation (1 drink per day for women and 2 drinks a day for men), is shown to have a positive affect on bone mineral density of spine and total body (Ilich et al. 2002), and is shown to benefit cholesterol and triglyceride levels (Freiberg et al. 2004).

Dietary Recommendations

The 2005 USDA Dietary Guidelines recommends Americans consume a variety of nutrient-dense foods and beverages within the basic food groups, and choosing foods limited in saturated fat, trans fat, cholesterol, added sugars, and salt (Dietary Guidelines for Americans 2005). Two eating patterns that exemplify the Dietary Guidelines are the *DASH* eating plan and the USDA *myPyramid* (Dietary Guidelines for Americans 2005). Both eating plans promote higher intake of fruits, vegetables, low-fat dairy products, whole grains, and legumes. The *myPyramid* provides intake recommendations based on individual weight, gender, and activity level. Intakes are given in serving sizes instead of ranges of intakes. The recommendations for macronutrient distribution include 22–29% of total energy from fat (only 5–7.8% of total energy from saturated fat), 18–21% of total energy from protein, and 50–60% of total energy from carbohydrates (Dietary Guidelines for Americans 2005). For fluid intake, there are no specific recommendations since it has been determined that the combination of thirst and normal drinking behavior is usually sufficient to maintain normal hydration (Dietary Guidelines for Americans 2005).

The current DRIs for adults are separated into three age categories, 19–30 years, 31–50 years, and >50 years. For all three age categories the estimated energy requirements are 2,403 kcal for females and 3,067 kcal for males; however, females should subtract 7 calories for each year above age 19, and males should subtract 10 calories for each year above 19 (2002). For example, a 35-year-old male would require an estimated 2,907 kcal a day. The recommended protein intake for males and females 19 and over is 0.8 g/kg/day (2002). For maintenance of bone mass, the calcium requirement for females and males 19–50 years is 1,000 mg/day, and vitamin D is 200 IU/day. For vision, reproduction, and immune function the requirement for vitamin A is 700 and 900 µg/day for females and males ages 19 and over, respectively. Another fat-soluble vitamin and important antioxidant, vitamin E, has the same DRI for males and females 19 and over, which is 15 mg/day.

Issues with Athletes

Proper nutrition is essential for optimal performance of athletes. With training, energy needs can double depending on the intensity, duration, and frequency of activities performed during training. The higher the body weight, the more calories will be expended per activity. Depending on the sport, a lighter weight may be desired. If athletes need to lose weight, they should do so when they are not competing in order not to affect the performance. Weight loss should be realistic resulting in a healthy body weight. Energy intake should be reduced by 200–500 kcal a day and combined with daily exercise to achieve a weight loss of 0.5–1 lb a week. To gain weight, 200–500 kcal should be added a day, accompanied with an exercise program designed to increase lean tissue.

During training, athletes need to consume food with adequate complex carbo-hydrates, such as whole grains and starchy vegetables as well as the food containing simple sugars such as milk and fruit to be able to replace muscle and glycogen stores that become depleted with physical activity, and at the same time, provide adequate vitamin and mineral supply (Burke et al. 2004). Percentage of carbohydrate, fat, and protein in the diet for athletes is the same as for the general population. Excess dietary fat should be avoided. There is no evidence that high-fat low-carbohydrate diets benefit performance (Burke et al. 2004). A protein intake of 0.8 g/kg body weight is usually sufficient for most athletes' training needs. Additional protein intake is shown to give only a minimal additional advantage in lean body mass (Tipton and Wolfe 2004). A slightly higher protein intake of 1.0–1.5 g/kg should only be used for endur-ance athletes and those in weight training.

Aging and the Aged

Physiological Aspects of Aging

There is a gradual decline in functioning on cellular and organ-tissue levels with aging. Oxidative stress due to free radicals, degeneration of the mito-chondrial repair and defense mechanisms contribute to the decline in cellular function and a decline in many organ systems. Oxidation also causes damage within the cells of the eye, which leads to poor vision. With aging, bone den-sity decreases, increasing the risk of fractures. Changes in hormone levels with aging can affect the body's ability to regulate body fluids, temperature, and blood glucose levels. Osteoarthritis, the most common cause of disability in the elderly, can limit mobility. In the stomach, the production of acid declines diminishing vitamin B_{12} absorption as well as proper digestive functions. As the kidneys' functioning declines, glomerular filtration rates diminish, as well as the ability to produce vitamin D in a usable form for the body. There is also a decline in mental and cognitive capacity, and an increase incidence of dementia. Dementia has been linked to poor nutrition, especially for the foods rich in folate and vitamin B_{12} (Brownbill and Ilich 2004).

Nutrient Requirements

As lean body mass decreases in older adults, so does the basal metabolic rate, meaning that the energy requirement decreases as well. An increase in body weight throughout adulthood will result if energy intake and physical activity continue at the same rate as in younger age.

The newest dietary recommendations for older adults are divided into two age categories, 51–70 years and over 70 years (2002). It is worth noting that several nutrient requirements are increased in the elderly. In males, the DRI for vitamin B_6 is increased from 1.3 mg/day in 19–50-year old to 1.7 mg/day males over 50 years (2001). For females, the DRI is increased from 1.3 mg/day for 19–50 years to 1.5 mg/day for females over 50 years (2001). The DRI for calcium is increased from 1,000 mg/day for the adults 19–50 to 1,200 mg/day for the adults over 50 years (1997). The iron requirement is reduced from 18 mg/day to 8 mg/day for females over 50 years (2001). The requirement for chromium is also decreased, from 35 μg to 30 μg, and 25 μg to 20 μg for males and females over 50, respectively (2001). Vitamin D seems to be the most critical nutrient. Males and females require 200 IU until age 50, which increases to 400 IU until age 70, and then to 600 IU after age 70 (1997). Basically, the requirement for vitamin D increases throughout the life due to the decreased ability of the skin to manufacture vitamin D.

Fluid needs for the elderly are the same as those for younger adults. However, with aging there are increased problems with urinary incontinence, which could limit fluid intake. The risk of dehydration is increased in individuals on laxatives and diuretics or certain chronic medical conditions. Inadequate fluid intake can also lead to problems with constipation.

There are many other factors that can contribute to malnutrition in the elderly. Poverty is the highest among very old, women, and persons who live alone. Many elderly live on fixed income or have limited access to food. Many medical conditions and medications are linked with malnutrition. Osteoarthritis and limited mobility as a result of a stroke can make it difficult to prepare or obtain food. Medications used to treat diabetes, hypertension, and heart disease may have nutrient interactions or require special diets. Certain medications can cause nausea or loss of appetite, making it difficult to consume a diet adequate in nutrients. Medications can also interfere with nutrient absorption. For example, anticonvulsants increase the need for vitamin D, and diuretics increase the need for potassium.

Nutrition and Health Issues During Menopause

As a woman reaches the end of her reproductive life, she will experience irregular ovarian and uterine cycles due to a shortage of primordial follicles and a decrease in estrogen levels. Menopause refers to the period during which female sex hormone levels greatly diminish. Women tend to gain more weight during this stage of life.

The cessation of ovarian functions is characterized by diminished estrogen production. This change causes LDL (bad cholesterol) levels to rise. The lack of estrogen also decreases the sensitivity to insulin that results in higher blood glucose levels. Probably the most profound consequence of estrogen cessation is an increased risk for osteoporosis. A woman can lose up to 20% of her bone mass in the 5–7 years following menopause. Due to the above changes, a woman would benefit from a diet low in fats and saturated fats, moderate intake of sugars, and the use of calcium supplements. Since the menstruation has ceased the requirement for iron is decreased (8 mg/day).

Chronic Diseases

Cardiovascular/Hypertension

The leading cause of death in the United States is cardiovascular disease (CVD) that affects 950,000 Americans per year (Center for Disease Control).

Hypertension is the elevation of blood pressure, which increases the risk of CVD. Various CVDs include stoke, atherosclerosis, coronary heart disease, and arteriosclerosis. Overall risk factors for CVD include high blood pressure, smoking, obesity, high LDL cholesterol, HDL levels that are lower than normal, high glucose levels, lack of physical exercise, diet, and family history (Smith et al. 2004). A diet including complex carbohydrates, low in sodium, saturated fats, trans fats, and cholesterol may help reduce the risk of having cardiovascular disease.

Diabetes

According to the Center for Disease Control, as of 2006, 16.8 million people were diagnosed with diabetes. Approximately 550,000 new cases are diagnosed per year (Center for Disease Control, accessed 09/09). Type 2 diabetes mellitus (adult-onset diabetes) is generally noninsulin dependant. Those diagnosed with type 2 usually have blood sugar levels of >200 mg/dl and a fasting glucose of 126 mg/dl or higher. Diabetes leads to complications such as high blood pressure, heart disease, stroke, amputations, and inadequate ability for wound healing (Center for Disease Control, accessed 09/09).

Overweight/Obesity

The National Health and Nutritional Examination Survey from 2003 to 2004, estimates that 65% of adults are overweight or obese (Center for Disease Control, accessed 09/09). Overweight and obesity are defined as having a body mass index (BMI) greater than 25 and 30 kg/m^2, respectively. Factors contributing to overweight or obesity are hormone levels, genetic factors, and an accumulation of adipocytes during childhood. However, imbalance in energy intake versus energy expenditure is the most dominant factor leading to increased weight. Overweight/obesity leads to about 30 different impairments and disease and the most prevalent and serious ones are diabetes, osteoarthritis, heart problems, and certain cancers.

Cancer

Cancer is the second leading cause of death and it is estimated that one of every four deaths in the US is due to some form of cancer (Center for Disease Control, accessed 09/09). Factors that influence the development of cancer are smoking, environmental causes, genetics, and diet. A compilation of statistical data was analyzed from nine different studies and the most promising nutritional strategies for site-specific cancer prevention were: vitamin E and selenium for prostate cancer, the combination of beta-carotene, vitamin E, and selenium for stomach cancer and retinal (plus zinc) for gastric cancer and squamous cell carcinoma of the skin (Patterson et al. 2004). Prudent recommendation for the prevention of various kinds of cancer are to eat plenty of fruits and vegetables, drink alcohol in moderation, consume meat in moderation, maintain a healthy weight, and limit overexposure to sunlight.

Osteoporosis

Osteoporosis is characterized with the decreased bone mass and impaired bone quality that leads to an increase in susceptibility to fractures. Osteoporosis accounts for 1.5 million fractures per year and its rate in women is about four times higher than in men (http://www.osteo.org). Risk factors for osteoporosis include sedentary lifestyle, life-long low calcium intake, low vitamin D intake, current smoking, excessive alcohol intake, low body weight, low estrogen levels, certain medications, and chronic medical conditions, as well as being Caucasian or Asian. Prevention of bone loss includes achieving the highest genetically predisposed peak bone mass during adolescence, leading an active lifestyle and consuming nutrient adequate diet. For postmenopausal women who have osteoporosis or low bone mass, there are various treatment options such as bisphosphanates, calcitonin, and hormone therapy.

References

Brownbill, R. A., Ilich, J. Z. (2004). Cognitive function in relation with bone mass and nutrition: Cross sectional association in postmenopausal women BMC Women's Health. 4:2. http://www.biomedcentral.com/1472-6874/4/2.

Burke, L. M., Kiens, B., & Ivy, J. L. (2004). Carbohydrates and fat for training and recovery. *Journal of Sports Sciences, 22,* 15–30.

Butte, N., Cobbs, K., Dwyer, J., Graney, L., Heird, W., & Rickhard, K. (2004). The start healthy feeding guidelines for infants and toddlers. *Journal of the American Dietetic Association, 104,* 442–54.

Center for Disease Control. http://www.cdc.gov/cancer/ accessed, 09/09.

Center for Disease Control: http://www.cdc.gov/diabetes/, accessed 09/09.

Center for Disease Control: http://www.cdc.gov/obesity/index.html, accessed 09/09.

Cheruku, S. R., Montgomery-Downs, H. E., Farkus, S. L., Thoman, E. B., & Lammi-Keefe, C. J. (2002). Higher maternal plasma docosahexaenoic acid during pregnancy is associated with more mature neonatal sleep-state patterning. *The American Journal of Clinical Nutrition, 76,* 608–13.

Crespo, C. J., Smit, E., Troiano, R. P., Bartlett, S. J., Macera, C. A., & Anderson, R. E. (2001). Television watching, energy intake, and obesity in US children. *Archives of Pediatrics & Adolescent Medicine, 155,* 360–365.

Diagnostic and Statistical Manual of Mental Disorders – Fourth Edition (DSM-IV) (1994). Washington DC: American Psychiatric Association.

Dietary Guidelines for Americans (2005). HHS/USDA.

Dietary Reference Intakes for Calcium, Phosphorous, Magnesium, Vitamin D and Fluoride (1997). Copyright 1997 by the National Academies. www.nap.edu.

Dietary Reference Intakes for Energy, Carbohydrate, Fiber, Fat, Fatty Acids, Cholesterol, Protein, and Amino Acids (2002). Copyright 2002 by the National Academies www.nap.edu.

Dietary Reference Intakes for Thiamin, Niacin, Vitamin B6, Folate, Vitamin B12, Pantothenic Acid, Biotin and Choline (1998). Copyright 2001 by the National Academies. www.nap.edu.

Dietary Reference Intakes for Vitamin A, Vitamin K, Arsenic, Boron, Chromium, Copper, Iodine, Iron, Manganese, Molybdenum, Nickel, Silicon, Vanadium and Zinc (2001). Copyright 2001 by the National Academies. www.nap.edu.

Freiberg, M. S., Cabral, H. J., Heeren, T. C., Vassan, R. S., & Curtis, E. R. (2004). Alcohol consumption and the prevalence of the metabolic syndrome in the US: A cross-sectional analysis of data from the Third National Health and Nutrition Examination Survey. *Diabetes Care, 27,* 2954–9.

Gross, S. M., Bronner, Y., Welch, C., Dewberry-Moore, N., & Paige, D. M. (2004). Breakfast and lunch meal skipping patterns among fourth-grade children from selected public schools in urban, suburban, and rural Maryland. *Journal of the American Dietetic Association, 104,* 420–3.

Hornstra, G. (2000). Essential fatty acids in mothers and their neonates. *The American Journal of Clinical Nutrition, 71,* 1262S–1269S.

Ilich, J. Z., Brownbill, R. A., Tamborini, L., & Crncevic-Orlic, Z. (2002). To drink or not to drink: How are alcohol, caffeine and past smoking related to bone mineral density in elderly women? *Journal of the American College of Nutrition, 21,* 536–544.

National Institute of Health: Osteoporosis and Related Bone Disease National Resource Center. http://www.osteo.org.

Nehlig, A., & Debry, G. (1994). Potential teratogenic and neurodevelopmental consequences of coffee and caffeine exposure: A review of human and animal data. *Neurotoxicology and Teratology, 16*, 531–43.

Nutrition During Lactation. Institute of Medicine, 1991.

Ogden, C. L., Flegal, K. M., Carrol, M. D., & Johnson, C. L. (2002). Prevalence and trend in overweight among US children and adolescents, 1999–2000. *The Journal of the American Medical Association, 288*, 1728–32.

Patterson, R. E., Frank, L. L., Kristal, A. R., & White, E. (2004). A comprehensive examination of health conditions associated with obesity in older adults. *American Journal of Preventive Medicine, 27*, 385–390.

Pike, K. M., Walsh, B. T., Vitousek, K., Wilson, G. T., & Bauer, J. (2003). Cognitive behavior therapy in the posthospitalization treatment of anorexia nervosa. *The American Journal of Psychiatry, 160*, 2046–2049.

Ravaldi, C., Vannacci, A., Zucchi, T., Mannucci, E., Cabras, P. L., Boldrini, M., et al. (2003). Eating disorders and body image disturbance among ballet dancers, gymnasium users and body builders. *Psychopathology, 36*, 247–54.

Rothman, K. J., Moore, L. L., Singer, M. R., Nguyen, U.-S. D. T., Mannino, S., & Milunsky, A. (1995). Teratogenicity of high vitamin A intake. *The New England Journal of Medicine, 333*, 1369–73.

Schnoll, R., Burshteyn, D., & Cea-Aravena, J. (2003). Nutrition in the treatment of attention-deficit hyperactivity disorder: A neglected but important aspect. *Applied Psychophysiology and Biofeedback, 28*, 63–75.

Simopoulos, A. P., Leaf, A., & Salem, N. (1999). Workshop on the essentiality of and recommended dietary intakes for omega-6 and omega-3 fatty acids. *Journal of the American College of Nutrition, 18*, 487–9.

Smith, S. C., Jackson, R., Pearson, T. A., Fuster, V., Yusuf, S., Faergeman, O., et al. (2004). Principles for national and regional guidelines on cardiovascular disease prevention. *Circulation, 109*, 3112–3121.

St-Onge, M., Keller, K. L., & Heymsfield, S. B. (2003). Changes in childhood food consumption patterns: A cause for concern in light of increasing body weights. *The American Journal of Clinical Nutrition, 78*, 1068–73.

Sullivan, C. S., Beste, J., Cummings, D. M., Hester, V. H., Holbrook, T., Kolasa, K. M., et al. (2004). Prevalence of hyperinsulinemia and clinical correlates in overweight children referred for lifestyle intervention. *Journal of the American Dietetic Association, 104*, 433–6.

Tipton, K. D., & Wolfe, R. R. (2004). Protein and amino acids for athletes. *Journal of Sports Sciences, 22*, 65–79.

Tolstrup, J. S., Kjaer, S. K., Munk, C., Madsen, L. B., Ottesen, B., Bergholt, T., et al. (2003). Does caffeine and alcohol intake before pregnancy predict the occurrence of spontaneous abortion? *Human Reproduction, 18*, 2704–10.

U.S. Department of Health and Human Services. The Health Consequences of Smoking: A Report of the Surgeon General. U.S. Department of Health and Human Services, Centers for Disease Control and Prevention, National Center for Chronic Disease Prevention and Health Promotion, Office on Smoking and Health, 2004.

Wen, W., Shu, X. O., Jacobs, D. R., Jr., & Brown, J. E. (2001). The associations of maternal caffeine consumption and nausea with spontaneous abortion. *Epidemiology, 12*, 38–42.

Chapter 32

The Role of Animals and Animal-Assisted Therapy in Stressful Life Transitions

Jeanine M. Miller Adams

Animals and pets have often played a significant role in the lives of humans. Animal-assisted therapy (AAT) has touched the lives of many people experiencing stressful life transitions. It is a growing form of therapy that benefits both the humans and the animals involved. This chapter describes AAT and how it impacts people and animals, provides case examples of how it has affected individuals during the stressful life transitions they have experienced, and explores theoretical perspectives applicable to this form of therapy.

Historically, William Tuke was the first to document the use of animal therapy in the eighteenth century. He believed the people in asylums received inhumane treatment and helped to make their lives better by encouraging them to take care of animals (Moore 1984). More recently, Boris Levinson (1962, 1969) began documenting therapeutic benefits for individuals receiving contact with pets and discussed the use of animals as adjuncts to his psychology practice. Currently, there are animal therapy programs across the country, and national and local organizations to sponsor and provide them, such as Therapy Dogs, Incorporated; the Delta Society; Therapy Dogs, International; and the National Center for Equine Facilitated Therapy.

In formal therapeutic situations, AAT is defined as an "interaction between patients and a trained animal, along with its human handler, with the intent of facilitating individuals' progress toward therapeutic goals" (Barker and Dawson 1998). However, in a broader sense, AAT is a process that simply "brings animals and people with physical and/or emotional needs together" (Carmack 1984). AAT has an interdisciplinary base and is viewed as an adjunct to other therapies, such as occupational, physical, speech, and psychological therapy. It has also been termed "animal-facilitated therapy" (AFT; Moore 1984), "pet-facilitated therapy" (PFT; Altschuler 1999), "pet therapy" (Zisselman et al. 1996), and "animal therapy" (Willis 1997).

AAT can occur in groups (Reichert 1994) or individual (Reichert 1998) settings. Programs have been implemented with a wide variety of populations, including those with psychiatric/emotional disturbance and behavioral disorders (Bardill and Hutchinson 1997; Banman 1995; Granger et al. 1998);

From: *Handbook of Stressful Transitions Across the Lifespan,*
Edited by: T.W. Miller, DOI 10.1007/978-1-4419-0748-6_32,
© Springer Science+Business Media, LLC 2010

elderly people in homebound (Harris et al. 1993), outpatient, institutional (nursing home/long-term care: Katsinas 2000; Crowley-Robinson and Blackshaw 1998; Fick 1993; Taylor et al. 1994; Gammonley and Yates 1991), and adult day care (Holcomb et al. 1997) situations; hospitalized individuals in psychiatric settings (Barker and Dawson 1998; Holcomb and Meacham 1989), cancer centers, children's hospitals, rehabilitation, hospice (Doyle and Kukowski 1989), coronary care, intensive care (Cole and Gawlinski 1995), and acute care settings (Barba 1995; Counsell et al. 1997); people with mild to severe physical and cognitive disabilities of all ages (Farias-Tomaszewski et al. 2001; Law & Scott 1995; Nathanson et al. 1997); individuals with autism and autism spectrum disorders (Law and Scott 1995) and learning disabilities (Limond et al. 1997); prison inmates (Cushing and Williams 1995; Walsh and Mertin 1994); people with HIV/AIDS (Allen et al. 2000; Angulo et al. 1996); those in therapy for sexual abuse (Reichert 1994, 1998) and anger management (Hanselman 2001); individuals with depression (Holcomb et al. 1997; Folse et al. 1994); and individuals undergoing dental/medical procedures (Havener et al. 2001; Hansen et al. 1999).

The Influence of Animals on Humans

Baker (1992) studied the effects of animals on human blood pressure levels to compare risk factors for cardiovascular disease in pet owners and nonowners. Accepted risk factors for cardiovascular disease were measured in 5,741 participants attending a free, screening clinic at the Baker Medical Research Institute in Melbourne. Blood pressure, plasma cholesterol, and triglyceride values were compared in pet owners ($n = 784$) and nonowners ($n = 4,957$).

On the basis of the results obtained, pet owners had significantly lower systolic blood pressure and plasma triglycerides than nonowners. In men, pet owners had significantly lower systolic but not diastolic blood pressure than nonowners, and significantly lower plasma triglyceride levels and plasma cholesterol levels. In women over 40 years old, systolic but not diastolic pressure was significantly lower in pet owners and plasma triglycerides also tended to be lower. There were no differences in body mass index and self reported smoking habits were similar, but pet owners reported that they took significantly more exercise than nonowners, and ate more meat and "takeaway" foods. The socioeconomic profile of pet owners and nonowners appeared to be comparable.

On the basis of the results of this study, findings suggest that pet owners had lower levels of accepted risk factors for cardiovascular disease, and this was not explicable on the basis of cigarette smoking, diet, body mass index, or socioeconomic profile. The possibility that pet ownership reduces cardiovascular risk factors was inferred.

Similarly, Crosby (2006) indicates that the bond between pets and humans can be an intervening variable in reducing cholesterol, lower blood pressure, reduced stress levels, and better mental health for those living with pets. Pets require attention. The physical activity they require in humans may be a significant factor and be exemplified in going for a walk, dropping everything for a game of Frisbee or hide and seek, going on a trail ride, and providing the everyday pet care encourages owners to interact and get out.

Pet therapy often involves small animals most often dogs and cats but there is a role for large animals as well. Horses and horse riding is also part of pet therapy. Riding horses teaches balance and flexibility to the handicapped, and gives a sense of accomplishment and companionship to those involved. Some programs are related to the care of horses as well, teaching responsibility and horsemanship skills. Services provided by dogs for humans include: dogs that guide the blind, assist the deaf, assist the mobility-impaired, even alert epileptic owners that a seizure is imminent, so the owners can sit down/take their medications before the seizure strikes. Dogs can be trained to turn on/off lights, pick up objects, and even pull wheel chairs for those who are disabled. Police dogs serve as protection for officers, as well as for sniffing out drugs, explosives, and other dangerous chemicals long before a human can. Search and Rescue dogs use their powerful sense of smell to locate people lost or injured.

Various types of animals and people work in or are involved with AAT. Researchers have studied the effects of therapeutic relationships between humans and dogs (Katsinas 2000; Barker and Dawson 1998; Limond et al. 1997; Cole and Gawlinski 1995; Folse et al. 1994; Walsh and Mertin 1994), horses (Farias-Tomaszewski et al. 2001), cats (Turner and Rieger 2001; Rieger and Turner 1999; Wells et al. 1997), birds (Holcomb et al. 1997), monkeys (Ianuzzi and Rowan 1991), fish (Law and Scott 1995), dolphins (Lukina 1999; Nathanson 1998), rabbits (Law and Scott 1995), Guinea pigs (Nielson and Delude 1994; Carmack and Fila 1989), cows (Mallon 1994), and snakes (Shalev and Ben-Mordehai 1996). Also involved are the animals' handlers or trainers and professionals, such as occupational (Allen et al. 2000; Fick 1993; Taylor et al. 1994; Fine (2000)), physical (Nathanson et al. 1997), and speech (Adams 1997) therapists (Dossey 1997), activities directors/therapists (Wilkes et al. 1989), recreation therapists (Wilkes et al. 1989), psychologists/psychiatrists (Barker and Dawson 1998; Zisselman et al. 1996; Walsh et al. 1995), social workers (Hanselman 2001; Reichert 1994, 1998; Mallon 1994), health educators (Doyle and Kukowski 1989), teachers (Granger et al. 1998; Limond et al. 1997; Law and Scott 1995), nurses (Willis 1997; Carmack and Fila 1989), doctors and other health care practitioners (Hansen et al. 1999), dentists (Havener et al. 2001), and veterinarians (Crowley-Robinson and Blackshaw 1998).

There are four major categories involving therapeutic approaches with the use of animals: visiting animal programs, residential programs, service animal programs, and nondomesticated animal programs. Visiting animal programs involve animals entering an institution, home, or other facility to visit participants for a short period of time. Popular programs include those using dogs. The animals may simply be visiting to provide companionship and cheer, or they may be involved in a more structured therapy session with, for example, an occupational, physical, or speech therapist. Not only do the animals positively affect the *patients*, but family members and staff also reap the benefits (Carmack and Fila 1989).

Residential programs involve animals living where the therapy occurs. In this situation, the animals reside on the unit or in the facility in which the program participants are housed, such as in a psychiatric unit (Bardill and Hutchinson 1997), a prison (Walsh and Mertin 1994), or a nursing home (Crowley-Robinson and Blackshaw 1998). This type of program differs from a visiting animal program in that the individuals involved may have more contact with the animals and greater responsibilities for them, such as grooming, training, exercising, and feeding.

Service animals provide therapy in various ways to humans. There are several types of assistance dogs. *Guide dogs* work for people with visual impairments; *hearing dogs* are trained to help people with hearing impairments in awareness of certain important sounds, such as a fire alarm, a knock at the door, or a baby crying; *service dogs* are trained to assist individuals with disabilities, such as spinal cord injury, multiple sclerosis, or cerebral palsy, with mobility enhancement and object retrieval (Sachs-Ericsson et al. 2002).

Nondomesticated animal programs include hippotherapy, or therapeutic horseback riding, dolphin assisted therapy, and the use of farm animals in AAT. Wells et al. (1997) used feral cats as adjuncts to psychotherapy. Regardless of the category of AAT, these programs impact participants in many positive ways.

The therapeutic use of animals impacts humans' health and wellness. There are several dimensions to our health and wellness and researchers have documented benefits of AAT in every area:

- *Physical/physiological* wellness involves the health of our physical self, eating well, exercising, recognizing symptoms of disease, and monitoring physical disorders. Benefits of AAT in this area include sensory stimulation (Counsell et al. 1997); satisfying the universal need for physical touch; improved gross and fine motor skills (Nathanson 1997); significant increases in neurochemicals (prolactin, oxytocin, B-endorphin, phenylacetic acid, and dopamine) in both the humans and dogs involved (Odendaal 2000); decreased muscle rigidity, blood pressure (Harris et al. 1993), triglyceride levels, and heart rate (Walsh et al. 1995; Harris et al. 1993); and stress reduction (Nielson and Delude 1994).

- *Social* wellness includes having satisfying interpersonal relationships, good communication skills, and a supportive network. Researchers have found that AAT has contributed to increased communication, speech/language (Nathanson 1997), responsiveness (Adams 1997), laughter, conversation (Bernstein et al. 2000; Nielson and Delude 1994), smiles (Marr et al. 2000), interaction (Adams 1997; Fick 1993), eye contact (Granger et al. 1998); speech elicited from nonverbal individuals; decreased social isolation (Adams 1997; Holcomb and Meacham 1989), and noise levels (psychiatric ward; Walsh et al. 1995); companionship, comfort, break down of social barriers; and AAT has acted as a catalyst for positive social behavior.

- *Emotional/psychological* wellness involves how we feel about ourselves, self-esteem, having healthy emotional relationships. Benefits of AAT include unconditional acceptance/positive regard (Bardill and Hutchinson 1997), no fear of rejection; increased positive mood, feelings of love, self-esteem (Gammonley and Yates 1991), self-worth (Walsh and Mertin 1994), self-efficacy (Farias-Tomaszewski et al. 2001), compassion, security; improved attitude, self-concept, feelings of relaxation and pleasure; reactions from those who have been withdrawn; sustaining our emotional balance (Banman 1995); providing something to look forward to (Harris et al. 1993), memories of former pets (Banman 1995), emotional support for staff/family (Dossey 2005; Carmack and Fila 1989), building staff morale and decreasing turnover rates; decreased anxiety (Barker and Dawson 1998), depression (Holcomb et al. 1997), learned helplessness (Granger et al. 1998); the animals are viewed as nonjudgmental, friends, listeners, therapists, distracters, and uniquely sensitive (Bardill and Hutchinson 1997).

- *Cognitive/mental* wellness involves critical and creative thinking, mastering new skills, being open to new ideas, and learning and storing new information. AAT has benefited individuals in this area by acting as a catalyst for teaching and learning; contributing to increased concentration/focusing skills, attention span (Limond et al. 1997), knowledge, self-respect, and control of environment (Gammonley and Yates 1991); decreased distractibility (Granger et al. 1998); and relief from boredom.
- *Environmental* health involves the quality of our surroundings. AAT deinstitutionalizes a facility, making it feel more home-like (Bardill and Hutchinson 1997).
- *Spiritual* health is having a purpose or meaning in life, believing in a higher power, or in oneness with nature. AAT provides a feeling of oneness with life and creation (Gammonley and Yates 1991), fosters the human–animal bond, and provides the healing power of a pet's presence (Banman 1995; Harris et al. 1993).
- *Occupational/vocational* wellness involves being satisfied with ones daily activities. In AAT studies, pet ownership and care have been found to be an avenue for enabling meaningful occupation (Allen et al. 2000).
- From a *behavioral* perspective, benefits include increased play and laughter (Banman 1995); decreased disciplinary reports for violent offenders (Cushing and Williams 1995); decreased aggressiveness (Walsh and Mertin 1994), violent behavior, and drug use (Moneymaker and Strimple 1991); reduced behavioral distress (Hansen et al. 1999); increased calmness and outward expressions of happiness (Walsh and Mertin 1994); learning nurturance and caring/responsibility (Banman 1995; Mallon 1994); and nurturing and affection have been elicited from violent-prone individuals.

The following case studies provide a glimpse of the impact that the therapeutic use of animals has had on three people and those involved in their lives.

Case Study 1

Harris et al. (1993) reported on the case of Mr. H, a 73-year-old man with severe arthiritis in one shoulder, legal blindness, and in recovery from a stroke, who lives alone and receives home health aide service for basic activities of daily living. He was described as "abrupt, difficult, depressed, and lonely … frowning most of the time with a very flat affect" by the visiting nurses and aides. With the initiation of a visiting AAT program, Mr. H's blood pressure decreased and his shoulder mobility improved, as he stroked, kissed, played with, and focused on the dog, and anticipated and enjoyed the visits. The aides stated that the only time they saw him smile was when the dog visited (Harris et al. 1993).

Case Study 2

Clarence is confined to a wheelchair and until he received a dog trained through the Prison PUP Partnership, he had to wait for help for simple tasks, such as retrieving fallen objects, turning on lights, and opening doors.

His dog, "Blitz," has greatly improved his quality of life (Gardner 1998). In these types of programs, dogs are paired full-time with carefully selected prison inmates and trained for 8–18 months. The dogs are later placed as assistance dogs with a person with disabilities. The inmates who train the dogs feel as though they're giving something back to the community they once violated. They gain skills training, boarding, and grooming the dogs. In addition, they learn valuable pet industry-related vocational skills to use when seeking employment after prison (Prison Pet Partnership Program 2003).

Case Study 3

Adams (1997) described the case of "WA," a 72 year-old woman recovering from two strokes and battling diabetes, epilepsy, right hemiplegia (paralysis), dementia, and apraxia, a speech problem in which one knows what they want to say, but cannot actually say it. She had good speech comprehension. Her writing abilities were moderately impaired, as she was required to change her dominant hand from right to left due to her hemiplegia. She became frustrated as she struggled to verbalize her thoughts and recognized the errors and distortions in her speech. A visiting AAT program was initiated with her in her facility during speech therapy sessions to work mainly on appropriate and correct word initiation. WA showed improvement with one-word answers, object identification tasks, and verbalization behaviors. Her behavior and outlook markedly improved, and her desire to interact increased, as noted by her increased participation in facility activities and spending more time outside of her own room. She held the leash of one dog as she was pushed in her wheelchair through the facility and spontaneously answered questions from interested staff and residents. Also noted were mild sensations and limited spontaneous use of her hemiplegic side and extremities (Adams 1997).

In order to understand how AAT provides the benefits discussed in this chapter, it is important to explore theoretical perspectives applicable to this form of therapy. One is *attachment theory*, which holds that emotional well-being is largely affected by personal relationships throughout life. In this theory, individuals who do not form secure attachments develop negative ideas about themselves and the world, seeing themselves as powerless and worthless and their caregivers as unreliable, unavailable, and rejecting. Pets can be considered a significant attachment figure in the promotion of general mental health and in the treatment of disturbed populations (Hanselman 2001). For example, in Bardill and Hutchinson's (1997) study with a residential therapy dog and adolescents hospitalized in a psychiatric unit, the dog was found to "reach unreachable kids" as he was described as being a friend, listener, and distracter from problems. The adolescents viewed him as "touchable," calm, and having a unique sensitivity to them. The adolescents did not have to worry about being rejected in the relationship and found him to be available and reliable. The dog helped the adolescents have increased feelings of self-worth and less emptiness in their lives. In this case, the adolescents formed a meaningful *attachment* to the dog, which helped them to feel trust, safety, and comfort.

Abraham Maslow (1970) discussed the importance of and need for *self-esteem*, which is satisfaction with, confidence in, and the valuing of oneself. Animal assisted therapy contributes to the development or enhancement of self-esteem. Examples of this include the use of AAT in prisons (Gardner 1998) and with farm animals (Mallon 1994). In these situations, program participants not only receive the benefits of having the animals as companions, but also learn about nurturing and caring for other living creatures through their responsibilities to train, groom, feed, and/or care for the animals. The skills they learn contribute to increased self-esteem for the participants.

From a *biomechanical* perspective, animals working in AAT with, for example, an occupational or physical therapist, can help a patient recovering from a stroke as the patient pets or brushes the animal to increase movement in an affected arm or holds the dog's leash for motivation as walking is addressed. From a *sensory* perspective, animals provide sensory stimulation and satisfy the universal need for touch.

Animal assisted therapy (AAT) helps many individuals in a wide variety of situations. It is a growing form of therapy with benefits for both the humans and the animals involved. It is hoped that this field continues to grow and flourish, touching the lives of many people and animals, helping them to better cope with the stressful life transitions they experience.

References

Adams, D. L. (1997). Animal-assisted enhancement of speech therapy: A case study. *Anthrozoos, 10*(1), 53–56.

Allen, J. M., Kellegrrew, D. H., & Jaffe, D. (2000). The experience of pet ownership as meaningful occupation. *Canadian Journal of Occupational Therapy, 67*(4), 271–278.

Altschuler, E. L. (1999). Pet-facilitated therapy for posttraumatic stress disorder. *Annals of Clinical Psychiatry, 11*(1), 29–30.

Angulo, F. J., Siegel, J. M., & Detels, R. (1996). Pet ownership and the reliability of the companion animal bonding scale among participants of the multicenter AIDS cohort study. *Anthrozoos, IX*, 5–9.

Baker, A. (1992). Pet ownership and risk factors for cardiovascular disease. *Medical Journal Australia, 157*, 298–301.

Banman, J. K. (1995). Animal-assisted therapy with adolescents in a psychiatric facility. *The Journal of Pastoral Care, 49*(3), 168–172.

Barba, B. E. (1995). The positive influence of animals: Animal assisted therapy in acute care. *Clinical Nurse Specialist, 9*(4), 199–202.

Bardill, N., & Hutchinson, S. (1997). Animal-assisted therapy with hospitalized adolescents. *Journal of Child and Adolescent Psychiatric Nursing, 10*(1), 17–24.

Barker, S. B., & Dawson, K. S. (1998). The effects of animal-assisted therapy on anxiety ratings of hospitalized psychiatric patients. *Psychiatric Services, 49*(6), 797–801.

Bernstein, P. L., Friedmann, E., & Malaspina, A. (2000). Animal-assisted therapy enhances resident social interaction and initiation in long-term care facilities. *Anthrozoos, 13*(4), 213–224.

Carmack, B. J. (1984). Animal-assisted therapy. *Nurse Educator, 9*(4), 40–41.

Carmack, B. J., & Fila, D. (1989). Animal-assisted therapy: A nursing intervention. *Nursing Management, 20*(5), 96–101.

Cole, K. M., & Gawlinski, A. (1995). Animal-assisted therapy in the intensive care unit. *Nursing Clinics of North America, 30*(3), 529–536.

Counsell, C. M., Abram, J., & Gilbert, M. (1997). Animal assisted therapy and the individual with spinal cord injury. *Scinursing, 14*(2), 52–55.

Crosby, J. T. (2006) The human-animal bond. *Your Guide to Veterinary Medicine.* Retrieved June 06, 2006, from http://vetmedicine.about.com/cs/diseasesall/a/humananimalbond.htm

Crowley-Robinson, P., & Blackshaw, J. K. (1998). Nursing home staffs' empathy for a missing therapy dog, their attitudes to animal-assisted therapy programs and suitable dog breeds. *Anthrozoos, 11*(2), 101–104.

Cushing, J. L., & Williams, J. D. (1995). The wild mustang program: A case study in facilitated inmate therapy. *Journal of Offender Rehabilitation, 22*(3/4), 95–112.

Delta Society. http://www.deltasociety.org

Dossey, L. (1997). The healing power of pets: A look at animal-assisted therapy. *Alternative Therapies in Health and Medicine, 3*(4), 8–16.

Dossey, L. (2005). Resident and therapist views of animal-assisted therapy: Implications for occupational therapy practice. *Australian Occupational Therapy Journal, 52*(1), 43–50.

Doyle, K., & Kukowski, T. (1989). Utilization of pets in a hospice program. *Health Education, 20,* 10–11.

Farias-Tomaszewski, S., Jenkins, S. R., & Keller, J. (2001). An evaluation of therapeutic horseback riding programs for adults with physical impairments. *Therapeutic Recreation Journal, 35*(3), 250–257.

Fick, K. M. (1993). The influence of an animal on social interactions of nursing home residents in a group setting. *The American Journal of Occupational Therapy, 47*(6), 529–534.

Fine, A. (2000). *Animal-assisted therapy. Theoretical foundations and guidelines for practice.* San Diego, CA, US: Academic Press.

Folse, E. B., Minder, C. C., Aycock, M. J., & Santana, R. T. (1994). Animal-assisted therapy and depression in adult college students. *Anthrozoos, 7*(3), 188–194.

Gammonley, J., & Yates, J. (1991). Pet projects: Animal assisted therapy in nursing homes. *Journal of Gerontological Nursing, 17*(1), 12–15.

Gardner (1998). A con's best friend: State program pairs pups with prisoners to provide companions for the disabled. North Central Massachusetts, MA: Sentinel & Enterprise.

Granger, B. P., Kogan, L., Fitchett, J., & Helmer, K. (1998). A human-animal intervention team approach to animal-assisted therapy. *Anthrozoos, 11*(3), 172–176.

Hanselman, J. L. (2001). Coping skills interventions with adolescents in anger management using animals in therapy. *Journal of Child and Adolescent Group Therapy, 11*(4), 159–195.

Hansen, K. M., Messinger, C. J., Baun, M. M., & Megel, M. (1999). Companion animals alleviating distress in children. *Anthrozoos, 12*(3), 142–148.

Harris, M. D., Rinehart, J. M., & Gertsman, J. (1993). Animal-assisted therapy for the homebound elderly. *Holistic Nursing Practice, 8*(1), 27–37.

Havener, L., Gentes, L., Thaler, B., Megel, M. E., Baun, M. M., Driscoll, F. A., et al. (2001). The effects of a copmanion animal on distress in children undergoing dental procedures. *Issues in Comprehensive Pediatric Nursing, 24,* 137–152.

Holcomb, R., Jendro, C., Weber, B., & Nahan, U. (1997). Use of an aviary to relive depression in elderly males. *Anthrozoos, 10*(1), 32–36.

Holcomb, R., & Meacham, M. (1989). Effectiveness of an animal-assisted therapy program in an inpatient psychiatric unit. *Anthrozoos, 2*(4), 259–264.

Ianuzzi, D., & Rowan, A. N. (1991). Ethical issues in animal-assisted therapy programs. *Anthrozoos, 4*(3), 154–163.

Katsinas, R. P. (2000). The use and implications of a canine companion in a therapeutic day program for nursing home residents with dementia. *Activities, Adaptation, and Aging, 25*(1), 13–30.

Law, S. & Scott, S. (1995). Tips for practitioners: Pet care: A vehicle for learning. *Focus on Autistic Behavior, 10*(2), 17–18.

Levinson, B. (1962). The dog as "co-therapist". *Mental Hygiene, 46,* 59–65.

Levinson, B. (1969). Pets and old age. *Mental Hygiene, 53*(3), 364–368.

Limond, J. A., Bradshaw, J. W. S., & Cormack, K. F. M. (1997). Behavior of children with learning disabilities interacting with a therapy dog. *Anthrozoos, 10*(2/3), 84–89.

Lukina, L. N. (1999). Influence of dolphin-assisted therapy sessions on the functional state of children with psychoneurological symptoms of diseases. *Human Physiology, 25*(6), 56–60.

Mallon, G. P. (1994). Cow as co-therapist: Utilization of farm animals as therapeutic aides with children in residential treatment. *Child and Adolescent Social Work Journal, 11*(6), 455–474.

Marr, C. A., French, L., Thompson, D., Drum, L., Greening, G., Mormon, J., et al. (2000). Animal-assisted therapy in psychiatric rehabilitation. *Anthrozoos, 13*(1), 43–47.

Maslow, A. (1970). *Motivation and Personality* (2nd ed.). New York: Harper & Row.

Moneymaker, J., & Strimple, E. (1991). Animals and inmates: A sharing companionship behind bars. *Journal of Offender Rehabilitation, 16*(3–4), 133–152.

Moore, D. (1984). Animal-facilited therapy: A review. *Children's Environments Quarterly, 1*(3), 37–39.

Nathanson, D. E. (1998). Long-term effectiveness of dolphin-assisted therapy for children with severe disabilities. *Anthrozoos, 11*(1), 22–32.

Nathanson, D. E., de Castro, D., Friend, H., & McMahon, M. (1997). Animal-Assisted Therapy for Children with Pervasive Developmental Disorder. *Western Journal of Nursing Research, 24*(6), 657–670.

Nathanson, D. E., de Castro, D., Friend, H., & McMahon, M. (1997). Effectiveness of short-term dolphin-assisted therapy for children with severe disabilities. *Anthrozoos, 10*(2/3), 90–100.

National Center for Equine Facilitated Therapy. http://www.nceft.com.

Nielson, J. A., & Delude, L. A. (1994). Pets as adjunct therapists in a residence for former psychiatric patients. *Anthrozoos, 7*(3), 166–171.

Odendaal, J. S. J. (2000). Animal-assisted therapy: Magic or medicine? *Journal of Psychosomatic Research, 49*, 275–280.

Prison Pet Partnership Program (2003). http://members.tripod.com/~prisonp.

Reichert, E. (1994). Play and animal-assisted therapy: A group-treatment model for sexually abused girls ages 9–13. *Family Therapy, 21*(1), 55–62.

Reichert, E. (1998). Individual counseling for sexually abused children: A role for animals and storytelling. *Child and Adolescent Social Work Journal, 15*(3), 177–185.

Rieger, G., & Turner, D. C. (1999). How depressive moods affect the behavior of singly living persons toward their cats. *Anthrozoos, 12*(4), 224–233.

Sachs-Ericsson, N., Hansen, K., & Fitzgerald, S. (2002). Benefits of assistance dogs: A review. *Rehabilitation Psychology, 47*(3), 251–277.

Shalev, A., & Ben-Mordehai, D. (1996). Snakes: Interactions with children with disabilities and the elderly – some psychological considerations. *Anthrozoos, IX*(4), 182–187.

Taylor, E., Maser, S., Yee, J., & Gonzalez, S. M. (1994). Effect of animals on eye contact and vocalizations of elderly residents in a long term care facility. *Physical and Occupational Therapy in Geriatrics, 11*(4), 61–71.

Therapy Dogs, Incorporated. http://www.therapydogs.com

Therapy Dogs, International. http://www.tdi-dog.org

Turner, D. C., & Rieger, G. (2001). Singly living people and their cats: A study of human mood and subsequent behavior. *Anthrozoos, 14*(1), 38–46.

Walsh, P. G., & Mertin, P. G. (1994). The training of pets as therapy dogs in a women's prison: A pilot study. *Anthrozoos, 7*(2), 124–128.

Wells, E. S., Rosen, L. W., & Walshaw, S. (1997). Use of feral cats in psychotherapy. *Anthrozoos, 10*(2/3), 125–130.

Wilkes, A. N., Shalko, T. K., & Trahan, M. (1989). Pet Rx: Implications for good health. *Health Education, 20*, 6–9.

Willis, D. A. (1997). Animal therapy. *Rehabilitation Nursing, 22*(2), 78–81.

Zisselman, M. H., Rovner, B. W., Shmuely, Y., & Ferrie, P. (1996). A pet therapy intervention with geriatric psychiatry inpatients. *The American Journal of occupational Therapy, 50*(1), 47–51.

Chapter 33

The Role of Humor in Transforming Stressful Life Events

Clifford C. Kuhn, Michael R. Nichols, and Barbara L. Belew

Life Transitions

There often seems to be only one constant in life – change! And change comes in all sizes, shapes, and colors. Life changes can be so major that they overwhelm us, or so minor as to be hardly noticeable. They can be very subtle or dramatic, happy or sad, welcomed or feared. Change can be a cause for celebration or sorrow. Change can provide new opportunities to reach for our greatest potential, or change can diminish our capacities and cause us to redefine ourselves. Change sometimes brings us face to face with the prospect of death – our own or a loved one's. Change can take many forms:

Earning a promotion at work
Receiving a medical diagnosis that alters a life forever
Seeing parents grow older and possibly become dependent
Seeing children grow older and hopefully become independent
Coming to the time of retirement
Moving to a new city
Divorcing
Marrying or remarrying
Friends moving away
Adding a new child to the family
The passing of a friend or a loved one

And for the most part, change is nonnegotiable. As the bumper sticker says:

Change is inevitable – except from a vending machine.

And change, even a positive one, causes us stress. Label it growth or progress, change still takes a toll on us emotionally and physically. We long for the safe, familiar, and predictable. We fear change because we know it involves some kind of loss – loss of control, loss of respect, loss of comfort, loss of freedom, choice, security, function, status, connection to others, pleasure, ability to cope, and perhaps even the loss of love. The fear and pain of loss is what makes change hard to accept.

From: *Handbook of Stressful Transitions Across the Lifespan*,
Edited by: T.W. Miller, DOI 10.1007/978-1-4419-0748-6_33,
© Springer Science+Business Media, LLC 2010

When faced with inevitable change, we can resist it, blame others, or (probably the worst case scenario) ignore it and pretend that everything is just the same. There are many ways of coping with change that help us bring some control back into our lives and put events into perspective, but we would like to focus on a resource that might not readily come to mind: humor.

By humor, we don't mean an arsenal of good jokes, although those can help sometimes. Nor do we mean laughing off a situation that demands and deserves attention and action; that is denial and usually makes the situation worse. We certainly don't advocate the use of cruel humor that belittles the people who may have caused the change.

Our definition of humor refers to an attitude that allows us to see life in better perspective, to transcend our current situation, to seek out and enjoy all the absurdities that present themselves to us on a daily basis, to gain control of our destinies, and to live in the present without fear of change. This definition is better understood as lived out by the remarkable example of Darla, a young cancer patient who was seen by one of the authors, who used humor positively and constructively to help deal with the changes that her diagnosis produced.

The Case of Darla

Less than a month after she learned the persistent pain in her right leg was a tumor called a sarcoma, 15-year-old Darla sought our help. Her oncologist had told her she had only about 18 months, but she was determined to outlive that "sentence." Our work together spanned more than five years until her death at age twenty. Those years were filled with many incredible moments for Darla – high school graduation, college, romance, marriage, a much dreamed of honeymoon in Hawaii and lots of laughter.

The most important lesson Darla taught us during those years was the value of laughter during serious moments. She thought laughter's place was every-where and its time, any time. She had an inherent understanding of her sense of humor – what it was and what it was for.

In a term paper written for her English Composition course during freshman year in college, Darla wrote:

> … a sense of humor goes beyond the ability to tell an amusing anecdote and includes a capacity to see the positive aspects of otherwise adverse situations. I use my own sense of humor to help me remain sane through the difficult times in my battle with cancer.

Darla's sense of humor was audacious and spontaneous. When she shared it with us, her eyes would sparkle and a triumphant grin would beam from her face. Hers was not an example of laughing away fears and burdens or making light of pain. Darla's cancer was very real and serious to her. Instead of giving in to it, however, she counted on humor to help her rise above the pain and fear.

Neither should we confuse her tactics with avoidance. Avoidance involves ignoring or denying an unwelcome experience. Darla never shrank from confronting the harsh realities of her medical condition. By transcending them with humor, she was able to acknowledge pain and fear without allowing those elements to dominate or disable her.

How Darla figured all this out at such a tender age, we do not know. All we can say is that she was a brilliant example of how humor sustains resilience and energy. Her humor strategies are not restricted to the task of battling a dire disease, but can be generalized to address the challenges we face in the stress and angst of normal daily life.

Here are a few examples as quoted: in her own words:

- *"Don't waste time on self pity."* Instead of sitting around pondering "why me?" move on to the more important question, "what's next?"
- *"Find the funny side."* Instead of assigning blame for your situation, lighten its impact by taking note of some of life's ironic twists and its amusing incongruities.
- *"Understand the difference between acceptance and approval."* Darla never approved of her cancer, but she accepted it as her personal challenge, almost from day one of her diagnosis.

Humor and Healing: A Brief History

There is certainly nothing new about the notion that humor is a worthy tool for getting through tough times. The Bible's Old Testament contains the words, "A happy heart is good medicine; and a cheerful mind works healing." (Proverbs 17:22). Throughout history, all who have undertaken to understand human beings at their best have echoed similar sentiments.

Our modern understanding of humor's beneficial power was ushered in during the twentieth century by scientific research linking the experience of frequent laughter to measurable and sometimes dramatic improvements in physical, mental, social, and even spiritual well-being. Humor has now been shown to effectively reduce stress, boost immunity, relieve pain, decrease anxiety, stabilize mood, rest the brain, enhance communication, inspire creativity, maintain hope, bolster morale, sustain resilience, and provide a healthy long-term perspective – an impressive array of benefits by any measure.

One of the pioneers who made the study of humor so popular and so respectable was Norman Cousins. In his classic, *The Anatomy of an Illness as Perceived by the Patient: Reflections on Healing and Regeneration* (1979), Cousins describes his own battle with ankylosing spondylitis, a disease of the connective tissues. The major theme of the book is that patients should take some responsibility for their own recovery of illness, but Cousins also describes the importance of using humor as a therapeutic tool. While he was still hospitalized, Cousins began a systematic program of "exercising the affirmative emotions as a factor in enhancing body chemistry" (p. 39). He secured episodes of Allen Funt's "Candid Camera" series and Marx Brothers films. He found that 10 minutes of solid, belly laughter gave him 2 hours of pain-free sleep. He also read anthologies of humor with similar results. He concluded:

> How scientific was it to believe that laughter – as well as the positive emotions in general – was affecting my body chemistry for the better? If laughter did in fact have a salutary effect on the body's chemistry, it seemed at least theoretically likely that it would enhance the system's ability to fight the inflammation. So we took sedimentation rate readings just before as well as just after the laughter episodes. Each time, there was a drop of at least five points. The drop by itself was not substantial,

but it held and was cumulative. I was greatly elated by the discovery that there is physiological basis for the ancient theory that laughter is good medicine. (p. 40)

In a later work, *Head First: the Biology of Hope and the Healing Power of the Human Spirit*, (1989), Cousins describes his career as a lecturer in a medical school and even provides the reader with a list of humorous books, movies, and audio presentations that help patients at the Comprehensive Cancer Center at Duke University, (pp. 150–153). Practicing what he preached, Cousins also describes how, as an editor at *The Saturday Review*, he and writers enjoyed concocting absurd notices for the "Personals" section of the magazine. Among the spoofs he cited is this particularly funny public apology:

We wish to apologize publicly to the 796 members of the World Stamp Collector's Society who went to Norwalk, Connecticut, instead of Norwalk, California, for our annual convention because of printer's error on the invitation. M. G. Stuckey, President, WSCS, SR Box AC. (p. 147)

Spurred on by Cousins' writing and the pioneering work of William Fry, Jr. M. D., Department of Psychiatry, Stanford University, the popular press has produced a number of worthwhile volumes devoted to the power of humor to deal with change in everyday life. Among these are:

Humor Works by John Morreall, Ph.D. (1997)
Compassionate Laughter by Patty Wooten, R.N. (1996)
The Healing Power of Humor by Allen Klein (1989)
It All Starts with a Smile by Clifford Kuhn, M.D. (2007)
And many others

Interest in studying humor led in 1987 to the establishment of The Association for Applied and Therapeutic Humor (AATH), an international community of professionals who help disseminate evidence-based information about current research and practical applications of humor. Based in Aliso Viejo, California, the Association states as its mission:

To advance the understanding and application of humor and laughter for their positive benefits.

In addition, a number of specialized scholarly journals are devoted to the advancement of knowledge and humor research and include *Humor: International Journal of Humor Research* and the *International Journal for Humor and Health*.

Scientific research has produced an impressive array of findings that support the positive effects of humor at a physiological level. For example, a series of studies by Berk, Tan, et al. (beginning in 1988) reveal that laughter influences levels of cortisol, immunoglobulins, and natural killer cell activity. Among their findings is that cortisol levels were diminished significantly for subjects who viewed what they dubbed a "laughter video," both during the viewing of the video and for a period of time following the viewing. Additionally, immunoglobulins (IgA, IgG and IgM) as well as natural killer cell activity and gamma interferon levels increased both during and following the viewing of laughter videos.

These substances are important in maintaining physical health, for the following reasons:

- Elevated cortisol levels are considered immunosuppressive and are associated with reductions in immunoglobulins, circulating lymphocytes and natural killer cell activity;
- Immunoglubulins, better known as antibodies, help to fight infections and serve as one of the body's primary defense systems;
- Natural killer cells function to seek out and destroy abnormal cells, and represent a key mechanism for what has been termed immunosurveillance; and
- Gamma interferon is one of the best known substances that regulate anticellular activities and act to enhance immune functions. To sum up, laughter was found to improve functioning of the immune system, our primary defense from invasive and harmful organisms: the healthier the immune system, the healthier the physical body.

Studies conducted at the University of Maryland Medical Center (2005, 2007: see http://www.umm.edu/features/laughter.htm and http://www.umm.edu/news/releases/laughter2.htm) also suggest that a good sense of humor and the ability to laugh at stressful situations help mitigate the damaging physical effects of distressing emotions often associated with stress. They report that a good hearty laugh can reduce the experience of stress while boosting immune functioning, lowering blood pressure and elevating mood; in addition, laughter has been shown to improve brain functioning, protect the heart, foster instant relaxation and generally make you feel good. They also note that humor essentially changes our biochemical state by decreasing stress hormones and increasing infection fighting antibodies, as well as increasing our attentiveness, heart rate and pulse.

Laughter, along with an active sense of humor, may even help protect you against a heart attack; exactly how laughter may protect the heart is not entirely understood, although reductions in stress responses are suggested. People with healthy hearts are more likely to use humor to cope with difficulty, while people with heart disease have been found to be 40 percent less likely to laugh in a variety of situations.

In addition, laughter gives your body a good workout because it massages abdominal organs, tones intestinal functioning and strengthens the muscles that hold the abdominal organs in place. It can benefit digestion and absorption of nutrients, and a hearty laugh can burn calories equivalent to several minutes on a rowing machine or exercise bike. Furthermore, laughter stimulates the release of endorphins, which may have a role in decreasing the experience of pain and increasing pain tolerance. And finally, humor improves brain function and relieves stress by stimulating both sides of the brain, easing muscle tension associated with psychological stress, and keeping the brain alert, thereby allowing us to retain more information.

Benefits of Humor During Change

Every change represents a transition and every transition requires three basic actions:

1. *Letting go* of the old
2. *Expressing* painful emotions
3. *Accepting* the new.

In order to accomplish these behaviors, human beings go through a natural process called grief. It's important to recognize that grief is an inevitable part of change. We develop strong affinities for and attachments to the status quo, which create in us a natural, built-in resistance to change, even when it appears to be for the better. Therefore every transition involves grieving because it requires us to let go of the familiar and accept the unfamiliar.

Generally speaking, we all grieve in pretty much the same pattern. In the 1960s Kubler-Ross and her associates published their landmark study of grief, in which they described a pattern for normal grief that remains the standard today (Kubler-Ross 1969). The pattern moves through five stages – denial, anger, bargaining, depression (sadness), and acceptance. The first three stages (denial, anger and bargaining) serve the mechanism of letting go of the old. The fourth stage (sadness) meets the challenge of expressing, and thus healing, the pain of our loss. The final stage (acceptance) assists us in facing new circumstances and moving ahead with our lives.

Letting Go

It shouldn't surprise us that 60% (three out of five stages) of the grieving process is devoted to only one of the three change behaviors – letting go. This is by far the biggest challenge in accommodating any change. We are creatures of habit and our attachments are strong. For most of us, letting go of anything short of a hot frying pan is a last resort, after we've tried everything else. Denying reality, raging at fate and bargaining for an "exemption" must first fail before we will consider loosening our grip.

This is precisely where humor can help dramatically. Humor, after all, is nothing if not a highly effective and efficient way to let go. In fact it is impossible to experience humor without letting go. A mere smile, which is the most basic expression of humor, has the power to silently release tension and lift the person with a smile above the paralyzing grip of a single moment. At the other extreme, many of us are well acquainted with the capacity of hearty laughter to at times compromise our decorum and dissemble our physical continence.

> A hiker was enjoying an early morning trek along the edge of the Grand Canyon, when he stumbled, lost his balance and fell into the ravine. Tumbling in free-fall, he desperately reached out and managed to grab a stout branch growing out of the canyon wall. This broke his fall, and there he dangled.

Thousands of feet below was the Colorado River. He was too far down the wall to scramble back to the top. He was stuck.

> So, he began to yell, "Help! Help! Is there anybody up there?"
> He heard a voice. "How can I help you?"
> "Oh, thank God!" he exclaimed. "Who is it?"
> "It's the Lord," the voice answered reassuringly.
> "I knew you would never forsake me," cried the hiker. "You know I've been faithful. What shall we do?"
> "Let go, and I'll catch you," came the reply.
> "What did you say?"
> "I said let go and I will catch you," repeated the soothing voice.
> "That's what I thought you said," exclaimed the hiker.
> He looked down and gasped several times. Then, at the top of his lungs, he shouted, "Is there anybody else up there?"

We know how he felt. It's tough to let go, especially when we can't be certain of the outcome. Humor can overcome our fears in the same way that light overcomes darkness. Fear simply cannot prevail in the presence of humor.

Expressing

If letting go is the focus of denial, anger and bargaining, the fourth stage of grief (sadness and despair) helps us express emotions, which serves to heal the pain and fear that follow the loss of something dear to us. Once our hiker lets go, he's going to need to scream out his feelings until his benefactor makes good on the promise of "catching" him. As we ventilate our pain and give voice to our fears, we become open to the willingness of others to understand and share our feelings. Over a period of time we recognize that we are not alone and this comforts us.

Once again, it is humor "to the rescue." The essence of humor is its spontaneous expression of emotion and attitude. Whenever we smile or laugh, we are expressing feelings for which we might not have words. Holding emotions in is the worst strategy for healing from our losses and humor makes it virtually impossible to fall into this trap.

Connecting with others is a major objective in this stage of grief. Our emotions are not always rational and words may not adequately express what we feel. A smile or a shared laugh can connect us even more deeply than words, and offer the reassuring comfort of silent understanding.

Humor can also lessen the intensity of our pain and suffering.

> Steven, a 52-year-old gentleman suffering from chronic, unremitting back pain, was reporting on a recent trip he had taken to visit his 10-week-old grandson for the first time.
>
> "The first morning, I was sitting in the living room, having a second cup of coffee, when my daughter brought the little fellow in to see me. She put him in my arms."
>
> "He was so small. It had been a long time since I had last held a baby."
>
> "I was staring down at his sweet face when he opened his eyes and looked directly back at me. Then he smiled. It was like the roof had opened up to let sunshine directly into the room. I felt a wonderful warmth all through me. I smiled back and we really connected."
>
> "Then I noticed something. My pain was gone. That pain never subsides, but, just for an instant, it disappeared completely. It was a miracle."

We do not know the exact mechanism by which humor changes pain, but the experience of Steven is not an isolated one. Humor and laughter can offer dramatic relief to our painful emotions, even as we struggle to express them. Humor expert Allen Klein puts it this way: "Humor doesn't diminish pain – it makes the space around it get bigger." Whatever the mechanism, humor deserves recognition as a valuable asset during the fourth stage of grief.

Accepting

Finally we come to acceptance, the last stage of grief and the action that signals the completion of a successful transition. Note that acceptance does not necessarily mean approval or endorsement. It is simply a recognition that change is a reality and can no longer be resisted or ignored. Accepting new ideas and new experiences means we acknowledge that they are upon us, like it or not. This is our first step toward embracing the possibilities they represent.

Surviving a transition gives us the opportunity to weave a new tapestry out of the changed elements in our lives. The beauty and durability of any tapestry depends to a great extent on the strength as well as the flexibility of its fibers. If the fibers are not strong and resilient, the cloth will be weak and easily torn. On the other hand, if the fibers lack flexibility they will not blend smoothly and may produce a brittle and fragmented fabric.

It is easy to see how humor is a valuable resource at this phase of the process. As with the proverbial "spoonful of sugar" that helps us take our medicine, one of the chief functions of humor is to help us make unacceptable things a little more acceptable. Moreover, humor can act as a shock absorber that lessens the jolt of absorbing new and unfamiliar things.

Returning to the metaphor of our new tapestry, we discover that humor produces both of the qualities we need. In addition to giving us resilience, endurance, and hope during times of uncertainty, by gently acquainting us with alternative points of view, it assists our flexibility as well.

> Grady, a physician specializing in internal medicine, was diagnosed with insulin-dependent diabetes at the age of 45. Eighteen months later he described his progress in adjusting to the demands of his disease.
>
> "For the first several months I was furious at God and myself, and jealous of everybody else," he recalled. "It didn't seem fair. I had worked hard to develop my practice and to reach the status and life-style I was enjoying. Nobody handed it to me. I had earned it, and suddenly it was being taken away. I remember thinking, 'What's the use,' if that was all it would come to. Then, I began to listen to my patients, many of whom had even more severe restrictions than I, and I felt ashamed for all my whining."
>
> "So, I decided I had to make a choice. Either I could go on being resentful, angry, resistant and reluctant about my fate, or I could give in to the positive perspective, which is that I had a game plan for managing my illness and a way to monitor my day-to-day success in following it. I could be grateful for what I still had, rather than obsessing over what I'd lost. As soon as I surrendered to the more positive perspective, I noticed I immediately had more energy and enthusiasm for everything, and my family seemed to find me easier to be around."
>
> "Don't get me wrong," he added. "I still would rather not have diabetes. It's just a little easier to live with since I decided to accept it as an opportunity, instead of a defeat."

Summing up: Maybe Openness is the Key

Humor is an important ally in our struggle to cope and adjust to life's inevitable transitions – both positive and negative. When we take ourselves and our situation less seriously, search for the humor that is in everyday life, and gain perspective and distance, we rally inner resources that give us strength and courage to deal constructively and even joyfully with change.

Scholars have provided us with a research that supports the value of humor in:

- Relaxing tense muscles (Fry 1989)
- Boosting the immune response (Berk & Tan 1995; Berk et al. 2001)
- Increasing pain tolerance (Cogan et al. 1987)
- Decreasing anxiety (Lefcourt and Martin 1995)
- Stabilizing mood fluctuations (Martin and Lefcourt 1983)

- Resting the brain (George et al. 1995)
- Enhancing communication (Balzer 1993)
- Inspiring creativity (Miller 1988)
- Bolstering morale (Provine 2000)

Why does humor work? Why do we laugh? Certainly, that is the question that has been asked by philosophers, scientists, literary critics, and others for all of human history. In his classic text, *Taking Humor Seriously* (State University of New York Press, 1983), John Morreall devotes considerable effort to outlining a number of theories:

> The Superiority Theory: "Wow, am I ever glad that didn't happen to me."
> The Incongruity Theory: "I sure didn't expect that!"
> The Relief Theory: "When I laugh, I vent all those negative emotions and feel better."

Morreal suggests his own theory that laughter works because it provides "a pleasant psychological shift" (p. 39). This seems to explain the range of humor from highly abstract satire to a baby's laughter when a foot is tickled.

Maybe the key to humor's benefits is an openness to allowing laughter and humor to permeate all of life's transitions. Maybe we can just remember Darla and ask, "What's next?" rather than "Why me?"

References

Balzer, J. W. (1993). Humor-A missing ingredient in collaborative practice. *Holistic Nursing Practice, 7*, 28–35.

Berk, L., Felten, D., Tan, S., Bittman, S., & Westengard, J. (2001). Modulation of neuroimmune parameters during the eustress of humor-associated mirthful laughter. *Alternative Therapies in Health and Medicine 7*, 62–72, 74–76

Berk, L., & Tan, S. (1995). Eustress of mirthful laughter modulates the immune system lymphokine interferon-gamma. In *Annals of Behavioral Medicine Supplement, Proceedings of the Society of Behavioral Medicine's 16th Annual Scientific Sessions* (Vol. 17, p. C064)

Berk, L., Tan, S., & Fry, W. (1993). Eustress of humor associated laughter modulates specific immune system components. In *Annals of Behavioral Medicine Supplement, Proceedings of the Society of Behavioral Medicine's 16th Annual Scientific Sessions* (Vol. 15, p. S111)

Berk, L., Tan, S., Fry, W. F., Napier, B. J., Lee, J. W., Hubbard, R. W., et al. (1989a). Neuroendocrine and stress hormone changes during mirthful laughter. *American Journal of Medical Science, 298*, 391–396.

Berk, L., Tan, S., Napier, B. J., & Eby, W. C. (1989b). Eustress of mirthful laughter modifies natural killer cell activity. *Clinical Research, 37*, 115A.

Berk, L., Tan, S., Nehlsen-Cannarella, S., Napier, B., Lewis, J., Lee, J., et al. (1988). Humor associated laughter decreases cortisol and increases spontaneous lymphocyte blastogenesis. *Clincal Research, 36*, 435A.

Cogan, R., Cogan, D., Waltz, W., & McCue, M. (1987). Effects of laughter and relaxation on discomfort thresholds. *Journal of Behavioral Medicine, 10*, 139–144.

Cousins, N. (1979). *Anatomy of an illness as perceived by the patient*. New York, NY: W. W. Norton & Company, Inc.

Cousins, Norman. (1989). *Head first: The biology of hope*. New York, NY: E. P. Dutton.

Fry, W. E. (1989). Humor, physiology, and the aging process. In L. Nahemow, K. A. McCluskey-Fawcett & P. E. McGhee (Eds.), *Humor and aging*. New York, NY: Academic Press.

George, M. S., Ketter, T. A., Parekh, P. I., Horwitz, B., Herscovitch, P., & Post, R. M. (1995). Brain activity during transient sadness and happiness in healthy women. *Journal of Psychiatry, 152*, 341–351.

Klein, A. (1989). *The healing power of humor.* New York, NY: Jeremy P. Tarcher/ Putnam Book.

Kubler-Ross, E. (1969). *On death and dying.* New York, NY: Macmillan.

Kuhn, C. (2007). *It all starts with a smile: Seven steps to being happier right now.* Louisville, KY: Butler Books.

Lefcourt, H. M., & Martin, R. A. (1995). *Humor and life stress: An antidote to adversary.* New York, NY: Springer-Verlag.

Martin, R. A., & Lefcourt, H. M. (1983). Sense of humor as a moderator between stressor and moods. *Journal of Personality and Social Psychology, 45*, 1313–1324.

Miller, J. (1988). Jokes and joking: A serious laughing matter. In J. Durant & J. Miller (Eds.), *Laughing matters: A serious look at humor.* Essex, England: Longman Scientific and Technical.

Morreall, J. (1983). *Taking humor seriously.* Albany, NY: State University of New York Press.

Morreall, J. (1997). *Humor works.* Amherst, MA: HRD Press, Inc.

Provine, R. R. (2000). *Laugher: A scientific investigation.* New York, NY: Viking Penguin.

Wooten, P. (1996). *Compassionate laughter: Jest for your health!.* Salt Lake City, UT: Commune-A-Key Publishing.

Chapter 34

Concluding Comments and Future Considerations for Stressful Life Events and Transitions Across the Life Span

Thomas W. Miller

Life itself is a process of beginnings and endings, of transitions and transformations. Within the natural course of life, there are periods when there are multiple transitions, or so it seems and then there are other times when life events move slowly and do not seem to change at all. Within the course of life, many of these transitions are stressful for some and at least require adaptation and adjustment for most. Transitions in the life span are as natural as the changing seasons.

Life transitions are often stressful, because they require shifts and changes in our lives Dohrwend and Dohrwend (1974). Rahe (1989) along with his colleague Holmes led the research on rating the degree of stress related to several life events and transitions. The challenge for any individual involves letting go of the established and the familiar and confronting the change and the new aspects of life. The shifts involve the future and the unexpected aspects of what the future brings with a sense of vulnerability to what is unexpected. Whether it is the economy, a health-related condition, or mass trauma, it requires effective coping skills and adaptation to the change and the conditions associated with it.

We live in the 21st century, which recognizes a culture that has taught us to be very uncomfortable with uncertainty, so we become stressed and anxious when a shift is required and our lives are disrupted. It is however these transitions that give us a chance to learn about our strengths as human beings, to understand that transformations may lead to a better or richer life experience and such transformations allow us to explore what one really wants and needs in our lives. This is for many a journey in time for reflection that can result in a sense of renewal, stability, and as Piaget suggested, a new equilibrium and accommodation.

Life transitions require the optimism and positivism that Seligman discusses in his latest writings on optimism and positivism. Each event in our life is tied to change and transitions can be stressful or stress free, or planned or unexpected. There are those transitions that happen without warning, and they may be quite dramatic, as in cases of accidents, death, divorce, job loss, or serious illness. Other life transitions come from more favorable experiences such as

From: *Handbook of Stressful Transitions Across the Lifespan,*
Edited by: T.W. Miller, DOI 10.1007/978-1-4419-0748-6_34,
© Springer Science+Business Media, LLC 2010

birth, marriage, entering school or the freedom of going away to college, starting a new job, moving to a new home, or making a new friendship. Even though events like these are usually planned and anticipated, they can be just as life altering as the unexpected events. Whether positive or negative, life transitions cause us to leave behind the familiar and require us to adjust to new ways of living and this may well be the stressing part of transitions. They can leave one feeling completely inept and unprepared or provide the opportunity to use one's abilities to accommodate and accept the changes that we are confronted with in life.

There are numerous examples of life transitions that may be stressful. Among them are birth, death, having a baby, entering college, relocation, ,career changes, retirement, buying or selling a house, surviving being shot or an automobile accident, changing jobs, separation from a long friendship or partnership, divorce, developing a new friendship, losing friends for a spectrum of reasons, entering a marital relationship, receiving the unexpected diagnosis, being told of a loved one's terminal illness, or the loss of a person, a pet, or a significant other.

How Do We Process Life Transitions?

Conceptualizing stages of change in transitioning stressful life experiences became the early focus of Kubler-Ross (1969) who initially offered a model of the grieving process to transitions in general and stages of adaptation to death. These stages begin with the entry experience of surprise, shock, confusion, and emotional discomfort. Following this initial reaction is a brief period of anger, then sadness or despair, often alternating with relief and positive feelings that include bargaining and then acceptance.

Horowitz (1986) and others have generated paradigms for assessing the normal phases of processing stressful life experiences. Generally recognized in these paradigms include a series of stages or phases which first recognize the traumatic event, allow for the person to decipher both the psychological and physical impact of the traumatic stress, then leading to a stage of disorganization and denial which may then be followed by a peril of reevaluation wherein both the psychological and physical components of the disorder are revisited, which then leads to an eventual acceptance of the trauma or a resolution to the psychopathological impact of the trauma.

Miller and Veltkamp (1989, 1993) suggest that the victim processes the trauma by moving through a series of stages. The initial stage of the Trauma Accommodation Syndrome involves victimization which is recognized as a stressor and usually realizes an acute physical and/or psychological traumatic experience. The victim's response is usually one of feeling overwhelmed and intimidated. Loss of control is recognized, and it is not uncommon for the victim to think recurring of the stressful experience and focus upon the intimidating factors of the trauma.

The acute traumatic stage is followed by a stage involving more cognitive disorganization and confusion. This stage is marked by vagueness in understanding both the concept of trauma and the expectations associated with the adaptation, adjustment, or accommodation. The next stage involves a phase of avoidance, which can take two directions and may vary in its choice, depending on various considerations. The first is a conscious inhibition where an effort is made on the part of the victim to actively inhibit the thoughts and feelings related to the trauma. This may involve revisiting the traumatic experience itself or early memories through flashbacks to a more acute physical and psychological trauma. The second is avoidance involving unconscious denial, wherein the victim is not aware of the effort to avoid the psychological trauma associated with the traumatic event. Unconscious denial occurs, and less frequently allows a revisitation to the cognitive disorganization stage as well as the stressor and stressful life event itself. For the most part each of these theorists offers support that life transitions are predictable changes and result in a predictable adaptation process.

One goal is to let go of the past person, thing, job, or value and take hold of a new object or relationship. These attitudes and resources, combined with the passage of time, enable the person to regain self-confidence and self-esteem. The person begins to look to the future with optimism and hope. If this process of healing and taking hold is successful, this stage emerges in a renewal phase characterized by setting new goals, making plans, and initiating actions. Thus, growth is enhanced through continual renewal efforts.

Successfully transitioning through a lifecycle usually means experiencing a series of phases or stages of change not unlike childhood, adolescence, adulthood, and aging. Processing with care and detail the range of feelings one experiences in each one of these changes range from joy and sorrow, certainty to uncertainty, happiness to sadness, peace to anger, safety to anxiety, clarity to confusion, associated with the impact of this event on one's life. The impact of any of these transitions requires change to one's self image and one's self-esteem. It also involves the tendency to seek solitude in denial, withdrawal or disassociation when the changes are not desired. The temptation to revisit the change and how it will affect one's life becomes a part of the processing. Questions arise as to what ifs and what could I have done differently. The acknowledgment and eventual acceptance of the change and the pathway to survive the transition realizes a level of accommodation. The shift in feelings and the contemplation and plan for accepting the transition is the reassurance that adaptation has occurred. The accommodation and acceptance of the transition and the development of an optimistic view of the future are critical ingredients in resolving the trauma. The accommodation and acceptance of the transition and the development of an optimistic view of the future.

The process of moving through a transition does not always proceed in order, in predictable stages. People usually move through the process in different ways, often cycling back and forth among the stages and revisiting the implications of the stressful life transition. This figure depicts the process of accommodating change as part of stressful transitions and was discussed earlier in this volume (Fig. 34-1).

What Is the Nature of Stressful Life Transitions?

Twenty-first century science has viewed the impact of life stress events to mainly encompass the diagnostic entity that has come to be known as post-traumatic stress disorder. A more recent inquiry into this question suggests that it may be more important to look at the impact of stressful life events on health

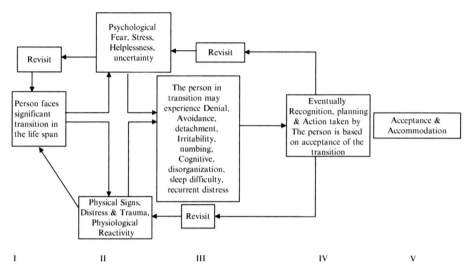

Fig. 34-1. Processing the Trauma of a Stressful Life Transition

as a spectrum disorder looks at the components and processing of anxiety, depression, somatization, and dissociation. Its components can include panic disorder, generalized anxiety, hypochondriasis, somatrization, and components of hysterical neurosis and multiple personality disorder. Its etiology may be nested in DSM-IV Axis II diagnoses suggesting personality disturbance as a predisposition to a major psychiatric disorder in the multiaxial system.

In viewing this as a spectrum disorder, we recognize that anxiety and depression are widely present in individuals with traumatic stress. The precise description is important for several reasons. The etiology and onset may be discernible from certain other psychological disturbances, most notably generalized anxiety disorder or major depressive disorder. Features relating to re-experiencing trauma including the assessment of the degree to which an individual ruminates and the ruminations' effect on daily functioning is extremely important. Furthermore, numbing of responsiveness is assessed as a core ingredient in traumatization. This feature may be intertwined with aspects of anxiety and depressive components and is most similarly diagnostically to the lack of interest or anhedonia and withdrawal often found on patients with clinical depression. The distinguishing features of the numbing found in traumatic stress often relate more to the unremitting severity, intensity, and chronicity of the symptoms, which often derive from situations or feelings reminiscent of the traumatic event.

Critical to the numbing and restricted range of emotional experiences found in traumatized individuals is the role of anger. For many, anger is a frequently expressed emotion that creates multiple interpersonal problems. For some, the control of anger and the accompanying fear of loss of control are major preoccupations that cause considerable distress and frequently lead to social withdrawal and isolation. The startle response seen in traumatized individuals may be similar to that found in generalized anxiety disorder. The exaggerated startle response may reflect a few psychophysiological arousals that are noticeably worsened in the presence of specific situational reminders and triggers.

Finally, the presence of dual diagnosis has been important in understanding the nine complexity of the impact of trauma on the individual's functioning. The presence of co-existing Axis I or Axis II disorders has considerable conical relevance in influencing formulation of the patient's problem in both an etiological and treatment perspective. Frequently traumatized individuals can meet the criteria for major depression, substance abuse/dependence, and various components of anxiety disorders including panic disorder. The identification of co-existing disorders at the onset of treatment can influence decision-making regarding the sequence and timing of specific interventions and strategies that can be potentially helpful in optimizing treatment outcome.

What Is the Best Way to Assess Stressful Life Transitions?

Several approaches have been utilized in the assessment of transitions and life stress. Included are such things as structured clinical interviews, diagnostic interview scales, and specific measures that have been helpful including several psychometric measures and psycho-physiological measures. All have been discussed elsewhere (Miller 1996). Kay (2009) has discussed elsewhere in this book the breakthroughs and trends in neuro-imaging hold promise in assessing adaptation to trauma and stress. Miller (2009a, b) and medical genetics have contributed to our understanding of the impact of genetic assessment and the implications of genetic predisposition to transitioning life events elsewhere in this volume.

The efforts of clinicians and researchers alike to assess biological markers of psychological disorders have focused considerable attention and interest on psychobiology and psycho-physiological assessment (Friedman 1991). Currently it is considered to be the best and most specific biological diagnostic test for traumatic stress. This diagnostic technique is based on the fact that traumatization and the stimuli there from elicit sympathetic hyper arousal. It has been found to be even more discriminatory when provocative stimuli are used an individualized autobiographical traumatic anecdote (Pitman 1988). The Dexamethasone Suppression Test has been recognized for its use in diagnosing major depressive disorders. Clinical researchers are finding that patients with traumatic stress disorder tend to have normal DST's and could therefore be classified as suppressors, whereas patients with traumatic stress disorder and major depressive disorder may well be seen as non-suppressors. Sodium lactate or yohimbine infusion and sodium amatol interviews have also been helpful in diagnosing traumatic stress in patients.

What Are the Coping Skills Needed in Transitions?

Perhaps the secrets held within the "Human Genome" hold for many of us a glimpse as to how we may most effectively cope with stressful transitions. The day is likely to come when each of us at birth will have the information to know our genetic makeup and will have the ability to correct genetic abnormalities in our gene structure. The life cycle in which one is currently provides for a spectrum of life transitions. Some are often more difficult for some than for others, but they have a positive side too. They provide us with an opportunity to assess the direction our lives are taking. They are a chance to grow and learn. Here are some ideas that may help make the process successful. We may begin by revisiting a stressful life event in an attempt to accept that change as a normal part of life. People who have this attitude seem to have the easiest time getting through life transitions. When transitions are negative experiences it is more difficult to navigate the acceptance and accommodation process. In the face of stressful transitions, Identify and redefine one's goals, objectives, and life values. If a person knows who they are and what they want from life, they may see the change as just another life challenge. These people are willing to take responsibility for their actions and do not blame others for the changes that come along without warning. Map your thoughts and feelings in accepting and adjusting to these transitions. Focus on identifying the images and thoughts and feelings the transition evokes. While it is normal to try to push away feelings of fear and anxiety, you will move through them more quickly if you acknowledge them. Make them real by writing them down and talking about them with trusted friends and family members. Life transitions can provide a productive time to introspectively understand ourselves. Such experiences provide for a reasonable transition that can allow one to accommodate and accept the transition. When life is disrupted, it takes time to adjust to the new realities of life. It is essential to acknowledge that which you are leaving behind and take one step at a time. This is the initial step to acceptance and accommodation. The transitions that we face in our lives offer us the opportunity to explore what our ideal life might be. When things are in disarray, you can reflect on the hopes and dreams you once had but perhaps forgot about. It is essential to take this time to write about them in a journal or talk about them with a trusted friend or therapist.

Are there Ethno-cultural, Religious and Spiritual Variants to Consider in Stressful Transitions?

Ethno cultural aspects of addressing stressful transitions across the life span are of significant importance in understanding the etiology, processing, and adaptation of individuals to the experience. Cross-cultural studies offer an opportunity to compare like populations who have experienced like stressors with the search for social and cultural correlates that may provide clues to the etiology of certain conditions, their onset, their maintenance, and their resolution. Boehnlein and Kinzie (1994) note that the study and diagnosis of psychiatric disorders cross-culturally remains an area of great opportunity and controversy and that traumatization and stress must be analyzed and assessed on a cross cultural basis. Westermeyer (1987) has noted that interpretations of stressful life experiences cross-culturally can have a variety of meanings and raises the question as to whether the clinician from one culture can understand and interpret the meaning and significance of transitioning for a patient from another culture. It becomes imperative that everyone including clinicians and researchers realize that understanding the entire socio-cultural milieu in which the patient functions is a critical factor in recognizing diagnostic symptomology consistent with stress related to life change.

Boehnlein et al. (1992) and Boehnlein and Kinzie (1994) have carefully examined the processing of trauma and subsequent bereavement and have determined that this is highly cultural in nature. Kinzie notes that culturally constituted symbols, communication patterns, and healing approaches vary considerably from culture to culture. In much the same way, these researchers argue that rituals that enable individuals to address the traumatization process are cultural-bound, spear-heading the answers to the many questions that have been raised within an ethno-cultural perspective. The authors encourage clinical researchers to show a significant sensitivity to social structures, cultural values, and self-identity of the individual within the ethno-cultural context. Other investigators including Mollica et al. (1990) and Boehnlein and Kinzie (1994) have examined cross-cultural samples and realized similar findings. This volume has drawn on an international group of scholars and devoted an entire section to cultural, religious, and spiritual influences in stressful life transitions. Further study and discussion from a global perspective focusing on these important dimensions of transitioning stressful life experiences is essential as we attempt to better understand the critical factors that contribute to adjustment to major shifts and changes in our lives.

What Are the Future Trends in Studying Stressful Life Transitions?

Future trends in assessing the impact of stressful life events and the transitions we confront in our lives will involve neurobiological, genetic, and biochemical markers. There are a multiplicity of factors that must be considered in understanding these life experiences. The growing body of information and clinical findings (Kay 2009; Miller 2009a, b) has expanded our theoretical understanding of trauma and stress from a purely psychological context to a biopsychosocial model in which many different factors contribute to the etiology, onset, and impact of life stress events on health and well being.

Several questions have emerged in our discussion for individuals as well as for clinicians and researchers that must be explored through further study, investigation, and research in order to help us understand critical issues in stressful life events and resulting transitions faced. How we approach this study is of critical importance. For example is it better to examine such transitions as a single event or within the context of a spectrum of factors that must be considered? We have used several forms of assessing the impact of significant life transitions. Are they better studied within a series of case examples or by a combination of evidence based research along with single subject design? Of even more significance, how does one process the transitions faced in life? What theory applies to each and what have we learned from the insights offered from both a research and the clinical perspective? What are the ethno cultural, religious, and spiritual perspectives that influence our base of understanding the influence of critical transitions that we face in the life span? And finally what interventions aid in our understanding of how individuals cope with, adapt, or accommodate to the most difficult and stressful life transitions. Encouragement towards a biopsychosocial model in which many different factors contribute to our understanding of transition and adaptation there is the realization that this diagnostic entity is not a single concept, but rather a more complex spectrum of factors.

What Are the Interventions of Choice in Coping with Stressful Transition?

There is considerable interest today in understanding models of coping with transitions in the life span. Several clinical and professional models are discussed elsewhere. The publication Briere and Scott (2006) has an extensive summary of a spectrum of treatment options for stressful transitions in the life span. In this volume, Nichols et al. (2009) argue that humor plays an important role in successfully transitioning stressful life changes. Illich and Brownbill (2009) provide excellent models for nutrition and dietary issues and Nyland and Abbott (2009) note the importance of functional fitness in adapting to certain traumas. Adams (2009) suggests the affection gained in pet therapy may be helpful in adaptation and adjustment.

As we have gained in our understanding of our genetic make-up, the role of genetic testing will be a critical element in the years ahead and has profound implications for our understanding of ourselves and our genetically disposed predisposition especially with respect to disease and illness (Miller 2009a, b). What is being realized, however, is that data from a number of studies have shown that various stressors can adversely affect immune function. The bodily immune system is a complex surveillance apparatus that functions to determine self from non-self. An immune reaction is activated in response to exposure to foreign antigens in an effort to maintain the body's homeostasis. There is ample evidence from human and animal studies that demonstrate the downward modulation of immune function concomitant with stressful life experiences. As a consequence of this, the possible enhancement of immune function by behavioral strategies has generated considerable interest. Clinicians and researchers have used a number of diverse strategies to modulate immune functioning including relaxation, hypnosis, exercise, classical conditions, self-disclosure, exposures to a phobic stress, and to enhance perceived coping self-efficacy and cognitive behavioral interventions.

What is clear is that the approach chosen to cope with transitions in the life span needs to be individualized. It is imperative that as we attempt to answer this question in the treatment of trauma and stress, we must take into consideration the bio-psycho-, social and cultural dimensions of the individual within the societal context. Finally, questions related to whether concurrent or sequential interventions are better must be answered through further study. All of these can be addressed within the context of tailor-made interventions for individuals who are transitioning stressful life experiences.

Twenty-first century science requires further research and clinical studies that uphold the following: A holistic perspective and bridge for the multicultural and multinational similarities and differences we have come to realize among the various countries and cultures of the world. Innovative models are needed that draw on science and best practices, ethics and moral judgment and assures quality of care. A willingness to engage with others is essential especially among empowered groups of educators, scientists, practitioners, and consumers to address the political, social, and environmental needs of the world community. International openness, understanding, and exchanges to eliminate the barriers and borders that currently limit the trans-nationalization of science, education, ethics, morality, and professional practice, to create an international body of professionals working to solve the traumas faced by so many worldwide. New models of diagnosis and treatment utilizing more complex analyses, systems, and networks which will analyze how genetic factors influence clinical markers that result in adaptation ,accommodation, and resolution of trauma. A greater understanding of the role and function of health, religion, economics, spirituality, politics, and personal beliefs and their effect on our world community.

Stressful life events and their impact on our health have traditionally focused on physical and mental health (Tennant 2006; Miller 1996; Dohrwend and Dohrwend 1974; Seligman 1975; Horowitz 1979; Quarantelli 1985; Veltkamp and Miller 1994). The world, as we know it at the dawn of the 21st century, realizes that recent economic, social, political, and environmental factors have had a profound impact on the health, healthcare available and the well being of our global population. Wars, military conflicts, famine, political violence, and climatic changes are among some of the factors that have traumatized some in this first decade of the twenty-first century. The presence of trauma resulting from exposure to violence will have increased the need for contemporary psychological interventions and prevention strategies in this era of change. From school based violence, work place stress, cultural, religious and climatic changes to the continuing threat from al Qaeda, the presence of violence, both domestically and internationally, will require a greater commitment and understanding from the psychological community toward meeting the needs of human beings facing trauma in their lives. It will require innovative research, new practice models, and ethical concern for our global community. Innovative models of treatment and intervention strategies must be able to accommodate and assimilate the biochemistry, genetics, and psychosocial domains which form the basis for science. Transitions, therefore, must be paced but also be deliberate and extensive, embodying a vision of a better future for all humankind, their communities, and their nations as an ultimate goal. Structural and political changes, backed hopefully by some attitudinal and behavior change, will be necessary to stabilize the external context.

As Seligman (2004) so ably argues, there are two factors in human potential, one is our ability and the other is our optimism. We're showing that there is a science to the interplay between our attitudes and our actions. The psychological community must take the action and in doing so provide the cornerstone to build through science and practice, the models for humanistic caring and support necessary to resolve many of these crises. They have to be complemented by the international community toward rooting out such structures within the social fabric so as to effect genuine social, psychological, and environmental transformation in the global community.

Visionary concepts such as these provide the baseline for which science and practice will need to address the shifts and changes which will likely occur during the first quarter of the 21st century. The issues confronting them today are increasingly complex and varied in content. We all must have clarity of vision for the future and the competency to adapt to the shifts and transitions that will occur for the benefit of our global community.

References

Adams, J. (2009). The role of animals and animal assisted therapy in stressful life transitions. In T. W. Miller (Ed.), *Stressful life events: Transitions in the life span*. New York: Springer Publications Incorporated

Boehnlein, J. K., & Kinzie, J. D. (1994). Cross-cultural assessment of traumatization. In T. W. Miller (Ed.), *Stressful life events*. Madison, CT: International Universities Press, Inc.

Boehnlein, J. K., Kinzie, J. D., & Fleck, J. (1992). DSM diagnosis of posttraumatic stress disorder and cultural sensitivity: A response. *Journal of Nervous and Mental Disease, 180*, 597–599.

Briere, J., & Scott, C. (2006). *Principles of trauma therapy: A guide to symptoms, evaluation, and treatment*. New York: SAGE.

Dohrwend, B. S., & Dohrwend, B. P. (1974). *Stressful life events: Their nature and effects*. New York: Wiley.

Kübler-Ross, E. (1969). *On Death and Dying*, Macmillan, NY.

Friedman, M. (1991). *Neurological alterations associated with post-traumatic stress disorder*. National Center for PTSD, Clinical Laboratory and Education Diversion, Teleconference Report, July, 1991

Horowitz, M. J. (1979). Stress response syndromes and their treatment. In L. Goldberger, & S. Breznitz, (Eds.), *Handbook of stress* (2nd ed.). New York: Free Press

Horowitz, M. J. (1986). Stress response syndromes: a review of posttraumatic and adjustment disorders. *Hospital and Community Psychiatry, 37*, 241–249.

Illich Ernst, J., & Brownbill, R. (2009). The influence of food on adapting to stressful life events. In T. W. Miller, (Ed.), *Stressful life events: Transitions in the life span*. New York: Springer Publications Incorporated

Kay, J. (2009). The neurobiology of stress within the life cycle. In T. W. Miller (Ed.), *Stressful life events: Transitions in the life span*. New York: Springer Publications Incorporated

Miller, D. (2009a). Psychological impact of genetic testing. In T. W. Miller (Ed.), *Stressful life events: Transitions in the life span*. New York: Springer Publications Incorporated

Miller, T. W. (2009b). Life stress and transitions in the life span. In T. W. Miller (Ed.), *Stressful life events: Transitions in the life span*. New York: Springer Publications Incorporated

Miller, T. W., & Veltkamp, L. J. (1989). The abusing family in rural America. *International Journal of Family Psychiatry, 9*(3), 259–275.

Miller, T. W. (1996). *Theory and Assessment of Stressful Life Events*, Madison, Connecticut: International Universities Press, Inc.

Mollica, R. F., Wyshak, G., Lavelle, J., Truong, T., Tor, S., & Yang, T. (1990). Assessing symptom of change in Southeast Asian refugee survivors of mass violence and torture. *American Journal of Psychiatry, 147*, 83–88.

Nichols, M., Kuhn, C., & Belew, B. (2009). Humor as a way of transitioning stressful life events. In T. W. Miller (Ed.), *Stressful life events: Transitions in the life span*. New York: Springer Publications Incorporated

Nyland, J., & Abbott, M. (2009). Functional fitness: Life stress and transitions in the life span. In T. W. Miller (Ed.), *Stressful life events: Transitions in the life span*. New York: Springer Publications Incorporated

Pitman, R. K. (1988). Post-traumatic stress disorder, conditioning, and network theory. *Psychiatric Annals, 18*, 182–189.

Quarantelli, E. L. (1985). An assessment of conflicting views on mental health: The consequences of traumatic events. In B. M. P. Stress (Ed.), *Trauma and its wake*: The study and treatment of post-traumatic stress disorder (Vol. 4, pp. 173–215). New York: Brunner/Mazel

Rahe, R. (1989). Recent life change and psychological depression. In T. W. Miller (Ed.), *Theory and assessment of stressful life events,* Madison, CT: International Universities Press, Inc

Seligman, M. E. P. (1975). *Helplessness: On depression, development and death.* San Francisco: Freeman.

Seligman, M. E. P. (2004) *Learned optimism: How to change your mind and your life.* http://www.amazon.com/Learned-Optimism-Change-Your-Mind/dp/0671019112

Tennant, C. (2006). Life events stress and depression. *Australian and New Zealand Journal of Psychiatry, 36*, 173–182.

Veltkamp, L., & Miller, T. (1994). *Clinical handbook of child abuse and neglect.* Madison, CT: International Universities Press Incorporated.

Westermeyer, J. (1987). Clinical considerations in cross-cultural diagnosis. *Hospital and Community Psychiatry, 38*, 160–165.

Index

Breinigsville, PA USA
31 January 2010
231600BV00002B/3/P